Adult Hydrocephalus

Adult Hydrocephalus

Edited by
Daniele Rigamonti
Professor of Neurosurgery, Radiology, and Radiation Oncology, Johns Hopkins University, Baltimore, MD, USA

CAMBRIDGE
UNIVERSITY PRESS

CAMBRIDGE
UNIVERSITY PRESS

University Printing House, Cambridge CB2 8BS, United Kingdom

Published in the United States of America by Cambridge University Press, New York

Cambridge University Press is part of the University of Cambridge.

It furthers the University's mission by disseminating knowledge in the pursuit of education, learning and research at the highest international levels of excellence.

www.cambridge.org
Information on this title: www.cambridge.org/9781107031777

First published 2014

Printing in the United Kingdom by TJ International Ltd, Padstow, Cornwall

A catalogue record for this publication is available from the British Library

Library of Congress Cataloguing in Publication data
Adult hydrocephalus / edited by Daniele Rigamonti.
p. ; cm.
Includes bibliographical references and index.
ISBN 978-1-107-03177-7 (hardback)
I. Rigamonti, Daniele, 1951– editor of compilation.
[DNLM: 1. Hydrocephalus–etiology. 2. Adult. 3. Cerebrospinal Fluid Pressure. 4. Hydrocephalus – physiopathology. 5. Hydrocephalus–therapy. WL 203]
RC391
616.85′8843–dc23
2013025680

ISBN 978-1-107-03177-7 Hardback

I dedicate this book to my wife Karen, to my children Eva, Luigi and Alessandra, to my parents Luigi and Santa, to Bunny and Charles Salisbury who have endowed a chair for me, and to Carol Swenson-Tanzola and her family for their support of my work on hydrocephalus.

In memory of Professor Tony Marmarou: a scientist, a teacher, and a friend

Contents

List of contributors ix
Prologue xii

Section 1 – Basic sciences

1 **Anatomy and physiology of the cerebrospinal fluid system** 1
Thomas A. Kosztowski, Aristotelis S. Filippidis, C. Rory Goodwin, Benjamin D. Elder, and Daniele Rigamonti

2 **Neuropathology of human hydrocephalus** 14
Marc R. Del Bigio

3 **Animal models of hydrocephalus** 28
Marianne Juhler

4 **Genetics of hydrocephalus** 36
Jun Zhang

5 **The epidemiology of hydrocephalus** 57
Are Brean and Per Kristian Eide

Section 2 – Pathophysiology

6 **Pathophysiology of gait dysfunction in normal pressure hydrocephalus** 63
Jonathan Pindrik, Amy Bastian, and Daniele Rigamonti

7 **The pathophysiologic basis of cognitive dysfunction in idiopathic normal pressure hydrocephalus** 70
Norman Relkin and Heather Katzen

8 **Incontinence and lower urinary tract symptoms in normal pressure hydrocephalus** 80
Adam P. Klausner and Samuel P. Robinson

9 **Normal pressure hydrocephalus grading scales** 91
Masatsune Ishikawa

Section 3 – Diagnosis

10 **The differential diagnosis of normal pressure hydrocephalus** 99
Daniele Rigamonti, Marianne Juhler, and Carsten Wikkelsø

11 **Core imaging in adult hydrocephalus** 110
Benjamin D. Elder, Patrick Bankah, Ari M. Blitz, C. Rory Goodwin, Thomas A. Kosztowski, Ignacio Jusué-Torres, and Daniele Rigamonti

12 **Imaging of the cerebrospinal fluid circulation** 121
Olivier Balédent

13 **Cerebrospinal fluid dynamics and infusion techniques** 139
Cemil Kayis and Gunes A. Aygok

14 **Monitoring of intracranial pressure and assessment of cerebrospinal fluid dynamics** 150
Marek Czosnyka, Martin U. Schuhmann, Stefano Signoretti, Zofia Czosnyka, and John D. Pickard

15 **Cerebrospinal fluid biomarkers in idiopathic normal pressure hydrocephalus** 164
Andrew A. Tarnaris

Section 4 – Treatment and outcomes

16 **Hydrocephalus shunt procedures** 175
Benjamin D. Elder, C. Rory Goodwin, Thomas A. Kosztowski, and Daniele Rigamonti

17 **Hydrocephalus shunts: principles, hardware, shunt testing** 190
Zofia Czosnyka, Krzysztof Cieslicki, Hugh K. Richards, John D. Pickard, and Marek Czosnyka

18 **Management of shunts in normal pressure hydrocephalus: follow-up and late complications** 207
Ahmed Mohyeldin, Ammar Shaikhouni, and John McGregor

19 **Endoscopic third ventriculostomy: indications, technique, outcome, and complications** 218
Steffen Fleck, Jörg Baldauf, and Henry W. S. Schroeder

20 **Outcome of idiopathic normal pressure hydrocephalus** 232
Gunes A. Aygok

Section 5 – Associated conditions

21 **Normal pressure hydrocephalus syndrome secondary to hemorrhage, infection, and malignancy** 247
C. Rory Goodwin, Benjamin D. Elder, Thomas A. Kosztowski, and Daniele Rigamonti

22 **Low-pressure syndromes and cerebrospinal fluid leaks: diagnosis and management** 256
Debraj Mukherjee and Wouter I. Schievink

23 **Management of the adult with congenital hydrocephalus** 264
Jonathan Pindrik and Edward S. Ahn

24 **Management of hydrocephalus with associated cerebrospinal fluid pathologies** 275
Petra Margarete Klinge

25 **Chiari malformation and hydrocephalus in adults** 291
Aristotelis S. Filippidis and Harold L. Rekate

26 **Pseudotumor cerebri syndrome** 296
John D. Pickard and Nicholas Higgins

Epilogue 304
Index 305

Color plates appear between pages 132 and 133.

Contributors

Edward S. Ahn, MD
Division of Pediatric Neurosurgery, Johns Hopkins University School of Medicine, Baltimore, MD, USA

Gunes A. Aygok, MD, PhD
Medical College of Virginia Commonwealth University, Department of Neurosurgery, Richmond, VA, and Department of Neurosurgery, North Shore Long Island Jewish Hospital School of Medicine, Manhasset, NY, USA

Jörg Baldauf, MD
Consultant, Department of Neurosurgery, University Medicine Greifswald, Germany

Olivier Balédent, PhD
Department of Magnetic Resonance Imaging Processing, University Hospital of Amiens, Amiens, France

Patrick Bankah, MBChB, FWACS
Neurosurgery Division, Department of Surgery, Korle Bu Teaching Hospital, Accra, Ghana

Amy Bastian, PhD
Professor, Department of Neuroscience, Johns Hopkins University School of Medicine, Kennedy Krieger Institute, Baltimore, MD, USA

Marc R. Del Bigio, MD, PhD, FRCPC
Department of Pathology, University of Manitoba, Diagnostic Services Manitoba, and Manitoba Institute of Child Health, Winnipeg, Canada

Ari M. Blitz, MD
Division of Neuroradiology, Department of Radiology and Radiologic Sciences, The Johns Hopkins Medical Institutions, Baltimore, MD, USA

Are Brean, MD, PhD
Senior Consultant in Neurology, Department of Neurology, Oslo University Hospital – Rikshospitalet, Oslo, and Journal of the Norwegian Medical Association, Oslo, Norway

Krzysztof Cieslicki, PhD
Faculty of Mechatronics, Warsaw University of Technology, Warsaw, Poland

Marek Czosnyka, PhD
Department of Clinical Neurosciences, University of Cambridge, Addenbrooke's Hospital, Cambridge, UK

Zofia Czosnyka, PhD
Department of Clinical Neurosciences, University of Cambridge, Addenbrooke's Hospital, Cambridge, UK

Per Kristian Eide, MD, PhD
Professor of Neurosurgery, Department of Neurosurgery, Oslo University Hospital – Rikshospitalet, Oslo, and Faculty of Medicine, University of Oslo, Oslo, Norway

Benjamin D. Elder, MD, PhD
Department of Neurosurgery, The Johns Hopkins Medical Institutions, Baltimore, MD, USA

Aristotelis S. Filippidis, MD, PhD
Fellow, Department of Neurosurgery, Boston Medical Center, Boston, MA, USA

Steffen Fleck, MD
Consultant, Department of Neurosurgery, University Medicine Greifswald, Germany

C. Rory Goodwin, MD, PhD
Department of Neurosurgery, The Johns Hopkins Hospital, Baltimore, MD, USA

Nicholas Higgins, FRCP, FRCR
Department of Neuroradiology, Addenbrooke's Hospital, Cambridge, UK

Masatsune Ishikawa, MD, PhD
Normal Pressure Hydrocephalus Center, Otowa Hospital, Rakuwakai, Kyoto, Japan

Marianne Juhler, MD, DMSc
Professor of Experimental Neurosurgery, Copenhagen University and University Clinic of Neurosurgery at Rigshospitalet, Copenhagen, Denmark

Ignacio Jusué-Torres, MD, PhD
Post-doctoral Fellow, Department of Neurosurgery, The Johns Hopkins Medical Institutions, Baltimore, MD, USA

Heather Katzen, PhD
Assistant Research Professor, Department of Neurology, University of Miami Miller School of Medicine, Miami, FL, USA

Cemil Kayis, PhD
Department of Neurosurgery, Medical College of Virginia Commonwealth University, Richmond, VA, USA

Adam P. Klausner, MD
Associate Professor, Division of Urology, Director, Neurology and Voiding Dysfunction, and Warren W. Koontz Professor of Urologic Research, Virginia Commonwealth University School of Medicine, Richmond, VA, USA

Petra Margarete Klinge, MD
Associate Professor of Neurosurgery, Warren Alpert Medical School of Brown University, Providence, RI, USA

Thomas A. Kosztowski, MD
Department of Neurosurgery, The Johns Hopkins Medical Institutions, Baltimore, MD, USA

John McGregor, MD
Department of Neurological Surgery, The Ohio State University Wexner Medical Center, Columbus, OH, USA

Ahmed Mohyeldin, MD, PhD
Department of Neurological Surgery, The Ohio State University Wexner Medical Center, Columbus, OH, USA

Debraj Mukherjee, MD, MPH
Maxine-Dunitz Neurosurgical Institute, Department of Neurosurgery, Cedars-Sinai Medical Center, Los Angeles, CA, USA

John D. Pickard, MD
Professor, Academic Neurosurgery Unit, Department of Clinical Neurosciences, University of Cambridge, Addenbrooke's Hospital, Cambridge, UK

Jonathan Pindrik, MD
Assistant Resident/Housestaff, Department of Neurological Surgery, Johns Hopkins University School of Medicine, Baltimore, MD, USA

Harold L. Rekate, MD
Director, The Chiari Institute and Professor of Neurosurgery, Hofstra Northshore LIJ College of Medicine, Great Neck, NY, USA

Norman Relkin, MD, PhD
Department of Neurology, Weill Cornell Medical College, New York, NY, USA

Hugh K. Richards, PhD
Academic Neurosurgery, Addenbrooke's Hospital, Cambridge, UK

Daniele Rigamonti, MD, FACS, FAHA
Professor of Neurosurgery, Radiology, and Radiation Oncology, Johns Hopkins University, Baltimore, MD, USA

Samuel P. Robinson, MD
Virginia Commonwealth University School of Medicine, Richmond, VA, USA

Wouter I. Schievink, MD
Maxine-Dunitz Neurosurgical Institute, Department of Neurosurgery, Cedars-Sinai Medical Center, Los Angeles, CA, USA

Henry W. S. Schroeder, MD, PhD
Professor and Chairman, Department of Neurosurgery, University Medicine Greifswald, Germany

Martin U. Schuhmann, MD, PhD
Department of Neurosurgery, Eberhard-Karls-Universität Tübingen, Germany

Ammar Shaikhouni, MD, PhD
Department of Neurological Surgery, The Ohio State University Wexner Medical Center, Columbus, OH, USA

Stefano Signoretti, MD, PhD
Division of Neurosurgery, Department of Head & Neck Surgery, Azienda Ospedaliera S. Camillo-Forlanini, Rome, Italy

Andrew A. Tarnaris, MD, MRCS
Department of Neurosurgery, University Hospitals Birmingham NHS Foundation Trust, Birmingham, UK

Carsten Wikkelsø, MD, PhD
Professor, Institute of Neuroscience and Physiology, Department of Clinical Neuroscience and Rehabilitation, University of Gothenburg, Gothenburg, Sweden

Jun Zhang, ScD, PhD
Associate Professor, Center of Excellence in Neurosciences, Texas Tech University Health Sciences Center, El Paso, TX, USA

Prologue

Solomon Hakim and colleagues, fifty years ago, described a new syndrome of reversible dementia, which they called normal pressure hydrocephalus (NPH).

Prior to the advent of CT and MRI the diagnosis was limited and depended greatly on the clinical acumen of the clinician to recognize the presence of the triad of symptoms and to notice improvement following a lumbar puncture.

CT and MRI have revolutionized the diagnostic process and document symptomatic and asymptomatic ventriculomegaly. The understanding of the pathophysiology has improved and we better understand the biology and the natural history of this syndrome.

The late Tony Marmarou led an effort to develop, in the last decade, a very useful set of guidelines to improve the diagnosis and treatment of this condition.

Currently, there is a general consensus that surgical intervention should be recommended when either a large volume spinal puncture or prolonged external lumbar drainage produces unequivocal improvement or an infusion test demonstrates an abnormal resistance to outflow. The recently published European multicenter study on hydrocephalus, however, confirmed that these diagnostic procedures have a significant false negativity.

The standard surgical intervention for NPH has been a shunt. Endoscopic third ventriculostomy (ETV) has been very effective in those cases of NPH where a clear obstruction to the CSF pathway is present. Several early reports advocating the use of ETV in cases of "idiopathic" NPH have not been reproduced.

Analysis of interventional outcomes in cases in which high definition MRI has ruled out any obstruction to CSF pathway confirms that a significant percentage of patients diagnosed with hydrocephalus do not improve following ETV.

The main purpose of this book is to provide an update on NPH, and more broadly on adult hydrocephalus, that will lead to better diagnosis and management for these patients.

I, therefore, asked internationally recognized scholars in the field to contribute their knowledge and experience to critically summarize knowledge gained in recent years and to create a common foundation for future patient care.

Section 1 discusses the pathology, epidemiology, anatomy, animal models, and genetics of hydrocephalus providing the foundation for the understanding of the nature of this condition.

Section 2 discusses the pathophysiology of hydrocephalus in the human disease and the mechanisms underlying gait, memory, and urinary dysfunction. It also looks at the NPH grading scales that are critical to improving patient selection.

Section 3 deals with the important elements of the differential diagnosis, imaging and physiological diagnostic modalities, as well as CSF biomarkers.

Section 4 reviews the therapeutic options and the outcomes.

Section 5 includes conditions that are frequently associated with or mentioned in the context of hydrocephalus.

My heartfelt thanks go to all the contributors, whose effort made this book possible; to Jamie Hoffberger, my research assistant; and to the team at Cambridge University Press, led by Nicholas Dunton, that shepherded the project through.

Chapter 1

Anatomy and physiology of the cerebrospinal fluid system

Thomas A. Kosztowski, Aristotelis S. Filippidis, C. Rory Goodwin, Benjamin D. Elder, and Daniele Rigamonti

Introduction

Water distribution of the brain

In the average human, the total body water is about 60% of the body weight [1]. The brain is highly sensitive to the amount and distribution of water in the intracranial space. The intracranial space enclosing the brain has a capacity of about 1600–1700 ml. About 100–150 ml of this capacity is occupied by cerebrospinal fluid (CSF) [1]. Other components in the intracranial cavity include blood (100–150 ml). The remaining volume is comprised of brain parenchyma and intracellular and interstitial spaces. The brain parenchyma, CSF, and blood all interact with one another in a pressure–volume relationship known as the Monro–Kellie doctrine. According to the Monro–Kellie doctrine, the volume inside the cranium is a fixed volume and the intracranial components are in equilibrium such that an increase in one component (i.e. brain parenchyma) must lead to a compensatory decrease in another component. Since the brain parenchyma is minimally compressible, the primary buffers for increased intracranial volumes are CSF and to a lesser extent blood. The total intracranial and extracranial volume of CSF is divided between the ventricular system (35 ml, 25%), the spinal canal (30–70 ml, 20–50%), and the cranial subarachnoid space (35–75 ml, 25–55%) [2,3]. Cerebrospinal fluid is formed at a rate of approximately 500 ml each day. This volume is three to four times as much as the total volume in the entire CSF system and reflects that CSF is constantly being replaced [1].

CSF function

CSF provides physical protection for the brain and spinal cord through buoyancy and thus by reducing the active weight of the nervous structures. Immersed in CSF, the active weight of the brain is reduced from 1500 g to as few as 50 g thus reducing tension on the nerve roots and vessels and the risk of injury in case of trauma [4]. More importantly, CSF functions as a reservoir to get rid of metabolites and toxins from the brain. It also plays a role in homeostatic hormonal signaling, chemical buffering, circulations of nutrients, and neurodevelopment [4–7].

CSF composition

Under normal conditions, CSF is a clear and colorless fluid with a density ranging from 1.003 to 1.008 g/cm^3. Compared to plasma, CSF has a lower concentration of glucose, protein, and potassium while having a higher concentration of chloride. The CSF protein concentration in adult mammals is 2–3 orders of magnitude lower than plasma, reflecting the degree of impermeability of the blood–CSF barrier to macromolecules [8]. Nevertheless, a great amount of research is being done on protein composition and the role it may play in disease states. β2-transferrin is a special iron-binding glycoprotein only found in CSF, perilymph, and ocular fluids that can be used to determine whether watery discharge from a patient is CSF [9,10].

Anatomy of the CSF system

The CSF system is a multi-compartmental large-cavity fluid system encompassing the ventricles, cisterns, and subarachnoid space (SAS), all serially linked with one another. The two lateral ventricles drain into the third ventricle through the foramina of Monro. The third ventricle subsequently drains into the fourth ventricle through the narrowest portion of the ventricular system called the cerebral aqueduct (of Sylvius). From there CSF enters the subarachnoid cisterns around the

Adult Hydrocephalus, ed. Daniele Rigamonti. Published by Cambridge University Press.

brain through the foramen of Magendie and the foramina of Luschka.

Although CSF is contained within the walls of the ventricular system, ventricular CSF is functionally interactive with the ependymal walls of the ventricles as well as the underlying brain capillary surfaces [11]. Bulk flow and diffusion promote water and solute distribution in and out of the brain, depending upon prevailing regional concentration gradients and hydrostatic pressure gradients.

Anatomy of the lateral ventricles

The two lateral ventricles are mirror images of one another, separated by the septum pellucidum and septal nuclei. The inferolateral portion of the frontal horn, body, and atrium of the lateral ventricles comes in contact with the caudate and then the thalamus more posteriorly. The portions of the lateral ventricles are bounded superiorly by the corpus callosum and forceps. Laterally, the lateral ventricles are bordered by the cerebral white matter between the caudate and thalamus below and the corpus callosum above [12].

The temporal horn of the lateral ventricles is surrounded by the hippocampus medially, the parahippocampal white matter inferiorly, and the temporal lobe white matter laterally and superiorly. The tail of the caudate nucleus also runs along the roof of the temporal horns. The amygdala also abuts the medial portion near the temporal horns.

The occipital horn of the lateral ventricles is completely encompassed by the white matter of the occipital lobe except when the calcarine fissure encroaches near the calcar avis.

Anatomy of the foramina of Monro

The anterior and medial border of the foramen of Monro is the fornix, whereas the posterior and lateral circumference of the foramen of Monro is bounded by the thalamus and choroid plexus. The choroid plexus courses anteriorly along the choroidal fissure (a cleft between the fornix medially, and the thalamus laterally) to reach the inferolateral aspect of the foramen of Monro. The thalamostriate vein runs in a sulcus that separates the caudate nucleus and thalamus. The confluence of the thalamostriate vein and the septal vein gives origin to the internal cerebral vein. The point of confluence is the venous angle – an angiographic landmark for the foramen of Monro on lateral view angiogram.

Anatomy of the third ventricle

The midline, normally slit-like third ventricle is bounded laterally by the thalami. On the anteroinferior border there is the hypothalamus. The interthalamic adhesion (massa intermedia) traverses the third ventricle. The floor of the third ventricle is comprised of the tuber cinereum anteriorly whereas the posterior portion is comprised of the mammillary bodies and the rostral portion of the midbrain. The lamina terminalis forms the anterior wall and contains the anterior commissure superiorly and the optic chiasm inferiorly. The optic recess is found on the anterior aspect of the floor of the third ventricle just above the optic chiasm. More posteriorly is the infundibular recess. The roof of the third ventricle is comprised of the tela choroidea, which contains the internal cerebral veins and the posteromedial choroidal arteries and is a continuation of the choroid plexus that runs across the lateral ventricles into the foramina of Monro and then along the roof of the third ventricle. The internal cerebral veins drain the choroid plexuses and join to form the great cerebral vein (of Galen).

Cerebral aqueduct

The cerebral aqueduct connects the third and fourth ventricles and is on average 15 mm in length in adults with a diameter varying from 0.5 to 2.8 mm along its course. It is surrounded by the periaqueductal gray matter of the midbrain. Anterior to the cerebral aqueduct lie the tegmental midbrain structures including the oculomotor and trochlear nuclei. Posterior to the cerebral aqueduct is the midbrain tectum comprised of the superior and inferior colliculi, which contribute to the strictures in the cerebral aqueduct [13].

Anatomy of the fourth ventricle

The fourth ventricle is located behind the pons (rostral half) and the medulla (caudal half). It is bounded laterally by the superior, middle, and inferior cerebellar peduncles. The roof of the fourth ventricle is bounded by the vermis of the cerebellum (superior half) and the fastigium (inferior half). The caudal portion of the roof of the fourth ventricle opens into the cisterna magna via the foramen of Magendie medially and the foramina of Luschka laterally. The inferior apex of the fourth ventricle is surrounded by the obex and is continuous with the central canal of the spinal cord.

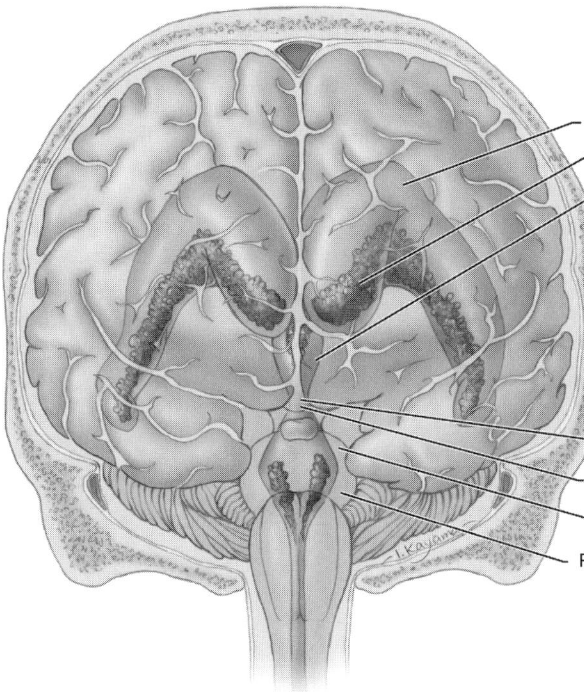

Figure 1.1 Overview of the ventricular system and cisterns. CSF is produced and flows from the lateral ventricles into the third and then fourth ventricles. From the fourth ventricle, CSF empties into the cisterns of the skull base, which will then flow into CSF cisterns of the cerebral convexities. A full-color version is included in the color plate section.

Overview of the cisterns

The cisterns are CSF spaces situated between the brain and skull separated from each other by trabeculated porous walls of arachnoid with various size openings. They typically contain traversing arteries, veins, or nerves. These cisterns are bounded by septations, which may become inflamed and fibrotic thus limiting circulation of CSF [12]. There is increasing research now suggesting that this pathology may contribute to some cases of communicating hydrocephalus. CSF empties into the cistern magna via the medial foramen of Magendie and the lateral foramina of Luschka (Figure 1.1). The CSF then circulates in the subarachnoid cisterns surrounding the brainstem (i.e. prepontine, interpeduncular, and ambient cisterns) to reach the cerebral convexities. Ultimately, CSF will diffuse passively into the venous sinuses via the arachnoid villi.

Cerebral convexity CSF spaces

The cerebral convexity CSF spaces are located over the cerebral cortex and within sulci as well as between the dura. Much of the CSF reabsorption will occur at the arachnoid granulations of the dural sinuses. The cerebral convexity CSF spaces are large in fetuses and become progressively smaller towards childhood and adolescence. However, they enlarge again in old age, most prominently over the parietal lobes.

Spinal CSF anatomy

The CSF spaces of the spine extend from the foramen magnum down to the filum terminale surrounding the spinal cord and the nerve roots. The CSF spaces extend laterally from the vertebral foramina to the nerve sheaths of the spinal sensory ganglions. These nerve sheath diverticula have mechanical purposes (e.g. sliding motion to the spinal nerves and elasticity to the meninges) as well as serving as sites for CSF reabsorption.

CSF production

About 500 ml of CSF is produced each day in the average human adult. The choroid plexus is responsible for 60–70% of CSF production. Another 30–40% comes from the interstitial fluid exudated from the pia from vessels as well as metabolism. CSF production is to a degree dependent on blood perfusion. In instances of increased intracranial pressure (ICP) with subsequent decreased cerebral perfusion, there will be a decrease in CSF production.

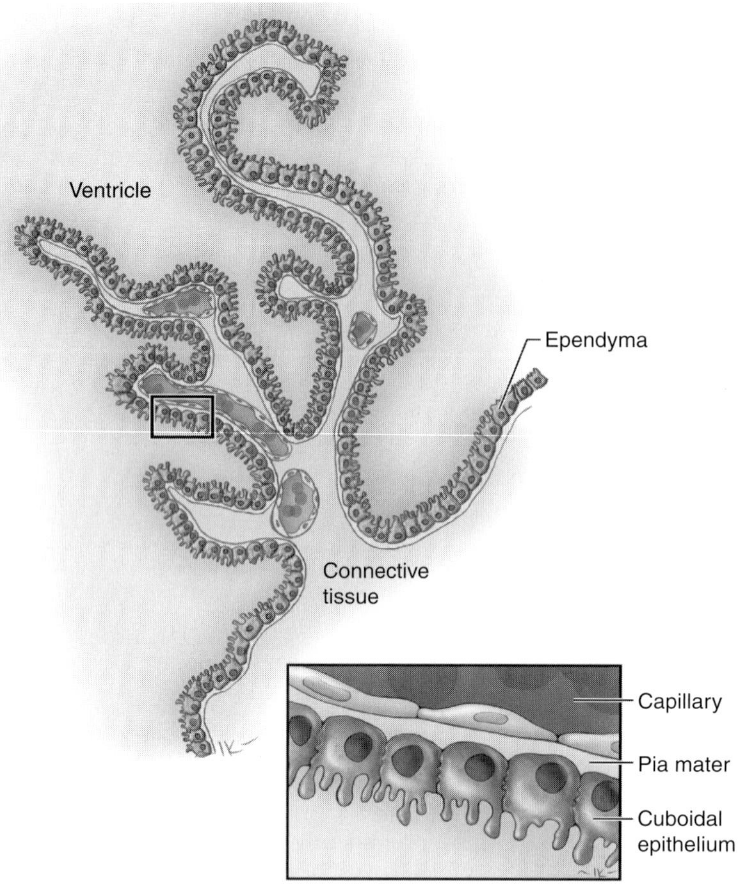

Figure 1.2 The choroid plexus has a "hobnail" appearance. It consists of a layer of cuboidal epithelial cells that surround an inner core comprised of connective tissue, pia mater, and capillaries. A full-color version is included in the color plate section.

Choroid plexus

Structure

The choroid plexus is located in the roof of the temporal horns of the lateral ventricle and the roof of the third and fourth ventricles and rests on the floor of the frontal horns and atriums of the lateral ventricles. It is comprised of vascular pial stroma covered by a choroidal epithelium (Figure 1.2). The choroid plexus contains a vascular endothelium that is fenestrated, unlike most vessels of the brain [4]. The zona occludens that connect the choroidal endothelial cells still permit most small hydrophilic molecules to pass [3]. The tight junctions present on the apical surface of choroid plexus epithelial cells, however, provide for tightly sealed junctions in contrast to the ventricular ependyma [4].

CSF secretion

The primary function of the choroid plexus is the secretion of CSF, which is accomplished by water ultrafiltrate following an osmotic gradient produced by ions such as Na^+, Cl^-, and HCO_3^-. Active transport with ATP hydrolysis occurs to create a unidirectional flux of these ions across the choroid plexus epithelial layer, in turn driving osmotic transcellular movement of water [14,15]. The aquaporin-1 channel located on the CSF-facing apical surface of the choroid epithelial cells allows for water movement [16]. Aquaporin-1 inhibition has been proposed as a method to treat hydrocephalus; however, studies with aquaporin-1 knockout mice still produce a normal amount of CSF, suggesting other mechanisms of water transport [17]. Nevertheless, CSF production is known to be reduced by acetazolamide, diuretics, changes in CSF osmolality, steroids, and low temperatures [18].

Other functions

In addition to its CSF secretory function, the choroidal epithelium synthesizes a large number of bioactive peptides [6]. These bioactive peptides include insulin-like growth factor II, transforming growth factor beta, fibroblast growth factor, human growth factor, arginine vasopressin, and some bone morphogenetic proteins [11]. These CSF peptides can act on brain structures such as the hypothalamus or chemosensitive structures of the medulla oblongata. They can also act on the choroid plexus itself in an autocrine fashion [11].

The choroid plexus may also be involved in eliminating endogenous waste and foreign substances from the CSF, thus cleansing the CSF and adjusting CSF and brain extracellular fluid [11,19,20]. On the apical surface of choroid plexus epithelial cells have been found peptide transporters, multidrug resistance-associated proteins, organic anion-transporting polypeptides, and organic ion transporters [11,20]. Furthermore, the continual turnover of CSF is a mechanism to rid the brain of metabolic wastes and also maintain optimal pH.

Interstitial fluid contribution to CSF production

Anywhere from 10% to 30% (but possibly as much as 60%) of CSF fluid is thought to arise from bulk flow of interstitial fluid that derives from transport across blood vessels and from endogenous metabolism that produces water byproducts [4,21]. One large contributor to this volume of fluid is oxidative metabolism of glucose leading to water production, which can produce as much as 12% of net volume of CSF.

CSF flow

CSF flows via net bulk flow from the lateral ventricles through the foramen of Monro into the third ventricle, then on into the fourth ventricle via the cerebral aqueduct. Ultimately, CSF empties out of the fourth ventricle via the midline foramen of Magendie and the lateral foramina of Luschka into the subarachnoid cisterns (there is also a minor amount of CSF that is thought to travel through the spinal central canal straight from the fourth ventricle). Once in the subarachnoid space, the CSF travels over the cortical convexity and skull base, and to a lesser extent into the spinal subarachnoid space until it is ultimately reabsorbed at the dural venous sinuses and around the neural sheaths [22].

Cellular composition of the ventricles

CSF circulation is influenced by the cells, junctional barriers, and membranes lining the ventricular and subarachnoid spaces. In addition to the choroid plexus, the ventricles and the central canal are lined by a continuous single layer of cuboidal and columnar ciliated epithelial cells called ependymal cells [23]. The zona adherens and the numerous gap junctions between these cells allow them to act as a barrier to water movement, although fluid still may permeate into the brain parenchyma. The cilia are believed to possibly contribute to the direction and quantity of CSF flow. Scattered in the layer of ependymal cells are specialized cells, called tanycytes, which have radially directed basal processes that extend into the neuropil where they come in contact with blood vessels. The tanycytes of the third ventricle are believed to help regulate neuroendocrine function as well as guiding functions for hypothalamic axons, and transport between ventricle and blood vessels of the portal system [24,25]. Directly beneath the cells of the ependyma is a basement membrane that forms labyrinths connecting the basement membrane to the perivascular basement membranes of the subependymal capillaries and veins. These glycoprotein and glycolipid basement membranes hold fluid by swelling [26].

CSF flow through the ventricles

CSF is thought to travel through the ventricles in a pulsatile manner with each cardiac systole and respiratory inhalation. There are data from human radiographic imaging studies as well as animal studies showing that cardiac pulsation plays a dominant role in CSF flow [27,28]. Animal data suggest that pressures in the subarachnoid space are also influenced by respiratory function to a great degree [29,30]. Coughing or Valsalva maneuver will cause CSF to flow cranially and then caudally. The cilia of the ependyma most likely play a lesser role in CSF movement; however, there are some animal data suggesting that cilia function is necessary for regulating ion transport and CSF production, as well as for CSF flow through the ventricles [31].

CSF flow through the cranial subarachnoid cisterns and Virchow–Robin spaces

Outside of the ventricles, the intracranial CSF exists within the subarachnoid space between the pia and arachnoid mater. The arachnoid cell layer contributes

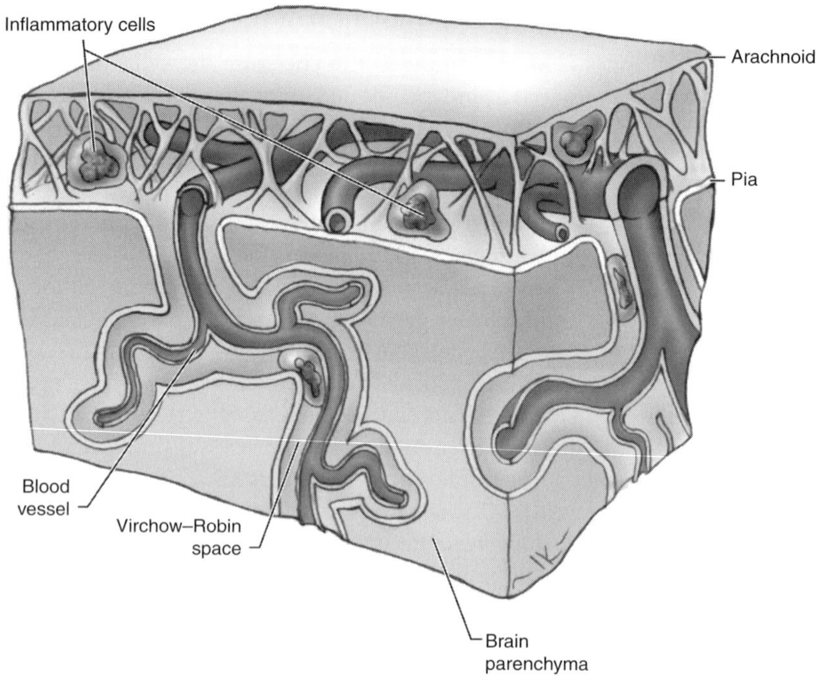

Figure 1.3 Virchow–Robin spaces are fluid-filled spaces surrounding perforating arteries and veins coming into and out of the brain parenchyma, respectively. They are found in the subarachnoid and subpial spaces. A full-color version is included in the color plate section.

to the blood–brain barrier and is composed of cells, cell junctions, and an internal basement membrane [32]. The arachnoid consists of an outer portion, the arachnoid barrier cell layer, and an inner part, the arachnoid trabeculae which span the subarachnoid space [33]. Arachnoid barrier cells are closely packed and joined by many cell junctions [33]. Arachnoid trabecular cells comprise the arachnoid trabeculae that span the subarachnoid space, have extracellular collagen associated with their flattened processes, and form cisternal structures of variable shapes and sizes [33]. Nerves and vessels traverse these cisterns. Under normal conditions, CSF flows through the cisterns. Obstruction of CSF flow through the cisterns may explain the development of communicating hydrocephalus in some conditions such as post-meningitic or hemorrhagic hydrocephalus [34].

Another location that has important implications in cerebral fluid movement is the perivascular Virchow–Robin spaces found between the blood vessels and the brain and spine (Figure 1.3). Virchow–Robin spaces are continuous with the subpial and subarachnoid spaces and thus provide a pathway for fluid flow from the subarachnoid space to the brain and spinal cord [35]. This perivascular flow of CSF has been shown in animal models [36,37]. The pulsation of arteries has been suggested as the driving force for perivascular flow [27].

CSF flow through the spinal central canal and subarachnoid space

The central canal plays little to no part in CSF flow. Human cadaver studies have demonstrated central canal stenosis or occlusion in 75–97% of people after the third decade of life [38,39].

Magnetic resonance imaging has suggested that spinal subarachnoid CSF is also greatly influenced by the cardiac cycle. Cardiac systole initiates an anterior and caudal spinal cord movement, followed by caudal CSF flow and then cranial flow during diastole [28,40].

Other possible routes of CSF circulation

Recent advances in molecular biology and ionic physiology provided a different prism for the understanding of biological fluid turnover and homeostasis in biological membranes. The discovery of aquaporins, by Peter Agre, solved a longstanding riddle related to water homeostasis and movement in biology and led to a Nobel Prize in 2003 [41]. Aquaporins, later on, were identified as the most important regulators of water movement and homeostasis in various organisms from bacteria, to plants, to mammals [42]. Interestingly, aquaporin-1 (AQP1) and aquaporin-4 (AQP4) can be identified in abundance in the central nervous system. AQP1 is predominantly identified at the apical

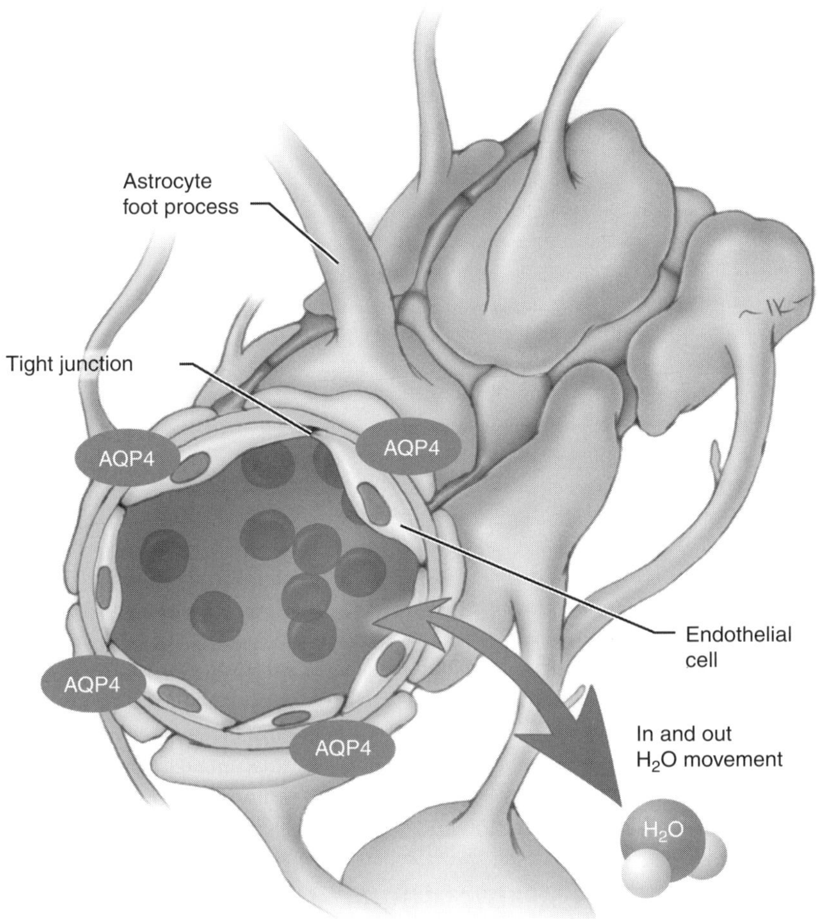

Figure 1.4 AQP4 can be identified at the astrocytic endfeet, at the level of the blood–brain barrier and plays a significant role in the movement of water into and out of the brain. A full-color version is included in the color plate section.

(CSF side) of the choroid plexus and the ependyma while AQP4 is found mainly at the brain cortical surface, at the glia limitans layer just below the pia matter, and also can be identified at the astrocytic endfeet, at the level of the blood–brain-barrier (BBB) [42, 43] (Figures 1.4 and 1.5). The presence of aquaporins at anatomical sites related to CSF production or outflow or sites where the brain interstitial fluid (ISF) meets the circulation (BBB) created a strong debate concerning their role in CSF turnover at these sites. Most evidence describing their role is obtained indirectly from studies related to hydrocephalus or AQP knockout mice [44]. In AQP1 knockout (KO) mice, ICP is lower and CSF production is lower too, although a systemic effect at the kidneys was also observed. This observation suggested a role for AQP1 in CSF production or turnover at the AQP1-rich sites such as the choroid plexus and the ependyma [45]. In AQP4 KO mice, kaolin-induced hydrocephalus, ICP, and brain water content were significantly worse than in the controls. These findings suggested that AQP4 could be a significant water channel related to the ISF-CSF drainage in extreme conditions and possibly the sites of drainage could be the AQP4-rich sites such as the BBB and the glia limitans at the subpial zone [46].

In the field of biological fluid turnover, especially in preformed spaces lined by biological membranes, water channels work in perfect harmony with ion channels to induce micro-osmotic gradients that create water flux. Ionic flux especially for Na^+ and Cl^- is translated to paired water flux and this process is well described as "solute-coupled" transport [47–49]. A common example related to CSF turnover is the additive effect of the ion channels at the apical side of the choroid plexus, governed mainly by the effect of the sodium-potassium-ATPase pump that drives sodium

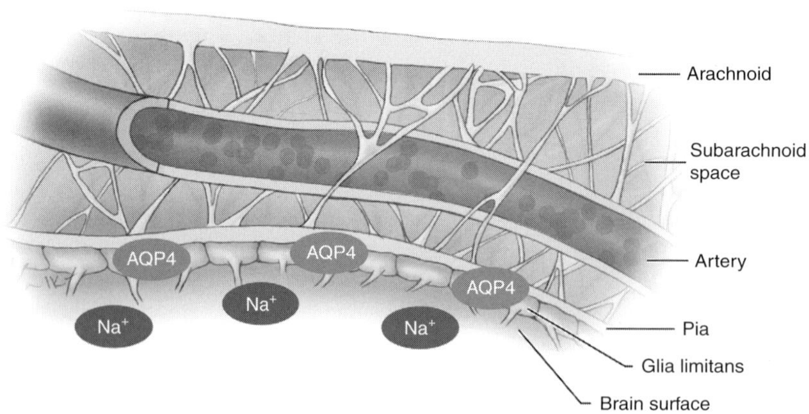

Figure 1.5 AQP4 is found mainly at the brain cortical surface, at the glia limitans layer just below the pia matter. A full-color version is included in the color plate section.

into the CSF side, paired with the effect of AQP1 that drives water from the basal site (bloodstream) through the choroid plexus cell to its apical site to the ventricle [50]. Ouabain, a specific sodium-potassium-ATPase inhibitor, can reduce CSF production by 70% [51,52], suggesting that the inhibition of "solute-coupled" transport is an important regulator of CSF turnover. The sodium-potassium-ATPase pump is the cornerstone of "solute-coupled" transport in epithelia [50,51,53,54]. It seems though that there are potentially more sites where "solute-coupled" transport related to CSF turnover occurs. In a seminal paper by Milhorat, CSF turnover was studied by observing the movement of ^{24}Na. Milhorat tried to identify differences between normal monkeys and monkeys that have undergone choroid plexectomy. Interestingly, in plexectomized monkeys, CSF production was reduced by 40%, while ^{24}Na, as an indirect water or CSF marker, was accumulated at brain sites around the ventricles and at sites bordering the subarachnoid space [55]. Thus, a potential avenue for CSF or water movement should also exist at the ventricular ependymal and the subarachnoid space. AQPs, such as AQP1 and AQP4, exist at these brain–CSF interfaces (Figure 1.5). In order to have a "solute-coupled" transport of water, polarized ion channels, and especially the presence of sodium-potassium-ATPAse, are needed at these interfaces. Filippidis et al. identified with membrane electrophysiology that the subarachnoid space behaves as a "leaky epithelium," an epithelium with high ionic movement and properties similar to mesothelial tissues with an essential role in fluid turnover such as the pleura, omentum, and pericardium [49]. Filippidis et al. also identified a polarized expression of sodium-potassium-ATPase at the subarachnoid space, which could be blocked with ouabain [56], suggesting that at the brain surface–glia limitans–subarachnoid space interface, water or CSF movement could potentially occur by the paired actions of the sodium-potassium-ATPase pump and aquaporins.

Cellular physiology and functional anatomy of the CSF spaces should be studied together to provide a holistic approach to the understanding of CSF physiology. It is coming to be understood that solute-coupled transport and bulk flow are the main forces governing the behavior of CSF flow in the central nervous system, both important at the micro and macro world of CSF production and outflow.

CSF absorption

The classic theory has been that the arachnoid granulations draining into the dural sinuses were the only site of CSF reabsorption but recent data are now suggesting that the mechanism of CSF reabsorption may be more complex than initially thought. There may be other pathways of CSF reabsorption such as the ependymal layer of the ventricular system, endothelial layer of the brain parenchyma, and the lymphatics [57–59].

Arachnoid granulations

Arachnoid villi consist of invaginations of arachnoid into the venous space called arachnoid granulations [60] (Figure 1.6). They are present in the cranial venous sinuses, and to a lesser extent in the venous angles in spinal nerve roots [22]. Arachnoid granulations are dilations of the subarachnoid space within a villus. Arachnoid granulations are more commonly found in adults over 18 years of age, while arachnoid villi have been found in younger infants [61]. Cords of arachnoid membrane penetrate the dura around a draining vein

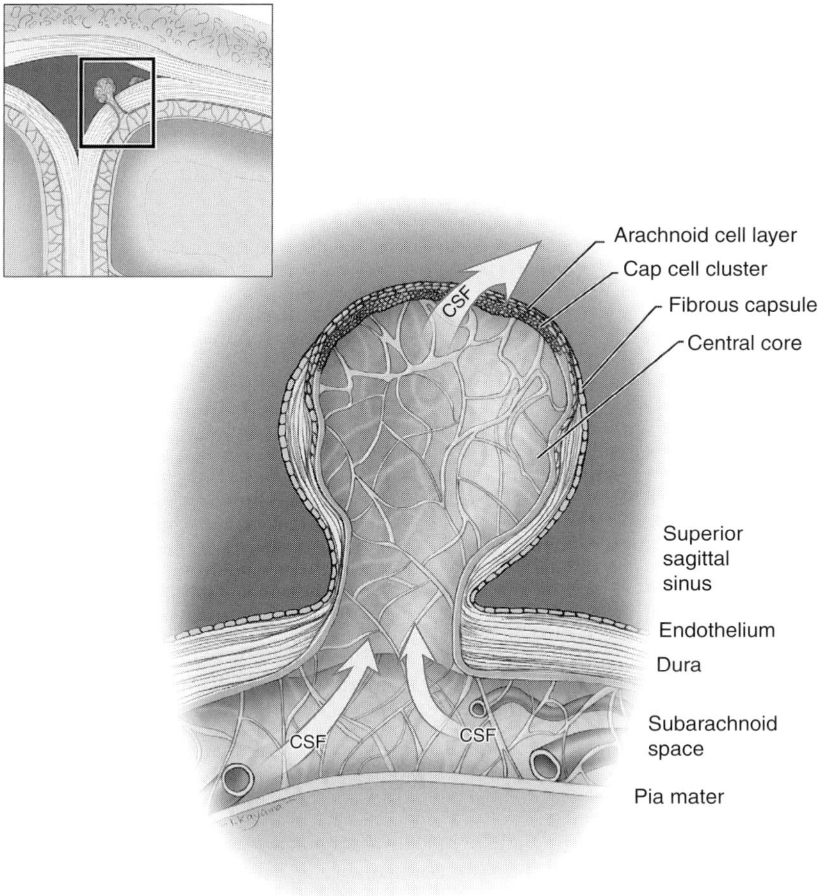

Figure 1.6 Arachnoid granulations consist of invaginations of arachnoid into the venous space. CSF from the subarachnoid space drains into the arachnoid villi and ultimately into the venous sinus. A full-color version is included in the color plate section.

and become a solid mass covered by arachnoid cells. CSF drains into the arachnoid villi from the neck of the villus, which is in contact with the subarachnoid space through dural defects allowing CSF to circulate into the arachnoid villi from the cranial subarachnoid space and ultimately into the venous sinus. CSF flow into the venous sinuses occurs passively via a pressure gradient [22]. Electron microscopy studies have shown that giant vacuoles form that communicate with both the subarachnoid and luminal parts of the cell simultaneously [60]. The greater the pressure gradient, the more vacuoles form.

Lymphatic drainage

Although lymphatics are not found within the central nervous system, there are experimental data suggesting connections between the brain tissue and cervical lymphatics [62]. One of the most prominent possible routes of lymphatic drainage is via the olfactory nerve rootlets at the cribriform plate with direct communication with lymphatic vessels [63,64]. In fact, some animal studies have suggested as much as 50% of CSF exits the cranium at the cribriform plate in various animal species [65,66]. Injection of various tracers (i.e. Microfil, ink tracers, labeled ink) into the brains of experimental animals or human cadavers had led to accumulation of tracer in the perivascular spaces, and eventually in the cervical and spinal lymph nodes, reaching a peak in 4 to 15 hours [63,67]. Obstruction of the lymphatics from the head in animal models resulted in elevated intracranial pressures [68].

The spinal lymphatic routes of CSF drainage have been proposed as another lymphatic drainage route.

In sheep as much as 25% of total CSF drainage can occur via this route. Radionucleotide testing in healthy human volunteers demonstrated that 0.11–0.23 ml/min of CSF could be absorbed from spinal routes, and more during exercise [69]. It has been hypothesized that CSF drainage from the spine occurs at spinal arachnoid granulations as well as at where the nerve sheaths merge with the perineurium at the arachnoid angle. CSF drainage may also occur as a result of direct CSF movement across dura into the epidural space into spinal lymphatic vessels.

Windkessel effect on CSF drainage

Our understanding of the mechanisms related to the absorption of intracranial arterial blood flow energy and how they relate to the absorption of CSF is continuing to evolve. The problem with relying on the Monro–Kellie doctrine is that it cannot explain CSF circulation and absorption in relation to cardiac function, which is why there has been interest in the Windkessel effect on CSF. The Windkessel effect is the energy transfer resultant from arterial blood flow energy formed by cardiac action that is transferred to the intracranial space as arterial blood flow, brain pulsation, and CSF pulsation and bulk flow. Arterial distension occurs during the systolic phase of blood pressure while arterial recoiling occurs during the diastolic phase of blood pressure. This provides for constant blood flow to arterioles and capillaries as a result of energy transferred from the force of arterial distension during the systolic phase to the recoil of the diastolic phase. A portion of this energy is also transferred to the brain in the form of brain pulsation and to the CSF in the form of CSF pulsation and bulk flow. The remaining energy finally dissipates as CSF passes through the arachnoid villi and exits via the venous system via a pressure gradient. The pulsatile flow kinetic energy of CSF is more than 100-fold greater than the bulk flow kinetic energy of CSF and would thus seem appropriate as the source of energy dissipation from arterial blood flow energy. It has been proposed that the CSF pulsation energy dissipates while maintaining a low intracranial pressure by the summation of a diverse array of CSF flow vectors that offset each other in direction and time [70]. This dispersion of CSF pulsation energy has been demonstrated radiographically by the diffuse, random mixing of CSF flow [71–73]. The dissipation of arterial blood flow energy by the CSF pulsation energy provides for the maintenance of a low ICP and subsequently high cerebral blood flow, which is the difference between mean arterial pressure and ICP. The Windkessel effect on CSF may explain why lateral ventricular dilation may occur in communicating hydrocephalus without changes in the mean ICP [70,74].

Conclusion

There is still a great amount that needs to be understood in regard to the dynamics between CSF production and absorption. Further understanding of the physiology and anatomy of the cerebrospinal fluid system will enable scientists and clinicians to develop better ways to approach and treat hydrocephalus.

References

1. Hall GA. *Medical Physiology*, 11th edn. Elsevier; 2006.
2. Kohn MI, Tanna NK, Herman GT, et al. Analysis of brain and cerebrospinal fluid volumes with MR imaging. Part I. Methods, reliability, and validation. *Radiology* 1991;178(1):115–22.
3. Redzic ZB, Segal MB. The structure of the choroid plexus and the physiology of the choroid plexus epithelium. *Adv Drug Deliv Rev* 2004;56(12):1695–716.
4. Kimelberg HK. Water homeostasis in the brain: basic concepts. *Neuroscience* 2004;129(4):851–60.
5. Redzic ZB, Preston JE, Duncan JA, Chodobski A, Szmydynger-Chodobska J. The choroid plexus-cerebrospinal fluid system: from development to aging. *Curr Top Dev Biol* 2005;71:1–52.
6. Chodobski A, Szmydynger-Chodobska J. Choroid plexus: target for polypeptides and site of their synthesis. *Microsc Res Tech* 2001;52(1):65–82.
7. Oldendorf WH, Davson H. Brain extracellular space and the sink action of cerebrospinal fluid. Measurement of rabbit brain extracellular space using sucrose labeled with carbon 14. *Arch Neurol* 1967;17(2):196–205.
8. Johanson CE, Stopa EG, McMillan PN. The blood-cerebrospinal fluid barrier: structure and functional significance. *Methods Mol Biol* 2011;686:101–31.
9. Papadea C, Schlosser RJ. Rapid method for beta2-transferrin in cerebrospinal fluid leakage using an automated immunofixation electrophoresis system. *Clin Chem* 2005;51(2):464–70.
10. Sloman AJ, Kelly RH. Transferrin allelic variants may cause false positives in the detection of cerebrospinal fluid fistulae. *Clin Chem* 1993;39(7):1444–5.

11. Smith DE, Johanson CE, Keep RF. Peptide and peptide analog transport systems at the blood-CSF barrier. *Adv Drug Deliv Rev* 2004;56(12):1765–91.
12. Raybaud C, Greenberg G. Imaging (normal and abnormal). In: Mallucci C, Sgouros S. (Eds.) *Cerebrospinal Fluid Disorders*. Informa Healthcare; 2010.
13. Longatti P, Fiorindi A, Perin A, Martinuzzi A. Endoscopic anatomy of the cerebral aqueduct. *Neurosurgery* 2007;61(3 Suppl):1–5; discussion 5–6.
14. Redzic ZB, Segal MB. The structure of the choroid plexus and the physiology of the choroid plexus epithelium. *Adv Drug Deliv Rev* 2004;56(12):1695–716.
15. Brown PD, Davies SL, Speake T, Millar ID. Molecular mechanisms of cerebrospinal fluid production. *Neuroscience* 2004;129(4):957–70.
16. Amiry-Moghaddam M, Ottersen OP. The molecular basis of water transport in the brain. *Nat Rev Neurosci* 2003;4(12):991–1001.
17. Gunnarson E, Zelenina M, Aperia A. Regulation of brain aquaporins. *Neuroscience* 2004;129(4):947–55.
18. McCarthy KD, Reed DJ. The effect of acetazolamide and furosemide on cerebrospinal fluid production and choroid plexus carbonic anhydrase activity. *J Pharmacol Exp Ther* 1974;189(1):194–201.
19. Emerich DF, Skinner SJ, Borlongan CV, et al. The choroid plexus in the rise, fall and repair of the brain. *Bioessays* 2005;27(3):262–74.
20. Kusuhara H, Sugiyama Y. Efflux transport systems for organic anions and cations at the blood-CSF barrier. *Adv Drug Deliv Rev* 2004;56(12):1741–63.
21. Cserr HF. Physiology of the choroid plexus. *Physiol Rev* 1971;51(2):273–311.
22. Brodbelt A, Stoodley M. CSF pathways: a review. *Br J Neurosurg* 2007;21(5):510–20.
23. Del Bigio MR. The ependyma: a protective barrier between brain and cerebrospinal fluid. *Glia* 1995;14(1):1–13.
24. Wittkowski W. Tanycytes and pituicytes: morphological and functional aspects of neuroglial interaction. *Microsc Res Tech* 1998;41(1):29–42.
25. Rodriguez EM, Blázquez JL, Pastor FE, et al. Hypothalamic tanycytes: a key component of brain-endocrine interaction. *Int Rev Cytol*, 2005;247:89–164.
26. Leonhardt H, Desaga U. Recent observations on ependyma and subependymal basement membranes. *Acta Neurochir (Wien)* 1975;31(3–4):153–9.
27. Stoodley MA, Brown SA, Brown CJ, Jones NR. Arterial pulsation-dependent perivascular cerebrospinal fluid flow into the central canal in the sheep spinal cord. *J Neurosurg* 1997;86(4):686–93.
28. Henry-Feugeas MC, Idy-Peretti I, Balédent O, et al. Origin of subarachnoid cerebrospinal fluid pulsations: a phase-contrast MR analysis. *Magn Reson Imaging* 2000;18(4):387–95.
29. Hall P, Turner M, Aichinger S, Bendick P, Campbell R. Experimental syringomyelia: the relationship between intraventricular and intrasyrinx pressures. *J Neurosurg* 1980;52(6):812–17.
30. Williams, B. On the pathogenesis of syringomyelia: a review. *J R Soc Med* 1980;73(11):798–806.
31. Banizs B, Pike MM, Millican CL, et al. Dysfunctional cilia lead to altered ependyma and choroid plexus function, and result in the formation of hydrocephalus. *Development* 2005;132(23):5329–39.
32. Alcolado R, Weller RO, Parrish EP, Garrod D. The cranial arachnoid and pia mater in man: anatomical and ultrastructural observations. *Neuropathol Appl Neurobiol* 1988;4(1):1–17.
33. Haines DE. On the question of a subdural space. *Anat Rec* 1991;230(1):3–21.
34. Li J, McAllister JP 2nd, Shen Y, et al. Communicating hydrocephalus in adult rats with kaolin obstruction of the basal cisterns or the cortical subarachnoid space. *Exp Neurol* 2008;211(2):351–61.
35. Zhang ET, Inman CB, Weller RO. Interrelationships of the pia mater and the perivascular (Virchow-Robin) spaces in the human cerebrum. *J Anat* 1990;170:111–23.
36. Ichimura T, Fraser PA, Cserr HF. Distribution of extracellular tracers in perivascular spaces of the rat brain. *Brain Res* 1991;545(1–2):103–13.
37. Stoodley MA, Jones NR, Brown CJ. Evidence for rapid fluid flow from the subarachnoid space into the spinal cord central canal in the rat. *Brain Res* 1996;707(2):155–64.
38. Milhorat TH, Kotzen RM, Anzil AP. Stenosis of central canal of spinal cord in man: incidence and pathological findings in 232 autopsy cases. *J Neurosurg* 1994;80(4):716–22.
39. Yasui K, Hashizume Y, Yoshida M, Kameyama T, Sobeu G. Age-related morphologic changes of the central canal of the human spinal cord. *Acta Neuropathol* 1999;97(3):253–9.
40. Greitz D, Greitz T, Hindmarsh T. A new view on the CSF-circulation with the potential for pharmacological treatment of childhood hydrocephalus. *Acta Paediatr* 1997;86(2):125–32.
41. Agre P, Nielsen S, Ottersen OP. Towards a molecular understanding of water homeostasis in the brain. *Neuroscience* 2004;129(4):849–50.
42. Verkman AS. Aquaporins at a glance. *J Cell Sci* 2011;124(Pt 13):2107–12.

43. Nielsen S, Nagelhus EA, Amiry-Moghaddam M, et al. Specialized membrane domains for water transport in glial cells: high-resolution immunogold cytochemistry of aquaporin-4 in rat brain. *J Neurosci* 1997;17(1):171–80.
44. Filippidis AS, Kalani MY, Rekate HL. Hydrocephalus and aquaporins: lessons learned from the bench. *Childs Nerv Syst* 2011;27(1):27–33.
45. Oshio K, Watanabe H, Song Y, Verkman AS, Manley GT. Reduced cerebrospinal fluid production and intracranial pressure in mice lacking choroid plexus water channel Aquaporin-1. *FASEB J* 2005;19(1):76–8.
46. Bloch O, Auguste KI, Manley GT, Verkman AS. Accelerated progression of kaolin-induced hydrocephalus in aquaporin-4-deficient mice. *J Cerebral Blood Flow Metab* 2006;26(12):1527–37.
47. Frömter E, Diamond J. Route of passive ion permeation in epithelia. *Nat New Biol* 1972;235(53):9–13.
48. Ussing HH, Zerahn K. Active transport of sodium as the source of electric current in the short-circuited isolated frog skin. *Acta Physiol Scand* 1951;23(2–3):110–27.
49. Filippidis A, Zarogiannis S, Ioannou M, et al. Transmembrane resistance and histology of isolated sheep leptomeninges. *Neurol Res* 2010;32(2):205–8.
50. Damkier HH, Brown PD, Praetorius J. Epithelial pathways in choroid plexus electrolyte transport. *Physiology (Bethesda)* 2010;25(4):239–49.
51. Pollay M, Curl F. Secretion of cerebrospinal fluid by the ventricular ependyma of the rabbit. *Am J Physiol* 1967;213(4):1031–8.
52. Segal MB, Pollay M. The secretion of cerebrospinal fluid. *Exp Eye Res* 1977;25(Suppl):127–48.
53. Hatzoglou CH, Gourgoulianis KI, Molyvdas PA. Effects of SNP, ouabain, and amiloride on electrical potential profile of isolated sheep pleura. *J Appl Physiol* 2001;90(4):1565–9.
54. Zarogiannis S, Gourgoulianis K, Molyvdas PA, Hatzoglou C. Existence of Na(+)-K(+) ATPase in sheep visceral and parietal pleura. *Respir Physiol Neurobiol* 2008;164(3):289; author reply 290.
55. Milhorat TH, Hammock MK, Fenstermacher JD, Levin VA. Cerebrospinal fluid production by the choroid plexus and brain. *Science* 1971;173(3994):330–2.
56. Filippidis AS, Zarogiannis SG, Ioannou M, et al. Permeability of the arachnoid and pia mater. The role of ion channels in the leptomeningeal physiology. *Childs Nerv Syst* 2012;28(4):533–40.
57. Sato O, Takei F, Yamada S. Hydrocephalus: is impaired cerebrospinal fluid circulation only one problem involved? *Childs Nerv Syst* 1994;10(3):151–5.
58. Pollay M. Overview of the CSF dual outflow system. *Acta Neurochir Suppl* 2012;113:47–50.
59. Oreskovic D, Klarica M. Development of hydrocephalus and classical hypothesis of cerebrospinal fluid hydrodynamics: facts and illusions. *Prog Neurobiol* 2011;94(3):238–58.
60. Tripathi BJ, Tripathi RC. Vacuolar transcellular channels as a drainage pathway for cerebrospinal fluid. *J Physiol* 1974;239(1):195–206.
61. Weed LH. Studies on cerebro-spinal fluid. No. III: The pathways of escape from the subarachnoid spaces with particular reference to the arachnoid villi. *J Med Res* 1914;31(1):51–91.
62. Mortensen OA, Sullivan WE. Cerebrospinal fluid and the cervical lymph nodes. *Anat Rec* 1933;56:356–63.
63. Cserr HF, Harling-Berg CJ, Knopf PM. Drainage of brain extracellular fluid into blood and deep cervical lymph and its immunological significance. *Brain Pathol* 1992;2(4):269–76.
64. Johnston M. The importance of lymphatics in cerebrospinal fluid transport. *Lymphat Res Biol* 2003;1(1):41–4; discussion 45.
65. Boulton M, Flessner M, Armstrong D, Hay J, Johnston M. Determination of volumetric cerebrospinal fluid absorption into extracranial lymphatics in sheep. *Am J Physiol* 1998;274(1 Pt 2):R88–96.
66. Boulton M, Flessner M, Armstrong D, et al. Contribution of extracranial lymphatics and arachnoid villi to the clearance of a CSF tracer in the rat. *Am J Physiol* 1999;276(3 Pt 2):R818–23.
67. Nagra G, Koh L, Zakharov A, Armstrong D, Johnston M. Quantification of cerebrospinal fluid transport across the cribriform plate into lymphatics in rats. *Am J Physiol Regul Integr Comp Physiol* 2006;291(5):R1383–9.
68. Mollanji R, Bozanovic-Sosic R, Zakharov A, Makarian L, Johnston MG. Blocking cerebrospinal fluid absorption through the cribriform plate increases resting intracranial pressure. *Am J Physiol Regul Integr Comp Physiol* 2002;282(6):R1593–9.
69. Edsbagge M, Starck G, Zetterberg H, Ziegelitz D, Wikkelso C. Spinal cerebrospinal fluid volume in healthy elderly individuals. *Clin Anat* 2011;24(6):733–40.
70. Min KJ, Yoon SH, Kang JK. New understanding of the role of cerebrospinal fluid: offsetting of arterial and brain pulsation and self-dissipation of cerebrospinal fluid pulsatile flow energy. *Med Hypotheses* 2011;76(6):884–6.
71. Greitz D, Wirestam R, Franck A, et al. Pulsatile brain movement and associated hydrodynamics studied by magnetic resonance phase imaging. The Monro-Kellie doctrine revisited. *Neuroradiology* 1992;34(5):370–80.

72. Greitz D. Radiological assessment of hydrocephalus: new theories and implications for therapy. *Neurosurg Rev* 2004;27(3):145–65; discussion 166–7.

73. Balédent O, Henry-Feugeas MC, Idy-Peretti I. Cerebrospinal fluid dynamics and relation with blood flow: a magnetic resonance study with semiautomated cerebrospinal fluid segmentation. *Invest Radiol* 2001;36(7):368–77.

74. Lee HS, Yoon SH. Hypothesis for lateral ventricular dilatation in communicating hydrocephalus: new understanding of the Monro-Kellie hypothesis in the aspect of cardiac energy transfer through arterial blood flow. *Med Hypotheses* 2009;72(2):174–7.

Chapter 2

Neuropathology of human hydrocephalus

Marc R. Del Bigio

Introduction

Hydrocephalus can be defined as a pathologic enlargement of the intracranial cerebrospinal fluid (CSF)-filled spaces. Usually this refers to the cerebral ventricles, but enlargement of the subarachnoid space can be an associated phenomenon. Most CSF is produced by the choroid plexus, while ~20% is water derived from brain as product of glycolysis [1] and movement of water across the blood–brain barrier [2]. Absorption of CSF is via arachnoid villi, which are mainly associated with venous sinuses, as well as via lymphatics associated with the exit sites of cranial and spinal nerves. The relative contribution of the two routes is likely species specific; the exact proportionate role in humans is not known [3,4]. CSF has multiple functions including cleansing of potentially noxious byproducts of brain metabolism, a route for molecular communication, and protection of brain by cushioning from vascular and extraneous shock waves [5,6]. It should be noted that the relative density of brain (1.036 g/cm^3) compared to CSF (1.006 g/cm^3) precludes the brain actually floating in CSF.

The monographs by Russell [7] and by Milhorat [8] summarize well the malformation, post-inflammatory, post-hemorrhagic, and tumor-associated causes of hydrocephalus. The author has reviewed the pathology and pathophysiology of hydrocephalus previously [9,10]; most of the recent reviews focus on developmental aspects particular to hydrocephalus in the immature brain including relationships to spina bifida and associated cerebellar changes, as well as potential pharmacologic interventions [11–13]. The reader is referred to these and other reviews [14,15] for a more comprehensive coverage of the subject. This chapter will focus on aspects of hydrocephalus that are common to all ages with a particular emphasis on the aging brain and the so-called normal pressure hydrocephalus (NPH) syndrome, which is a chronic disease that likely evolves over a period of years. It has been clear for decades that the rate of ventricular dilatation and the state of brain maturation have a significant impact on the pathology, and possibly the pathogenesis of brain damage. It is critical to recognize that the vast majority of experimental work related to hydrocephalus has utilized immature or young adult animals in which the ventricles dilate over a period of days to weeks. The extent to which this information can be generalized to a chronic disease of aging brain is not clear and the reader must use caution. Limitations and valid aspects of the animal models are revealed by autopsy descriptions of adults with chronic hydrocephalus including NPH [16–40].

Factors leading to ventricular enlargement

Idiopathic NPH has been distinguished from chronic adult hydrocephalus associated with prior meningitis, brain trauma, or subarachnoid hemorrhage (secondary NPH) [41]. This may be useful from a clinical and prognostic vantage, but from a pathophysiological perspective there is likely a spectrum rather than a boundary. Mild head trauma or "aseptic" meningitis, forgotten after decades, could create the basis for eventual impairment of CSF movement. Even mild subarachnoid hemorrhage causes inflammation and cellular proliferation in the subarachnoid compartment [42]; this, added to the gradual leptomeningeal fibrosis that occurs with aging [43], may eventually serve as a detriment to CSF movement. Brain biopsies on patients being investigated for NPH showed arachnoid fibrosis in approximately half the cases [44]. The fact that this did not correlate with CSF outflow resistance is not surprising given the limited sample.

In addition to changes in the subarachnoid compartment, another potential factor to explain the onset of symptoms in the elderly is the parallel accumulation of brain tissue and vascular changes associated with aging [45–47].

It is now apparent that some individuals with NPH have larger heads than unaffected individuals; they might have previously unrecognized congenital hydrocephalus that becomes symptomatic only late in life [48,49]. Discussion of the CSF forces that cause the ventricles to dilate is beyond the scope of this chapter although it should be noted that experimental studies show that very small pulsatile forces, only slightly greater than the normal pulse pressure, are capable of compressing the brain [50–52].

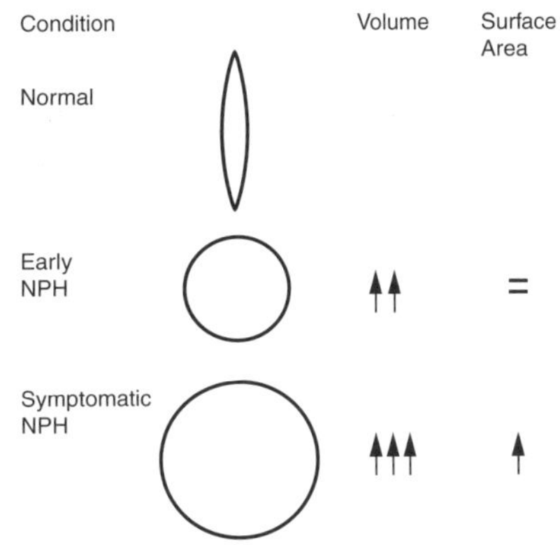

Figure 2.1 Diagram explaining the postulated threshold effect for tolerance to ventriculomegaly. In the normal state the ventricles are narrow. In the early presymptomatic stages of normal pressure hydrocephalus (NPH), the ventricle volume increases considerably by displacement of the ventricle walls but there is no stretching of the ventricle surface. In the symptomatic phase, the ventricles might be only marginally larger but the periventricular structures are stretched and experience decreased blood flow.

Consequences of ventricular enlargement and pathogenesis of brain damage in hydrocephalus

As the ventricles enlarge, adjacent brain tissue is displaced and later stretched or compressed (depending on the location). The initial displacement (e.g. elevation of the corpus callosum) may be at the expense of the subarachnoid compartment (especially if there is brain atrophy), the venous compartment, and the extracellular compartment with negligible damage to brain cells. Initially the opposite surfaces of the ventricles are spread apart but there is no change in the surface area. Beyond this threshold, when the surface area of the ventricles is forced to expand (Figure 2.1), periventricular white matter begins to sustain injury and functional changes become apparent. Atrophy of the ependymal lining of the ventricle surface is one of the first histopathological changes. However, this can be caused by a variety of factors and consequences in the adult brain are likely negligible [53].

NPH and white matter and cerebrovascular disease

Many imaging studies on NPH patients have shown decreased cerebral blood flow, especially in white matter [54]. Experimental studies in young adult dogs and rabbits suggest that this might be due to compression or constriction of the microvasculature [55,56]. This is likely more than a simple physical compression; regulation of blood flow at the local level is highly complex involving numerous signaling mediators, innervation, and interactions between astrocytes and blood vessels [57]. Calcium ion distribution and nitric oxide production are altered in experimental hydrocephalus [58,59]; although both could be involved in regulation of vascular tone, the hypothesis has not been directly tested in hydrocephalus. Studies of CSF from hydrocephalic humans provide evidence for hypoxic metabolism and lipid peroxidation [60,61]. As a consequence of these changes, oligodendrocytes, myelin, and axons are subject to hypoxic-ischemic stress and injury [59]. The molecular processes that damage axons are similar to those that follow ischemic stroke and head injury.

Imaging studies show atrophy of the fornix and corpus callosum in NPH patients [62]. We reported similar abnormalities in an autopsy study that included the full age spectrum of hydrocephalic patients [63]. Selective analysis of elderly brains from the same dataset shows that the corpus callosum and fornix are atrophic (Table 2.1). In general, however, the most severe ventricular enlargement and white matter atrophy associated with NPH are less than in the most severe chronic childhood-onset hydrocephalus cases. Compounding the situation in the aging brain is the accumulation of vascular changes associated with arterial hypertension and atherosclerosis. Many studies show an association between NPH and vascular disease [64–66], as well as diabetes [67]. However, the presence of white matter "vascular" abnormalities on imaging does not preclude a good response to shunting [68,69]. Although it is well known that rats with spontaneous arterial

Table 2.1 White matter changes in chronic adult hydrocephalus[a,b]

	Normal	Asymptomatic ventricle enlargement	Symptomatic hydrocephalus	Shunted hydrocephalus
Number of cases	8	10	5	1
Age range	60–81	66–87	68–90	67
Ventricle size cm[c]	1.5 ± 0.1	3.6 ± 0.2*	5.4 ± 1.1**	6.0
Corpus callosum thickness (mm)	4.1 ± 0.3	3.5 ± 0.3*	2.3 ± 0.6**	3.6
Area of fornix (mm^2)	6.0 ± 0.4	3.9 ± 1.0	4.2 ± 1.6	6.2

[a] The symptomatic hydrocephalus cases are compatible with a diagnosis of NPH. Most measurements were made on the coronal slice of the frontal lobes at the level of the caudate nucleus head. The data are shown as mean ± standard error of mean. Statistical comparison versus control used the Student *t* test; *$p < 0.05$, **$p < 0.01$.

[b] There was no difference between groups with respect to thickness of the periventricular layer of astrocytes (0.19 ± 0.05 mm), thickness of the alveus (0.31 ± 0.01 mm), or thickness of the frontal cortex (2.5 ± 0.1 mm). No case had more than minimal Alzheimer's disease neuropathologic change (i.e. senile plaque density sparse).

[c] Lateral ventricles were measured across the frontal horns at the horizontal level of the mid-caudate nucleus head.

hypertension (SHR strain) develop moderate enlargement of the ventricles [70], the additive effect between hydrocephalus and cerebrovascular disease has not been addressed experimentally.

Hydrocephalus and the extracellular fluid

In addition to the cascade of damage caused by diminished periventricular blood flow, alterations in fluid movements can cause changes in composition of the brain extracellular environment. Metabolic byproducts that cannot be recycled or moved across the blood–brain barrier normally flow to the ventricles whereupon they are washed away with CSF flow [6]. There is an accumulation of waste products, degeneration products, and neuromodulatory agents in CSF and brain tissue of hydrocephalic patients [60,71,72]. In hydrocephalic rats the cortical extracellular fluid flow is reduced [73,74], in rats and mice the extracellular spaces of gray matter are reduced in size [75,76], and in rabbits the cerebral cortex is compressed [77]. However, an electron microscopic study of the cortex from NPH patients showed enlargement of the extracellular space in 9/11 cases [78]. It is difficult to reconcile the discrepancy between the human and experimental animal findings. Morphologic and imaging studies indicate that the extracellular compartment is enlarged in periventricular white matter [79]. Disturbance of the extracellular volume and composition has the potential for impairing neuron and axon function. Reversal of this disturbance might account for some of the rapid improvement that occurs following shunting.

NPH and Alzheimer's disease

One of the main neuropathological features revealed in large series of NPH patients is the coexistence of Alzheimer's disease type changes, including senile (neuritic) plaques and neurofibrillary tangles. These have been demonstrated in cortical biopsies taken at the time of intracranial pressure monitoring or shunting [80,81], as well as in autopsies. This is the subject of an excellent recent review [23]. The biopsy studies and the larger series of autopsies (9–16 cases each) on NPH patients show that coexisting Alzheimer type changes and/or cerebrovascular changes do not necessarily predict failure of response to shunting [22,23,35]; however, moderate to severe Alzheimer type changes are associated with worse baseline cognitive performance and diminished postoperative improvement following shunting [82].

The only experiments that come close to investigating the combined effects of hydrocephalus and aging are those by Klinge, Silverberg, and coworkers. One-year-old rats were rendered hydrocephalic by injection of kaolin into the cisterna magna; over the following 10 weeks the brains had accumulations of amyloid beta protein and phosphorylated tau protein, both of which play a role in the pathogenesis of Alzheimer's disease [83,84]. Given that the average lifespan of rats is >2 years, these studies barely met their stated objective; nevertheless they do support the hypothesized interplay between extracellular fluid flow and the development of Alzheimer type pathological changes [85]. The relationship is not a simple one though. A prospective, randomized, double-blinded trial failed to show any benefit of a surgically implanted shunt in subjects with probable Alzheimer's disease [86].

NPH and autopsy findings

The question of disease coexistence with hydrocephalus was further addressed by retrospectively studying brains with ventricular enlargement in a population-based (rather than disease selected) autopsy series (Table 2.2 and Figure 2.2). From 1996 to 2012 the author has performed detailed brain examinations on 5 patients with a clinical diagnosis of idiopathic NPH, 3 patients with a clinical diagnosis of secondary NPH, and 20 patients in whom ventriculomegaly could not readily be explained by other disease processes identified. In the first two groups, 6/8 patients had been shunted; all had resolution of their gait abnormalities and incontinence, but not their cognitive deficits. Senile plaques were present in 6/8 cases, and cerebrovascular changes in 4/8. From the neuropathology perspective, there was no difference between the idiopathic and secondary NPH cases. Among the other 20 cases, the age and magnitude of ventricular enlargement was similar to those with a clinical diagnosis of NPH. As with the NPH groups, Alzheimer's disease type changes and cerebrovascular abnormalities were often present. The presence or absence of such changes could not explain the lack of symptoms in 9/20 individuals (although it must be noted that detailed histories were not always available). In retrospect, one individual who had ataxia and dementia might have had NPH (case C16 in Table 2.2). Considering all three groups together, 9/28 cases had prominent dorsal grooving of the corpus callosum caused by its elevation and impingement on the falx cerebri. Of interest is the identification of three patients (cases A2, C6, C8 in Table 2.2) with parkinsonism (in one developing 2 years after shunting); none had Lewy bodies or synuclein immunoreactive deposits characteristic of Parkinson's disease, nor evidence of other neurodegenerative disease associated with parkinsonism. It is known that the clinical distinction between NPH and Parkinson's disease can be difficult [87], and in some cases the parkinsonism can respond to shunting [88]. In this circumstance projections from the substantia nigra to the striatum might be compromised [89]. Three patients had abnormal narrowing of the cerebral aqueduct as the likely cause of hydrocephalus (cases A5, C13, C17 in Table 2.2), consistent with the current knowledge that some NPH patients might be delayed presentations of congenital anomalies [48]. In general, however, a structural cause for hydrocephalus was not always apparent despite careful inspection of the meninges and arachnoid granulations.

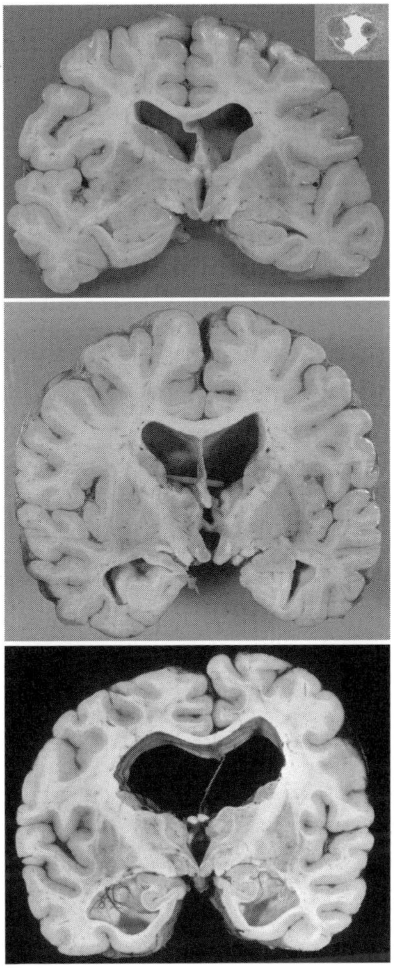

Figure 2.2 Photographs of coronal slices of hydrocephalic brains at the frontotemporal level highlighting the unpredictability of functional impairment. The upper slice is from a patient with clinical diagnosis of idiopathic NPH (case A5 in Table 2.2). The inset shows the cerebral aqueduct partially obstructed by granular extrusions, likely the consequence of an irritating process (possibly mild ventriculitis) many years earlier. The middle slice is from a patient with clinical diagnosis of secondary NPH (case B3 in Table 2.2). The shunt (piercing the septum pellucidum) was no longer functional and the symptoms had recurred. The lower slice is from an individual whose ventricles had enlarged considerably over the preceding 9 years but was asymptomatic (case C13 in Table 2.2). The septum pellucidum is destroyed and the corpus callosum thinned. A full-color version is included in the color plate section.

Table 2.2 Summary of neuropathologic autopsy findings in chronic adult hydrocephalus cases[a]

(A) Clinical diagnosis of idiopathic normal pressure hydrocephalus

Case #	Age	Sex	History	Shunted	Autopsy findings	Alzheimer type features	Cerebrovascular features
A1	73	M	Progressive weakness of the legs, ataxia, incontinence	No (died of metastatic cancer; brain not involved)	Leptomeningeal fibrosis; moderately enlarged lateral and third ventricles	Rare neurofibrillary tangles, no plaques	Nil
A2	84	M	Unsteady gait and enlarged ventricles at age 79	Yes (age 79) – improved for 2 years then developed parkinsonian tremor and dementia; fell from bed	Acute large and chronic subdural hematoma; large ventricles, shunt patent	Moderate senile plaques and scattered neurofibrillary tangles; substantia nigra degeneration (no Lewy bodies)	Atherosclerosis, arteriolosclerosis
A3	60	M	Unsteady gait and short-term memory loss at age 55 years; MRI showed enlarged ventricles with periventricular signal change	Yes (age 58) – gait improved but not memory	Ventricles large despite patent shunt, corpus callosum elevated with dorsal groove, resolved subdural hematoma	Moderate senile plaques	Nil
A4	82	M	Confusion, urinary incontinence and gait disturbance at age 76	Yes (age 76) – gait and incontinence normalized, residual recent memory deficit; headaches at age 82	Shunted ventricles small; no obvious meningeal fibrosis	Sparse senile plaques	Enlarged perivascular spaces, arteriolosclerosis
A5	72	M	Decreased mobility and truncal ataxia; CT showed enlarged ventricles and cisterna magna	No (died from pneumonia during investigations)	Large ventricles, aqueduct stenosis due to granular scarring of ependymal surface; damaged axons in corpus callosum	Sparse senile plaques	Nil

(B) Clinical diagnosis of normal pressure hydrocephalus secondary to known cause

Case #	Age	Sex	History	Shunted	Autopsy findings	Alzheimer type features	Cerebrovascular features
B1	80	M	Minor head injury age 79; 8 months later developed slow shuffling gait, frequent falling, urinary frequency, and memory disturbance; CT showed enlarged ventricles and chronic subdural hematomas	Yes (age 79) – all abnormalities resolved quickly; recurrent subdural hematomas with decreased level of consciousness	Chronic subdural hematomas; small shunted ventricles	Moderate senile plaques but no neurofibrillary tangles in neocortex	Mild arteriolosclerosis
B2	67	M	Age 57 TIA, CT scan showed large ventricles; age 58 mild cognitive deficit; age 62 aphasia, CT showed multifocal ischemic foci and larger ventricles; age 63 gait instability and incontinence	Yes (age 63) – opening pressure 23 cm water; gait improved but not cognitive	Moderate ventricle enlargement, corpus callosum thin (3 mm); shunt patent	Moderate plaques and tangles with amyloid angiopathy	Minimal atherosclerosis; infarct internal capsule and left parietal lobe; enlarged perivascular spaces
B3	58	M	Mild head injury decades earlier (unconscious for hours); at 56 years unsteadiness of gait, headache, transient vision loss, urinary incontinence, problems with recent memory	Yes (age 56) – all symptoms resolved for 14 months; recurrence of symptoms, no change ventricle size, shunt pressure adjusted, died suddenly 1 week later	Mild ventricle enlargement, shunt through septum, resolved subdural hematoma; abundant grumose degeneration in substantia nigra	Nil	Nil

Table 2.2 *(cont.)*

(C) Hydrocephalus at autopsy in adults with no neurologic complaints or atypical history (none were shunted)

Case #	Age	Sex	History	Autopsy findings	Alzheimer type features	Cerebrovascular features
C1	89	F	No neurological complaints	Moderate enlargement lateral and third ventricles, septum pellucidum focally disrupted	Moderate senile plaques in cortex, rare neurofibrillary tangles in hippocampus	Scattered atherosclerotic plaques
C2	72	M	No neurological complaints	Moderate enlargement lateral and third ventricles	Rare senile plaques and neurofibrillary tangles, frontal lobe and hippocampus	Moderate patchy atheroma; peripheral vascular disease, hypertension; enlarged perivascular spaces, arteriolosclerosis
C3	80	M	Occasional seizures since 70 years age; CT scan age 78 years showed infarct right superior cerebellum	Moderate enlargement lateral, third and fourth ventricles, and cerebral aqueduct	Nil	Old infarct cerebellum (<1 cm)
C4	70	M	No neurologic history	Moderately enlarged lateral and third ventricles, elevated corpus callosum with dorsal groove; mild meningeal fibrosis; rare varicose axons corpus callosum	Nil	Nil
C5	90	F	Dementia, depression	Moderately enlarged lateral and third ventricles, elevated corpus callosum with dorsal groove; mild meningeal fibrosis; rare varicose axons corpus callosum	No senile plaques, rare neurofibrillary tangles in temporal lobes; grumose bodies in substantia nigra	Nil
C6	85	M	Age 52 subarachnoid hemorrhage and anterior communicating artery aneurysm clipping; "Parkinson's disease"	Moderately enlarged lateral ventricles, holes in septum pellucidum; right inferior frontal lobe scar; leptomeningeal and arachnoid villi fibrosis	Moderate senile plaques in temporal lobes and rare neurofibrillary tangles; normal substantia nigra, no Lewy bodies	Nil
C7	68	M	Head injury age 58 years; mild left side weakness	Small old contusions inferior frontotemporal; moderately enlarged lateral and third ventricles, elevated corpus callosum with dorsal groove, holes in septum pellucidum	Many neurofibrillary tangles in temporal lobes, no plaques	Minimal atherosclerosis

C8	76	M	"Parkinson's disease" for several years	Moderately enlarged lateral and third ventricles, elevated corpus callosum with dorsal groove	No plaques; rare neurofibrillary tangles in hippocampus; normal substantia nigra	Nil
C9	58	F	No neurological complaints	Moderately enlarged lateral and third ventricles, elevated corpus callosum with dorsal groove; arachnoid fibrosis	Sparse diffuse plaques	Nil
C10	77	M	No neurologic complaints	Old contusion left temporal lobe; moderately enlarged lateral ventricles; septum pellucidum absent; focal arachnoid fibrosis	Sparse senile plaques	Nil
C11	74	M	Alcohol abuse; no neurologic complaints; cervical spine fracture after fall	Moderately enlarged lateral and third ventricles, elevated corpus callosum with dorsal groove	Moderate senile plaques	Nil
C12	80	F	Early dementia	Moderately enlarged lateral ventricles, elevated corpus callosum with dorsal groove; thin (<1 mm) subacute subdural hematoma	Moderate senile plaques	Nil
C13	44	F	Congenital heart defect; age 35 years TIA, CT scan showed mild ventricle enlargement; no recent neurologic complaints	Head normal size, severely enlarged ventricles, elevated corpus callosum, fornix normal, septum pellucidum absent; aqueduct stenosis	Nil	Mild neuron loss hippocampi (possibly hypoxic-ischemic)
C14	82	M	No known neurological complaints	Moderate ventricle enlargement and leptomeningeal fibrosis	Sparse to moderate senile plaques	Nil
C15	66	M	Mild dementia, tremor, depression	Moderate ventricle enlargement	Nil	Widened perivascular spaces
C16	77	M	Ataxia and dementia	Severely enlarged ventricles with elevation and thinning of corpus callosum; atrophy of fornix, aqueduct large, no obvious fibrosis	Sparse plaques temporal lobe and hippocampus	Nil
C17	76	M	Age 68 "stroke"	Severely enlarged ventricles with elevation of corpus callosum; aqueduct stenosis	Moderate senile plaques and scattered neurofibrillary tangles	Nil

Table 2.2 *(cont.)*

Case #	Age	Sex	History	Autopsy findings	Alzheimer type features	Cerebrovascular features
C18	70	M	Multiple infarcts	Moderately enlarged ventricles with elevation of corpus callosum and dorsal groove; diffuse leptomeningeal fibrosis	Neurofibrillary tangles in hippocampus and temporal lobe	Severe atherosclerosis, multiple small infarcts in frontal lobes and deep nuclei
C19	62	M	No known neurological history, alcohol abuse, suicide	Moderately enlarged ventricles with elevation of corpus callosum and fenestration of septum pellucidum	Nil	Arteriolosclerosis
C20	86	M	Dementia; CT scan showed ventricular enlargement out of proportion to cerebral atrophy – possible NPH	Enlarged lateral, third, and fourth ventricles	Abundant senile plaques; amyloid angiopathy; atrophy (1125 g)	Arteriolosclerosis; enlarged perivascular spaces

[a] Retrospective review of unselected autopsy cases with complete brain examination in Province of Manitoba 1996–2012 (approximately 300–350 adult brains per year, hospital and medicolegal cases). Excluded were those cases with overt malformation, neurologic problems dating back to childhood, history of severe head injury or cerebrovascular event, and acute causes. None of the cases presented here were included in a previously reported series [28]. Precise measurements of the ventricle sizes are not available.

Secondary reactive changes due to hydrocephalus

When the cerebral ventricles expand, damage to periventricular white matter stimulates prominent reactive changes among glial cell populations including activation and proliferation of astrocytes and microglia [9]. In chronic adult hydrocephalus including NPH, the rate of ventricular enlargement is slow (e.g. years) and such reactive changes are usually subtle. When varicose axons are identifiable (especially using immunohistochemical detection of neurofilament or amyloid precursor protein, which accumulates at sites of axonal compromise), one may also recognize reactive microglia using appropriate immunohistochemical labeling (e.g. HLA-DR, CD68, or Iba1). Rarely phagocytosed myelin debris can be demonstrated (e.g. with the Marchi silver precipitation method [90]). Reactive astrocytes increased their expression of the water channel protein aquaporin-4, especially in their endfeet where blood vessels are contacted. This has been demonstrated in many of the animal models and most recently in biopsies from NPH patients [91]. This is of potential relevance to compensatory water movements in the hydrocephalic brain.

Altered neurons and connections in the hydrocephalic brain

Brain function is ultimately determined by the integrity of connections between neurons. Axons in the periventricular white matter are the main target for damage due to hydrocephalus. Therefore, connections within the cerebrum, between the hemispheres, and to the brainstem and spinal cord are potentially compromised. The structure–dysfunction relationship in young hydrocephalic brains, about which there is considerable information, has been reviewed in detail recently [13]. The gait abnormality in NPH may be due to dysfunction of the supplementary motor cortex and possibly connections with the basal nuclei [92,93]. Functional MRI studies indicate that sensation related to urinary bladder filling occurs in the insular cortex, the anterior cingulate gyrus provides monitoring and control, and the prefrontal cortex makes voiding decisions [94]. Adults with hydrocephalus appear to have cognitive abnormalities attributable to changes in the septohippocampal circuit, while those with NPH seem to have dysfunction of prefrontal structures [95]. All of these dysfunctions can be explained by the periventricular white matter damage and subcortical disconnection. Long pathways extending to the brainstem and spinal cord can also be damaged [63,96,97].

Most histopathological studies of neuron changes in hydrocephalic brains have been conducted in young animals. Neuron death is infrequent unless the white matter is completely destroyed and the deep cortical layers exposed to the ventricles [98]; this seldom happens in NPH. Disconnected neurons have fewer synapses and their dendritic complexity is reduced. This too is likely subtle in NPH. In contrast to Alzheimer's disease patients, people with NPH do not have significant atrophy of the hippocampus [99]. Adult hydrocephalic rabbits have changes in monoamine neurotransmitter concentrations including decreased dopamine in the hypothalamus and medulla, decreased serotonin in the basal nuclei, and increased norepinephrine in the thalamus [100]. Although neuronal changes in the striatum are not typically identifiable at the microscopic level, positron emission tomography studies in NPH patients indicate a correlation between postsynaptic dopamine (D2) receptor hypoactivity in the putamen and the severity of gait impairment [101,102]. Autopsy studies have demonstrated nonspecific degenerative changes in the substantia nigra of adults with chronic hydrocephalus [28].

Summary

Neuropathological changes in NPH suggest that the pathogenesis of white matter damage (and secondary neuronal disconnection) is similar to that in young hydrocephalic brains, but in general less severe. Blood flow hypoperfusion leads to hypoxic-ischemic changes in the white matter, physical stretching compromises axon integrity, and retarded turnover of the CSF alters the extracellular microenvironment. The additive effects of age-related cerebrovascular disease and neurodegenerative disease (especially Alzheimer's) contribute to the brain dysfunction and perhaps help explain distinctive aspects of the clinical syndrome. There is potential for reversal of some symptoms, often without substantial reduction in ventricle size, likely through correction of white matter hypoperfusion and normalization of the extracellular environment. To gain a greater understanding of the brain damage in NPH, detailed analysis of autopsy material along with experimental studies in aged animals is required.

Conflict of interest disclaimer

The author has in the past received consulting fees from Codman and Medtronic, both in relation to development of shunt technology.

Funding support

Dr. Del Bigio holds the Canada Research Chair in Developmental Neuropathology.

References

1. Rapoport SI. *Blood-Brain Barrier in Physiology and Medicine*. New York: Raven Press; 1976.
2. Cao Y, Brown SL, Knight RA, Fenstermacher JD, Ewing JR. Effect of intravascular-to-extravascular water exchange on the determination of blood-to-tissue transfer constant by magnetic resonance imaging. *Magn Reson Med* 2005;53(2):282–93.
3. Johnston M, Zakharov A, Papaiconomou C, Salmasi G, Armstrong D. Evidence of connections between cerebrospinal fluid and nasal lymphatic vessels in humans, non-human primates and other mammalian species. *Cerebrospinal Fluid Res* 2004;1(1):2.
4. Foldi M. Prelymphatic-lymphatic drainage of the brain. *Am Heart J* 1977;93(1):121–4.
5. Johanson CE, Duncan JA, 3rd, Klinge PM, et al. Multiplicity of cerebrospinal fluid functions: New challenges in health and disease. *Cerebrospinal Fluid Res* 2008;5:10.
6. Schiller F. The cerebral ventricles. From soul to sink. *Arch Neurol* 1997;54(9):1158–62.
7. Russell DS. Observations on the pathology of hydrocephalus. *Med Res Council Special Report Ser* 1949;265:1–138.
8. Milhorat TH. *Hydrocephalus and the Cerebrospinal Fluid*. Baltimore: Williams & Wilkins; 1972.
9. Del Bigio MR. Neuropathological changes caused by hydrocephalus. *Acta Neuropathol (Berl)* 1993;85(6):573–85.
10. Del Bigio MR. Pathophysiologic consequences of hydrocephalus. *Neurosurg Clin N Am* 2001;12(4):639–49.
11. Del Bigio MR. Future directions for therapy of childhood hydrocephalus: a view from the laboratory. *Pediatr Neurosurg* 2001;34(4):172–81.
12. Del Bigio MR. Cellular damage and prevention in childhood hydrocephalus. *Brain Pathol* 2004;14(3):317–24.
13. Del Bigio MR. Neuropathology and structural changes in hydrocephalus. *Dev Disabil Res Rev* 2010;16(1):16–22.
14. McAllister JP, II, Chovan P. Neonatal hydrocephalus. Mechanisms and consequences. *Neurosurg Clin N Am* 1998;9(1):73–93.
15. McAllister JP, 2nd. Pathophysiology of congenital and neonatal hydrocephalus. *Semin Fetal Neonatal Med* 2012;17(5):285–94.
16. Akai K, Uchigasaki S, Tanaka U, Komatsu A. Normal pressure hydrocephalus. Neuropathological study. *Acta Pathol Jpn* 1987;37:97–110.
17. Ball MJ. Neurofibrillary tangles in the dementia of "normal pressure" hydrocephalus. *Can J Neurol Sci* 1976;3(4):227–35.
18. DeLand FH, James AE, Jr., Ladd DJ, Konigsmark BW. Normal pressure hydrocephalus: a histologic study. *Am J Clin Pathol* 1972;58(1):58–63.
19. Di Rocco C, Di Trapani G, Maira G, et al. Anatomo-clinical correlations in normotensive hydrocephalus. Reports on three cases. *J Neurol Sci* 1977;33:437–52.
20. Vessal K, Sperber EE, James AE. Chronic communicating hydrocephalus with normal CSF pressures: a cisternographic-pathologic correlation. *Ann Radiol (Paris)* 1974;17:785–93.
21. Koto A, Rosenberg G, Zingesser LH, Horoupian D, Katzman R. Syndrome of normal pressure hydrocephalus: possible relation to hypertensive and arteriosclerotic vasculopathy. *J Neurol Neurosurg Psychiatry* 1977;40(1):73–9.
22. Cabral D, Beach TG, Vedders L, et al. Frequency of Alzheimer's disease pathology at autopsy in patients with clinical normal pressure hydrocephalus. *Alzheimers Dement* 2011;7(5):509–13.
23. Leinonen V, Koivisto AM, Savolainen S, et al. Post-mortem findings in 10 patients with presumed normal pressure hydrocephalus and review of the literature. *Neuropathol Appl Neurobiol* 2012;38:72–86.
24. Derouesne C, Gray F, Escourolle R, Castaigne P. 'Expanding cerebral lacunae' in a hypertensive patient with normal pressure hydrocephalus. *Neuropathol Appl Neurobiol* 1987;13:309–20.
25. Earnest MP, Fahn S, Karp JH, Rowland LP. Normal pressure hydrocephalus and hypertensive cerebrovascular disease. *Arch Neurol* 1974;31(4):262–6.
26. Lorenzo AV, Bresnan MJ, Barlow CF. Cerebrospinal fluid absorption deficit in normal pressure hydrocephalus. *Arch Neurol* 1974;30(5):387–93.
27. Ball MJ, Vis CL. Relationship of granulovacuolar degeneration in hippocampal neurones to aging and to dementia in normal-pressure hydrocephalics. *J Gerontol* 1978;33(6):815–24.
28. Del Bigio MR, Cardoso ER, Halliday WC. Neuropathological changes in chronic adult

hydrocephalus: cortical biopsies and autopsy findings. *Can J Neurol Sci* 1997;24(2):121–6.

29. Jellinger K. Neuropathological aspects of dementias resulting from abnormal blood and cerebrospinal fluid dynamics. *Acta Neurol Belg* 1976;76(2):83–102.
30. Heinz ER, Davis DO, Karp HR. Abnormal isotope cisternography in symptomatic occult hydrocephalus. A correlative isotopic-neuroradiological study in 130 subjects. *Radiology* 1970;95(1):109–20.
31. Sohn RS, Siegel BA, Gado M, Torack RM. Alzheimer's disease with abnormal cerebrospinal fluid flow. *Neurology* 1973;23(10):1058–65.
32. Sypert GW, Leffman H, Ojemann GA. Occult normal pressure hydrocephalus manifested by parkinsonism-dementia complex. *Neurology* 1973;23(3):234–8.
33. Coblentz JM, Mattis S, Zingesser LH, et al. Presenile dementia. Clinical aspects and evaluation of cerebrospinal fluid dynamics. *Arch Neurol* 1973;29(5):299–308.
34. Newton H, Pickard JD, Weller RO. Normal pressure hydrocephalus and cerebrovascular disease: findings of postmortem. *J Neurol Neurosurg Psychiatry* 1989;52(6):804.
35. Esiri MM, Rosenberg GA. Hydrocephalus and dementia. In: Esiri MM, Lee VM-Y, Trojanowski JQ (Eds.) *The Neuropathology of Dementia*. Cambridge University Press; 2004: 442–56.
36. Brusa G, Piccardo A, Pizio N, Gambini C. Anatomopathological study of dementia syndrome linked with an abnormal cerebrospinal fluid flow. Report of literature and personal observations. *Pathologica* 1991;83(1085):351–8.
37. Constantinidis J, Yanniotis G, de Ajuriaguerra J. Syndrome dementiel senile avec dilatation des ventricules cerebraux sans autres lesions (a propos de 18 observations anatomo-cliniques). *Schweiz Arch Neurol Neurochir Psychiatr* 1977;121(2):229–48.
38. Crowell RM, Tew JM, Jr., Mark VH. Aggressive dementia associated with normal pressure hydrocephalus. Report of two unusual cases. *Neurology* 1973;23(5):461–4.
39. Ribadeau-Dumas JL, Ricou P, Verdure L, Rondot P, Escourolle R. Etude anatomique d'un cas d'hydrocephalie a pression normale. *Neurochirurgie* 1976;22:138–46.
40. Vanderkelen B, Brihaye J, Flament-Durand J. Constatations anatomo-pathologiques dans un cas d'hydrocephalie normotensive. *Acta Neurol Belg* 1975;75:279–87.
41. Relkin N, Marmarou A, Klinge P, Bergsneider M, Black PM. Diagnosing idiopathic normal-pressure hydrocephalus. *Neurosurgery* 2005;57(3 Suppl):S4–S16.
42. Massicotte EM, Del Bigio MR. Human arachnoid villi response to subarachnoid hemorrhage: possible relationship to chronic hydrocephalus. *J Neurosurg* 1999;91(1):80–4.
43. Bellur SN, Chandra V, McDonald LW. Arachnoidal cell hyperplasia. Its relationship to aging and chronic renal failure. *Arch Pathol Lab Med* 1980;104(8):414–16.
44. Bech RA, Juhler M, Waldemar G, Klinken L, Gjerris F. Frontal brain and leptomeningeal biopsy specimens correlated with cerebrospinal fluid outflow resistance and B wave activity in patients suspected of normal pressure hydrocephalus. *Neurosurgery* 1997;40:497–502.
45. Bradley WG, Jr., Bahl G, Alksne JF. Idiopathic normal pressure hydrocephalus may be a "two hit" disease: benign external hydrocephalus in infancy followed by deep white matter ischemia in late adulthood. *J Magn Reson Imaging* 2006;24(4):747–55.
46. Kalaria RN. Vascular basis for brain degeneration: faltering controls and risk factors for dementia. *Nutr Rev* 2010;68(Suppl 2):S74–S87.
47. Redzic ZB, Preston JE, Duncan JA, Chodobski A, Szmydynger-Chodobska J. The choroid plexus-cerebrospinal fluid system: from development to aging. *Curr Top Dev Biol* 2005;71:1–52.
48. Krefft TA, Graff-Radford NR, Lucas JA, Mortimer JA. Normal pressure hydrocephalus and large head size. *Alzheimer Dis Assoc Disord* 2004;18(1):35–7.
49. Wilson RK, Williams MA. Evidence that congenital hydrocephalus is a precursor to idiopathic normal pressure hydrocephalus in only a subset of patients. *J Neurol Neurosurg Psychiatry* 2007;78(5):508–11.
50. Di Rocco C, Pettorossi VE, Caldarelli M, Mancinelli R, Velardi F. Communicating hydrocephalus induced by mechanically increased amplitude of the intraventricular cerebrospinal fluid pressure: experimental studies. *Exp Neurol* 1978;59(1):40–52.
51. Shulyakov AV, Buist RJ, Del Bigio MR. Intracranial biomechanics of acute experimental hydrocephalus in live rats. *Neurosurgery* 2012;71(5):1032–40.
52. Bateman GA. Pulse-wave encephalopathy: a comparative study of the hydrodynamics of leukoaraiosis and normal-pressure hydrocephalus. *Neuroradiology*. 2002;44(9):740–8.
53. Del Bigio MR. Ependymal cells: biology and pathology. *Acta Neuropathol* 2010;119(1):55–73.
54. Chang CC, Asada H, Mimura T, Suzuki S. A prospective study of cerebral blood flow and cerebrovascular reactivity to acetazolamide in 162 patients with idiopathic normal-pressure hydrocephalus. *J Neurosurg* 2009;111(3):610–17.

55. Del Bigio MR, Bruni JE. Changes in periventricular vasculature of rabbit brain following induction of hydrocephalus and after shunting. *J Neurosurg* 1988;69(1):115–20.

56. Luciano MG, Skarupa DJ, Booth AM, et al. Cerebrovascular adaptation in chronic hydrocephalus. *J Cereb Blood Flow Metab* 2001;21(3):285–94.

57. Itoh Y, Suzuki N. Control of brain capillary blood flow. *J Cereb Blood Flow Metab* 2012;32(7):1167–76.

58. Del Bigio MR. Calcium-mediated proteolytic damage in white matter of hydrocephalic rats? *J Neuropathol Exp Neurol* 2000;59(11):946–54.

59. Del Bigio MR, Khan OH, da Silva Lopes L, Juliet PA. Cerebral white matter oxidation and nitrosylation in young rodents with kaolin-induced hydrocephalus. *J Neuropathol Exp Neurol* 2012;71(4):274–88.

60. Del Bigio MR. Hydrocephalus-induced changes in the composition of cerebrospinal fluid. *Neurosurgery*. 1989;25(3):416–23.

61. Krueger RC. Use of a novel double-sandwich enzyme-linked immunosorbent assay method for assaying chondroitin sulfate proteoglycans that bear 3-nitrotyrosine core protein modifications, a previously unrecognized proteoglycan modification in hydrocephalus. *Anal Biochem* 2004;325(1):52–61.

62. Hattori T, Sato R, Aoki S, Yuasa T, Mizusawa H. Different patterns of fornix damage in idiopathic normal pressure hydrocephalus and Alzheimer disease. *Am J Neuroradiol* 2012;33(2):274–9.

63. Del Bigio MR, Wilson MJ, Enno T. Chronic hydrocephalus in rats and humans: white matter loss and behavior changes. *Ann Neurol* 2003;53(3):337–46.

64. Graff-Radford NR, Godersky JC. Idiopathic normal pressure hydrocephalus and systemic hypertension. *Neurology* 1987;37:868–71.

65. Krauss JK, Regel JP, Vach W, et al. Vascular risk factors and arteriosclerotic disease in idiopathic normal-pressure hydrocephalus of the elderly. *Stroke* 1996;27:24–9.

66. Boon AJ, Tans JT, Delwel EJ, et al. Dutch Normal-Pressure Hydrocephalus Study: the role of cerebrovascular disease. *J Neurosurg* 1999;90(2):221–6.

67. Jacobs L. Diabetes mellitus in normal pressure hydrocephalus. *J Neurol Neurosurg Psychiatry* 1977;40(4):331–5.

68. Tullberg M, Hultin L, Ekholm S, et al. White matter changes in normal pressure hydrocephalus and Binswanger disease: specificity, predictive value and correlations to axonal degeneration and demyelination. *Acta Neurol Scand* 2002;105(6):417–26.

69. Tisell M, Tullberg M, Hellström P, et al. Shunt surgery in patients with hydrocephalus and white matter changes. *J Neurosurg* 2011;114(5):1432–8.

70. Ritter S, Dinh TT. Progressive postnatal dilation of brain ventricles in spontaneously hypertensive rats. *Brain Res* 1986;370(2):327–32.

71. Tarnaris A, Watkins LD, Kitchen ND. Biomarkers in chronic adult hydrocephalus. *Cerebrospinal Fluid Res* 2006;3:11.

72. Tarnaris A, Kitchen ND, Watkins LD. Noninvasive biomarkers in normal pressure hydrocephalus: evidence for the role of neuroimaging. *J Neurosurg* 2009;110(5):837–51.

73. Sykova E, Fiala J, Antonova T, Vorisek I. Extracellular space volume changes and diffusion barriers in rats with kaolin-induced and inherited hydrocephalus. *Eur J Pediatr Surg* 2001;11(Suppl 1):S34–7.

74. Shoesmith CL, Buist R, Del Bigio MR. Magnetic resonance imaging study of extracellular fluid tracer movement in brains of immature rats with hydrocephalus. *Neurol Res* 2000;22(1):111–16.

75. McLone DG, Bondareff W, Raimondi AJ. Brain edema in the hydrocephalic hy-3 mouse: submicroscopic morphology. *J Neuropathol Exp Neurol* 1971;30:627–37.

76. Del Bigio MR, Enno TL. Effect of hydrocephalus on rat brain extracellular compartment. *Cerebrospinal Fluid Res* 2008;5(1):12.

77. Del Bigio MR, Bruni JE. Cerebral water content in silicone oil-induced hydrocephalic rabbits. *Pediatr Neurosci* 1987;13(2):72–7.

78. Foncin JF, Redondo A, LeBeau J. Le cortex cérébral des malades atteints d'hydrocéphalie à pression normale: étude ultrastructurale. *Acta Neuropathol* 1976;34:353–7.

79. Ng SE, Low AM, Tang KK, Chan YH, Kwok RK. Value of quantitative MRI biomarkers (Evans' index, aqueductal flow rate, and apparent diffusion coefficient) in idiopathic normal pressure hydrocephalus. *J Magn Reson Imaging* 2009;30(4):708–15.

80. Leinonen V, Koivisto AM, Alafuzoff I, et al. Cortical brain biopsy in long-term prognostication of 468 patients with possible normal pressure hydrocephalus. *Neurodegener Dis* 2012;10:166–9.

81. Seppala TT, Nerg O, Koivisto AM, et al. CSF biomarkers for Alzheimer disease correlate with cortical brain biopsy findings. *Neurology* 2012;78(20):1568–75.

82. Hamilton R, Patel S, Lee EB, et al. Lack of shunt response in suspected idiopathic normal pressure hydrocephalus with Alzheimer disease pathology. *Ann Neurol* 2010;68(4):535–40.

83. Klinge PM, Samii A, Niescken S, Brinker T, Silverberg GD. Brain amyloid accumulates in aged rats with

kaolin-induced hydrocephalus. *Neuroreport* 2006;17(6):657–60.

84. Silverberg GD, Miller MC, Machan JT, et al. Amyloid and tau accumulate in the brains of aged hydrocephalic rats. *Brain Res* 2010;1317:286–96.

85. Weller RO. Pathology of cerebrospinal fluid and interstitial fluid of the CNS: significance for Alzheimer disease, prion disorders and multiple sclerosis. *J Neuropathol Exp Neurol* 1998;57(10):885–94.

86. Silverberg GD, Mayo M, Saul T, et al. Continuous CSF drainage in AD: results of a double-blind, randomized, placebo-controlled study. *Neurology* 2008;71(3):202–9.

87. Morishita T, Foote KD, Okun MS. INPH and Parkinson disease: differentiation by levodopa response. *Nat Rev Neurol* 2010;6(1):52–6.

88. Akiguchi I, Ishii M, Watanabe Y, et al. Shunt-responsive parkinsonism and reversible white matter lesions in patients with idiopathic NPH. *J Neurol* 2008;255(9):1392–9.

89. Racette BA, Esper GJ, Antenor J, et al. Pathophysiology of parkinsonism due to hydrocephalus. *J Neurol Neurosurg Psychiatry* 2004;75(11):1617–19.

90. Smith MC. The recognition and prevention of artefacts of the Marchi method. *J Neurol Neurosurg Psychiatry* 1956;19:74–83.

91. Skjolding AD, Holst AV, Broholm H, Laursen H, Juhler M. Differences in distribution and regulation of astrocytic aquaporin-4 in human and rat hydrocephalic brain. *Neuropathol Appl Neurobiol* 2012, Apr 13; doi: 10.1111/j.1365-2990.2012.01275.x.

92. Stolze H, Kuhtz-Buschbeck JP, Drücke H, et al. Comparative analysis of the gait disorder of normal pressure hydrocephalus and Parkinson's disease. *J Neurol Neurosurg Psychiatry* 2001;70(3):289–97.

93. Hiraoka K, Yamasaki H, Takagi M, et al. Is the midbrain involved in the manifestation of gait disturbance in idiopathic normal-pressure hydrocephalus? *J Neurol* 2011;258(5):820–5.

94. Griffiths D, Tadic SD. Bladder control, urgency, and urge incontinence: evidence from functional brain imaging. *Neurourol Urodyn* 2008;27(6):466–74.

95. Donnet A, Schmitt A, Dufour H, Giorgi R, Grisoli F. Differential patterns of cognitive impairment in patients with aqueductal stenosis and normal pressure hydrocephalus. *Acta Neurochir (Wien)* 2004;146(12):1301–18.

96. Shirai T, Ishii K. Postnatal changes of HRP-labeled corticospinal neurons in congenital hydrocephalic rats (HTX). In: Matsumoto S, Tamaki N (Eds.) *Hydrocephalus Pathogenesis and Treatment*. Tokyo: Springer-Verlag; 1991: 36–45.

97. Del Bigio MR, da Silva MC, Drake JM, Tuor UI. Acute and chronic cerebral white matter damage in neonatal hydrocephalus. *Can J Neurol Sci* 1994;21:299–305.

98. Ding Y, McAllister JP, II, Yao B, Yan N, Canady AI. Neuron tolerance during hydrocephalus. *Neuroscience* 2001;106(4):659–67.

99. Savolainen S, Laakso MP, Paljarvi L, et al. MR imaging of the hippocampus in normal pressure hydrocephalus: correlations with cortical Alzheimer's disease confirmed by pathologic analysis. *Am J Neuroradiol* 2000;21(2):409–14.

100. Del Bigio MR, Bruni JE, Vriend JP. Monoamine neurotransmitters and their metabolites in the mature rabbit brain following induction of hydrocephalus. *Neurochem Res* 1998;23(11):1379–86.

101. Ouchi Y, Nakayama T, Kanno T, et al. In vivo presynaptic and postsynaptic striatal dopamine functions in idiopathic normal pressure hydrocephalus. *J Cereb Blood Flow Metab* 2007;27(4):803–10.

102. Nakayama T, Ouchi Y, Yoshikawa E, et al. Striatal D2 receptor availability after shunting in idiopathic normal pressure hydrocephalus. *J Nucl Med* 2007;48(12):1981–6.

Chapter 3

Animal models of hydrocephalus

Marianne Juhler

Pulchra sunt, quae videntur pulchriora quae sciuntur longe pulcherrima quae ignorantur. (Beautiful is what we see, even more beautiful what we know, but most beautiful what is still unknown to us.)

Nicolaus Steno. From a 1673 speech for the Copenhagen Anatomical Theatre.

The purpose of any animal study in human medicine is in very general terms to learn about human conditions. Thus, considerations on transferring results from the laboratory to man – either to normal human physiology or to human disease depending on the purpose and design of the study – is pivotal to all studies of this kind. As details about particular models are easily accessible through goal-directed internet searches, the aim of this chapter is to convey an overview of the general principles in different types of animal models. In addition, some of the ethical and historic contributions are included, as they are important, but generally less present in our awareness when we search for scientific information.

In order to address these very general statements, this chapter will describe the following issues:

- ethics of animal models;
- formal requirements – general to any experimental model;
- specific requirements for models of hydrocephalus;
- existing and preferred models;
- recent and current research areas in experimental hydrocephalus.

Ethics of animal models

Ethical standards for experimental studies involving animals are legally set by laws and regulations. Although these may differ between individual countries, they all share the same mindset and purpose – i.e. to ensure animal welfare by reducing or if possible completely preventing suffering in animals used for experiments. Within the EU, this is also covered by EU directive No. 86/809.

The ethical mindset behind the legislation demands that animal models must provide new knowledge. The number of animals used and the inflicted suffering in a given experiment must be balanced against and justified by future progress in treatment of human diseases and definition of important issues for health improvement. As early as 1959, standards were coined in the publication *Principles of Humane Experimental Technique* by Russell and Burch [1]. They identified *replacement, reduction, and refinement* as important ethical principles, which are still the basis for present day legislation and ethics [2,3].

The replacement principle requires that alternative methods to animal experiments for obtaining the same knowledge must be exploited first. This entails techniques of cell, tissue, or organ cultures. Relative replacement is a recent modification of this principle, in which in vitro experiments and/or computer models are conducted in parallel to an animal study thus replacing part of the study. Alternatively animals with a lower phylogeny can also be included in such experimental designs [4]. In vitro studies generally can contribute knowledge at cellular and molecular levels, but are of limited use in elucidating integration between several biological factors and between organ systems in an entire organism. Experimental animals therefore fill the gap between in vitro research and studies in humans, where they typically are included in protocols designed to investigate pathogenesis and pathophysiology of diseases, to test toxicology in drug development, and in preclinical studies [5].

The reduction principle entails that planning and execution of an experimental study considers bringing the number of animals used to a statistically safe minimum by precision in study design and by meticulous pre-experiment analysis of statistical power. Technical improvements ensuring reliability in measurements thus reducing methodological error is another way to decrease random variation and thus make it possible to reduce the necessary sample size. In keeping with this principle, data for as many biological parameters as possible should be provided by each experiment if this can be done without increasing the exposure to suffering unnecessarily.

Refinement refers to improvement of experimental methods with the specific purpose of reducing distress. Inherently this comprises optimizing anesthesia and analgesia. Development of transgenic animal models removes the need for infliction procedures in order to induce a pathological condition post-partum and may thus be regarded as part of this principle.

Formal requirements – general to any experimental model

The advantage of laboratory investigations is the ability to create a biological system as simplified as possible by avoiding or eradicating factors with a confounding influence on the results. The cleanest setting in this respect is of course cell or organ cultures, where the biological environment can be maximally controlled. Naturally, such simplistic biological systems carry substantial inherent limitations, and investigations in entire vertebrate organisms are still the closest to replace investigations in the human body.

Animal models resemble human disease by conditions which are genetically determined, naturally acquired, or induced by the investigator. Apart from producing the desired disease or condition, a large number of physiological factors must be taken into account. Some may be obviously related to the disease in question (e.g. a female animal model in investigation of ovarian cancer); others may be less obvious, but nevertheless important to standardize in order to reduce variability and maximize reproducibility and reliability [6].

- Gender is important due to the influence of hormonal cycles and gender-related behavior. In addition, the possibility of gender-related disease effect and response to intervention must be considered. The usual solution is to use animals of male gender for initial experiments and continue with these unless the disease or question addressed requires female animals; e.g. if studying idiopathic intracranial hypertension (IIH), which is a condition related to hydrocephalus with a much higher incidence in young women.
- Weight and age of the experimental animals. The neonatal, infant, and juvenile organism is in many respects different from adults both in humans and animals. Particularly when studying diseases of the brain, it is relevant that there is a much higher degree of neuronal plasticity in younger individuals and that the response to disease or injury in the developing brain is different from that in the mature brain. Furthermore, pediatric hydrocephalus, either congenital or acquired at an early age, differs from hydrocephalus in the adult in almost every aspect of the disease including clinical presentation, underlying causes, treatment reactions, complications, and prognosis.
- The influence of external factors such as confinement, handling, nutrition, and physical environment (lighting, day/night cycles, temperature, humidity, sound and noise impact) may all influence the stress level and general biological responsiveness of laboratory animals.

Analogy with human pathology, and reproducibility and reliability of the pathological process are extremely important for the validity of the model. Consequently, a model subjected to defined conditions for testing, intervention, or observation must produce identical or closely comparable results regardless of time and place.

A system for evaluating the validity of a given model has been proposed by Tkacs and Thompson [6], who distinguish between predictive and construct validity. Predictive validity deals with the question of accuracy and predictability in transferring observations and data from interventions in the model to clinical intervention in the human organism. This principle is often evident in testing and predicting drug response and can also be used to observe and predict long-term consequences of a disease process with or without different types of intervention. Construct validity is a concept which questions the theoretical rationale behind the model. Clinical, pathological, and physiological similarities are the key issues used to address the congruence between the model and the human clinical condition. Another theoretical principle is the "bedside to bench" concept, according to which specific biological variables most prominent in the human disease must be identified and then "mimicked" in the desired animal model.

Animal models may be classified into the following main types:

- A living organism with a hereditary or naturally occurring disease/pathology resembling a similar disease in humans. The limitations are an often less than optimal resemblance to human disease.
- A living organism in which changes in one or more variables or in one or more organs are induced with the purpose of altering the normal condition to resemble human disease.
- Transgenic animals, in which a specific genetic or hereditary condition is induced by genetic manipulation.

Requirements and challenges for models of hydrocephalus

Creating new insight and hypotheses based on the original clinical problem is the hallmark of animal model research. From this point of view, it seems reasonable to define unanswered questions about hydrocephalus physiology and pathology, to address controversies in its treatment, to systematically collect knowledge on the incidence and types of clinical complications, and then consider which of all these questions and hypotheses can be answered in clinical protocols – and how studies in animal models can clarify those that cannot. Taking this approach, a group of clinicians and scientists with broad expertise in clinical and experimental hydrocephalus proposed ten unanswered questions about hydrocephalus which were most urgently in need of clarification [7].

(1) How do we define hydrocephalus?
(2) How is cerebrospinal fluid (CSF) absorbed normally and what are the causes of CSF malabsorption in hydrocephalus?
(3) Why do the ventricles dilate in communicating hydrocephalus?
(4) What happens to the structure and function of the brain when it is compressed and stretched by the expanding ventricles?
(5) What is the role of cerebrovenous pressure in hydrocephalus?
(6) What causes normal pressure hydrocephalus?
(7) What causes low pressure hydrocephalus?
(8) What is the pathophysiology of slit ventricle syndrome?
(9) What is the pathophysiological basis for neurological impairment in hydrocephalus, and to what extent is it reversible?
(10) How is the brain of a child with hydrocephalus different from that of a young or elderly adult?

This group further pointed out that, for many of the proposed questions, "medical factual knowledge" is based on very incomplete evidence and dogmatic beliefs. As clinical diagnosis, treatment decisions, and handling of complications all rest on this, the group concludes "our understanding of hydrocephalus is not nearly as sophisticated or complete as we might have imagined. Fifty years after the introduction of shunts for the treatment of this previously untreatable disorder, we must acknowledge that the shunt is not a cure for hydrocephalus; it is only a 'patch,' and an unreliable one at that. We know a lot about hydrocephalus, but much of what is true about hydrocephalus is strange, and is not necessarily the same as what we think we know. There is surprisingly little scientific basis for many of our commonly held opinions." They also address the need to think in contexts different to the previous mainstream and thus in reality set the challenge for hydrocephalus animal model research: "we must be willing to expand into an exciting, albeit more complex, scientific frontier of CSF physiology that relies less on bulk flow."

Existing and preferred models

In general, animal models are classified as rodent and non-rodent types, the background of course being that rodent models are by far the most commonly used because their small size makes handling considerably easier and cheaper. This is also true for animal models of hydrocephalus, where various types of rodent models, particularly rat models, are by far the most commonly used. The difference in size, cerebral phylogenic development, anatomy, cerebrovascular anatomy, and functional organization pose a problem when transferring results from rodent models to the human brain [5,6]. Anatomical differences frequently also imply differences in physiology and metabolism, and studies in "higher" animals are generally recommended to supplement rodent studies [6]. Primates are the closest to humans, but induction and studies of human-like diseases in these involve practical, economic, and ethical problems.

Naturally occurring hydrocephalus is quite rare in animals – exemplified by the fact that application of the search term "hydrocephalus" yields very few results in the veterinary literature [8]. The earliest scientific documentation in a modern sense is the paper written in the 1660s by the Danish scientist and scholar Nicolaus Steno on an anatomical study of a hydrocephalic calf [9]. The general belief at that time held since ancient Greece was that the "spiritus animalis" (CSF) was propagated from the brain through the cranial nerves into the muscles by pumping movements of the pineal gland. The motion of the pineal was determined by the will, and this pumping made the muscles swell and move voluntarily. By meticulous anatomical dissection and stringent scientific deduction based on his observations, Steno was able to disprove this theory by showing that the pineal gland cannot move. He further showed that the ventricles were blocked by a mass, which makes this the first scientific observation defining obstruction of the CSF pathways as a cause of hydrocephalus. This dispute between generally held opinion and rational analysis is still an inspiration for modern hydrocephalus research.

Apart from the study of a genetic predisposition to ventriculomegaly, Chiari malformation, and epilepsy in King Charles spaniels [10], the veterinary literature contains relatively few publications on hydrocephalus, consisting of single case reports on sporadically occurring hydrocephalus in different species including dog [11], cat [12], and parrot [13]. This implies that experimental studies on hydrocephalus are impractical to carry out on the naturally occurring condition, and such studies are thus based entirely on experimentally induced hydrocephalus. Basically, experimental hydrocephalus models are produced either by physical/surgical manipulation introducing an agent into CSF spaces or by genetic alteration of animals.

Hydrocephalus induced by physical or chemical agents

As early as 1914 W. S. Thomas published a paper describing a handful of published reports on sporadic cases of human hydrocephalus secondary to meningitis or mass lesions, concluding that systematic experimental studies require reliable induction by injection of substances capable of blocking the aqueduct or fourth ventricle outlets [14]. In his paper, he meticulously describes preparation of the substance (aleuronate granules), the surgical technique in dogs, and a time course experiment with gross anatomical and microscopic findings. The experiment was further divided into a group of adult and a group of juvenile animals. He was able to produce a severe inflammatory reaction, ependymal proliferation, ventriculomegaly as well as clinical and pathological evidence of increased ICP. Since then it has been recognized that injection of noxious substances into the CSF pathways can reliably cause inflammation and hydrocephalus.

As severe inflammation is not part of the picture in most types of human hydrocephalus except in relation to meningitis, substances which do not produce inflammation have been used and shown to obstruct the CSF pathways, e.g. silicone oil [15] or acrylic glue [16].

Induction of hydrocephalus by injection of kaolin into the basal cisterns was reported by Dixon and Heller in 1932 [17]. Currently, although other substances injected into the basal cisterns have been shown to produce hydrocephalus, kaolin remains the most commonly employed substance to produce hydrocephalus by injection into the CSF spaces. Kaolin is an inert silicate, and although there is no demonstrable inflammation distant from the injection site, it has been speculated whether a reaction to the injected substance could play a role in the biological response in addition to the mechanical obstruction at the injection site. Injection into the cisterna magna, fourth ventricle or both causing blockage of the fourth ventricle outlets and thus obstructive hydrocephalus is the original method, which has been shown to produce hydrocephalus in many different species including rodents, rabbits, cats, dogs, and sheep [17–19] (Figures 3.1 and 3.2). As obstructive hydrocephalus, particularly in adults, accounts for only a portion of human hydrocephalus cases, a method for kaolin deposition into the basal cisterns to create "communicating experimental hydrocephalus" with CSF passage through preserved anatomic fourth ventricle outlets has recently been described [20].

Inducing hydrocephalus by changing the composition of the CSF is an entirely different principle, and includes models of intra- or periventricular hemorrhage [21] or alteration of CSF osmolarity [22]. Intraventricular infusion of mock-CSF may be regarded a model of acute high pressure hydrocephalus analogous to these models [23].

Nonmechanical induction methods, such as viral and bacterial inoculations, can also produce communicating hydrocephalus. However, as these models involve the additional biological response to the infectious agent, they are not recommended for studies of the effects of hydrocephalus per se [18].

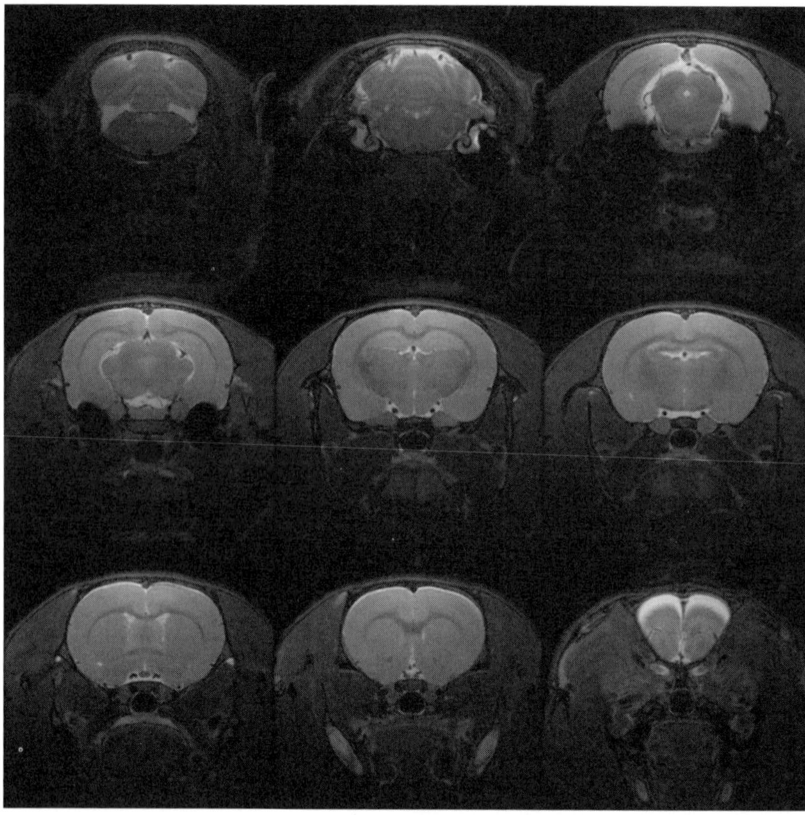

Figure 3.1 T2-weighted serial coronal sections of a normal rat. The ventricular system is very slim, and the uncompressed structures of the brain occupy most of the intracranial volume. Courtesy of Osama Abdullah, Imaging Core Facility, and James P. McAllister II, PhD, University of Utah, as well as Anders Skjolding, MD, Copenhagen University Hospital.

Genetically determined hydrocephalus in inbred strains or by genetic manipulation

The HTX rat is a genetically determined model with heterozygous disposition to congenital hydrocephalus due to stenosis of the aqueduct that develops in fetal life [24].

This strain develops very severe obstructive hydrocephalus soon after birth and is therefore the most widely used model for neonatal or juvenile hydrocephalus. Other less used models of inborn hydrocephalus are an inbred Wistar-Lewis rat strain with aqueductal stenosis and several mouse strains, e.g. hy1, hy2, and hyh mice [25–28].

Hydrocephalus can also be induced by transgenic manipulation, i.e. artificial insertion of DNA sequences. Transgenic animals can be produced by injection of foreign DNA into a fertilized egg or developing embryo. Several mouse hydrocephalus models are produced by genetic manipulation [19,28]. One such model is a transgenic mouse in which cytokine transforming growth factor-β1 (TGF-β1) is overexpressed [29]. Knockout models constitute another type of genetic manipulation, in which the function of a gene is removed by mutation or deletion. In hydrocephalus research, this technique has been utilized to remove subsets of the aquaporin water transport protein family (AQP-null mice) [30]. AQP4-null mice show accelerated progression of ventriculomegaly relative to wildtype controls following induction of hydrocephalus [31].

Recent and current research areas in experimental hydrocephalus

A published report of a meeting for hydrocephalus and CSF investigators to discuss advances in animal models highlights research areas in brain development, anatomical and functional characterization of choroid plexus and periventricular structures, biochemical and growth promoting constitution of CSF, and mechanical as well as biochemical tissue damage as main areas where animal research can contribute to the advancement of knowledge about the hydrocephalic brain [26].

The topics in recent publications direct us to areas which are presently regarded as most important in

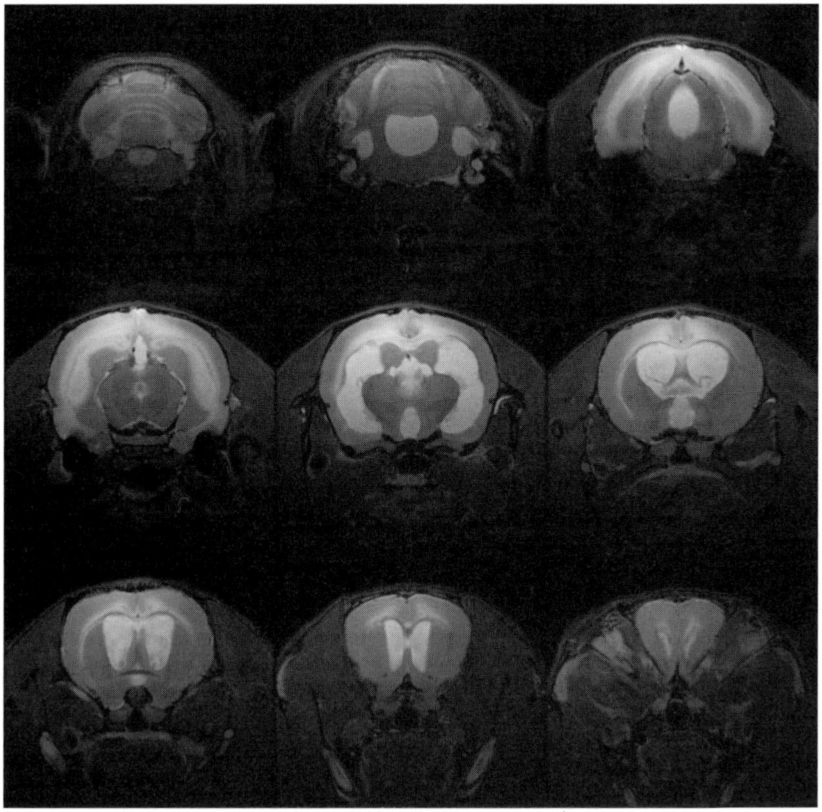

Figure 3.2 T2-weighted serial coronal sections of a rat 2 weeks after induction of hydrocephalus by kaolin injection into the basal cisterns. The ventricles and aqueduct are massively dilated. The cortex and subcortical white matter are severely thinned. Courtesy of Osama Abdullah, Imaging Core Facility, and James P. McAllister II, PhD, University of Utah, as well as Anders Skjolding, MD, Copenhagen University Hospital.

experimental hydrocephalus research, i.e. brain development and anatomy of CSF pathways and associated areas [32–35]; neuroinflammation, tissue damage and repair [36–44]; aquaporins and molecular water transport [45,46]; and biomechanical properties of hydrocephalic brain tissue [20,47,48].

An important advance in experimental studies has been the application of CSF shunting techniques in experimental hydrocephalus [18,42], which offers unique and much needed possibilities for systematic studies on factors in shunt complications – bearing in mind both the dismal actuarial shunt survival coupled with the fact that shunt insertion still accounts for treatment of the great majority of hydrocephalus cases. Shunted animal models also provide a unique potential for insight into questions concerning the destructive effects of hydrocephalus on the brain and its development, as it is rarely possible to obtain brain tissue from humans with hydrocephalus [45]. Which effects and which pathological processes are reversible? Is there a critical time limit for relieving CSF pressure beyond which the pathological effects become irreversible? Shunting was previously only technically possible in animals large enough for implantation of the tubing for clinical use in humans. Procedures and implants have recently been developed also for smaller animals, so that systematic studies on the effects of shunting can be applied to rodents, which remain the most widely used animal models for hydrocephalus research.

Normal pressure hydrocephalus (NPH)

Most of the hydrocephalus animal models are neonatal or juvenile animals and the majority of research is thus directed at congenital or pediatric hydrocephalus. There are, however, models in adult or aging animals that contain the possibility to address NPH-related issues in animal models. Kaolin injection in adult rats is thus proposed as a model of NPH [49,50]. In addition, a minority of HTX rats develop a mild and later occurring hydrocephalus which could also be a potential model for NPH [19].

References

1. Russell WMS, Burch RL. *The Principles of Humane Experimental Technique*. London: Methuen; 1959.

2. Manciocco A, Chiarotti F, Vitale A, et al. The application of Russell and Burch 3R principle in rodent models of neurodegenerative disease: the case of Parkinson's disease. *Neurosci Biobehav Rev* 2009;33(1):18–32.
3. Workman P, Aboagye EO, Balkwill F, et al. Guidelines for the welfare and use of animals in cancer research. *Br J Cancer* 2010;102(11):1555–77.
4. Festing S. On the necessity for animal experimentation. *Bioessay* 2008;30(1):94–5; author reply 6–7.
5. Musch TI, Carroll RG, Just A, Lane PH, Talman WT. A broader view of animal research. *Br Med J* 2007;334(7588):274.
6. Tkacs NC, Thompson HJ. From bedside to bench and back again: research issues in animal models of human disease. *Biol Res Nurs* 2006;8(1):78–88.
7. Bergsneider M, Egnor MR, Johnston M, et al. What we don't (but should) know about hydrocephalus. *J Neurosurg* 2006;104 (3 Suppl):157–59.
8. Thrusfield M. The application of epidemiological techniques to contemporary veterinary problems. *Br Vet J* 1988;144(5):455–69.
9. Kardel T. On a calf with hydrocephalus. A scientific letter dated June 1669 to Ferdinand II, Grand Duke of Tuscany. By Niels Stensen, Royal Anatomist. *J Hist Neurosci* 1993;2(3):179–202.
10. Driver CJ, Chandler K, Walmsley G, Shihab N, Volk HA. The association between Chiari-like malformation, ventriculomegaly and seizures in cavalier King Charles spaniels. *Vet J* 2013;195(2):235–7.
11. Vural SA, Besalti O, Ilhan F, Ozak A, Haligur M. Ventricular ependymoma in a German shepherd dog. *Veterinary J* 2006;172:185–7.
12. Bestbier ME, Blunden AS, Abramson C, Vondenbusch T. Unusual intraventricular neoplasm in a cat. *Research in Vet Sci* 2003;74(Suppl 1):10.
13. Keller KA, Guzman DS, Muthuswamy A, et al. Hydrocephalus in a yellow-headed Amazon parrot (*Amazona ochrocephala oratrix*). *J Avian Med Surg* 2011;25(3):216–24.
14. Thomas WS. Experimental hydrocephalus. *J Exp Med* 1914;19:106–20.
15. James AE, Flor WJ, Novak GR, et al. Experimental hydrocephalus. *Exp Eye Res* 1977;25(Suppl):435–59.
16. Park JH, Park YS, Suk JS, et al. Cerebrospinal fluid pathways from cisterns to ventricles in N-butyl cyanoacrylate-induced hydrocephalic rats. *J Neurosurg Pediatr* 2011;8(6):640–46.
17. Dixon WE, Heller H. Experimentelle Hypertonie durch Erhohung des intrakraniellen Druckes. *Arch Exp Pathol Pharmacol* 1932;166:265–75.
18. McAllister JP. Experimental hydrocephalus. In: Winn HR (Ed.) *Youman's Textbook of Neurological Surgery*. New York: Elsevier; 2011: 2002–8.
19. McAllister JP. Pathophysiology of congenital and neonatal hydrocephalus. *Semin Fetal Neonatal Med* 2012;17(5):285–94.
20. Wagshul ME, McAllister JP, Rashid S, et al. Ventricular dilation and elevated aqueductal pulsations in a new experimental model of communicating hydrocephalus. *Exp Neurol* 2009;218(1):33–40.
21. Aquilina K, Chakkarapani E, Love S, Thoresen M. Neonatal rat model of intraventricular haemorrhage and post-haemorrhagic ventricular dilatation with long-term survival into adulthood. *Neuropathol Appl Neurobiol* 2011;37(2):156–65.
22. Krishnamurthy S, Li J, Schultz L, Jenrow KA. Increased CSF osmolarity reversibly induces hydrocephalus in the normal rat brain. *Fluids Barriers CNS*. 2012;9(1):13.
23. Hauerberg J, Juhler M. Cerebral blood flow autoregulation in acute intracranial hypertension. *J Cereb Blood Flow Metab* 1994;14:519–25.
24. Jones HC, Chen GF, Yehia BR, et al. Single and multiple congenic strains for hydrocephalus in the H-Tx rat. *Mamm Genome* 2005;16(4):251–61.
25. Kohn DF, Chinookoswong N, Chou SM. A new model of congenital hydrocephalus in the rat. *Acta Neuropathol* 1981;54:211–18.
26. Johanson C, Del Bigio MR, Kinsman S, et al. New models for analysing hydrocephalus and disorders of CSF volume transmission. *Br J Neurosurg* 2001;15:281–3.
27. Miller JM, Kumar R, McAllister JP, Krause GS. Gene expression analysis of the development of congenital hydrocephalus in the H-Tx rat. *Brain Res* 2006;1075:36–47.
28. Zhang J, Williams MA, Rigamonti D. Genetics of human hydrocephalus. *J Neurol* 2006;253:1255–66.
29. Crews L, Wyss-Coray T, Masliah E. Insights into the pathogenesis of hydrocephalus from transgenic and experimental animal models. *Brain Pathol* 2004;14:312–16.
30. Verkman AS, Yang B, Song Y, Manley GT, Ma T. Role of water channels in fluid transport studied by phenotype analysis of aquaporin knockout mice. *Exp Physiol* 2000;85(Supp1):233–41.
31. Bloch O, Auguste KI, Manley GT, Verkman AS. Accelerated progression of kaolin-induced hydrocephalus in aquaporin-4-deficient mice. *J Cereb Blood Flow Metab* 2006;26:1527–37.
32. Watanabe M, Miyajima M, Nakajima M, et al. Expression analysis of high mobility group box-1 protein (HMGB-1) in the cerebral cortex,

hippocampus, and cerebellum of the congenital hydrocephalus (H-Tx) rat. *Acta Neurochir Suppl* 2012; 113:91–6.

33. Rammling M, Madan M, Paul L, Behnam B, Pattisapu JV. Evidence for reduced lymphatic CSF absorption in the H-Tx rat hydrocephalus model. *Cerebrospinal Fluid Res* 2008;5:15.
34. Cains S, Shepherd A, Nabiuni M, Owen-Lynch PJ, Miyan J. Addressing a folate imbalance in fetal cerebrospinal fluid can decrease the incidence of congenital hydrocephalus. *J Neuropathol Exp Neurol* 2009;68(4):404–16.
35. Chen X, Huang X, Li B, et al. Changes in neural dendrites and synapses in rat somatosensory cortex following neonatal post-hemorrhagic hydrocephalus. *Brain Res Bull* 2010;83(1–2):44–8.
36. Xu H, Zhang SL, Tan GW, et al. Reactive gliosis and neuroinflammation in rats with communicating hydrocephalus. *Neuroscience* 2012;218:317–25.
37. Lekic T, Manaenko A, Rolland W, et al. Rodent neonatal germinal matrix hemorrhage mimics the human brain injury, neurological consequences, and post-hemorrhagic hydrocephalus. *Exp Neurol* 2012;236(1):69–78.
38. Simard PF, Tosun C, Melnichenko L, et al. Inflammation of the choroid plexus and ependymal layer of the ventricle following intraventricular hemorrhage. *Transl Stroke Res* 2011;2(2):227–31.
39. Deren KE, Forsyth J, Abdullah O, et al. Low levels of amyloid-beta and its transporters in neonatal rats with and without hydrocephalus. *Cerebrospinal Fluid Res* 2009;6:4.
40. McAllister JP 2nd, Miller JM. Minocycline inhibits glial proliferation in the H-Tx rat model of congenital hydrocephalus. *Cerebrospinal Fluid Res* 2010;7:7.
41. Nonaka Y, Miyajima M, Ogino I, Nakajima M, Arai H. Analysis of neuronal cell death in the cerebral cortex of H-Tx rats with compensated hydrocephalus. *J Neurosurg Pediatr* 2008;1(1):68–74.
42. Miller JM, McAllister JP 2nd. Reduction of astrogliosis and microgliosis by cerebrospinal fluid shunting in experimental hydrocephalus. *Cerebrospinal Fluid Res* 2007;4:5.
43. Chu SH, Feng DF, Ma YB, et al. Expression of HGF and VEGF in the cerebral tissue of adult rats with chronic hydrocephalus after subarachnoid hemorrhage. *Mol Med Rep* 2011;4(5):785–91.
44. Li X, Miyajima M, Arai H. Analysis of TGF-beta2 and TGF-beta3 expression in the hydrocephalic H-Tx rat brain. *Childs Nerv Syst* 2005;21(1):32–8.
45. Skjolding AD, Holst AV, Broholm H, Laursen H, Juhler M. Differences in distribution and regulation of astrocytic aquaporin-4 in human and rat hydrocephalic brain. *Neuropathol Appl Neurobiol* 2012, Apr 13; doi: 10.1111/j.1365-2990.2012.01275.x.
46. Skjolding AD, Rowland IJ, Søgaard LV, et al. Hydrocephalus induces dynamic spatiotemporal regulation of aquaporin-4 expression in the rat brain. *Cerebrospinal Fluid Res* 2010;7:20.
47. Shulyakov AV, Cenkowski SS, Buist RJ, Del Bigio MR. Age-dependence of intracranial viscoelastic properties in living rats. *J Mech Behav Biomed Mater* 2011;4(3):484–97.
48. Yuan W, McAllister JP 2nd, Lindquist DM, et al. Diffusion tensor imaging of white matter injury in a rat model of infantile hydrocephalus. *Childs Nerv Syst* 2012;28(1):47–54.
49. Silverberg GD, Miller MC, Machan JT, et al. Amyloid and tau accumulate in the brains of aged hydrocephalic rats. *Brain Res* 2010;1317:286–96.
50. Kondziella D, Sonnewald U, Tullberg M, Wikkelsø C. Brain metabolism in adult chronic hydrocephalus. *J Neurochem* 2008;106:1515–24.

Chapter 4

Genetics of hydrocephalus

Jun Zhang

Introduction

Hydrocephalus is a common human neurological abnormality that requires medical intervention, yet remains an elusive pathological condition which scientists and physicians aim to understand. Improvements in both diagnostic techniques and surgical treatments of hydrocephalus have led to better long-term outcomes and increased prevalence of patients harboring this disease, however our knowledge of hydrocephalus is still very limited [1,2]. Human hydrocephalus can be classified as syndromic versus nonsyndromic, and congenital versus acquired [3]. Syndromic hydrocephalus is usually associated with other major developmental and structural abnormalities such as intraventricular hemorrhage, congenital neoplasia, Chiari malformation, Dandy–Walker malformation, prenatal and perinatal infections, and other severe developmental syndromes. This chapter focuses on nonsyndromic or uncomplicated hydrocephalus, which can be further subclassified into congenital or acquired. Congenital hydrocephalus is defined as being present at birth with or without associated anomalies while acquired hydrocephalus is defined as cases that occur after normal development of the brain and ventricles.

Hydrocephalus is a heterogeneous disease with multiple possible causes [4,5]. A growing body of evidence suggests that the pathogenesis of hydrocephalus is a complex interaction of genetic and environmental factors. Known environmental factors such as maternal alcohol abuse [6], X-ray radiation [7,8], infection [9], nutritional deficiencies [10], and side effects of antibiotic and antineoplastic drugs [11,12] have all been linked to hydrocephalus. It is estimated that about 40% of hydrocephalus cases may have a significant genetic component [13]; we previously have described at least 43 mutants/loci linked to hereditary hydrocephalus in animal models and humans [14]. Among these 43 loci, 10 causative genes in the pathogenesis of hydrocephalus have been defined, 9 of which have been identified in animal models [14]. In humans, only the *L1CAM* gene localized to Xq28 encoding L1 protein and comprising approximately 5–15% of congenital hydrocephalus cases has been positively associated with this condition (X-linked, HSAS1, OMIM) [15–18].

Several reports in human kindreds harboring an autosomal recessive, autosomal dominant, additional X-linked, and mitochondrial patterns of inheritance have been reported; however, the genes and loci responsible for these forms of transmission have not been clearly identified [19–27]. Differential expressivity in gene or gene products has also been implicated as a causative factor.

Genetic epidemiology

Although significant progress has been made in our understanding of molecular pathophysiology of hydrocephalus, the genetic study of hydrocephalus has been hindered by a lack of sufficient epidemiological evidence. The genetic etiology for the majority of hydrocephalus cases remains elusive.

Twin studies

Comparative twin studies have been performed to analyze the genetic influences in congenital structural defects including hydrocephalus [28,29]. Familial inheritance of hydrocephalus was first suggested almost sixty years ago by comparing the concordance in collective pairs of monozygotic twins [30,31]; however, the presence of hydrocephalus was later challenged in some of these twins [32]. In a follow-up study, after eliminating twin pairs in which the hydrocephalus was found to be secondary to some other etiological factor, congenital hydrocephalus in seven pairs of monozygotic twins was found, supporting the notion that genetic factors may play a major role in some cases of congenital hydrocephalus [32]. Recently in a single-institution 3-year retrospective study, a possible concordance for congenital hydrocephalus was observed among three twin pairs, one monozygotic twin pair both with hydrocephalus and two dizygotic twin pairs in each of which only one had hydrocephalus, suggesting a potential genetic influence in hydrocephalus [33]. Moreover, another report showing that a dizygotic twin pair, each with hydrocephalus, were homozygous for the FAC gene mutation, which provides molecular proof that VACTERL with hydrocephalus may be the result of severe Fanconi anemia [34]. This report also raises the possibility that dizygotic twin pairs, each with hydrocephalus, may be caused by genetic concordance due to homogeneity in a certain genomic region.

Epidemiology

It has been suggested that the majority of congenital hydrocephalus (CHC) is caused by some kind of a genetic defect [35]. A study of 74 patients with uncomplicated CHC found that there was a significant increase (five times the population frequency) of CHC among first cousins. Once X-linked inheritance has been excluded in uncomplicated CHC, the overall empirical risk of recurrence is approximately 1 in 50 [36]. In a prospective study, results suggest that couples who have had one child with hydrocephalus have a recurrence risk of 4% [5]. Our group performed a 10-year retrospective study (1997–2007) in Mississippi with a total of 4312 hydrocephalic patients, 710 with congenital hydrocephalus. Among those with CHC, we identified 47 congenital hydrocephalus patients with siblings or first to third degree relatives who also have hydrocephalus, which we further subcategorized into familial cases. Of these familial hydrocephalus cases, we found 14 siblings including 6 sets of twins and 1 set of triplets, 9 first cousins, 22 second cousins, and 6 third cousins. Four of these families had three affected members with hydrocephalus. The pedigrees of each of these 47 families were developed, with the largest cohort consisting of 29 members. However, only two families showed an X-linked inheritance pattern, indicating that most of them were pedigrees with inheritance patterns other than X-linked [2].

One recent study examined familial aggregation of primary CHC in an unselected, nationwide population in Denmark from the Danish Central Person Register. This study identified all children born in Denmark between 1978 and 2008 and their family members (up to third degree relatives). Recurrence risk ratios (RRRs) of congenital hydrocephalus were estimated and a log-linear regression model was used to quantify the genetic effect and the maternal effect. The data showed that among nearly two million live births, 2194 had a diagnosis of idiopathic congenital hydrocephalus (1.1%). Of those, 75 (3.4%) had at least one other family member with CHC. Significantly increased RRRs of CHC were observed for same-sex twins, and for first and second degree relatives. A maternal component was supported by the facts that RRRs for opposite-sex twins (37.3, 95% CI 11.9–116.7) were significantly higher than for other first degree relatives, and that RRRs for maternal half-siblings (8.4, 95% CI 3.7–18.7) were significantly higher than for paternal half-siblings (3.0, 95% CI 0.8–12.2). This is the first large-scale genetic epidemiology study in an unselected, nationwide population. Taking advantage of extensive and detailed records from the national database in a relatively homogeneous population, this study provided the strongest evidence so far of familial aggregation of CHC, supporting the existence of a genetic component to the etiology. In addition, the pattern of association suggests a strong maternal component contributing to the familial aggregation [37].

Genetics in hydrocephalus

Human hydrocephalus

Familial hydrocephalus has long been suggested as a heritable disease [38,39], with heterogeneous causes [40,41], which may result from distinct monogenic or multifactorial disorders [14]. However, limited knowledge exists about the genetic and molecular mechanisms that may cause human hydrocephalus. Identification of large numbers of heritable forms of hydrocephalus would pave the way for elucidation of cellular functions of gene products that lead to alteration in cerebrospinal fluid (CSF) dynamics. Clarification of perturbed cellular pathways may lead clinicians to improved genetic counseling for patients, prenatal diagnosis, and in developing potential novel therapeutic approaches for hydrocephalus.

Idiopathic normal pressure hydrocephalus

Acquired hydrocephalus is also termed adult-onset or idiopathic normal pressure hydrocephalus (iNPH). In contrast to CHC, familial cases of iNPH are not well identified and the genetic basis is totally unknown [42]; only a few familial iNPH cases have been reported to date [26,43–45]. We first reported a large five-generation kindred with essential tremor (ET) presenting during the teen years and the subsequent appearance of iNPH when elderly (>65 years), in an autosomal dominant fashion. Through clinical and genetic analysis, we defined this kindred as a new essential tremor–idiopathic normal pressure hydrocephalus (ETINPH) disorder [43]. We then performed genome-wide linkage scans using two different genotyping microarrays and two- or multipoint linkage analysis strategies and mapped the ETINPH locus to chromosome 19q12–13.31. Fine-mapping in this region revealed a maximum two-point LOD score of 2.8 at rs2023865 and a maximum multipoint LOD score of 17.9 at rs9304878. By haplotype construction, an approximately 17-cM critical region was defined for ETINPH locus. This region contains several neuronal genes that constitute tantalizing etiological candidates for ETINPH [44]. Currently we have deep-sequenced this entire interval with next generation sequencing technology and are analyzing data to identify the genetic variant that causes this ETINPH phenotype. Another large family consisting of four patients with adult-onset iNPH in three generations has been reported recently, supporting the existence of familial iNPH and the genetic components of iNPH [45]. Interestingly, a recent report using a candidate gene approach identified a small familial case of two sisters with iNPH who were homozygous for the apolipoprotein E (ApoE) e3 allele on chromosome 19 [46]. Similarly, another recent study with 15 iNPH patients found that iNPH is associated with the homozygous ApoE 3/3 genotype [47].

Another report has suggested a genetic association between iNPH and the ApoE e4 allele [48]. Building on previous finding that homozygosity of the A allele of the alpha-1-antichymotrypsin (ACT) gene and of allele 1 of the presenilin-1 (PS-1) gene are associated with an increased risk for late-onset Alzheimer's disease (AD), the distribution of ApoE, ACT, and PS-1 genotypes and the corresponding allele frequencies in 13 iNPH patients were analyzed. Only an increased ApoE e4 allele frequency was observed in iNPH patients versus controls, thus suggesting that the ApoE e4 allele may also be involved in the pathogenesis of iNPH [49].

Congenital hydrocephalus

Congenital hydrocephalus (CHC) is far more common than iNPH and its incidence has been estimated to be 3–5 cases per 1000 live births [50]. CHC is usually the consequence of deficient brain development and perturbed cellular function, implicating the important roles that CHC genes play during brain development. Since there is heterogeneity among clinical phenotypes, more genetic loci are expected in CHC. In general, the recurrence risk for CHC excluding X-linked hydrocephalus is low. Empiric risk rates range from <1% to 4% [51–53], demonstrating the rarity of heritable congenital hydrocephalus [13,17,20,21]. However, multiple human kindreds with CHC have been reported [13,17,19–27,38,54–67]. One kindred was reported in which congenital hydrocephalus was transmitted in an autosomal dominant fashion. This condition was associated with aqueductal stenosis but was not associated with mental retardation or pyramidal tract dysfunction. The lack of mental retardation and pyramidal tract dysfunction was in contrast to X-linked or recessive CHC with stenosis of the aqueduct of Sylvius where these abnormalities are commonly seen [60]. Another study identified a kindred with a microdeletion of 8q12.2–q21.2 that subsequently developed hydrocephalus. This trait was also transmitted in an autosomal dominant fashion [68]. One genetic mutation associated with human CHC has been identified so far, that is for X-linked human congenital hydrocephalus. Molecular genetic studies have revealed that the responsible gene for this X-linked human congenital hydrocephalus is *L1CAM* (L1 protein) at Xq28 [69]. The mutations are distributed over the functional protein domains. The exact mechanisms by which these mutations cause a loss of L1 protein function are still under investigation. In addition to the *L1CAM* gene at Xq28, there is another form of X-linked hydrocephalus linked to the proximal region at Xq27.3 [70]. Interestingly, in another three-generation pedigree of hydrocephalus (with megacisterna magna [MCM]) with autosomal or X-linked dominant inheritance, *L1CAM* and *FOXC1* gene involvement in the pathogenesis of the disease was excluded, suggesting a different locus for CHC [62]. Uncomplicated CHC due to obstruction of the third ventricle has been found in two separate familial cases, one of which presented as an autosomal

Table 4.1 Summary of current known loci of hydrocephalus in humans

Clinical form[a]	Trait[b]	Locus	Chromosome	Gene	References
C	AR	Unknown	Unknown		19–24, 26, 27, 54, 56–59, 63, 65
C	AD	Unknown	8q12.2–21.2 or unknown		38, 60, 62, 64, 66, 68
C	MIT	Unknown	Unknown		25
C	X-linked	L1cam	Xq28	*L1CAM*	69
C	X-linked	Unknown	Xq27.3		70
AO	X-linked	Unknown	X		62
AO	AD	iNPH	Unknown		26, 43–45
AO	AD	ETINPH	19		43, 44
AO	Unknown	iNPH	19	*ApoE*	46–48

[a] Clinical form: C, congenital; AO, adult-onset.
[b] Genetic trait: AR, autosomal recessive; AD, autosomal dominant; MIT, mitochondria.

recessive trait [20,59]. Current known loci of hydrocephalus in humans are summarized in Table 4.1.

Animal hydrocephalic models

To date, the majority of identified hydrocephalus loci and genes are from genetic analysis in hydrocephalic animal models. Relative easy access and manipulation in animal models has led to the identification of large numbers of heritable forms of hydrocephalus.

Quantitative trait locus (QTL)

The hydrocephalic Texas strain (HTX) rat model of inherited congenital hydrocephalus demonstrates a complex mode of inheritance and associated ventricular dilatation with abnormalities in the subcommissural organ. The severity of hydrocephalus in the HTX rat seems to be influenced by different genetic loci [71–73]. One study suggested that the HTX strain is a homozygous carrier of an autosomal recessive hydrocephalus gene with incomplete penetrance [74]. In another study, through backcrossing the HTX rat with the non-hydrocephalic Fischer F344 strain, with quantitative trait locus (QTL) mapping, potential CHC loci were identified on chromosome (Chr) 9 (peak markers D9Rat2), 10 (between markers D10Rat136 and D10Rat135), 11 (peak markers D11Arb2 and D11Rat46), and 17 (peak markers D17Mit4 and D17Rat154).

The genetics of hydrocephalus in an inbred strain of Wistar-Lewis rats (LEW/Jms) suggests genetic traits as an autosomal recessive [75] or semidominant or multigenic (possible QTL) trait with a possible locus on sex chromosomes [76], but none of the loci have been localized. In inbred mouse models by back-crossing strains (A/J and C57BL/6J), three QTL loci associated with congenital hydrocephalus have been identified and labeled as Vent8a, Vent4b, and Vent7c. As a major QTL controlling variance in ventricular size, Vent8a is located on Chr 8 (near the markers D8Mit94 and D8Mit189). The other two loci, Vent4b and Vent7c, show strong epistatic interactions affecting ventricular size in the developing embryo. Vent4b is located on Chr 4 (near D4Mit237 and D4Mit214), and Vent7c is located on Chr 7 (between D7Mit178 and D7Mit191) [77].

Monogenic congenital hydrocephalus

The autosomal recessive congenital hydrocephalus-1 (hy1) mouse has a dome-shaped head seen at birth or during the first 2 weeks due to dilatation of the entire ventricular system [78,79]. A more severe phenotypic form, the hydrocephalus-2 (hy2) mouse [80,81], and an obstructive hydrocephalus (oh) mouse with communicating hydrocephalus and secondary aqueductal stenosis have also been described [82,83]. Genetic loci on these non-inbred mouse strains have not been identified yet.

The transgenic mouse line OVE459 is generated by a Bdnf transgene-induced insertional mutation on a single locus on mouse chromosome 8 (near marker D8Mit152), and suggests an autosomal recessive trait in congenital hydrocephalus. The OVE459 insertion locus overlapped with that of autosomal recessive hydrocephalus-3 (hy3) mouse and phenotypically shows lethal communicating hydrocephalus with perinatal onset [84,85]. This transgene insertion resulted in a rearrangement of *Hydin* exons in OVE459 mice. Subsequently, a single CG base-pair deletion in exon

15 of *Hydin* was also identified in hy3 mice, implicating *Hydin* as *hy3* gene [86,87].

An autosomal recessive congenital hydrocephalus (ch) mouse strain was identified many decades ago [84,85,88]. The mutation on winged helix/forkhead transcription factor gene, *Foxc1* (*Mf1*), on chromosome 13 has been identified in ch mouse [89,90]. This finding is supported by another report of six children with hydrocephalus from three different families that have sub-telomeric deletions from chromosome 6p. Three forkhead genes within this region (*FOXF1* and *FOXQ1*) or proximal to it (*FOXC1*) were evaluated as potential candidate disease genes but no disease causing mutations were identified [91]. A recent report indicates that one of the three forkhead genes, *FOXC1*, is required for normal cerebellar development. *FOXC1* mutations have been shown to contribute to chromosome 6p sub-telomere deletion hydrocephalic phenotype, such as Dandy–Walker malformation [92].

The autosomal recessive hydrocephalus with hop gait (hyh) mouse exhibits dramatic dilation of the ventricles at birth and invariably develops a hopping gait. The hyh mouse shows a markedly small cerebral cortex at birth, which indicates altered development of the neuronal cells, and dies postnatally from progressive enlargement of the ventricular system. It has been hypothesized that the small cortex phenotype is the result of developmental events in which neural progenitor cells withdraw prematurely from the cell cycle, producing more early-born, deep-layer cerebral cortical neurons but depleting the cortical progenitor pool. Genetic linkage analysis localized the *hyh* locus on mouse Chr 7, and subsequently the *hyh* gene was identified as α-Snap (soluble NSF attachment protein α). α-Snap protein is essential for apical protein localization and cell fate determination in neuroepithelial cells [93]. Homozygous mutant mice harbor a missense mutation, M105I, in a conserved residue in one of the α-helical domains. The *hyh* mutant is not a null allele and is expressed; however, the mutant protein is 40% less abundant in hyh mice, suggesting a possible haploinsufficiency mechanism [94].

The autosomal recessive hemorrhagic hydrocephalus (hhy) homozygous mutant mouse has dilated lateral ventricles and a patent aqueduct, with no histological abnormalities either in the subarachnoid space or in the choroid plexus. Multiple hemorrhages in the meninges and throughout the brain parenchyma have also been observed in the advanced stages of hydrocephalus. The hhy locus has been localized on mouse Chr 12 [95], and *hhy* gene has been identified as Ccdc85c encoding a protein at apical junctions of radial glia [96]. Several loci on chromosomes 4, 5, 7, 11, 15, and 17 of mouse MSM strain were recently identified as having a significantly higher incidence of hydrocephalus, by using a congenic technique of backcrossing MSM with the C57BL/6J (B6) strain [97]. Current known loci of hydrocephalus in animal models are outlined in Table 4.2.

Genetic basis for pathophysiology of hydrocephalus

The neuropathology of hydrocephalus has been extensively explored. Cerebral ventricle dilatation secondary to disturbed CSF flow has been observed as an inheritable trait in a variety of laboratory animals (as well as in humans) as mentioned previously. In most cases, defective development of the cerebral aqueduct of the subarachnoid space has been observed [98]. Affected individuals have severe developmental delay and may have radiographic findings of hydrocephalus [40]. The pathophysiology of hydrocephalus in the ventricular system has been extensively studied through either down- or up-regulation of certain targeted gene expression, followed by comparative morphological and molecular studies.

Loss of the key molecular cues during early development

In all forms of hydrocephalus, the majority of phenotypic abnormalities are caused by a loss of function of certain genetic components. Below we discuss the effects of those deficient molecular cues on the initial pathogenic tissue/organs that eventually lead to hydrocephalus.

Subcommissural organ (SCO) defects

The subcommissural organ (SCO), a small gland in the diencephalic plate inferior to the pineal organ, is located on the ventral side of the posterior commissure and affects the opening of the cerebral (sylvian) aqueduct. The SCO facilitates the patency of the sylvian aqueduct and normal CSF circulation/metabolism through its secretory activity [99]. Stenosis of the sylvian aqueduct is a common form of CHC in humans. Some mouse models of CHC indicate that aqueduct stenosis is associated with abnormal development of the SCO [100]. The HTX rat shows a reduction in the

Table 4.2 Summary of current known loci (or mutants) of hydrocephalus in animal models

Species	Strain	Trait	Locus	Chromosome	Human syntenic region	Human gene	References
Rat	HTX	QTL	D9Rat2	9q38	5q21.1, 18p11.22–31		71–74
Rat	HTX	QTL	D10Rat136, D10Rat135	10q32.1–10q32.3	17q21.3–q25.3		71–74
Rat	HTX	QTL	D11Arb2, D11Rat46	11q23	3q27–28, 22q11.21, 10p12.2		71–74
Rat	HTX	QTL	D17Mit4, D17Rat154	17q12.1	1q43, 10p11.21–p13		71–74
Rat	LEW/Jms	AR, (QTL)	Unknown	Unknown			75,76
Mouse	C57BL/6J	QTL	Vent8a	8	8p11–23, 13q11–34		77
Mouse	C57BL/6J	QTL	Vent4b	4	6p, 9		77
Mouse	C57BL/6J	QTL	Vent7c	7	19q10–13		77
Mouse	C57BL/MSM			17			97
Mouse	C57BL/MSM			4			97
Mouse	C57BL/MSM			5			97
Mouse	C57BL/MSM			7			97
Mouse	C57BL/MSM			11			97
Mouse	C57BL/MSM			15			97
Mouse	hy1	AR	Unknown	Unknown			78, 79
Mouse	hy2	AR	Unknown	Unknown			80, 81
Mouse	hy3	AR	Hydin	8	16q22.2	*HYDIN*	84–87
Mouse	oh	AR					82, 83
Mouse	hhy	AR	hhy	12	14q32.31	*CCDC85C*	95, 96
Mouse	C57BL/10J	AR	hyh	7	19q13.3	*α-SNAP*	93, 94
Mouse	129/Sv X C57BL/6	AR		19	9q24.2	*RFX3*	109
Mouse	C57BL6/J	AD	Rfx4	10	12q24	*RFX4*	110
Mouse	ch	AR	Mf1	13	6p25	*FREAC-3*	89, 90
Mouse	C57BL/6*CBA/J	AR	Mdnah5	15	5p15.2	*DNAH5*	131
Mouse	C57BL/CBA	AD	Otx2	14	14q21–q22	*OTX2*	201
Mouse	qkv/C57BL/6	AD	Ptch1	13	9q22.3	*PTCH1*	133, 134
Mouse	129P2/OlaHsd	AR	Msx1	5	4p16.3–p16.1	*MSX1*	111–115
Mouse	C57BL/6	AR	Socs7	11	17q12	*SOCS7*	194

Table 4.2 *(cont.)*

Species	Strain	Trait	Locus	Chromosome	Human syntenic region	Human gene	References
Mouse	C57BL/6J	AR	Nmhc-b	11	17q13	*MYH10*	202
Mouse	Sey/Sey	AR	Pax6	2	11p13	*PAX6*	108
Mouse	129/SvJ/C57BL/6J	AR	Spag6	16	10p12.2	*SPAG6*	129
Mouse	C57BL/6 X CBA	AR	Hfh4	11	17q25.1	*FOXJ1*	144
Mouse	TgN737Rpw	AR	Ift88	14	13q12.1	*IFT88*	118, 121, 143
Mouse	C57BL/6	AR	PolL	19	10q23	*POLL*	130
Mouse	C57BL/6J X 129S6/SvEvTac	AR	Pcdp1	1	2q14.2	*PCDP1*	132
Mouse	C57BL/6	AR	wnt1	15	12q13	*WNT1*	142
Mouse	C57BL/6	AR	Dlg5	14	10q23	*DLG5*	117
Mouse	C57BL/6	X-linked	Ophn1	X	Xq12	*OPHN1*	149
Mouse	C57BL/6 or F129/Svj	AR	Slc39a4	15	8q24.3	*SLC39A4*	199
Mouse	C57BL/6	AR	Gli2	1	2q14	*GLI2*	136
Mouse	C57BL/6	AR	Gli3	13	7p13	*GLI3*	137, 138
Mouse	129/Sv × C57BL/6	AR	Itgb8	12	7p21.1	*ITGB8*	147
Mouse	129X1/SvJ	AR	Hif1a	12	14q23.2	*HIF1A*	196
Mouse	129/Sv × C57BL/6	AR	Cdon	9	11q23–q24	*CDON*	193
Mouse	C57BL/6	AR	NfiA	4	1p31.3–p31.2	*NFIA*	198
Mouse	C57BL/6	AR	NfiX	8	19p13.3	*NFIX*	199
Mouse	C57BL/6 X 129	AR	Nrp2	1	2q33.3	*NRP2*	197
Mouse	C57BL/6 X 129	AR	Stk36	1	2q35	*STK36*	152
Mouse	C57BL/6 X 129	AR	Ulk4	9	3p22.1	*ULK4*	152
Mouse	C57BL/6 X 129	AR	Nme5	18	5q31	*NME5*	152
Mouse	C57BL/6 X 129	AR	Nme7	1	1q24	*NME7*	152
Mouse	C57BL/6 X 129	AR	Kif27	13	9q21.32	*KIF27*	152
Mouse	C57BL/6 X 129	AR	Dpcd	19	10q24.32	*DPCD*	152
Mouse	C57BL/6 X 129	AR	Ak7	12	14q32.2	*AK7*	152
Mouse	C57BL/6 X 129	AR	Ak8	2	9q34.13	*AK8*	152

Mouse	Wnt1-Cre/+ X C57BL/6	AR	Htt	5	4p16.3	*HTT*	105
Mouse	C57BL/6J	AR	Mtf2	5	1p22.1	*MTF2*	139
Mouse	C57BL/6	AR	Msi1	5	12q24	*MSI1*	116
Mouse	Cre/Kip2[+]/F X C57BL/6	AR	Cdkn1c	7	11p15.5	*CDKN1C*	106
Mouse	C57BL/6J X 129	AR	Psen1	12	14q24.3	*PSEN1*	107
Mouse	Aqp4 mice	AR	Aqp4	18	18q11.2–q12.1	*AQP4*	154
Mouse	Aqp1 mice	AR	Aqp1	6	7p14	*AQP1*	153
Mouse	C57BL/6x129Sv	AR	Pkd1	17	16p13.3	*PKD1*	146
Mouse	Celsr2	AR	Celsr2	3	1p21	*CELSR2*	133, 145
Mouse	Celsr3	AR	Celsr3	9	3p21.31	*CELSR3*	133, 145
Mouse	C57BL/6	AR	stumpy	7	19q13.2	*B9D2*	151
Mouse	C57BL/6 X 129	AR	Mboat7	7	19q13.4	*MBOAT7*	152
Mouse	C57BL/6 X 129	AR	Fzd3	14	8p21	*FZD3*	152
Mouse	C57BL/6 X 129	AR	Sgk196	8	8p11.21	*SGK196*	152
Mouse	B6C3Fe a/a-Qkqk/J	AR	Pacrg	17	6q26	*PACRG*	135
Mouse	C57/Bl6X129/FBV/N	AD	Fgfr3	5	4p16.3	*FGFR3*	176–178
Mouse	C57BL/6Jx129SvJ	AR	Trp53bp2	1	1q41	*ASPP2*	170
Mouse	C57BL/6J	AR	Casp3	8	4q34	*CASP3*	171, 172
Mouse	C57BL/6J	AR	Casp9	4	1p36.21	*CASP9*	171, 172
Mouse	129/Sv	AR	Apaf1	10	12q23	*APAF1*	174, 175

AR, autosomal recessive; AD, autosomal dominant; QTL, quantitative trait locus.

secretory cells of the SCO. Comparative analysis on serial brain sections through aqueduct regions containing the SCO from HTX rats and normal Fischer F344 rats has found that reduced SCO glycoprotein immunoreactivity precedes both aqueduct closure and expansion of the lateral ventricles in the HTX rat [101,102]. The LEW/Jms and HTX mutant rat models were identical with regard to the form of presentation and progression of hydrocephalus in the postnatal period; the pathogenesis of these two conditions in the fetal period was different. The LEW/Jms rats showed primary congenital aqueductal stenosis in early prenatal life and the hydrocephalic state appeared before pulmonary maturation was completed [76,103,104]. Several cases of autosomal recessive or autosomal dominant CHC due to aqueductal stenosis have been reported in humans [13,19,27,60,63], although the genes causing this type of hydrocephalus are currently still unknown.

Huntingtin (htt) protein, which causes Huntington's disease (HD) primarily by a gain-of-function trinucleotide repeat expansion, plays a major role during embryogenesis through its interaction with multiple cellular partners. Conditional removal of mouse htt protein in Wnt1 cell lineages using the Cre-loxP system results in congenital hydrocephalus associated with abnormalities in the choroid plexus (CP) and SCO and an increase in CSF production by the CP [105]. The cyclin-dependent kinase inhibitor (CKI) p57 regulates the activities of E2F1 and p53 to ensure the proper proliferation and survival of cells in the SCO. Conditional disruption of p57 gene in the brain results in severe nonobstructive hydrocephalus [106]. Likewise, presenilin-1 (PS1), which is responsible for the development of early-onset familial Alzheimer's disease, regulates metabolism of several important brain molecules during neurogenesis, including APP, Notch, cadherins, and β-catenin. Mice conditionally lacking PS1 in Wnt1 cell lineages with the Cre–loxP system also showed congenital hydrocephalus and SCO abnormalities [107]. Pax6, a developmentally regulated transcription factor, is expressed in secretory cells of the SCO. Mice functionally lacking Pax6 protein (homozygous knockout) failed to develop the SCO. Mice with decreased Pax6 protein level (heterozygous knockout) have defective development of the SCO, indicating that development of the SCO requires normal Pax6 gene-dosage [108]. Regulatory factor X3 (RFX3), a winged helix transcription factor, is expressed in the ciliated ependymal cells of the SCO and CP. Rfx3-deficient mice suffer from congenital hydrocephalus of variable severity resulting from ependymal cell defects of the SCO and CP perturbing CSF production or circulation [109]. The CYP2J2 transgene interferes with the expression of a brain-specific isoform of the regulatory factor X4 (RFX4). This brain-specific isoform is called variant transcript 3 or RFX4_v3 and is crucial for normal brain development as well as for the genesis of the SCO. Loss of a single allele prevents formation of the SCO and leads to congenital hydrocephalus in an autosomal dominant fashion. This obstructive hydrocephalus appears to be secondary to failure of development of the SCO [110]. Msx1, a homeobox gene that is strongly expressed in the SCO and CP [111,112], controls a genetic hierarchy involving bone-morphogenetic-protein (BMP) and sonic hedgehog (Shh) signals [113]. Msx1-deficient mice showed absence or malformation of the SCO and of the posterior commissure (PC), collapse of the cerebral aqueduct, and development of hydrocephalus [114,115]. Msi1 (Musashi 1), a member of the Musashi family of RNA-binding proteins, is strongly expressed in neural precursor cells. Homozygous Msi1 mutant mice developed obstructive hydrocephalus with aberrant proliferation of ependymal cells surrounding the sylvian aqueduct [116]. Dlg5, a conserved coiled-coil MAGUK protein, binds to syntaxin 4, a t-SNARE protein that regulates fusion of transport vesicles. Therefore, Dlg5 may facilitate interaction with the t-SNARE transport vesicle fusion machinery. Dlg5-deficient mice had closure of the aqueduct, accompanied by loss of ependymal cells and cilia, leading to severe hydrocephalus with hopping gait, similar to hydrocephalic hyh mice [117].

Ciliopathies

Cilia are complex cellular organelles protruding from the apical surface of cells with the polarized microtubule backbone (axoneme), through intraflagellar transport (IFT). Cilia play major roles in cell locomotion and fluid movement. Defects in cilia, or ciliopathies that are caused mainly by mutations in IFT genes [118], are associated with a range of human diseases, including hydrocephalus [119–121]. The hydrocephalus can be caused by the malfunction of cilia in ependymal cells [122–125]. Within the neonatal brain, ependymal cells form the epithelial lining of cerebral ventricles and cilia move coordinately on the apical surface to facilitate circulation of the CSF. The mouse hydrocephalus-3 (hy3) protein, hydin, is confined to the ciliated ependymal cell layer lining the lateral, third, and fourth ventricles. Hydin is a large protein that localizes in cilia/flagella and is not closely related to any previously known protein. Interestingly, a 314 amino acid domain identified within hydin shows a strong homology to caldesmon, an actin-binding protein [126], suggesting its potential interaction with the cytoskeleton [86,87]. The hydin-associated projection may play an important role in regulating switching of dynein activity [126]. Cilia are impaired in motility and incapable of generating fluid flow in *hydin* mutants [127,128]. Likewise, mutations in sperm-associated antigen 6 (Spag6) [129] also show lack of ependymal cell cilia, resulting in hydrocephalus. PolL (DNA polymerase λ) plays an essential role in the maintenance of genome integrity during development. Homologous PolL mutant mice developed hydrocephalus due to defective inner dynein arms of cilia from the ependymal cell layer [130].

The protein of axonemal heavy chain 5 gene (Mdnah5) as the hydrocephalus inducing gene, dynein, is also specifically expressed in ependymal cells. Mdnah5 is essential for ultrastructural and functional integrity of ependymal cilia. In Mdnah5 mutant mice, lack of ependymal flow causes closure of the aqueduct resulting in a defective ependymal flow and hydrocephalus [131]. The higher incidence of aqueduct stenosis and hydrocephalus formation in patients with ciliary defects proves the relevance of this mechanism in humans [131]. Pcdp1 (primary ciliary dyskinesia protein 1) protein localizes the cilia of brain ependymal cells and plays an important role in ciliary and flagellar biogenesis and motility. Loss of Pcdp1 results from ciliary dysfunction and leads to hydrocephalus [132].

Hedgehog signaling. Hedgehog (Hh) signaling requires the IFT machinery to shuttle GLI proteins and SUFU to the ciliary tip. Mutations in Hh signaling, anterograde and retrograde IFT motors (such as *Kif3a* [kinesin family member-3A], *Dync2h1* [dynein cytoplasmic-2 heavy chain-1], ptch1 (Hh receptor patched-1]) would result defective cilia [133]. It was found that deficiency of ptch1 leads to defective cilia function in ependymal cells, resulting in hydrocephalus, through crossing quaking viable mouse (qkv/v) with ptch1+/− mice [134]. However, the qkv mouse contains a deletion of ~1.1 Mb in the proximal region of chromosome 17, affecting the expression of three genes: quaking (Qk), Parkin-coregulated gene (Pacrg) and parkin (Park2). One experiment showed that transgenic expression of Pacrg was necessary and sufficient to rescue the CHC phenotype in the qkv mutant, implicating the role of Pacrg in the pathogenesis of hydrocephalus [135]. Pacrg protein in the mouse has been localized to the motile ependymal cilia lining the ventricles of the brain as a component of the flagella axoneme. Loss of Pacrg in defective cilia is associated with impaired ciliary mediated CSF flow and the development of hydrocephalus [135]. Sonic hedgehog (Shh) signaling correlates spatially and temporally with fissure formation through its activators, *GLI2* and *GLI3*, and its receptor, smoothened (SMO). Conditional removal of Gli2 [136] and Gli3 [137] leads to hydrophilic phenotypes; furthermore, hydrocephalus is one of the clinical diagnostics of patients with *GLI3* mutation [138]. Mtf2 plays essential roles during early embryogenesis through its genetic interaction with Shh signaling; *Mtf2* mutant mice exhibit several neurological defects including hydrocephalus [139].

Wnt signaling. Wnt signaling not only regulates neurogenesis itself, but also coordinates with sonic hedgehog (Shh) signaling to regulate the development of the brain [140,141]. Deletion of Wnt1 in mice revealed severe abnormalities in the development of brain, including hydrocephalus-like phenotype [142]. Abnormal cilia and impaired CSF movement in the brain are also observed in mutations in *Ift88* gene (*Tg737* or *Polaris* mutant mouse), due to altered function of the CP epithelium, as evidenced by hydrocephalus [118, 121,143]. The winged helix family of transcription factors has also been found to play an important role in ciliary development in CP. Hydrocephalic phenotype was observed in the forkhead homologue (hfh)-4 (Foxj1) mutant mouse due to lack of ependymal cell cilia [144]. The planar cell polarity (PCP) signaling pathway, also known as non-canonical Wnt pathway, has genetic interaction with BBS gene mediated signaling. Both PCP and BBS proteins are colocalized to the basal body and ciliary axoneme, indicating the involvement of their signaling in cilia [133]. Deficiency of mammalian PCP proteins, *Celsr2* and *Celsr3*, the murine orthologs of the *Drosophila* core PCP gene *Flamingo*, disrupts the genesis of ependymal cilia, leading to hydrocephalus [145].

Cilia receptor signaling. Polycystin-1 (PC-1), the product of the PKD1 gene, also plays some roles in ciliary function or signaling. Deficiency of PC-1 in ependyma and CP results in dysfunctional cilia and hydrocephalus [146]. β8-integrin transcripts are localized in periventricular cells of the neuroepithelium in the brain, and integrin-β8-deficient mice have characteristics of hydrocephalus [147]. Another recent study reported that the disruption of β1-integrin–matrix interactions in the brain through the injection of β1-integrin antibodies generates ventricular pressure, leading to hydrocephalus development in rats [148]. OPHN1 (oligophrenin1), a RhoGAP protein, binds to the cellular membrane through interaction with phosphoinositides. Ophn1-deficient mice developed hydrocephalus [149].

Ciliopathies are commonly associated with the SCO defect in the pathogenesis of hydrocephalus; thus primary ciliary dyskinesia–associated aqueductal stenosis should be considered as a possible cause for congenital hydrocephalus [150]. *Stumpy* is a conditional deficient mouse of B9d2 (B9 protein domain 2) in brain and kidney with perinatal hydrocephalus. B9d2 protein, a cellular interacting partner of γ-tubulin, is localized with ciliary basal bodies along ciliary axonemes, suggesting that it plays a role in ciliary axoneme extension [151]. Mutant mice with autosomal recessive congenital hydrocephalus caused by deficient cilia were also found in Ulk4, Nme5, Nme7, Kif27, Stk36, Dpcd, Ak7, and Ak8 gene knockout lines [152].

Deficient water channels

Water channel aquaporin-1 (AQP1), which is expressed at the apical membrane of CP, facilitates CSF production and balance. Membrane-bound AQP1 was reduced following kaolin-induced hydrocephalus, suggesting that CSF accumulation is rooted in AQP1 inhibition or down-regulation in hydrocephalus [153]. Aquaporin-4 (AQP4) is also highly expressed in ependymal cells in brain. Aqp4-null mice developed progressive obstructive hydrocephalus as a consequence of accelerated ventricular enlargement and elevation in intracranial pressure (ICP) due to accumulation of CSF [154]. However, another study found that AQP4-deficient mice did not produce any hydrocephalus or hydrocephalus-like abnormalities in the brain [155]. Interestingly, increased AQP4 expression was observed in congenital hydrocephalus in the HTX rat [156] and kaolin-induced hydrocephalus in Sprague-Dawley rats while no changes in AQP1 or AQP9 were observed [157]. Up-regulated AQP4 expression was interpreted as a compensatory response to maintain water homeostasis in hydrocephalus [154,157]. Another report indicates that AQP4 levels are significantly altered in a spatiotemporal-dependent manner in kaolin-induced hydrocephalus, suggesting the total amount of AQP4 in the brain is irrelevant to the pathogenesis of hydrocephalus [158]. While the role of AQP1 as a regulator of CSF production is proposed in the pathophysiology of hydrocephalus [159], the role of AQP4 in the pathophysiology of hydrocephalus is still debatable [160–162]. Further research is needed to clarify these controversial findings.

Disrupted apoptotic pathways

Precisely controlled apoptosis is essential for normal brain morphogenesis during development [163]. The HTX fetus demonstrates secondary closure of the aqueduct in the perinatal period [164]. This secondary closure of the aqueduct in HTX rats is believed to be due to retrograde degeneration of the thalamus caused by apoptotic cell death [165,166] and failure of cell proliferation, indicating the involvement of altered apoptotic and biogenic events [167,168]. ASPP2 enhances the apoptotic function of p53 [169], and *ASPP2*-null pups develop hydrocephalus [170]. Caspases (cysteine-containing, aspartate-specific proteases) play key roles in apoptotic signaling in neuronal apoptosis. Hydrocephalic phenotypes have been reported in both caspase-3 and caspase-9 null mice, while a more severe phenotype was observed in the caspase-9 null mice [171,172]. Fas is a member of the tumor necrosis factor/nerve growth factors. In a clinical study, an increased level of the soluble form of the anti-apoptotic regulator Fas (sFas) in the CSF of infants with hydrocephalus was observed, while no difference was found in activated caspase 3 [173]. Apoptotic protein, Apaf1 (human homologue of *Caenorhabditis elegans* CED-4), plays a central role in the caspase-9-dependent activation of caspase 3 through mitochondrial pathways in embryonic brain. Apaf1-deficient mice show enlarged brains caused by hydrocephalus [174,175]. FGFR3 is a member of membrane tyrosine kinases, fibroblast growth factor (FGF) receptors. FGFR3 affects brain size by modulating neuronal cell proliferation and apoptosis during embryonic development. Mice with the K644E kinase domain mutation in Fgfr3 showed enlargement of the brain [176], while the same mutation in human patients results in neurological anomalies during embryonic development including hydrocephalus [177,178].

Neural tube defects

A longitudinal study on the family history in humans indicates that uncomplicated CHC has a genetic base akin to neural tube defects. The two conditions, at least in a large proportion of cases, might be caused by the same genetic etiology [179,180]. Many cases of CHC associated with neural tube defects have been reported [181–189]. Likewise, 20% of neural tube defects were found to be associated with CHC [190]. Surprisingly, one report found that there is not an obvious additional genetic risk for neural tube defects for CHC patients [191].

Altered immune response

Although some studies reported the activation of macrophages and microglia within the brain in animal hydrocephalus models, little is known of the dynamics of immune response in human congenital hydrocephalus. In one study, brain tissue samples of 10 human fetal cases with hydrocephalus and 10 non-hydrocephalic controls were analyzed immunohistochemically with antibodies directed against MHC class II and CD68 antigens, and tomato lectin. Hydrocephalus samples showed focal collections of CD68 and tomato lectin-positive macrophages along the ependymal lining of the lateral ventricles, particularly within the occipital horn. By comparison, brain tissue samples from controls showed few or no ependymal or supra-ependymal macrophages and the few macrophages that were present were not as intensely immunoreactive as in the hydrocephalus cases. The macrophage response detected at the ependymal lining of the ventricles and within the periventricular area in hydrocephalus may be related both to the severity of hydrocephalus and to the age of the fetus [192]. Unexpectedly, hydrocephalic cases also showed focal regions of hypovascularization or alterations in the structure and orientation of capillaries within periventricular areas, compared to controls [192]. CDO is a cell surface protein, a member of the immunoglobulins (Ig), that is highly expressed in the central nervous system. *Cdo* knockout mice have developmental defects in brain, including hydrocephalus [193]. SOCS7, a member of the suppressor of cytokine signaling (SOCS) proteins, prominently expresses *Socs7* in the brain; mice lacking SOCS7 developed hydrocephalus [194].

Unknown causes

Some hydrophilic mice have been well characterized, but the likely underlying causes in those mutant lines are still undetermined. Those hydrophilic mouse lines are caused by genes mutated in *Mboat7*, *Sgk196*, and *Fzd3* [152]. Hif-1α, a hypoxia inducible factor response to low oxygen condition, is expressed in the developing brain and contributes to brain development. Disruption of the mouse *Zic5* gene, a zinc finger protein, results in hydrocephalus [195]. Neural cell-specific ablation of the *Hif-1α* gene in mice results in hydrocephalus [196]. Mice with homozygous mutation of molecular cues involving neuronal development, such as *NP2* (neuropilin-2) [197], *NfiA* [198] and *NfiX* [199] (nuclear factor Ia and nuclear factor Ix), *Slc39a4* [200], *Otx2* [201], and *Myh10* [202], also have a hydrocephalic phenotype.

Enhanced expression during early development

Many cellular mechanisms involved in down-regulation of certain cellular factors, as occur in mutant animal lines, are critical for neural development. Their down-regulation may lead to hydrocephalus. However, many efforts have recently been made to up-regulate certain cellular factors that can also induce hydrocephalus or hydrocephalus-like characteristics, including enlarged ventricles, thinned cortex, agenesis of the corpus callosum, and significantly reduced subcommissural organ in animal models, indicating that elevated expressions of these cellular factors are important parts of the pathogenesis of hydrocephalus.

Kruppel-like factor 4 (KLF4) is a member of the KLF family of transcription factors which are highly expressed in mouse embryonic stem cells (ESCs) and during the early phases of mouse development [203]. Mice with increased expression of KLF4 in neural stem cells (NSCs) and NSC-derived ependymal cells had elevated glial fibrillary acidic protein (GFAP) expression and astrocyte hypertrophy accompanied by defective ventricular cilia, resulting in hydrocephalus [204]. Overexpression of an X-linked transcription factor, Sox3, which is expressed in the murine SCO throughout its development and in the mature organ, disrupts the development of the SCO primordium through inhibition of diencephalic roof plate identity without inducing programmed cell death, therefore generating congenital hydrocephalus [100]. Mice overexpressing the human PAC1 receptor, which is selectively activated by the neuropeptide PACAP, and expressed predominantly in the brain during early development of the CNS, showed marked reductions in the cerebral cortex, corpus callosum, and SCO together with decreased neuronal proliferation and accelerated apoptosis, and shorter, inefficient and disorganized cilia [205]. Those combined defects likely result in reduced CSF flow within the cerebral aqueduct, thereby promoting hydrocephalus [206]. *En1 (Engrailed 1)*, a homeodomain-containing protein that is an early target of *Wnt1* signaling during embryonic development, regulates the differentiation of the CP, the main site of production and secretion of CSF. Ectopic expression of *En1* gene induced prenatal hydrocephalus in mouse. Ectopically

Table 4.3 Current known hydrocephalic animal models caused by overexpression of certain genes

Species	Strain	Fold increase	Locus	Chromosome	Human syntenic region	Human gene	References
Mouse	FVB/N	2–6×	Klf4	4	9q31	*KLF4*	203, 204
Mouse	UKU302F	6×	Dbi	1	2q12–q21	*DBI*	208
Mouse	CBA × C57BL/6J	Variable	Adcyap1r1	6	7p14	*ADCYAP1R1*	205
Mouse	BALB/c × SJL	2–6×	Tgfb1	7	19q13.1	*TGFB1*	209
Mouse	WEXPZ.En1	Variable	En1	1	2q14.2	*EN1*	207
Mouse	C57BL/6XCBA	2–3×	Sox3	X	Xq27.1	*SOX3*	100

expressed *En2* gene in the developing chick embryo developed an identical phenotype to hydrocephalus [207]. Diazepam binding inhibitor (DBI) is a negative allosteric modulator of $GABA_A$ receptors; higher DBI levels have been associated with multiple neurological conditions. A hydrocephalic phenotype was developed in the transgenic mouse line with 6-fold higher expression levels of Dbi [208]. Transforming growth factor β (TGF-β) serves broad regulatory roles through its modulation of cell growth and differentiation. The development of severe hydrocephalus was found to be associated with high levels of TGF-β1 mRNA expression in the brain of a transgenic mouse line [209].

Ectopically overexpression of certain cellular factors can induce a phenotype of hydrocephalus, indicating that these cellular factors are involved in the signaling pathways, which when perturbed (could be caused by the loss of function of one of the upstream suppressors in the signaling pathway), leads to pathogenesis of hydrocephalus. Current known hydrocephalic animal models caused by overexpression of certain genes are described in Table 4.3.

Conclusion

Genetic studies in animal models have started to open new ways for understanding the underlying molecular pathophysiology of hydrocephalus. Based on data from animal models, current understanding of the pathophysiology of congenital hydrocephalus is that CHC is the result of abnormal brain development which sequentially leads to disrupted CSF secretion, circulation, absorption, and drainage [210].

Ironically, in contrast to the exciting research advances in genetic studies in animal models, human hydrocephalus genetic research has lagged far behind. In the first National Institutes of Health (NIH)-sponsored research conference on hydrocephalus (Bethesda, 2005), the topic "genetic cause" was "very fortunately" added to the future research tasks at the last minute. Amazingly, in the third NIH-sponsored research conference on hydrocephalus (Seattle, 2013) entitled "Opportunities in Hydrocephalus Research: Pathways to Better Outcomes," the very first session was about the genetic causes of hydrocephalus. This dramatic change partly reflects our current understanding, rapid research progress, and changing focus on the molecular etiology of hydrocephalus.

In summary, the pathological evidence of hydrocephalus clearly indicates that impaired and abnormal brain development in the early development stage is caused by altered neural cell fate and perturbed regulation of cellular events due to altered molecular cues during development. The abnormal brain development subsequently leads to the accumulation of CSF in cerebral cavities. All these cellular and developmental events are driven by certain genetic determinants, which eventually lead to congenital hydrocephalus accompanied by possible secondary inflammatory reaction and neurovascular pathogenesis.

References

1. Chi JH, Fullerton HJ, Gupta N. Time trends and demographics of deaths from congenital hydrocephalus in children in the United States: National Center for Health Statistics data, 1979 to 1998. *J Neurosurg* 2005;103:113–18.
2. Van Landingham M, Nguyen TV, Roberts A, Parent AD, Zhang J. Risk factors of congenital hydrocephalus: a 10 year retrospective study. *J Neurol Neurosurg Psychiatry* 2009;80:213–17.
3. Schrander-Stumpel C, Fryns JP. Congenital hydrocephalus: nosology and guidelines for clinical approach and genetic counselling. *Eur J Pediatr* 1998;157:355–62.

4. Varadi V, Toth Z, Korodi I, Papp Z. [Risk of heterogeneity and recurrence in congenital hydrocephalus (ventriculomegaly)]. *Orvosi hetilap* 1987;128:1349–52, 1356.

5. Varadi V, Toth Z, Torok O, Papp Z. Heterogeneity and recurrence risk for congenital hydrocephalus (ventriculomegaly): a prospective study. *Am J Med Genet* 1988;29:305–10.

6. Bearer CF. L1 cell adhesion molecule signal cascades: targets for ethanol developmental neurotoxicity. *Neurotoxicology* 2001;22:625–33.

7. Aolad HM, Inouye M, Hayasaka S, Darmanto W, Murata Y. Congenital hydrocephalus caused by exposure to low level x-radiation at early gestational stage in mice. *Uchu Seibutsu Kagaku* 1998;12:256–7.

8. Aolad HM, Inouye M, Darmanto W, Hayasaka S, Murata Y. Hydrocephalus in mice following x-irradiation at early gestational stage: possibly due to persistent deceleration of cell proliferation. *J Radiation Res* 2000;41:213–26.

9. Johnson RT, Johnson KP. Hydrocephalus following viral infection: the pathology of aqueductal stenosis developing after experimental mumps virus infection. *J Neuropathol Exp Neurol* 1968;27:591–606.

10. Adeloye A, Warkany J. Experimental congenital hydrocephalus. A review with special consideration of hydrocephalus produced by zinc deficiency. *Child's Brain* 1976;2:325–60.

11. Kazy Z, Puho E, Czeizel AE. Teratogenic potential of vaginal metronidazole treatment during pregnancy. *Eur J Obstet Gynecol Reprod Biol* 2005;123:174–8.

12. Orioli IM, Castilla EE. Epidemiological assessment of misoprostol teratogenicity. *BJOG* 2000;107:519–23.

13. Haverkamp F, Wolfle J, Aretz M, et al. Congenital hydrocephalus internus and aqueduct stenosis: aetiology and implications for genetic counselling. *Eur J Pediatr* 1999;158:474–8.

14. Zhang J, Williams MJ, Rigamonti D. Genetics of human hydrocephalus. *J Neurol* 2006; 253:1255–66.

15. Shannon MW, Nadler HL. X-linked hydrocephalus. *J Med Genet* 1968;5:326–8.

16. Jansen J. Sex-linked hydrocephalus. *Dev Med Child Neurol* 1975;17:633–40.

17. Halliday J, Chow CW, Wallace D, Danks DM. X linked hydrocephalus: a survey of a 20 year period in Victoria, Australia. *J Med Genet* 1986;23:23–31.

18. Rosenthal A, Jouet M, Kenwrick S. Aberrant splicing of neural cell adhesion molecule L1 mRNA in a family with X-linked hydrocephalus. *Nat Genet* 1992;2:107–12.

19. Vanlieferinghen P, Chazal J, Francannet C, Malpuech G, Storme B. [Congenital stenosis of the aqueduct of Sylvius transmitted in an autosomal recessive mode (5 cases in 2 families)]. *J Genet Hum* 1987;35:251–8.

20. Chow CW, McKelvie PA, Anderson RM, et al. Autosomal recessive hydrocephalus with third ventricle obstruction. *Am J Med Genet* 1990;35:310–13.

21. Barros-Nunes P, Rivas F. Autosomal recessive congenital stenosis of aqueduct of Sylvius. *Genet Couns* 1993;4:19–23.

22. Zlotogora J, Sagi M, Cohen T. Familial hydrocephalus of prenatal onset. *Am J Med Genet* 1994;49:202–4.

23. Zlotogora J. Genetic disorders among Palestinian Arabs. 2. Hydrocephalus and neural tube defects. *Am J Med Genet* 1997;71:33–5.

24. Chudley AE, McCullough C, McCullough DW. Bilateral sensorineural deafness and hydrocephalus due to foramen of Monro obstruction in sibs: a newly described autosomal recessive disorder. *Am J Med Genet* 1997;68:350–6.

25. Castro-Gago M, Alonso A, Pintos-Martinez E, et al. Congenital hydranencephalic-hydrocephalic syndrome associated with mitochondrial dysfunction. *J Child Neurol* 1999;14:131–5.

26. Chalmers RM, Andreae L, Wood NW, Durai Raj RV, Casey AT. Familial hydrocephalus. *J Neurol Neurosurg Psychiatry* 1999;67:410–11.

27. Hamada H, Watanabe H, Sugimoto M, et al. Autosomal recessive hydrocephalus due to congenital stenosis of the aqueduct of Sylvius. *Prenat Diagn* 1999;19:1067–9.

28. Schinzel A. [Congenital structural defects in twins: diversity, etiology and genetic counseling]. *Schweiz Rundsch Med Prax* 1985;74:351–7.

29. Berker E, Goldstein G, Lorber J, Priestley B, Smith A. Reciprocal neurological developments of twins discordant for hydrocephalus. *Dev Med Child Neurol* 1992;34:623–32.

30. Klein D, Bersot H, Borle A. [Familial hydrocephalus with concordant manifestation in univitelline twins]. *Confin Neurol* 1953;13:158–60.

31. Borle A. [The etiology of congenital hydrocephalus with regard to a case of concordant hydrocephalus in monozygotic twins]. *J Genet Hum* 1953;2:157–202.

32. Gellman V. Congenital hydrocephalus in monovular twins. *Arch Dis Child* 1959;34:274–6.

33. Idowu OE, Anga AL. Congenital hydrocephalus in mono and dizygotic twins. *East Central Afr J Surg* 2009;14:64–8.

34. Cox PM, Gibson RA, Morgan N, Brueton LA. VACTERL with hydrocephalus in twins due to Fanconi anemia (FA): mutation in the FAC gene. *Am J Med Genet* 1997;68:86–90.

35. Habib Z. Genetics and genetic counselling in neonatal hydrocephalus. *Obstet Gynecol Surv* 1981;36:529–34.

36. Adams C, Johnston WP, Nevin NC. Family study of congenital hydrocephalus. *Dev Med Child Neurol* 1982;24:493–8.
37. Munch TN, Rostgaard K, Rasmussen ML, et al. Familial aggregation of congenital hydrocephalus in a nationwide cohort. *Brain* 2012;135(Pt 8):2409–15.
38. Larson CA. Hydrocephalus and incomplete fusion of fetal clefts; report on a kindred. *Am J Hum Genet* 1954;6:16–25.
39. Martin C, Got M, Babin JP, Cazauran JM. [Familial hydrocephalus, a hereditary disease]. *Arch Fr Pediatr* 1971;28:787–8.
40. Sheen VL, Basel-Vanagaite L, Goodman JR, et al. Etiological heterogeneity of familial periventricular heterotopia and hydrocephalus. *Brain Dev* 2004;26:326–34.
41. Willems PJ. Heterogeneity in familial hydrocephalus. *Am J Med Genet* 1988;31:471–3.
42. Portenoy RK, Berger A, Gross E. Familial occurrence of idiopathic normal-pressure hydrocephalus. *Arch Neurol* 1984;41:335–7.
43. Zhang J, Williams MA, Rigamonti D. Heritable essential tremor-idiopathic normal pressure hydrocephalus (ETINPH). *Am J Med Genet A*. 2008;146A:433–9.
44. Zhang J, Carr CW, Rigamonti D, Badr A. Genome-wide linkage scan maps ETINPH gene to chromosome 19q12–13.31. *Hum Her* 2010;69:262–7.
45. Takahashi Y, Kawanami T, Nagasawa H, et al. Familial normal pressure hydrocephalus (NPH) with an autosomal-dominant inheritance: a novel subgroup of NPH. *J Neurol Sci* 2011;308:149–51.
46. Cusimano MD, Rewilak D, Stuss DT, et al. Normal-pressure hydrocephalus: is there a genetic predisposition? *Can J Neurol Sci* 2011;38:274–81.
47. Gudmundsson G, Kristjansdottir G, Cook E, Olafsson I. Association of ApoE genotype with clinical features and outcome in idiopathic normal pressure hydrocephalus (iNPH): a preliminary report. *Acta Neurochir* 2009;151:1511–12.
48. Casmiro M, D'Alessandro R, Cacciatore FM, et al. Risk factors for the syndrome of ventricular enlargement with gait apraxia (idiopathic normal pressure hydrocephalus): a case-control study. *J Neurol Neurosurg Psychiatry* 1989;52:847–52.
49. Nacmias B, Tedde A, Guarnieri BM, et al. Analysis of apolipoprotein e, alpha1-antichymotrypsin and presenilin-1 genes polymorphisms in dementia caused by normal pressure hydrocephalus in man. *Neurosci Lett* 1997;229:177–80.
50. Wiswell TE, Tuttle DJ, Northam RS, Simonds GR. Major congenital neurologic malformations. A 17-year survey. *Am J Dis Child* 1990;144:61–7.
51. Bay C, Kerzin L, Hall BD. Recurrence risk in hydrocephalus. *Birth Defects Orig Art Ser*. 1979;15:95–105.
52. Burton BK. Recurrence risks for congenital hydrocephalus. *Clin Genet*. 1979;16:47–53.
53. Burton BK. Empiric recurrence risks for congenital hydrocephalus. *Birth Defects Orig Art Ser* 1979;15:107–15.
54. Abdul-Karim R, Iliya F, Iskandar G. Consecutive hydrocephalus: report of 2 cases. *Obstet Gynecol* 1964;24:376–8.
55. Teebi AS, Naguib KK. Autosomal recessive nonsyndromal hydrocephalus. *Am J Med Genet* 1988;31:467–70.
56. Game K, Friedman JM, Paradice B, Norman MG. Fetal growth retardation, hydrocephalus, hypoplastic multilobed lungs, and other anomalies in 4 sibs. *Am J Med Genet* 1989;33:276–9.
57. Moog U, Bleeker-Wagemakers EM, Crobach P, Vles JS, Schrander-Stumpel CT. Sibs with Axenfeld-Rieger anomaly, hydrocephalus, and leptomeningeal calcifications: a new autosomal recessive syndrome? *Am J Med Genet* 1998;78:263–6.
58. Castro-Gago M, Alonso A, Eiris-Punal J. Autosomal recessive hydrocephalus with aqueductal stenosis. *Childs Nerv Syst* 1996;12:188–1.
59. Mungen E, Atay V, Ertekin AA. Autosomal recessive hydrocephalus due to third ventricle obstruction. *Int J Gynaecol Obstet* 2005;91:168–9.
60. Verhagen WI, Bartels RH, Fransen E, et al. Familial congenital hydrocephalus and aqueduct stenosis with probably autosomal dominant inheritance and variable expression. *J Neurol Sci* 1998;158:101–5.
61. Mochizuki Y, Suyehiro Y, Ihara Y, et al. Congenital hydrocephalus and clasped thumbs: Two cases of brothers in a family. *Brain Dev* 1981;3:407–9.
62. Basel-Vanagaite L, Raas-Rotchild A, Kornreich L, et al. Familial hydrocephalus with normal cognition and distinctive radiological features. *Am J Med Genet A* 2010;152A:2743–8.
63. Lapunzina P, Delicado A, de Torres ML, et al. Autosomal recessive hydrocephalus due to aqueduct stenosis: report of a further family and implications for genetic counselling. *J Matern Fetal Neonatal Med* 2002;12:64–6.
64. Nova HR. Familial communicating hydrocephalus, posterior cerebellar agenesis, mega cisterna magna, and port-wine nevi. Report on five members of one family. *J Neurosurg* 1979;51:862–5.
65. Lammer EJ, Scholes T, Abrams L. Autosomal recessive tetralogy of Fallot, unusual facies, communicating hydrocephalus, and delayed language development: A new syndrome? *Clin Dysmorphol* 2001;10:9–13.

66. Bogucki J, Taraszewska A, Baraniecka J, Czernicki Z. Familial incidence of obstructive hydrocephalus due to posterior fossa tumours leading to the diagnosis of Von Hippel-Lindau disease – a case report. *Folia Neuropathol* 2002;40:219–22.

67. Cardoso ER. A familial coincidence of pseudotumor cerebri and communicating hydrocephalus. *Neurosurgery* 1991;29:796.

68. Vincent C, Kalatzis V, Compain S, et al. A proposed new contiguous gene syndrome on 8q consists of branchio-oto-renal (bor) syndrome, Duane syndrome, a dominant form of hydrocephalus and trapeze aplasia; implications for the mapping of the bor gene. *Hum Mol Genet* 1994;3:1859–66.

69. Jouet M, Feldman E, Yates J, et al. Refining the genetic location of the gene for X linked hydrocephalus within Xq28. *J Med Genet* 1993;30:214–17.

70. Strain L, Gosden CM, Brock DJ, Bonthron DT. Genetic heterogeneity in X-linked hydrocephalus: linkage to markers within Xq27.3. *Am J Hum Genet* 1994;54:236–43.

71. Jones HC, Depelteau JS, Carter BJ, Lopman BA, Morel L. Genome-wide linkage analysis of inherited hydrocephalus in the H-Tx rat. *Mamm Genome* 2001;12:22–6.

72. Jones HC, Depelteau JS, Carter BJ, Somera KC. The frequency of inherited hydrocephalus is influenced by intrauterine factors in H-Tx rats. *Exp Neurol* 2002;176:213–20.

73. Jones HC, Yehia B, Chen GF, Carter BJ. Genetic analysis of inherited hydrocephalus in a rat model. *Exp Neurol* 2004;190:79–90.

74. Cai X, McGraw G, Pattisapu JV, et al. Hydrocephalus in the H-Tx rat: a monogenic disease? *Exp Neurol* 2000;163:131–5.

75. Sasaki S, Goto H, Nagano H, et al. Congenital hydrocephalus revealed in the inbred rat, LEW/Jms. *Neurosurgery* 1983;13:548–54.

76. Jones HC, Carter BJ, Morel L. Characteristics of hydrocephalus expression in the LEW/Jms rat strain with inherited disease. *Childs Nerv Syst* 2003;19:11–18.

77. Zygourakis CC, Rosen GD. Quantitative trait loci modulate ventricular size in the mouse brain. *J Comp Neurol* 2003;461:362–69.

78. Lark FH. Hydrocephalus, a hereditary character in the house mouse. *Proc Natl Acad Sci USA* 1932;18:654–6.

79. Lark FH. Anatomical basis of a hereditary hydrocephalus in the house mouse. *Anat Rec* 1934:225–33.

80. Immermann K. Eine neue Mutation der Hausmaus: "Hydrocephalus". *Z Indukt Abstamm Vererbungsl* 1933:176–80.

81. Lark FH. Two hereditary types of hydrocephalus in the house mouse (*Mus musculus*). *Proc Natl Acad Sci USA* 1935;21:150–52.

82. Dickie M. Obstructive hydrocephalus. *Mouse News Lett* 1968:27.

83. Borit A, Sidman RL. New mutant mouse with communicating hydrocephalus and secondary aqueductal stenosis. *Acta Neuropathol* 1972;21:316–31.

84. Gruneberg H. Two new mutant genes in the house mouse. *J Genet* 1943:22–8.

85. Raimondi AJ, Bailey OT, McLone DG, Lawson RF, Echeverry A. The pathophysiology and morphology of murine hydrocephalus in hy-3 and ch mutants. *Surg Neurol* 1973;1:50–5.

86. Robinson ML, Allen CE, Davy BE, et al. Genetic mapping of an insertional hydrocephalus-inducing mutation allelic to hy3. *Mamm Genome* 2002;13:625–32.

87. Davy BE, Robinson ML. Congenital hydrocephalus in hy3 mice is caused by a frameshift mutation in hydin, a large novel gene. *Hum Mol Genet* 2003;12:1163–70.

88. Green MC. The developmental effects of congenital hydrocephalus (ch) in the mouse. *Dev Biol* 1970;23:585–608.

89. Kume T, Deng KY, Winfrey V, et al. The forkhead/winged helix gene mf1 is disrupted in the pleiotropic mouse mutation congenital hydrocephalus. *Cell* 1998;93:985–96.

90. Hong HK, Lass JH, Chakravarti A. Pleiotropic skeletal and ocular phenotypes of the mouse mutation congenital hydrocephalus (ch/mf1) arise from a winged helix/forkhead transcription factor gene. *Hum Mol Genet* 1999;8:625–37.

91. Descipio C, Schneider L, Young TL, et al. Subtelomeric deletions of chromosome 6p: molecular and cytogenetic characterization of three new cases with phenotypic overlap with Ritscher-Schinzel (3c) syndrome. *Am J Med Genet A* 2005;134A:3–11.

92. Aldinger KA, Lehmann OJ, Hudgins L, et al. Foxc1 is required for normal cerebellar development and is a major contributor to chromosome 6p25.3 Dandy-Walker malformation. *Nat Genet* 2009;41:1037–42.

93. Chae TH, Kim S, Marz KE, Hanson PI, Walsh CA. The *hyh* mutation uncovers roles for alpha Snap in apical protein localization and control of neural cell fate. *Nat Genet* 2004;36:264–70.

94. Hong HK, Chakravarti A, Takahashi JS. The gene for soluble n-ethylmaleimide sensitive factor attachment protein alpha is mutated in hydrocephaly with hop gait (hyh) mice. *Proc Natl Acad Sci USA* 2004;101:1748–53.

95. Kuwamura M, Kinoshita A, Okumoto M, Yamate J, Mori N. Hemorrhagic hydrocephalus (hhy): a novel mutation on mouse chromosome 12. *Brain Res Dev Brain Res* 2004;152:69–72.

96. Mori N, Kuwamura M, Tanaka N, et al. Ccdc85c encoding a protein at apical junctions of radial glia is disrupted in hemorrhagic hydrocephalus (hhy) mice. *Am J Pathol* 2012;180:314–27.

97. Takahashi A, Shiroishi T, Koide T. Multigenic factors associated with a hydrocephalus-like phenotype found in inter-subspecific consomic mouse strains. *Mamm Genome* 2008;19:333–8.

98. Bruni JE, Del Bigio MR, Cardoso ER, Persaud TV. Hereditary hydrocephalus in laboratory animals and humans. *Exp Pathol* 1988;35:239–46.

99. Galarza M. Evidence of the subcommissural organ in humans and its association with hydrocephalus. *Neurosurg Rev* 2002;25:205–15.

100. Lee K, Tan J, Morris MB, et al. Congenital hydrocephalus and abnormal subcommissural organ development in sox3 transgenic mice. *PloS One* 2012;7:e29041.

101. Somera KC, Jones H. Subcommissural organ dysfunction in H-Tx rats with early-onset hydrocephalus. *Eur J Pediatr Surg* 2002;12(Suppl 1):S45–7.

102. Somera KC, Jones HC. Reduced subcommissural organ glycoprotein immunoreactivity precedes aqueduct closure and ventricular dilatation in H-Tx rat hydrocephalus. *Cell Tissue Res* 2004;315:361–73.

103. Jones HC, Totten CF, Mayorga DA, Yue M, Carter BJ. Genetic loci for ventricular dilatation in the LEW/Jms rat with fetal-onset hydrocephalus are influenced by gender and genetic background. *Cerebrospinal Fluid Res* 2005;2:2

104. Yamada H, Oi S, Tamaki N, Matsumoto S, Sudo K. Histological changes in the midbrain around the aqueduct in congenital hydrocephalic rat LEW/Jms. *Childs Nerv Syst* 1992;8:394–8.

105. Dietrich P, Shanmugasundaram R, Shuyu E, Dragatsis I. Congenital hydrocephalus associated with abnormal subcommissural organ in mice lacking huntingtin in wnt1 cell lineages. *Hum Mol Genet* 2009;18:142–50.

106. Matsumoto A, Susaki E, Onoyama I, et al. Deregulation of the p57-e2f1-p53 axis results in nonobstructive hydrocephalus and cerebellar malformation in mice. *Mol Cell Biol* 2011;31:4176–92.

107. Nakajima M, Matsuda K, Miyauchi N, et al. Hydrocephalus and abnormal subcommissural organ in mice lacking presenilin-1 in wnt1 cell lineages. *Brain Res* 2011;1382:275–81.

108. Estivill-Torrus G, Vitalis T, Fernandez-Llebrez P, Price DJ. The transcription factor pax6 is required for development of the diencephalic dorsal midline secretory radial glia that form the subcommissural organ. *Mech Dev* 2001;109:215–24.

109. Baas D, Meiniel A, Benadiba C, et al. A deficiency in rfx3 causes hydrocephalus associated with abnormal differentiation of ependymal cells. *Eur J Neurosci* 2006;24:1020–30.

110. Blackshear PJ, Graves JP, Stumpo DJ, et al. Graded phenotypic response to partial and complete deficiency of a brain-specific transcript variant of the winged helix transcription factor RFX4. *Development* 2003;130:4539–52.

111. Satokata I, Maas R. Msx1 deficient mice exhibit cleft palate and abnormalities of craniofacial and tooth development. *Nat Genet* 1994;6:348–56.

112. Ramos C, Martinez A, Robert B, Soriano E. Msx1 expression in the adult mouse brain: Characterization of populations of beta-galactosidase-positive cells in the hippocampus and fimbria. *Neuroscience* 2004;127:893–900.

113. Zhang Z, Song Y, Zhao X, et al. Rescue of cleft palate in Msx1-deficient mice by transgenic Bmp4 reveals a network of BMP and Shh signaling in the regulation of mammalian palatogenesis. *Development* 2002;129:4135–46.

114. Fernandez-Llebrez P, Grondona JM, Perez J, et al. Msx1-deficient mice fail to form prosomere 1 derivatives, subcommissural organ, and posterior commissure and develop hydrocephalus. *J Neuropathol Exp Neurol* 2004;63:574–86.

115. Ramos C, Fernandez-Llebrez P, Bach A, Robert B, Soriano E. Msx1 disruption leads to diencephalon defects and hydrocephalus. *Dev Dyn* 2004;230:446–60.

116. Sakakibara S, Nakamura Y, Yoshida T, et al. RNA-binding protein Musashi family: roles for CNS stem cells and a subpopulation of ependymal cells revealed by targeted disruption and antisense ablation. *Proc Natl Acad Sci USA* 2002;99:15194–9.

117. Nechiporuk T, Fernandez TE, Vasioukhin V. Failure of epithelial tube maintenance causes hydrocephalus and renal cysts in dlg5-/- mice. *Dev Cell* 2007;13:338–50.

118. Pazour GJ, Dickert BL, Vucica Y, et al. *Chlamydomonas IFT88* and its mouse homologue, polycystic kidney disease gene *Tg737*, are required for assembly of cilia and flagella. *J Cell Biol* 2000;151:709–18.

119. Cardenas-Rodriguez M, Badano JL. Ciliary biology: understanding the cellular and genetic basis of human ciliopathies. *Am J Med Genet C Semin Med Genet* 2009;151C:263–280.

120. Badano JL, Mitsuma N, Beales PL, Katsanis N. The ciliopathies: an emerging class of human genetic disorders. *Ann Rev Genomics Hum Genet.* 2006;7:125–48.

121. Banizs B, Pike MM, Millican CL, et al. Dysfunctional cilia lead to altered ependyma and choroid plexus function, and result in the formation of hydrocephalus. *Development* 2005;132:5329–39.

122. Takano T, Mekata Y, Yamano T, Shimada M. Early ependymal changes in experimental hydrocephalus after mumps virus inoculation in hamsters. *Acta Neuropathol* 1993;85:521–5.

123. Takano T, Rutka JT, Becker LE. Overexpression of nestin and vimentin in ependymal cells in hydrocephalus. *Acta Neuropathol* 1996;92:90–7.

124. Jimenez AJ, Tome M, Paez P, et al. A programmed ependymal denudation precedes congenital hydrocephalus in the hyh mutant mouse. *J Neuropathol Exp Neurol* 2001;60:1105–19.

125. Wagner C, Batiz LF, Rodriguez S, et al. Cellular mechanisms involved in the stenosis and obliteration of the cerebral aqueduct of hyh mutant mice developing congenital hydrocephalus. *J Neuropathol Exp Neurol* 2003;62:1019–40.

126. Smith EF. Hydin seek: finding a function in ciliary motility. *J Cell Biol* 2007;176:403–4.

127. Lechtreck KF, Delmotte P, Robinson ML, Sanderson MJ, Witman GB. Mutations in hydin impair ciliary motility in mice. *J Cell Biol* 2008;180:633–43.

128. Lechtreck KF, Witman GB. *Chlamydomonas reinhardtii* hydin is a central pair protein required for flagellar motility. *J Cell Biol* 2007;176:473–82.

129. Sapiro R, Kostetskii I, Olds-Clarke P, et al. Male infertility, impaired sperm motility, and hydrocephalus in mice deficient in sperm-associated antigen 6. *Mol Cell Biol* 2002;22:6298–305.

130. Kobayashi Y, Watanabe M, Okada Y, et al. Hydrocephalus, situs inversus, chronic sinusitis, and male infertility in DNA polymerase lambda-deficient mice: possible implication for the pathogenesis of immotile cilia syndrome. *Mol Cell Biol* 2002;22:2769–76.

131. Ibanez-Tallon I, Pagenstecher A, Fliegauf M, et al. Dysfunction of axonemal dynein heavy chain mdnah5 inhibits ependymal flow and reveals a novel mechanism for hydrocephalus formation. *Hum Mol Genet* 2004;13:2133–41.

132. Lee L, Campagna DR, Pinkus JL, et al. Primary ciliary dyskinesia in mice lacking the novel ciliary protein pcdp1. *Mol Cell Biol* 2008;28:949–57.

133. Fliegauf M, Benzing T, Omran H. When cilia go bad: cilia defects and ciliopathies. *Nat Rev Mol Cell Biol* 2007;8:880–93.

134. Gavino C, Richard S. Patched1 haploinsufficiency impairs ependymal cilia function of the quaking viable mice, leading to fatal hydrocephalus. *Mol Cell Neurosci* 2011;47:100–7.

135. Wilson GR, Wang HX, Egan GF, et al. Deletion of the Parkin co-regulated gene causes defects in ependymal ciliary motility and hydrocephalus in the quakingviable mutant mouse. *Hum Mol Genet* 2010;19:1593–602.

136. Corrales JD, Blaess S, Mahoney EM, Joyner AL. The level of sonic hedgehog signaling regulates the complexity of cerebellar foliation. *Development* 2006;133:1811–21.

137. Rachel RA, Wellington SJ, Warburton D, Mason CA, Beermann F. A new allele of gli3 and a new mutation, circletail (crc), resulting from a single transgenic experiment. *Genesis* 2002;33:55–61.

138. Naruse I, Ueta E, Sumino Y, Ogawa M, Ishikiriyama S. Birth defects caused by mutations in human *GLI3* and mouse *Gli3* genes. *Congenit Anom* 2010;50:1–7.

139. Wang S, He F, Xiong W, et al. Polycomblike-2-deficient mice exhibit normal left-right asymmetry. *Dev Dyn* 2007;236:853–61.

140. Gulacsi AA, Anderson SA. Beta-catenin-mediated wnt signaling regulates neurogenesis in the ventral telencephalon. *Nat Neurosci* 2008;11:1383–91.

141. Tang M, Villaescusa JC, Luo SX, et al. Interactions of wnt/beta-catenin signaling and sonic hedgehog regulate the neurogenesis of ventral midbrain dopamine neurons. *J Neurosci* 2010;30:9280–91.

142. Thomas KR, Capecchi MR. Targeted disruption of the murine int-1 proto-oncogene resulting in severe abnormalities in midbrain and cerebellar development. *Nature* 1990;346:847–50.

143. Banizs B, Komlosi P, Bevensee MO, et al. Altered ph(i) regulation and na(+)/hco3(-) transporter activity in choroid plexus of cilia-defective tg737(orpk) mutant mouse. *Am J Physiol Cell Physiol* 2007;292:C1409–16.

144. Chen J, Knowles HJ, Hebert JL, Hackett BP. Mutation of the mouse hepatocyte nuclear factor/forkhead homologue 4 gene results in an absence of cilia and random left-right asymmetry. *J Clin Invest* 1998;102:1077–82.

145. Tissir F, Qu Y, Montcouquiol M, et al. Lack of cadherins celsr2 and celsr3 impairs ependymal ciliogenesis, leading to fatal hydrocephalus. *Nat Neurosci* 2010;13:700–7.

146. Wodarczyk C, Rowe I, Chiaravalli M, et al. A novel mouse model reveals that polycystin-1 deficiency in ependyma and choroid plexus results in dysfunctional cilia and hydrocephalus. *PloS One* 2009;4:e7137.

147. Zhu J, Motejlek K, Wang D, et al. Beta8 integrins are required for vascular morphogenesis in mouse embryos. *Development* 2002;129:2891–903.

148. Nagra G, Koh L, Aubert I, Kim M, Johnston M. Intraventricular injection of antibodies to beta1-integrins generates pressure gradients in the brain favoring hydrocephalus development in rats. *Am J Physiol Regul Integr Comp Physiol* 2009;297:R1312–21.

149. Khelfaoui M, Denis C, van Galen E, et al. Loss of X-linked mental retardation gene oligophrenin1 in mice impairs spatial memory and leads to ventricular enlargement and dendritic spine immaturity. *J Neurosci* 2007;27:9439–50.

150. Vieira JP, Lopes P, Silva R. Primary ciliary dyskinesia and hydrocephalus with aqueductal stenosis. *J Child Neurol* 2012;27:938–41.

151. Town T, Breunig JJ, Sarkisian MR, et al. The stumpy gene is required for mammalian ciliogenesis. *Proc Natl Acad Sci USA* 2008;105:2853–8.

152. Vogel P, Read RW, Hansen GM, et al. Congenital hydrocephalus in genetically engineered mice. *Vet Pathol* 2012;49:166–81.

153. Wang D, Nykanen M, Yang N, et al. Altered cellular localization of aquaporin-1 in experimental hydrocephalus in mice and reduced ventriculomegaly in aquaporin-1 deficiency. *Mol Cell Neurosci* 2011;46:318–24.

154. Feng X, Papadopoulos MC, Liu J, et al. Sporadic obstructive hydrocephalus in Aqp4 null mice. *J Neurosci Res* 2009;87:1150–5.

155. Saadoun S, Tait MJ, Reza A, et al. AQP4 gene deletion in mice does not alter blood-brain barrier integrity or brain morphology. *Neuroscience* 2009;161:764–72.

156. Shen XQ, Miyajima M, Ogino I, Arai H. Expression of the water-channel protein aquaporin 4 in the H-Tx rat: possible compensatory role in spontaneously arrested hydrocephalus. *J Neurosurg* 2006;105:459–64.

157. Mao X, Enno TL, Del Bigio MR. Aquaporin 4 changes in rat brain with severe hydrocephalus. *Eur J Neurosci* 2006;23:2929–36.

158. Skjolding AD, Rowland IJ, Sogaard LV, et al. Hydrocephalus induces dynamic spatiotemporal regulation of aquaporin-4 expression in the rat brain. *Cerebrospinal Fluid Res* 2010;7:20.

159. Kalani MY, Filippidis AS, Rekate HL. Hydrocephalus and aquaporins: the role of aquaporin-1. *Acta Neurochir Suppl* 2012;113:51–4.

160. Aghayev K, Bal E, Rahimli T, et al. Aquaporin-4 expression is not elevated in mild hydrocephalus. *Acta Neurochir* 2012;154:753–9; discussion 759.

161. Filippidis AS, Kalani MY, Rekate HL. Hydrocephalus and aquaporins: the role of aquaporin-4. *Acta Neurochir Suppl* 2012;113:55–8.

162. Paul L, Madan M, Rammling M, et al. Expression of aquaporin 1 and 4 in a congenital hydrocephalus rat model. *Neurosurgery* 2011;68:462–73.

163. Roth KA, D'Sa C. Apoptosis and brain development. *Ment Retard Dev Disabil Res Rev* 2001;7:261–6.

164. Oi S, Yamada H, Sato O, Matsumoto S. Experimental models of congenital hydrocephalus and comparable clinical problems in the fetal and neonatal periods. *Childs Nerv Syst* 1996;12:292–302.

165. Miyan JA, Khan MI, Kawarada Y, Sugiyama T, Bannister CM. Cell death in the brain of the HTx rat. *Eur J Pediatr Surg* 1998;8(Suppl 1):43–8.

166. Mori F, Tanji K, Yoshida Y, Wakabayashi K. Thalamic retrograde degeneration in the congenitally hydrocephalic rat is attributable to apoptotic cell death. *Neuropathology* 2002;22:186–93.

167. Draper CE, Owen-Lynch PJ, Bannister CM, Miyan J. Proliferation of cerebral cortical cells from the hydrocephalic HTx rat: an in vitro study. *Eur J Pediatr Surg.* 2001;11(Suppl 1):S51–2.

168. Mashayekhi F, Bannister CM, Miyan JA. Failure in cell proliferation in the germinal epithelium of the HTx rats. *Eur J Pediatr Surg* 2001;11(Suppl 1):S57–9.

169. Samuels-Lev Y, O'Connor DJ, Bergamaschi D, et al. ASPP proteins specifically stimulate the apoptotic function of p53. *Mol Cell* 2001;8:781–94.

170. Vives V, Su J, Zhong S, et al. ASPP2 is a haploinsufficient tumor suppressor that cooperates with p53 to suppress tumor growth. *Genes Dev* 2006;20:1262–7.

171. Cowan CM, Roskams AJ. Caspase-3 and caspase-9 mediate developmental apoptosis in the mouse olfactory system. *J Comp Neurol* 2004;474:136–48.

172. Hakem R, Hakem A, Duncan GS, et al. Differential requirement for caspase 9 in apoptotic pathways in vivo. *Cell* 1998;94:339–52.

173. Felderhoff-Mueser U, Buhrer C, Groneck P, et al. Soluble fas (cd95/apo-1), soluble fas ligand, and activated caspase 3 in the cerebrospinal fluid of infants with posthemorrhagic and nonhemorrhagic hydrocephalus. *Pediatr Res* 2003;54:659–64.

174. Yoshida H, Kong YY, Yoshida R, et al. Apaf1 is required for mitochondrial pathways of apoptosis and brain development. *Cell* 1998;94:739–50.

175. Cecconi F, Alvarez-Bolado G, Meyer BI, Roth KA, Gruss P. Apaf1 (ced-4 homolog) regulates programmed cell death in mammalian development. *Cell* 1998;94:727–37.

176. Inglis-Broadgate SL, Thomson RE, Pellicano F, et al. FGFR3 regulates brain size by controlling progenitor cell proliferation and apoptosis during embryonic development. *Dev Biol* 2005;279:73–85.

177. Zankl A, Elakis G, Susman RD, et al. Prenatal and postnatal presentation of severe achondroplasia with developmental delay and acanthosis nigricans (saddan) due to the fgfr3 lys650met mutation. *Am J Med Genet A* 2008;146A:212–18.

178. Bellus GA, Bamshad MJ, Przylepa KA, et al. Severe achondroplasia with developmental delay and acanthosis nigricans (saddan): phenotypic analysis of a new skeletal dysplasia caused by a lys650met mutation in fibroblast growth factor receptor 3. *Am J Med Genet* 1999;85:53–65.

179. Lorber J. The family history of uncomplicated congenital hydrocephalus: an epidemiological study based on 270 probands. *Br Med J (Clin Res Ed)* 1984;289:281–4.

180. Lorber J. The family history of "simple" congenital hydrocephalus. An epidemiological study based on 270 probands. *Z Kinderchir* 1984;39(Suppl 2):94–5.

181. Di Rocco C, Rende M. Neural tube defects. Some remarks on the possible role of glycosaminoglycans in the genesis of the dysraphic state, the anomaly in the configuration of the posterior cranial fossa, and hydrocephalus. *Childs Nerv Syst* 1987;3:334–41.

182. Donnai D, Farndon PA. Examination of fetuses with a pre-termination diagnosis of neural tube defect or hydrocephalus. *Z Kinderchir* 1985;40(Suppl 1):51–2.

183. Gilbert JN, Jones KL, Rorke LB, Chernoff GF, James HE. Central nervous system anomalies associated with meningomyelocele, hydrocephalus, and the Arnold-Chiari malformation: reappraisal of theories regarding the pathogenesis of posterior neural tube closure defects. *Neurosurgery* 1986;18:559–64.

184. Grillo E, da Silva RJ. [Neural tube defects and congenital hydrocephalus. Why is prevalence important?]. *J Pediatr (Rio J)* 2003;79:105–6.

185. Penso C, Redline RW, Benacerraf BR. A sonographic sign which predicts which fetuses with hydrocephalus have an associated neural tube defect. *J Ultrasound Med* 1987;6:307–11.

186. Rajab A, Vaishnav A, Freeman NV, Patton MA. Neural tube defects and congenital hydrocephalus in the sultanate of Oman. *J Trop Pediatr* 1998;44:300–3.

187. Robertson RD, Sarti DA, Brown WJ, Crandall BF. Congenital hydrocephalus in two pregnancies following the birth of a child with a neural tube defect: aetiology and management. *J Med Genet* 1981;18:105–7.

188. Schlatter D, Sanseverino MT, Schmitt JM, et al. Severe fetal hydrocephalus with and without neural tube defect: a comparative study. *Fetal Diagn Ther* 2008;23:23–9.

189. Warf BC. Hydrocephalus associated with neural tube defects: characteristics, management, and outcome in sub-Saharan Africa. *Childs Nerv Syst* 2011;27:1589–94.

190. Hadzagic-Catibusic F, Maksic H, Uzicanin S, et al. Congenital malformations of the central nervous system: clinical approach. *Bosnian J Basic Med Sci* 2008;8:356–60.

191. Laurence KM. Genetic aspects of "uncomplicated" hydrocephalus and its relationship to neural tube defect. *Z Kinderchirur* 1984;39(Suppl 2):96–9.

192. Ulfig N, Bohl J, Neudorfer F, Rezaie P. Brain macrophages and microglia in human fetal hydrocephalus. *Brain Dev* 2004;26:307–15.

193. Zhang W, Yi MJ, Chen X, et al. Cortical thinning and hydrocephalus in mice lacking the immunoglobulin superfamily member CDO. *Mol Cell Biol* 2006;26:3764–72.

194. Krebs DL, Metcalf D, Merson TD, et al. Development of hydrocephalus in mice lacking socs7. *Proc Natl Acad Sci USA* 2004;101:15446–51.

195. Inoue T, Hatayama M, Tohmonda T, et al. Mouse zic5 deficiency results in neural tube defects and hypoplasia of cephalic neural crest derivatives. *Dev Biol* 2004;270:146–62.

196. Tomita S, Ueno M, Sakamoto M, et al. Defective brain development in mice lacking the hif-1alpha gene in neural cells. *Mol Cell Biol* 2003;23:6739–49.

197. Walz A, Rodriguez I, Mombaerts P. Aberrant sensory innervation of the olfactory bulb in neuropilin-2 mutant mice. *J Neurosci* 2002;22:4025–35.

198. das Neves L, Duchala CS, Tolentino-Silva F, et al. Disruption of the murine nuclear factor i-a gene (Nfia) results in perinatal lethality, hydrocephalus, and agenesis of the corpus callosum. *Proc Natl Acad Sci USA* 1999;96:11946–51.

199. Driller K, Pagenstecher A, Uhl M, et al. Nuclear factor I X deficiency causes brain malformation and severe skeletal defects. *Mol Cell Biol* 2007;27:3855–67.

200. Shenolikar S, Voltz JW, Minkoff CM, Wade JB, Weinman EJ. Targeted disruption of the mouse NHERF-1 gene promotes internalization of proximal tubule sodium-phosphate cotransporter type IIa and renal phosphate wasting. *Proc Natl Acad Sci USA* 2002;99:11470–5.

201. Makiyama Y, Shoji S, Mizusawa H. Hydrocephalus in the otx2+/- mutant mouse. *Exp Neurol* 1997;148:215–21.

202. Tullio AN, Bridgman PC, Tresser NJ, et al. Structural abnormalities develop in the brain after ablation of the gene encoding nonmuscle myosin II-B heavy chain. *J Comp Neurol* 2001;433:62–74.

203. Parisi S, Russo T. Regulatory role of Klf5 in early mouse development and in embryonic stem cells. *Vitam Horm* 2011;87:381–97.

204. Qin S, Liu M, Niu W, Zhang CL. Dysregulation of kruppel-like factor 4 during brain development leads to hydrocephalus in mice. *Proc Natl Acad Sci USA* 2011;108:21117–21.

205. Lang B, Song B, Davidson W, et al. Expression of the human PAC1 receptor leads to dose-dependent hydrocephalus-related abnormalities in mice. *J Clin Invest* 2006;116:1924–34.

206. Picketts DJ. Neuropeptide signaling and hydrocephalus: Sco with the flow. *J Clin Invest* 2006;116:1828–32.

207. Louvi A, Wassef M. Ectopic engrailed 1 expression in the dorsal midline causes cell death, abnormal differentiation of circumventricular organs and errors in axonal pathfinding. *Development* 2000;127:4061–71.

208. Siiskonen H, Oikari S, Korhonen VP, et al. Diazepam binding inhibitor overexpression in mice causes hydrocephalus, decreases plasticity in excitatory synapses and impairs hippocampus-dependent learning. *Mol Cell Neurosci* 2007;34:199–208.

209. Wyss-Coray T, Feng L, Masliah E, et al. Increased central nervous system production of extracellular matrix components and development of hydrocephalus in transgenic mice overexpressing transforming growth factor-beta 1. *Am J Path*ol 1995;147:53–67.

210. Zhang J, Williams MA, Rigamonti D. Genetics of human hydrocephalus. *J Neurol* 2006;253:1255–66.

Chapter 5

The epidemiology of hydrocephalus

Are Brean and Per Kristian Eide

Introduction

Assessing the epidemiology of a given disease should theoretically be an easy undertaking, by simply seeking out the population in question and counting the occurrence of the disease in question. While this might be the case for some clearly defined and easily delimited conditions, many diseases show particularities that complicate simple counting. The case of hydrocephalus illustrates this simple fact.

Hydrocephalus is not one, but several diseases. It occurs in all age groups, with probable predilection for the very young and the very old. The clinical signs are extremely diverse, ranging from acute and dramatic onsets with rapidly deteriorating courses to slow and insidious courses, clinically almost indistinguishable from the effects of normal aging. In line with this, the epidemiology of the more dramatic forms of hydrocephalus should be more easily discerned, yielding more consistent epidemiological numbers, while the more insidious forms of hydrocephalus, such as normal pressure hydrocephalus (NPH), should be more difficult to count. This, as we shall see, is the case in the scarce epidemiological literature on hydrocephalus, which yields highly divergent numbers as to the "true" occurrence of NPH.

In this chapter, we present the existing data concerning the epidemiology of selected forms of hydrocephalus, concentrating on congenital and infantile hydrocephalus and idiopathic and secondary NPH.

Epidemiology of specific types of hydrocephalus

Congenital and infantile hydrocephalus

The epidemiology of congenital and infantile hydrocephalus has been explored in several studies. In a Swedish epidemiological study, the mean crude prevalence was 0.60 per 1000 live births in the period 1973–1990 [1], excluding cases due to neural tube defects. This compares well to a population-based retrospective American cohort from 1991 to 2000, where the prevalence of congenital hydrocephalus was 0.59 per 1000 [2]. Data from four European registries of congenital malformations also approximate this, showing a prevalence of 0.47 per 1000 children born in the period 1996–2003 [3]. A Danish study including data from a local register of congenital malformations from the period 1986–1998 showed a prevalence of 0.4 per 1000 births, but 8 out of the 29 cases were stillbirths [4].

As to time trends of congenital hydrocephalus, the Swedish study showed a significant increase in prevalence from 1973–78 to 1979–82, considered due to the enhanced survival of very and extremely preterm infants [1]. However, this increase did not continue from 1983 to 1990, indicating an improved outcome in preterm infants in this period. In line with this trend, an Italian single-institution study showed a significant 8.8% decrease of the incidence between the periods 1985–90 and 2000–05 [5], and an epidemiological study from China showed a significant downward trend in the incidence of congenital hydrocephalus from 1998 to 2009 [6].

Idiopathic normal pressure hydrocephalus (iNPH)

The epidemiology of iNPH varies widely between the published studies, probably reflecting both inconsistent definitions of iNPH, differences between the populations sampled, and differences in the methodological approach towards the populations in question. As we shall see, many studies on the epidemiology of NPH do not differentiate between idiopathic and secondary NPH, something that makes the results even more

Adult Hydrocephalus, ed. Daniele Rigamonti. Published by Cambridge University Press.

Table 5.1 Occurrence of NPH in some epidemiological studies

Country	Clinically and radiologically defined NPH	iNPH/sNPH	Prevalence	Incidence	Reference
San Marino	Yes	iNPH	0.5% of all individuals <65 years	–	7
The Netherlands	Yes, with shunt response	Not defined	–	2.2/million/year	8
Germany	Yes	Not defined	0.4% of all individuals >65 years	–	9
Brazil	Not defined	Not defined	5.38% of dementia population	–	10
Germany	Yes, multiple centers, different criteria	Not defined	–	1.8/100 000/year	11
USA	Not defined	Not defined	3/560 cases of dementia. None responded to shunting	–	12
USA	Yes, "suspected iNPH"	iNPH	–	9–14% of residents in nursing homes	13
Norway	Yes, "probable iNPH"	iNPH	21.9/100 000/year	5.5/100 000/year	14
Japan	Yes	iNPH	2.9% of all individuals <65 years	–	16
Japan	Yes, "possible iNPH"	iNPH	1.4% of all individuals <65 years	–	17
Japan	Yes, "possible iNPH"	iNPH	0.51% of all individuals aged 61 years and 70–72 years		18
USA	Yes, "clinically suspected NPH"	Not defined	–	3.74/100 000/year, 0.36 sustained improvement after shunting	19
Thailand	Not defined	Not defined	0.9% of all patients with dementia in outpatient geriatric clinic		20

difficult to evaluate. An overview of some studies is given in Table 5.1.

In the earliest epidemiological study, Casmiro et al. examined five age cohorts over the age of 65 in the state of San Marino in 1985 [7]; 396 inhabitants out of a sample of 488 (81%) participated. The authors based the diagnosis on (1) absence of known causes of secondary NPH, (2) impaired gait, and (3) CT scans showing findings indicative of NPH. They found two cases of NPH, yielding a prevalence of 0.5%.

Vanneste et al. conducted a retrospective study in 1992, including only patients admitted to neurosurgical centers and having a good clinical response from treatment with shunt insertion [8]. This yielded an incidence of 2.2 per million inhabitants per year. However, the authors did not differentiate between idiopathic and secondary NPH, and the prevalence could also not be estimated from this design.

In a study from 1995 by Trenkwalder et al., 982 out of a total population of 1192 inhabitants over the age of 65 years in two German villages were examined primarily for parkinsonism [9]; 45 had clinical signs of parkinsonism. Out of these, 4 patients were diagnosed as having NPH, making the prevalence of NPH 0.41%.

The diagnostic criteria in this study included "typical gait disorder, bladder incontinence, dementia to a variable extent, and corresponding periventricular lucencies with ventricular enlargement." The authors did not distinguish between idiopathic and secondary NPH.

Vale and Miranda reported in 2002 the features of 168 patients with dementia, all admitted to a tertiary-care outpatient clinic in Brazil from 1997 to 1999 [10]. The patients were examined 18 months after their initial assessment. All patients underwent CT and/or MRI, but no results from these examinations relevant for the diagnosis of NPH are stated. The authors reported that 10 patients (5.4%) had NPH. Neither diagnostic nor clinical criteria for NPH are defined, and the authors do not distinguish between idiopathic and secondary NPH.

Krauss and Halve in 1997 conducted a questionnaire survey of 82 neurosurgical centers in Germany, out of which 65% responded [11]. The estimated annual incidence of NPH was 1.8/100 000. It is not clearly defined in the questionnaire whether shunt insertion and shunt response was necessary to confirm the diagnosis, and the diagnostic criteria varied from center to center. The authors estimated that "about two thirds of patients suffered from iNPH, and one third from sNPH," but no further data are given on this point.

As part of a local epidemiology project, Knopman et al. ascertained retrospectively incident cases of dementia in Rochester, Minnesota from 1990 to 1994 [12]. They found 560 cases of dementia. In 5 out of these, NPH was initially suspected. 3 underwent shunt placement, but none responded to therapy.

In contrast to this study stands a retrospective study among residents of assisted-living and extended-care facilities in four nursing homes [13]. Using a retrospective chart analysis, the authors included 147 patient records and found an estimated incidence of suspected iNPH ranging from 9% to 14%, depending on the diagnostic criteria used.

The authors of this chapter prospectively explored the epidemiology of iNPH in a Norwegian county of 220 000 inhabitants, by actively informing the public and professional health workers about the condition, asking for referral of suspected individuals on a broad clinical basis [14]. This yielded 86 referrals, of which 63 fulfilled the diagnostic criteria for "probable iNPH" [15] and 48 fulfilled the diagnostic criteria for "possible iNPH" [15]. From this, the prevalence of "probable iNPH" could be calculated as 21.9/100 000, with an incidence of 5.5/100 000/year. The prevalence of "possible iNPH" could be calculated as 28.7/100 000, with an incidence of 7.3/100 000/year. Most importantly, the prevalence of "probable iNPH" showed clear age dependency, ranging from 3.3/100 000 in the age group 50–59 years, 49.3/100 000 in the age group 60–69 years, 181.7/100 000 in the age group 70–79 years, to 93.3/100 000 in the age group ≥80 years.

Three studies from Japan assess the prevalence of iNPH in a general population. Hiraoka et al. analyzed retrospectively data from a community-based study of 170 randomly selected residents aged 65 years or older, finding that 2.9% showed clinical and radiological features consistent with iNPH [16]. Tanaka et al. analyzed data from 1645 people aged 65 years and older in Tajiri, Japan [17], 497 of whom underwent MRI. Using radiological and clinical criteria, the authors identified 7 individuals with "possible iNPH," yielding a prevalence of "possible iNPH" of 1.4% in this age group. No participants had the complete clinical triad. In an interesting prospective study, aiming to identify individuals having a preclinical stage of iNPH, 1142 residents aged 61 years and 70–72 years in two Japanese communities were invited to have brain MRI [18]; 790 (69.2%) participated. Four participants (0.51%) met the clinical and radiological criteria of "possible iNPH." In addition, two out of eight participants with asymptomatic ventriculomegaly later developed dementia and/or gait disturbance during a follow-up of 4–8 years.

In a retrospective study, reviewing the Mayo Clinic's medical records and available individual medical records from 1995 to 2003, Klassen and Ahlskog found 41 patients who had undergone an invasive diagnostic procedure for evaluation of suspected NPH [19]. This corresponds to an incidence of clinically suspected NPH of 3.74/100 000/year for the whole population, and 15.2/100 000/year for the population older than 50 years. Thirteen of these patients received shunts, yielding an incidence of NPH of 1.19/100 000/year when using "shunt insertion" as the final diagnostic criterion. The incidence of sustained definite improvements 3 years after shunting was 0.36/100 000/year. The authors did not differentiate between iNPH and secondary NPH (sNPH).

A study from Bangkok retrospectively reviewed the medical records of 293 patients with dementia or mild cognitive impairment assessed in an outpatient geriatric clinic. NPH was diagnosed in two patients (0.9%) [20]. The authors did not state the diagnostic criteria used for the diagnosis, nor did they differ between iNPH and sNPH.

Taken together, no firm conclusion can be drawn as to the true epidemiology of iNPH. The definition of the condition varies widely in the studies, ranging from no clearly specified definition [10,11], to strict definitions based on a good response from shunt insertion [8,12]. Many studies do not distinguish between iNPH and sNPH [8–10,12,19]. Also, several studies have taken into account only patients who have been admitted or evaluated for NPH [11,19], something that most certainly will underestimate the occurrence in the community-dwelling population. This is even more so in the studies that only take into account patients with a good response to shunt insertion [8,12]. On the other hand, the studies that estimate the occurrence of clinically and radiologically defined iNPH at a population or care facility level [7,9,13,14,16,17] will most certainly overestimate the occurrence of iNPH as long as a good response from shunt insertion is defined as a diagnostic criterion. This is because not all patients with clinically and radiologically defined iNPH will have a good response to shunt insertion. It can, however, be argued that a classification based only upon shunt response is a tautology, inherently excluding patients who have concomitant diseases that hinder a good shunt response, as well as patients in whom the pathological process has come too far to be reversed.

In line with all these difficulties in ascertaining the true epidemiology of iNPH, the estimates still differ widely in recent literature, leaving room for personal standpoints as to which epidemiological figures to emphasize from the international literature [19,21].

Secondary normal pressure hydrocephalus

The exact distribution of patients between the two conditions iNPH and sNPH is not fully known. In the previously cited multicenter study from Amsterdam constituting a total of 152 patients, 127 (84%) were classified as having iNPH, and 25 (16%) as having sNPH [8]. In a later Dutch multicenter study with 101 patients, 89% were classified as having iNPH, and 12% as having sNPH [22]. Nevertheless, some authors claim that the distribution between iNPH and sNPH is approximately 50/50 [23–25].

In vestibular schwannoma, the incidence of preoperative hydrocephalus has been reported to be as high as 18% (28/157) [26]. The hydrocephalus in this study was radiologically defined as mild in 11/28 (39%), moderate in 15/28 (54%), and severe in 2/28 (7%). Communicating hydrocephalus was present in 17/28 (61%) and noncommunicating in 11/28 (39%).

As to secondary hydrocephalus related to cerebral aneurysms, a nationwide American study conducted from 2002 to 2007 found hydrocephalus resulting in shunt placement in 9.3% of patients who underwent clipping after ruptured aneurysms, as compared to 10.5% in patients who underwent coiling [27]. The difference was not statistically significant. The frequency of hydrocephalus resulting in shunt placement after clipping or coiling in non-ruptured aneurysms was very much lower, 0.4% and 0.5%, respectively.

The frequency of surgery for iNPH and sNPH

In a Swedish study, the total incidence of surgery for adult hydrocephalus varied from 2.3 to 3.6/100 000/year between regions in Sweden during a 3-year period [28]. iNPH was listed as cause for operation in 243 out of a total of 891 operations, which equals an incidence of operation for iNPH of 0.91/100 000/year.

This figure is in line with the findings from a retrospective study conducted by the authors of this chapter and colleagues [29]. In this study, all operations for iNPH in Norway from 2002 to 2006 were registered, excluding patients who only underwent shunt revisions. A total of 252 patients were operated, giving a total incidence of 1.09/100 000/year. There was no clear trend as to whether the number of operations increased or decreased during the five-year period. The 5-year incidence was highest in the age group 70–79 years, reaching 52.1/100 000.

Finally, the previously cited work by Klassen and Ahlskog found an incidence of shunt insertion for NPH of 1.91/100 000/year, probably including both iNPH and sNPH [19].

These three studies all demonstrate a frequency of surgery for NPH that is far lower than the occurrence of iNPH found in most of the community-based studies with clinical and radiological criteria for iNPH. This discrepancy might have several explanations. iNPH is generally less known than many other diseases of the elderly, among both the public and general practitioners as well as other healthcare workers. The results from the information campaign we conducted in Vestfold, Norway, supports this, as it gave a total of 86 referrals and 20 shunted patients in one year, as opposed to a total of 18 shunted patients from the same region during the previous 10 years. This probably reflects a previous lack of awareness of the existence of the syndrome among healthcare workers. Adding to this is the fact that the symptoms of iNPH (gait problems, urinary incontinence, and dementia) are abundant in the elderly. Hence, even when they are aware of the syndrome, it is not necessarily evident for neither patients nor healthcare workers when and whom to refer. The lack of universally accepted guidelines for the diagnosis of iNPH, and the lack of powerful tests to predict shunt success, probably also contribute to the relative low rate of diagnosis, and consequently, of surgery. Lastly, iNPH mostly impinges on an age group where indeterminate, insidious symptoms often are considered an inevitable part of normal aging. A shuffling gait, or a gradual cognitive decline, might be inferred as a part of normal aging, and not as part of a treatable disease. The existence of iNPH thus reminds us that this is not always the case, and that such symptoms must be investigated in the individual patient, regardless of what one considers the "true" occurrence of hydrocephalic conditions.

References

1. Fernell E, Hagberg G, Hagberg B. Infantile hydrocephalus epidemiology: an indicator of enhanced survival. *Arch Dis Child* 1994;70:F123–8.
2. Jeng S, Gupta N, Wrensch M, et al. Prevalence of congenital hydrocephalus in California, 1991–2000. *Pediatr Neurol* 2011;45:67–71.
3. Garnel E, Loane M, Addor MC, et al. Congenital hydrocephalus – prevalence, prenatal diagnosis and outcome of pregnancy in four European regions. *Eur J Paediatr Neurol* 2010;14:150–5.
4. Christensen JH, Hansen LK, Garne E. Medfødt hydrocephalus – forekomst og prognose. Mortalitet og morbiditet i en populationsbaseret opgørelse. *Ugeskr Laeger* 2003;165:466–9.
5. Massimi L, Paternoster G, Fasano T, et al. On the changing epidemiology of hydrocephalus. *Childs Nerv Syst* 2009;25:795–800.
6. Sun G, Xu ZM, Liang JF, et al. Twelve-year prevalence of common neonatal congenital malformations in Zhejiang Province, China. *World J Pediatr* 2011;7:331–6.
7. Casmiro M, Benassi G, Cacciatore FM, et al. Frequency of idiopathic normal pressure hydrocephalus. *Arch Neurol* 1989;46:608.
8. Vanneste J, Augustijn P, Dirven C, et al. Shunting normal-pressure hydrocephalus: do the benefits outweigh the risks? A multicenter study and literature review. *Neurology* 1992;42:54–9.
9. Trenkwalder C, Schwarz J, Gebhard J, et al. Starnberg trial on epidemiology of Parkinsonism and hypertension in the elderly. Prevalence of Parkinson's disease and related disorders assessed by a door-to-door survey of inhabitants older than 65 years. *Arch Neurol* 1995;52:1017–22.
10. Vale FA, Miranda SJ. Clinical and demographic features of patients with dementia attended in a tertiary outpatient clinic. *Arq Neuropsiquiatr* 2002;60:548–52.
11. Krauss JK, Halve B. Normal pressure hydrocephalus: survey on contemporary diagnostic algorithms and therapeutic decision-making in clinical practice. *Acta Neurochir (Wien)* 2004;146:379–88.
12. Knopman DS, Petersen RC, Cha RH, et al. Incidence and causes of nondegenerative nonvascular dementia. A population-based study. *Arch Neurol* 2006;63:218–21.
13. Marmarou A, Young HF, Aygok GA. Estimated incidence of normal pressure hydrocephalus and shunt outcome in patients residing in assisted-living and extended-care facilities. *Neurosurg Focus* 2007;22:E1.
14. Brean A, Eide PK. Prevalence of probable idiopathic normal pressure hydrocephalus (iNPH) in a Norwegian population. *Acta Neurol Scand* 2008;118:48–53.
15. Marmarou A, Bergsneider M, Relkin N, et al. Development of guidelines for idiopathic normal-pressure hydrocephalus: introduction. *Neurosurgery* 2005;57:S1–S3.
16. Hiraoka K, Meguro K, Mori E. Prevalence of idiopathic normal pressure hydrocephalus in the elderly population of a Japanese rural community. *Neurol Med Chir (Tokyo)* 2008;48:197–9.
17. Tanaka N, Yamaguchi S, Ishikawa H, et al. Prevalence of possible idiopathic normal-pressure hydrocephalus in Japan: the Osaki-Tajiri project. *Neuroepidemiology* 2009;32:171–5.
18. Iseki C, Kawanami T, Nagasawa H, et al. Asymptomatic ventriculomegaly with features of idiopathic normal pressure hydrocephalus on MRI (AVIM) in the elderly: a prospective study in a Japanese population. *J Neurol Sci* 2009;277:54–7.
19. Klassen BT, Ahlskog JE. Normal pressure hydrocephalus. How often does the diagnosis hold water? *Neurology* 2011;77:1119–25.
20. Muangpaisan W, Petcharat C, Srinonprasert V. Prevalence of potentially reversible conditions in dementia and mild cognitive impairment in a geriatric clinic. *Geriatr Gerontol Int* 2012;12:59–64.
21. Conn HO. Normal pressure hydrocephalus (NPH): more about NPH by a physician who is also the patient. *Clin Med* 2011;11:162–5.

22. Boon AJ, Tans JT, Delwel EJ, et al. Dutch normal-pressure hydrocephalus study: prediction of outcome after shunting by resistance to outflow of cerebrospinal fluid. *J Neurosurg* 1997;87:687–93.
23. Pujari S, Kharkar S, Metellus P, et al. Normal pressure hydrocephalus: long-term outcome after shunt surgery. *J Neurol Neurosurg Psychiatry* 2008;79:1282–6.
24. McGirt MJ, Woodworth G, Coon AL, et al. Diagnosis, treatment, and analysis of long-term outcomes in idiopathic normal-pressure hydrocephalus. *Neurosurgery* 2005;57:699–705.
25. Woodworth GF, McGirt MJ, Williams MA, et al. Cerebrospinal fluid drainage and dynamics in the diagnosis of normal pressure hydrocephalus. *Neurosurgery* 2009;64:919–25.
26. Rogg JM, Ahn SH, Tung GA, et al. Prevalence of hydrocephalus in 157 patients with vestibular schwannoma. *Neuroradiology* 2005;47:344–51.
27. Hoh BL, Kleinhenz DT, Chi YY, et al. Incidence of ventricular shunt placement for hydrocephalus with clipping versus coiling for ruptured and unruptured cerebral aneurysms in the Nationwide Inpatient Sample database: 2002 to 2007. *World Neurosurg* 2011;76:548–54.
28. Tisell M, Höglund M, Wikkelsø C. National and regional incidence of surgery for adult hydrocephalus in Sweden. *Acta Neurol Scand* 2005;112:72–5.
29. Brean A, Fredø HL, Sollid S, et al. Five-year incidence of surgery for idiopathic normal pressure hydrocephalus in Norway. *Acta Neurol Scand* 2009;120:314–16.

Chapter 6

Pathophysiology of gait dysfunction in normal pressure hydrocephalus

Jonathan Pindrik, Amy Bastian, and Daniele Rigamonti

Introduction

Normal pressure hydrocephalus (NPH) presents in adult patients with gait dysfunction, cognitive decline, and urinary incontinence. Gait dysfunction typically represents the first or most prominent of these symptoms, and commonly exhibits greatest improvement following cerebrospinal fluid (CSF) drainage [1–4]. Despite their importance and debilitating effect on NPH patients, gait abnormalities remain unexplained by a unified, accepted theory. In contrast, more appears to be known regarding the mechanism of urinary dysfunction in idiopathic NPH. In this context, bladder irregularity appears to arise from detrusor overactivity in relation to aberrant cerebral autonomic control and exaggerated micturition reflexes [5].

Older theories regarding gait dysfunction in NPH targeted the pyramidal tracts controlling lower extremity movement. These hypotheses conjectured that third ventricular dilation compressed descending motor tracts within the internal capsule. Such compression could cause demyelination and/or axonal loss, resulting in amplitude reduction and latency prolongation [4]. However, later research using motor evoked potentials (MEPs) showed no evidence of aberrant conduction along the central motor pathway [4]. Furthermore, ventricular compression upon descending motor tracts in the internal capsule also should profoundly impact arm and hand movements. Nowak and Topka showed the hypokinetic movement disorder in NPH extends to upper limb motor control, specifically with grasp-lift synergy and force overshooting [6]. Nonetheless, upper limb involvement remains secondary to the hypokinetic gait disorder in the primary symptoms of NPH. These multiple findings have raised questions regarding the role of pyramidal tracts in the pathophysiology of NPH gait dysfunction. Additionally, the typical lack of lower extremity weakness in NPH patients might argue against pyramidal tract dysfunction. No commonly accepted theory regarding the mechanism of gait impairment in NPH has been otherwise formulated.

There are several anatomic substrates that can affect gait, posture, and balance, complicating the exact localization of this deficit in NPH [1]. For instance, balance control depends on the interaction between many areas that could be affected by NPH, including the frontal lobes, basal ganglia, midbrain, or brainstem postural control centers [1]. As such, several mechanisms to explain the pathophysiology of gait dysfunction in NPH have been proffered and corroborated by small cohort or research studies. This chapter presents objective measures of gait dysfunction that have been used clinically and highlights some of the major theories postulated to explain gait dysfunction in NPH.

Objective measures of gait dysfunction in NPH

Gait dysfunction in NPH has characteristic features that include a slow pace, short stride length, wide stance, and low foot-floor elevation [7,8]. Often, patients show hesitation with initiation of walking and turning. Both subjective and objective measures can be used to evaluate gait dysfunction in NPH and improvement following CSF drainage. Subjective rating scales are often used for clinical assessment. These may vary from broad categorical ratings often used in large cohorts (e.g. patient bedridden, patient ambulates but is unstable) [9], to more specific ratings (e.g. tandem walking disturbed, start hesitation) [10]. These types of evaluations are simple and represent an efficient manner of assessing gait. However, objective measures may provide more rigorous and reproducible assessments for comparison. Importantly, use of specific objective

Adult Hydrocephalus, ed. Daniele Rigamonti. Published by Cambridge University Press.

measures may allow for hypothesis testing regarding the pathophysiology of gait dysfunction in NPH.

Objective measures of gait can be used to quantify the pattern of walking and step-taking, focusing on walking speed, stride length, cadence, equilibrium, and posture. In general, the characteristic gait in patients with NPH reflects hypokinetic movement – steps tend to be short and hesitant. Several other neurodegenerative conditions including Parkinson's disease (PD), progressive supranuclear palsy (PSP), subcortical arteriosclerotic encephalopathy (SAE), and corticobasal degeneration involve hypokinetic gait. This has led to speculation that there may be some common neural substrates involved in these different conditions. Specific measures of gait that have been useful in characterizing NPH include speed, stride length, step height or floor-to-foot clearance, and gait equilibrium [1,8]. In the typical NPH patient, all of these variables are decreased or aberrant in the case of dynamic equilibrium [1]. Other measurable variables of gait in neurodegenerative conditions include postural and turning stability [2]. It is interesting that CSF drainage in NPH patients correlates with improvements in some measures of walking (e.g. walking speed and turning), but not necessarily all those that characterize the disorder [1,10]. Several authors and research groups have used objective gait parameters in the evaluation of NPH patients following therapeutic CSF drainage to develop and test various hypotheses regarding this enigmatic pathophysiology.

Tentative theories to explain gait dysfunction in NPH

Midbrain atrophy or compression

Located in the dorsolateral region of the midbrain, the mesencephalic locomotor region (MLR) plays an important role in the initiation of locomotion in humans and other animal species [1,3]. Based on animal studies correlating abnormalities in this anatomic region to gait disturbance in PD, the MLR has been implicated in gait dysfunction of NPH patients [1]. Lee et al. conducted a retrospective review of 21 NPH patients and age-matched controls showing significantly smaller baseline midbrain diameter in NPH patients [1]. Furthermore, midbrain diameter (measured anteroposteriorly in the midsagittal plane) related inversely to the severity of gait disturbance (Figure 6.1) [1]. These findings were partially supported

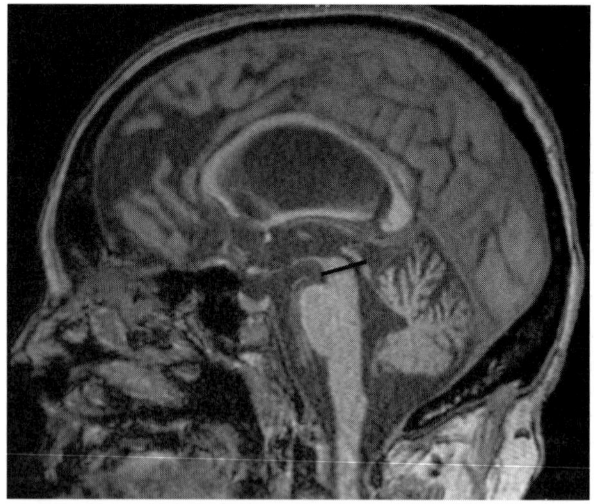

Figure 6.1 Measurement of midbrain maximal anteroposterior diameter (as demonstrated by the black bar) based on sagittal MRI in an NPH patient preoperatively.

by separate research showing increased diameters and wider angles between the cerebral peduncles of NPH patients based on magnetic resonance imaging (MRI) [11]. These combined results suggest that midbrain atrophy or compression potentially contribute to gait dysfunction in NPH.

Other studies evaluating midbrain size following CSF diversion corroborate the potential role of midbrain cytoarchitecture on gait dysfunction in NPH. Mocco et al. showed that increases in postoperative midbrain anteroposterior and transverse diameters in shunted NPH patients correlated with gait improvement [2] (Figure 6.2). The authors further postulated two mechanisms to explain the beneficial role of midbrain expansion on gait disturbance following ventricular shunt placement in NPH. One theory respects the adverse effect of ventricular pressure on descending MLR efferent tracts contacting the medullary reticular formation. These tracts help modulate reticulospinal fibers within the ventromedial medulla that contribute to gait and balance control. Interruption of modulatory input into the medullary reticular formation could cause locomotion and balance disturbance [2]. Furthermore, axonal decompression and reversal of this attenuated MLR input may account for the rapid gait improvement exhibited by NPH patients following CSF drainage [2]. In an alternate theory, the mechanical effects of hydrocephalus may adversely affect MLR synapses within the medulla. Therapeutic CSF drainage may restore synaptic integrity and allow reversal of

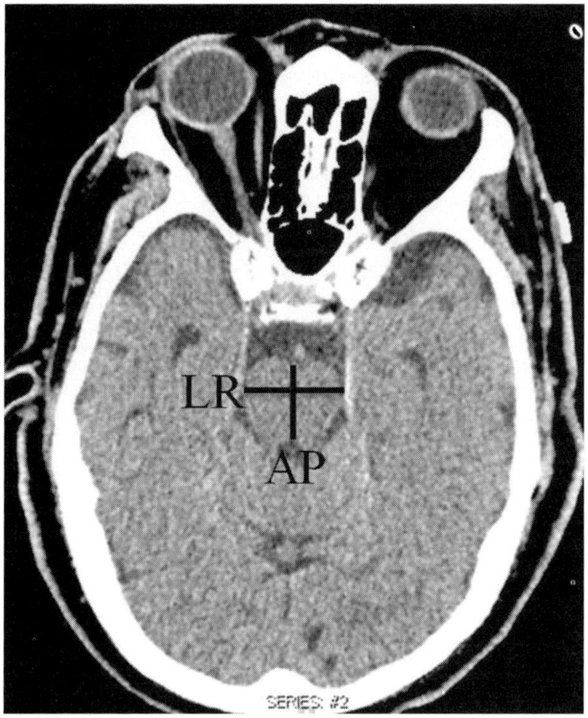

Figure 6.2 Measurement of anteroposterior (AP) and transverse left–right (LR) diameters of the midbrain at the pontomesencephalic junction based on head CT in an NPH patient preoperatively.

symptoms [2]. These theories focus on midbrain compression, rather than atrophy, as a potential culprit in gait dysfunction in NPH.

The correlation between decreasing midbrain anteroposterior diameter and gait dysfunction in NPH may alternatively result from midbrain atrophy. However, potential locations or mechanisms of midbrain atrophy remain unclear. Growing evidence suggests the pedunculopontine nucleus (PPN), located within the midbrain tegmentum, plays an important functional role in human locomotion [1]. In disease processes such as PSP and PD, the PPN exhibits significant degeneration of cholinergic neurons. This measurable loss of neurons has been linked to gait freezing and postural instability in neurodegenerative conditions [1]. Additionally, focal lesions within the midbrain tegmentum housing the MLR may precipitate gait and postural dysfunction [1,2]. As an integral part of the MLR, the PPN represents a potential pathological substrate for gait disequilibrium in NPH. However, other authors challenge the role of PPN degeneration in NPH owing to lack of supporting evidence [11]. Further research may help elucidate the potential roles of PPN and MLR underlying midbrain atrophy in NPH.

Other potential explanations for midbrain volume loss in NPH focus on chemical and mechanical mechanisms. One theory postulates that hydrocephalus induces abnormalities in the dopaminergic system of the substantia nigra, resulting in decreased dopamine levels [1]. Alternatively, mechanical compression from an expanding third ventricle on the rostral midbrain may induce volume loss or atrophy [1]. By whatever mechanism, midbrain atrophy or compression represent attractive targets potentially correlated to gait disequilibrium in NPH.

General consensus does not exist to fully support the correlation between midbrain size and gait dysfunction in NPH, however. At least one prospective study conducted in Sendai, Japan, refuted the role of the MLR in NPH gait disequilibrium. Hiraoka et al. [3] showed that baseline measurements of midbrain anteroposterior and lateral dimensions and cross-sectional areas in NPH patients did not correlate with baseline gait severity. Furthermore, this study reported no significant relationship between gait improvement and changes in midbrain parameters following shunt insertion [3]. The authors of this study questioned the measurement techniques employed by the earlier studies of Lee et al. [1] and Mocco et al. [2], citing the inaccuracy of midbrain diameter measurements on routine computed tomography (CT) and MRI. The authors claimed that ventricular deformation and brainstem tilting invalidated midbrain parameters measured on routine imaging [3]. To combat these limitations, Hiraoka et al. instituted advanced reconstruction techniques to obtain cross-sectional areas of the midbrain on consistent axial images through the top of the inferior colliculus and the PPN [3] (Figure 6.3). Their findings seriously questioned the role of midbrain size and the MLR in gait dysfunction of NPH patients. The presence of conflicting views regarding the contribution of midbrain abnormalities to NPH gait disturbance warrants further investigation.

Cortical dysfunction

Recognition of cortical involvement in locomotion stems from multiple research efforts evaluating gait in healthy individuals and those with cognitive disturbances. Prior notions described gait as an automated motor activity with minimal cortical input. However, more recent analysis supports the contribution of

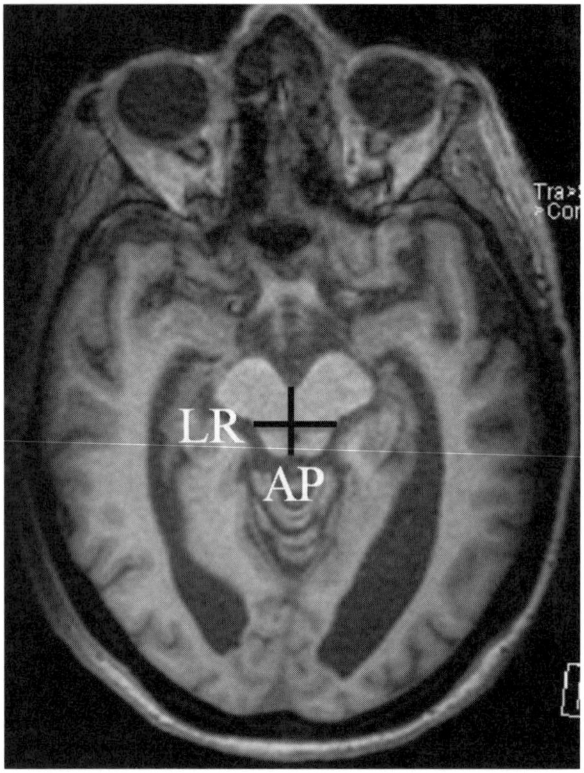

Figure 6.3 Measurement of anteroposterior (AP) and transverse left–right (LR) diameters of the midbrain based on MRI in an NPH patient preoperatively. Advanced reconstruction techniques were used to acquire an axial image through the pedunculopontine nucleus and top of the inferior colliculus. These techniques are described in Hiraoka et al. [3].

higher level cognitive function to walking [12]. The specific facets of cognition relevant to gait control include executive function and attention. Anatomically, executive function largely localizes to the frontal lobes, with input from other cerebral distributions [12]. The anatomic regions primarily involved include the dorsolateral prefrontal cortex (DLPFC; Brodmann's area 9) and anterior cingulate cortex (ACC; Brodmann's areas 24, 32) [12]. Abnormalities in executive function and attention may contribute to gait impairment in neurological disorders such as Parkinson's disease, cerebral infarction, and NPH [12].

Several research endeavors have focused on dual-tasking experiments to portray the effects of abnormal executive function and attention on gait control. Dual-tasking represents the ability to perform two separate tasks simultaneously. The performance of both tasks requires higher-level function and the executive balance of competing attention demands. Multiple research efforts incorporate dual-task assessment to investigate the attention-demanding properties of ambulation [12]. For instance, executive dysfunction has been correlated to decreased gait speed and increased gait variability under dual-task conditions [12]. As idiopathic NPH represents a disorder of both gait and cognition, dual-tasking represents a useful experimental paradigm to evaluate these patients [12–14].

Impaired cortical and executive function may negatively impact gait, especially during dual-task ambulation. In experiments performed on non-demented and demented subjects with or without impaired executive function (IEF), Allali et al. showed the importance of cortical contributions to gait stability and dual-tasking [13]. Patients with dementia and IEF exhibited significantly greater stride times than demented patients without IEF and non-demented patients. Dementia (with or without IEF) correlated to greater stride times during dual-tasking and to greater stride time variability as compared to non-demented patients [13]. Additionally, the deleterious effect of IEF on gait heightened during dual-tasking. As frontal lobe function worsened, stride time variability increased. The authors of this study linked stride time variability to loss of dynamic stability in gait [13]. Therefore, cortical and executive dysfunction may contribute to gait impairment and instability in demented patients, including those with cognitive deterioration as in NPH. In PD, executive dysfunction likely contributes to abnormal gait as well. Clinical trials have reported the successful use of methylphenidate in these patients to improve executive function and gait speed, and decrease gait variability [12].

Other studies support the potential role of cortical dysfunction in NPH gait impairment, highlighting the relationship between gait and cognition [14]. For instance, Armand et al. reported the enhancement of gait parameters during dual-tasking in NPH patients following CSF drainage. Importantly, gait speed and stride length significantly improved only during dual-tasking, without improvements observed for single-task ambulation [14]. Aberrant integration or distribution of attention to simultaneous thoughts or tasks may negatively impact gait equilibrium. Furthermore, the authors of this study argue that dual-tasking, rather than single-tasking, better evaluated gait improvement in NPH patients following CSF drainage – dual-tasking may represent a more sensitive test [14]. The exact role of cortical dysfunction in the pathogenesis of abnormal gait requires further analysis.

Cortical-subcortical and intracortical circuit abnormalities

Several research studies target cortical-subcortical circuit pathology as the culprit in NPH gait dysfunction. Neighboring the lateral ventricles, multiple tracts descend from cortical regions to synapse upon groups of neurons within the basal ganglia, cerebellum, brainstem, and spinal cord. These tracts include fronto-ponto-cerebellar fibers, corticospinal tracts controlling lower extremity movement, and the frontal cortical-subcortical basal ganglia loop [1,14]. Compression from ventricular enlargement may temporarily damage these tracts and produce gait disequilibrium with frontal-like disturbances [1,2]. Therapeutic CSF drainage may alleviate the pressure affecting descending tracts, improving gait control and equilibrium. Specifically, beneficial modifications of periventricular regional hydrostatic pressure may relieve compression of frontal-subcortical tracts [14]. Subsequent gait improvement, especially during dual-tasking that involves executive function, could represent restoration of frontal cortical-subcortical tract physiology [14].

Aberrant circuitry responsible for NPH gait impairment alternatively may lie within the motor cortex. Recent studies have implicated intracortical connections, rather than subcortical tracts, in the development of gait dysfunction in NPH. Under this premise, the correlation between frontal lobe dysfunction and gait impairment occurs due to elevated corticospinal excitability in the setting of disinhibition [15]. Chistyakov et al. stimulated the leg representation of motor cortex using transcranial magnetic stimulation (TMS) and monitored motor evoked potentials (MEPs) in patients with NPH gait dysfunction before and after shunting. They found reduced resting motor threshold (rMT) at baseline, which indicates increased corticospinal excitability, and reduced short intracortical inhibition (SICI), which is thought to reflect abnormal function of GABAergic interneurons [15]. Ventricular shunting significantly increased both of these variables (rMT, SICI) in NPH patients exhibiting dramatic improvement in ambulation [15]. The authors concluded that motor cortex disinhibition and abnormally increased corticospinal excitability result in reduced control of motor output, contributing to NPH gait impairment [15].

Several studies have evaluated the potential role of abnormal cortical and subcortical connections in the pathophysiology of NPH gait dysfunction. Aberrant circuitry may involve reduced intracortical inhibition within motor cortex, decreased inhibitory control from pre-motor regions, dysfunction of the frontal-subcortical basal ganglia loop, or abnormal function of other frontal-subcortical tracts (including the corticospinal tract) [14,15]. Regardless of the exact mechanism, aberrant functional connectivity within or between frontal, prefrontal, and basal ganglia regions likely contributes to NPH gait dysfunction.

Postural dysfunction

In addition to gait impairment, mental deterioration, and urinary incontinence, postural instability represents another frequent symptom of idiopathic NPH [7,8]. Posture control relies upon integration of three types of input: visual, vestibular, and somatosensory. While younger adults may rely more heavily upon proprioceptive than visual input, elderly individuals appear to depend on visual input for balance [7]. Given the partial dependence of motor function on balance, several studies have attempted to correlate postural disturbance to gait impairment in NPH. Following shunt insertion, NPH patients typically exhibit improvements in balance as well as gait [7]. Therefore, postural dysfunction may contribute to NPH gait abnormalities while balance improvement might account for enhanced gait following therapeutic CSF drainage.

The postural dysfunction observed in NPH patients includes a larger sway area, higher backward directed velocity while standing, and neutral or forward directed inclination [7]. Practically, this results in a forward leaning posture but with spontaneous or provoked backward falling [8]. Blomsterwall et al. showed a correlation between balance and motor tasks in NPH patients both before and after shunt surgery. Interestingly, NPH patients exhibited greater improvement in balance tasks than motor function [7]. Poor performance in balance and ambulation preoperatively coupled with improved posture and gait postoperatively suggested a relationship between gait and balance disturbance [7]. The authors conjectured that vertical axis distortion or misinterpretation within the pontine postural center may account for postural dysfunction [7]. Alternatively, aberrant higher cortical function responsible for both balance and motor function may contribute to NPH gait impairment [7].

Dopamine signaling abnormalities

Given certain similarities of symptomatic presentation and gait disturbance in NPH and PD, recent efforts have targeted dopamine signaling as a potential culprit in the pathophysiology of NPH. Abnormal pulsatile CSF flow might adversely affect dopaminergic pathways within the substantia nigra and/or striatum, degrading motor planning [8]. Alternatively, abnormalities in presynaptic or postsynaptic dopamine activity within the basal ganglia might relate to NPH gait impairment [11]. The striatum, incorporating the caudate and putamen, contains dopaminergic D2 receptors integral in the regulation of cortical motor input. While the caudate nucleus chiefly connects to the frontal eye fields, the dorsal putamen receives input from the sensorimotor cortex [11]. Within the dorsal putamen resides a somatotopically organized region representing the foot [11]. Derangements of dopamine signaling within the dorsal putamen might underlie the pathophysiologic gait in NPH.

Utilizing positron emission tomography (PET) and radioactive tracers for presynaptic transporters and postsynaptic receptors of dopamine, Ouchi et al. investigated dopamine signaling in NPH patients. This research exhibited postsynaptic D2 receptor hypoactivity within the dorsal putamen, due either to downregulation or to loss of receptors [11]. The reduction of postsynaptic D2 receptors correlated inversely with severity of gait impairment in NPH patients as measured by navigation times [11]. Presynaptic dopamine activity remained unchanged with respect to healthy subjects, indicating preservation of nigrostriatal dopamine function. The authors concluded that aberrant postsynaptic dopamine activity within the striatum, specifically the dorsal putamen, might reflect NPH pathophysiology [11]. However, few research studies have been conducted to corroborate these findings and further explore the role of dopamine in NPH gait dysfunction.

Decreased regional cerebral blood flow

Research investigating the potential role of regional cerebral blood flow (rCBF) variation in NPH has shown correlations between NPH symptoms and decreased perfusion. For instance, prior research endeavors have displayed decreased baseline perfusion in regions of the thalamus and basal ganglia in NPH patients [1]. Dumarey et al. reported significant increases of rCBF within bilateral frontal middle gyri and the left temporal parahippocampal cortex in NPH patients exhibiting gait improvement following lumbar puncture [16]. Potential mechanisms to explain enhanced perfusion include reduced stretch of the anterior cerebral arteries, downstream capillaries, and veins following CSF drainage. Decreased rCBF in NPH may also result from impaired autoregulatory mechanisms. Reflex vasoconstriction and stretching of cholinergic fibers projecting from the nucleus basalis of Meynert may interfere with normal restorative, homeostatic mechanisms to control rCBF [16]. Research investigating rCBF variation in NPH has mainly displayed correlations to gait impairment and improvement following CSF drainage, but has not elucidated a direct causal relationship between decreased perfusion and gait pathophysiology.

Conclusion

Several theories have been proposed to explain the pathophysiology of gait dysfunction in NPH. The variety of potential targets includes midbrain compression or atrophy, cortical dysfunction, cortical-subcortical or intracortical circuit abnormalities, postural disturbance, dopamine signaling abnormalities, and rCBF depression. Currently, no single theory boasts adequate scientific proof or agreement among physicians and practitioners caring for NPH patients. Further research and investigation may help corroborate proposed explanations or elucidate other mechanisms responsible for gait dysfunction in NPH.

References

1. Lee PH, Yong SW, Ahn YH, Huh K. Correlation of midbrain diameter and gait disturbance in patients with idiopathic normal pressure hydrocephalus. *J Neurol* 2005;252:958–63.

2. Mocco J, Tomey MI, Komotar R, et al. Ventriculoperitoneal shunting of idiopathic normal pressure hydrocephalus increases midbrain size: a potential mechanism for gait improvement. *Neurosurgery* 2006;59(4):B47–9.

3. Hiraoka K, Yamasaki H, Takagi M, et al. Is the midbrain involved in the manifestation of gait disturbance in idiopathic normal-pressure hydrocephalus? *J Neurol* 2011;258:820–25.

4. Zaaroor M, Bleich N, Chistyakov A, et al. Motor evoked potentials in the preoperative and postoperative assessment of normal pressure hydrocephalus. *J Neurol Neurosurg Psychiatry* 1997;62:517–21.

5. Sakakibara R, Kanda T, Sekido T, et al. Mechanism of bladder dysfunction in idiopathic normal pressure hydrocephalus. *Neurourol Urodyn* 2008;27:507–10.
6. Nowak DA, Topka HR. Broadening a classic clinical triad: the hypokinetic motor disorder of normal pressure hydrocephalus also affects the hand. *Exp Neurol* 2006;198:81–7.
7. Blomsterwall E, Svantesson U, Carlsson U, et al. Postural disturbance in patients with normal pressure hydrocephalus. *Acta Neurol Scand* 2000;102:284–91.
8. Tsakanikas D, Relkin N. Normal pressure hydrocephalus. *Semin Neurol* 2007;27(1):58–65.
9. Poca MA, Solana E, Martinez-Ricarte FR, et al. Idiopathic normal pressure hydrocephalus: results of a prospective cohort of 236 shunted patients. *Acta Neurochir Suppl* 2012;114:247–53.
10. Ravdin LD, Katzen HL, Jackson AE, et al. Features of gait most responsive to tap test in normal pressure hydrocephalus. *Clin Neurol Neurosurg* 2008;110(5):455–61.
11. Ouchi Y, Nakayama T, Kanno T, et al. In vivo presynaptic and postsynaptic striatal dopamine functions in idiopathic normal pressure hydrocephalus. *J Cereb Blood Flow Metab* 2007;27:803–10.
12. Yogev-Seligmann G, Hausdorff JM, Giladi N. The role of executive function and attention in gait. *Mov Disord* 2008;23(3):329–42.
13. Allali G, Assal F, Kressig R, et al. Impact of impaired executive function on gait stability. *Dement Geriatr Cogn Disord* 2008;26:364–69.
14. Armand S, Allet L, Landis T, et al. Interest of dual-task-related gait changes in idiopathic normal pressure hydrocephalus. *Eur J Neurol* 2011;18:1081–4.
15. Chistyakov AV, Hafner H, Sinai A, et al. Motor cortex disinhibition in normal-pressure-hydrocephalus. *J Neurosurg* 2012;116:453–9.
16. Dumarey NE, Massager N, Laureys S, et al. Voxel-based assessment of spinal tap test-induced regional cerebral blood flow changes in normal pressure hydrocephalus. *Nucl Med Commun* 2005;26:757–63.

Chapter 7

The pathophysiologic basis of cognitive dysfunction in idiopathic normal pressure hydrocephalus

Norman Relkin and Heather Katzen

Introduction

In nearly a half century since idiopathic normal pressure hydrocephalus (iNPH) was first identified, the origins of its symptoms have remained obscure. A fundamental question is how ventricular enlargement and alterations in cerebrospinal fluid (CSF) dynamics in iNPH disturb the function of neurons in the brain. Most theories of pathogenesis have fallen short of fully explaining why iNPH is associated with the specific triad of gait, urinary, and cognitive disturbances rather than any other constellation of symptoms. There are also remaining uncertainties about the mechanisms responsible for the temporary remission of iNPH symptoms after external drainage of CSF and the more lasting improvement that follows shunt placement. Although many advances have been made in its diagnosis and treatment over the past 45 years, iNPH is still an enigmatic syndrome on many levels.

Given these limits to the present state of knowledge, it may seem quixotic to attempt to explain the pathophysiology of the cognitive deficits encountered in iNPH. However, the cognitive symptoms of iNPH have certain features that have made them amenable to study. The distinctive profile of cognitive deficits in iNPH provides clues to their localization in light of the brain's established functional neuroanatomy. Structural and functional brain imaging have helped to elucidate the neural pathways involved in hydrocephalic cognitive impairment. In addition, studies of brain metabolism and blood flow, molecular imaging, and cerebrospinal fluid (CSF) physiology have provided novel windows into the pathogenesis of dementia in iNPH. While there is still much to be learned, there is considerable information available that is salient to understanding the origins of cognitive symptoms in iNPH.

Putative pathogenic mechanisms of iNPH

A number of pathophysiologic mechanisms have been identified that are potentially relevant to the pathogenesis of the cognitive symptoms of iNPH:

- *Mechanical distortion.* Stretching of white matter and mechanical compression of subcortical gray matter caused by ventricular enlargement may be a cause of cerebral dysfunction in iNPH [1,2]. Progressive ventricular expansion distorts the corpus callosum and periventricular corona radiata [3]. It also compresses subcortical gray structures such as the hippocampus, caudate nucleus, and thalamus. The importance of subcortical mechanical distortion as a pathogenic mechanism has been questioned because cognitive impairment and other symptoms of iNPH can progress without gross expansion of the ventricles [1] and cognitive recovery can occur without visible reductions in ventricular size [4,5]. Mechanical distortion is therefore unlikely to be the sole cause of cognitive impairments in iNPH, but could well be a contributing factor.
- *Pressure effects.* The modest increases in static intracranial pressure (ICP) of up to 240 mmH_2O that occur in iNPH are insufficient to cause neuronal dysfunction. Higher pressures can be recorded in iNPH patients as B waves (CSF pressure oscillations with a frequency of 0.5 to 2/min) that tend to occur transiently during sleep. B waves have not been directly linked to cognitive impairment nor would they be expected to cause the kind of persistent symptoms that iNPH patients typically experience. Increased CSF pulsatility (dynamic pressure changes that occur across the cardiac cycle) also occurs in iNPH and

may secondarily impact on cognition through effects on cerebral perfusion and induction of hyperdynamic CSF flow.

- *Flow phenomenon*. Hyperdynamic flow of CSF through the aqueduct of Sylvius is frequently observed in patients with iNPH [6]. The driving force for CSF flow is the systolic arterial pulsations that generate CSF in the choroid plexus and secondarily in the brain parenchyma. During systole, there is outward radial movement of the ventricular walls followed by flow of CSF through the cerebral aqueduct. However, owing to ventricular enlargement and decreased elasticity of the brain in iNPH, there is a reduced capacity for radial ventricular wall movement. This energy of the arterial pulsation is instead converted into a translational force driving CSF through the aqueduct at a greater than normal velocity and a hydrodynamic force driving transependymal CSF resorption. The rapid downward movement of CSF flow can exert a hammer-like effect on the roof of the brainstem causing damage to the nuclei such as the substantia nigra (SN). Nigral depigmentation and neuronal degeneration can result in parkinsonism as well as cognitive impairment. Since not all iNPH patients exhibit parkinsonism, this mechanism is most likely not a universal cause for iNPH symptoms but may be a factor in some cases.
- *Toxin accumulation*. CSF production has been reported to be reduced in iNPH when measured by bulk flow protocols such as the Masserman technique [7]. Since the circulation of CSF plays an important role in removal of the byproducts of brain metabolism, decreased CSF production in iNPH could lead to accumulation of toxic metabolites that cause neuronal dysfunction. Decreased clearance of beta amyloid in this context may be a factor in the association between iNPH and Alzheimer's disease (AD). It has been suggested that cerebral metabolic derangement in iNPH begins in conjunction with derangements in CSF dynamics but eventually becomes uncoupled and self-sustaining.
- *Neurochemical disturbances*. Disturbances in dopaminergic, glutaminergic, GABAergic, cholinergic, and serotoninergic neurotransmission have been found in kaolin models of hydrocephalus and may also be associated with iNPH (see Kondziella et al. [8]). Unlike AD, in which selective degeneration in the cholinergic system is a relatively early manifestation of neurodegeneration, neurochemical deficiencies are more likely late effects of iNPH and reflect compromise to the integrity of structures juxtaposed to the CSF spaces, such as the substantia nigra, striatum, thalamus, and hippocampus as well as their white matter projections.
- *Interstitial edema*. Interstitial edema occurs in the brain parenchyma in iNPH. This fluid accumulation is often visible in the periventricular regions on brain MRIs as T1 hyperintensities or T2 hypointensities that can often be reversed by shunt placement. The occurrence of interstitial edema may be a consequence of increased transependymal flow of CSF from the ventricles into the brain parenchyma and/or hydrostatic forces within the brain related to increased cerebrovascular resistance. Cerebral edema is a known cause of cerebral dysfunction and it represents a likely factor in the development of cognitive deficits and other neurological symptoms in iNPH. In experimental models, interstitial edema has been shown to decrease cerebrovascular reserve and cause other disturbances in regulation of cerebral blood flow [9]. These vascular mechanisms are also potential precipitant factors for iNPH's cognitive symptoms (see below). Successful shunt placement can result in reduction in interstitial edema that parallels improvements in iNPH symptoms.
- *Cerebrovascular compromise*. Cerebral blood flow (CBF) studies in iNPH have found global decreases but no clear correlation between resting perfusion and response to shunt [10,11]. Focal decreases in CBF involving mesial frontal and anterior temporal regions have also been documented with some correlation to shunt responsiveness [12]. While decreases in resting CBF do not seem sufficient to explain symptoms of iNPH, decreased cerebrovascular reserve (CVR), as can be documented by a diminished response to an acetazolamide challenge test, could contribute to inadequate cerebral perfusion during periods of heightened brain activity. Possible causes of altered CBF and CVR in iNPH include all of the above-mentioned mechanisms (mechanical distortion, pulsatile pressure increases, toxins, or interstitial edema) as well as other factors that compromise cerebral blood flow.

It seems likely that a combination of these and possibly other mechanisms are contributing factors in the pathogenesis of cognitive symptoms in iNPH. A possible synthesis of these mechanisms would be that an imbalance of CSF production and clearance leads to progressive ventricular enlargement. Resultant increases in CSF pulsatility and reflux of CSF into the ventricle drive the roof of the lateral ventricles upward, trapping the sagittal sinus between the hemispheric convexities and the skull. This further compromises CSF clearance and fosters the generation of alternative pathways for CSF movement through the brain parenchyma, particularly by transependymal resorption. As CSF moves across the ventricular ependyma into the interstitial spaces of the brain, interstitial edema develops in periventricular structures. This edema compounds the compressive effects of ventricular expansion and leads to reductions in cerebral perfusion and cerebrovascular reserve. Diminished CSF clearance may also foster accumulation of toxic metabolites which further disturb cerebrovascular autoregulation and cause neuronal dysfunction and secondary neurochemical disturbances. Unless iNPH is treated, vascular insufficiency eventually causes periventricular white matter infarction, at which point the symptoms become irreversible.

Based on the most commonly observed pattern of interstitial edema in cases of iNPH, it can be hypothesized that the early cognitive symptoms of iNPH reflect the development of interstitial edema and vascular compromise in the white matter pathways that pass near the anterior and posterior horns of the lateral ventricle. These regions are mechanically prone to reverse transependymal fluid movements which appear as ventricular "capping" on MR images. Gray matter structures juxtaposed to the ventricles, such as the caudate, thalamus, and hippocampus, may also be affected. The cognitive symptoms would therefore be considered manifestations of pathophysiological processes that are relatively circumscribed spatially and predominantly subcortical in nature.

Involvement of the cerebral cortex in the symptoms of iNPH is suggested by the results of some metabolic and perfusion imaging studies. Decreased cerebral blood flow and/or metabolism documented by imaging in the cortex of iNPH patients can be reversed by shunt treatment [13,14]. However, these imaging studies do not distinguish between a primary disturbance within the cerebral cortex and the distal effects of dysfunction (diaschisis) in the white matter tracts connecting to these regions. Diaschisis seems a more likely explanation since postmortem studies have failed to provide direct evidence of cortical pathology in iNPH.

General features of cognitive impairment in iNPH

The profile of cognitive impairments in iNPH is recognizably that of a subcortical pathological process. In this respect, iNPH resembles Huntington's or Parkinson's disease in which dysfunction in subcortical frontostriatal circuits leads to impairments of complex attention, speed of information processing, phonemic verbal fluency, and executive functions. In contrast, the pathology of Alzheimer's disease more directly involves neocortical areas, resulting in disturbances of semantic language, calculation abilities, and other cortical functions that are relatively spared or only secondarily affected in iNPH.

The extent of impairment in cognition in iNPH can range from subtle neuropsychological dysfunction to a frank dementia [15]. Early cognitive symptoms can readily go undetected in iNPH or can mistakenly be attributed to normal aging. In our experience, many high functioning patients do not report subjective cognitive changes early in the disease course. While these patients perform well on global screening measures (e.g. MMSE), they frequently exhibit some form of cognitive compromise when more detailed neuropsychological testing is performed. Therefore, even when the patient denies cognitive symptoms, formal cognitive evaluation is recommended. This should be pursued in any patient with suspected iNPH, even in patients who perform well on global screening measures during neurological work-up. The components of a neuropsychological battery useful for serially assessing patients with suspected or confirmed iNPH are presented in Table 7.1 [16–25].

In the early stages the presentation can include mild decrements in psychomotor speed, reduced information processing, and inefficiency in aspects of learning and memory [15,26–28]. Reaction time and psychomotor speed are also typically impaired at early stages. The cognitive symptoms of iNPH are more likely to be reversible when the disease is in its early stages.

Over the course of several months to years cognitive symptoms of iNPH typically progress. As a result, patients may show more severe reductions in

Table 7.1 Sample neuropsychological battery for serial assessments in iNPH

Global cognitive measures (i.e. MMSE or 3MS) [16,17]*
Boston Naming Test [18]
Controlled Oral Word Association [19]
Hopkins Verbal Learning Test – Revised [20]
Wechsler Adult Intelligence Scale IV (Digit Span) [21]
Trail Making Test A and B [22]*
Symbol Digit Modalities Test [23]*
Grooved Pegboard Test [22]*
Finger Tapping Test [22]*
Line Tracing Test [24]*
Serial Dotting Test [24]*
Gait scale [25]*

Note: * measures repeated to assess change

psychomotor speed, information processing, executive functioning, complex attention, and memory. In later stages, speech output may be reduced secondary either to dysexecutive syndrome or motivational problems. Pragmatic aspects of language may also be affected.

With progression of disease in the absence of treatment, cognitive and other symptoms of iNPH can become intractable. Delays in diagnosis and/or treatment can lead to the development of a syndrome that strongly resembles the late stages of Binswanger's disease [29]. The occurrence of confluent periventricular ischemic changes in untreated and late stage iNPH suggests that cerebrovascular compromise is one of the key mechanisms underlying the cognitive symptoms of iNPH.

Changes in gait impairment are commonly used to monitor improvements after drainage of CSF and shunt placement in cases of iNPH. While gait symptoms can provide sensitive measures of response, cognitive symptoms are also amenable to treatment. Specific tests that measure arousal, affect, and cognition before and after drainage of CSF have been shown to be a useful adjunct to gait testing in assessing candidacy for shunt [30]. Improvements in cognition can occur very rapidly after shunt placement and these gains may increase over the subsequent weeks to months. Evidence from serial phase-contrast MRI studies [31] suggests that iNPH symptoms may improve as aqueductal CSF flow normalizes after shunt placement, a process that can take several weeks with a fixed pressure shunt valve and longer with a programmable valve that requires serial adjustments.

Neuropsychological evaluation in iNPH

The neuropsychological examination is an extended mental status evaluation that assesses a broad range of cognitive skills and employs measures that are more sensitive to early changes than global cognitive screening measures. The general domains that are assessed as part of a neuropsychological evaluation include attention, memory, executive functions, visuospatial skills, psychomotor and motor skills, mood and other aspects of psychological functioning. The length of an evaluation varies based on the specific questions that are being asked. A typical battery that is focused on differential diagnosis of dementia ranges from 1.5 to 3 hours. The battery may be tailored slightly for iNPH patients to include a greater number of motor and psychomotor tasks, since these skills will likely be reassessed as part of the diagnostic process and as a gauge of outcome if patients undergo treatment. The initial evaluation serves both as the differential diagnostic work-up and as a means to establish a baseline level of functioning. In specialty centers, post-drainage testing is also performed. These evaluations are typically much shorter and focus on a subset of baseline tests that are helpful in prognosticating regarding candidacy for treatment. Patients who undergo treatment will also be seen for follow-up evaluation at regular intervals to track improvement and monitor response to treatment. In a clinical setting, the frequency and length of the follow-up evaluation will depend on the particular circumstances and questions that need to be addressed. A sample baseline neuropsychological battery is presented in Table 7.1 and measures that are repeated with diagnostic testing (e.g. drainage) and after treatment are noted.

Localization of neuropsychological deficits in iNPH

Attention/Executive/Psychomotor

Deficiencies in attention, working memory, set shifting, response inhibition and other aspects of executive functioning are commonly observed in iNPH and can be seen early in the disease course. In a recent large European trial, impairment at baseline compared to controls was observed in iNPH patients on the Stroop Color and Word Test, a test of complex attention and response inhibition [32]. Other researchers have demonstrated impairments in complex attention and set shifting on Trail Making A and B [30,33], Symbol Digit

Modalities [30], and other measures of executive skills such as verbal fluency and recitation of digits backwards [33]. These tests are weighted towards detection of functions mediated by pathways involving the dorsolateral prefrontal cortex and anterior cingulate. Dysfunction in these areas likely reflects pathological involvement of their subcortical projections in white matter pathways passing anterior and lateral to the frontal horns of the lateral ventricles as well as the caudate nucleus.

Comparison of iNPH and AD groups across several different attentional and executive tasks has shown that there is generally a greater executive deficit observed in iNPH. Ogino et al. [34] showed poorer performance in iNPH compared to AD on tests of attention, concentration and executive functioning, as well as impairment in calculation. Kanno et al. [35] compared iNPH and AD on a test of counting backwards and showed that iNPH patients showed greater deficits in response suppression. They also demonstrated that iNPH patients have greater impairment on tests of phonemic verbal fluency, motor sequencing, go/no/go paradigms, the Stroop Color and Word Test, and digit recall than patients with AD. Overall, these deficits were interpreted as an indication of difficulties with sequential motor learning, attention and working memory, response inhibition and suppression and are consistent with the majority of literature indicating executive skills and attention are disproportionately affected in iNPH. Motor learning and sequencing deficits in iNPH may relate to involvement of the subcortical projections of the supplementary motor area, the activity of which was recently shown by fMRI to improve in correlation with measures of gait after shunting [14].

Memory

Memory deficits observed in early stages of iNPH are characterized predominantly by difficulty acquiring new information and retrieval as opposed to rapid forgetting of information. This is typically secondary to deficits in the organization and efficient processing of information. Learning of new information can be impaired in iNPH, but performance typically improves with repeated trials and when organizational strategies are provided [36]. Delayed recall can be impaired, but is often facilitated by cueing. Performance on recognition memory paradigms (forced choice) is usually spared, suggesting preserved memory storage.

Most available data on memory impairment in iNPH is gleaned from word list learning tasks in which performance on the learning trials and delayed recall of the material is examined. Comparison of iNPH patients and controls has revealed decrements in learning and delayed recall on word list learning tasks such as the Rey Auditory Verbal Learning Test (RAVLT) [32, 33,37] and the Hopkins Verbal Learning Test – Revised [30]. Other studies have examined memory for verbal contextual material (story recall), and have shown evidence of impaired story memory [38]. Visual memory skills have not been widely studied, but investigations including nonverbal memory paradigms have demonstrated impaired learning and recall of visual stimuli [33,37].

Comparison of verbal memory profiles in iNPH and AD has revealed an overall greater degree of memory impairment in AD [34,39]. A differential pattern of performance has also been reported, with the iNPH group making fewer false positive errors on a discrimination trial of a word list learning test [39]. This pattern is a characteristic feature of frontal type memory impairments and can be used clinically to dissociate between AD and subcortical processes. It again points to predominant involvement of midline, fornical, and frontal pathways involved in memory with relative preservation of memory storage mediated by the hippocampal formation and associated mesial temporal structures.

Visuospatial

Few studies have examined visuospatial and visuoconstructive skills in iNPH. A recent investigation demonstrated that iNPH patients had greater difficulty than both normal controls and AD patients on tasks of visual counting and visual discrimination, suggesting impairment in visual form perception or constructive function [39]. Ogino et al. [34] compared a group of AD and iNPH patients and showed poorer performance in the iNPH group on a block design test, which measures visuoconstructional skills. However, this task is timed and the motor impairment in iNPH may partially explain the decrement.

Otani and colleagues [40] reported an interesting case in which higher-order visual functions such as facial recognition, spatial orientation, and object recognition were presenting symptoms of iNPH and proved to be reversible after shunt placement. Involvement of white matter pathways near the optical radiations was found on MRI, suggesting that posterior white matter involvement may play a role in the visuospatial symptoms sometimes observed in iNPH patients.

Although no systematic studies have been reported, we have observed impairment in iNPH patients when asked to perform clock drawing. Their performance is indicative of both visuospatial disturbances and frontal dysfunction that affects planning, fund of knowledge, and self monitoring.

Taking together, these observations may suggest some involvement of posterior brain regions and are consistent with previous neuroimaging findings that have shown reduced cerebral blood flow in the parietal cortex in iNPH [41,42]. However, more work is needed in this area to further determine whether visuospatial deficits are secondary to motor and executive impairment or reflect a true underlying impairment in the processing of visual information.

Motor skills

Given that motor impairment is one of the cardinal features of iNPH, it is not surprising that these patients exhibit deficits in motor speed, fine motor coordination, and motor precision. Deficits in fine motor coordination on measures such as the Grooved Pegboard and Perdue Pegboard tests have been widely documented [30,32,33]. Impairments in simple motor speed on standardized tests of tapping ability have also been shown [30]. In addition, two nonstandardized tests of motor precision, Serial Dotting and Line Tracing, have revealed impairments in this skill in iNPH patients [13,30]. These symptoms may reflect involvement of the basal ganglia and/or white matter projections to supplementary motor and other areas of the frontal cortex involved in motor sequencing.

Response to CSF drainage (tap test, external lumbar drainage, shunt)

While iNPH has been described as a reversible form of dementia, for many years, little was known about the recovery of cognitive functions following treatment. Quite a few studies had documented improvement in overall mental status (see Klinge [43]), but there was a lack of agreement about whether specific cognitive deficits responded to treatment. Other studies have found no improvement in cognition following shunting [26,44]. There was a notion set forth that more globally demented patients showed the most dramatic recovery following shunt placement [15], with less affected patients being less likely to improve cognitively after shunt. However, recent studies employing more detailed cognitive test batteries have not supported this finding [30,32,33,38].

In recent years there has been an increasing interest in studying outcome in iNPH, and several well-designed studies have clearly documented that many aspects of the cognitive syndrome can be improved with successful treatment [30,32,33,38]. There have also been investigations looking at initial response following CSF removal as a way to predict who will respond to shunt placement. The mechanisms that underlie the immediate, early improvement in motor and in some psychomotor tasks are not well understood. Tsakanikas et al. [45] demonstrated that tests of upper extremity motor functions improved following tap test and may be utilized to predict response to shunt. A recent study examining response to external lumbar drainage [5] showed clinical improvement in gait and also in psychomotor speed and attention in 50% of the patients. Interestingly, these clinical gains were not associated with changes in ventricular volume. These authors point to an "inverted hysteresis" as an explanation for the occasional phenomenon of prolonged improvement following drainage, suggesting that the alterations in neuronal integrity seen following CSF removal endure even after the CSF is replaced, "before the pathological mechanism gets control again."

There is mounting evidence that there are real and lasting improvements in cognition in carefully selected iNPH cases that undergo shunt placement. Duinkerke et al. [38] examined cognition following shunt placement in 10 iNPH patients and found that 6 of the 10 patients showed improvement in at least 50% of the tests administered, with the greatest improvement seen in verbal memory for both word lists and contextual information (story memory). Although a number of early investigations found no improvement in complex executive functions following treatment [15,26], multiple recent studies have shown clear gains in aspects of executive skills following treatment. Hellström et al. [32] showed an improvement in performance on the Stroop test following shunt, suggesting gains in attention and inhibitory control. Katzen et al. [30] showed that after controlling for practice effects in a small iNPH cohort, improvements were observed following shunt in Trail Making B, a test of complex attention and set shifting. A trend was also observed for symbol digit modalities (SDMT). The post-shunt performance at 6 months was improved for several of the other measures of processing speed and motor functions, but the differences were not significant after controlling for the practice effects in the control group in this small sample. Others have argued that there may not be an expected practice effect in iNPH or that practice effects may only be observed on certain measures [46]. The use of reliable change indices to address these issues has been suggested.

Several other investigators have also shown improvement in Trail Making B, Trail Making A, and SDMT after treatment [13,38,39]. One study of 185 iNPH patients conducted in Spain found that performance on Trail Making B was unchanged despite observed improvements in Trail Making A [33]. In that investigation, less than half of the subjects completed Trail Making B at baseline (n = 70) and only 13 additional patients performed the test at follow-up (n = 83), which suggests that this test may be too difficult for severely impaired patients. The presence of a floor effect on Trail Making B makes it challenging to assess changes following treatment in more impaired samples. Modifications to test administration and scoring procedure may be required to adequately capture performance gains in NPH. Further, additional measures of psychomotor and executive skills should be developed in order to better capture these changes.

Few investigations have examined changes in visuospatial skills and visual memory. One study that demonstrated baseline visuospatial impairment did not show improvements in these skills after successful treatment [39]. With regard to visual memory, the results are mixed with some studies showing that visual memory improves with shunting [33] and others not showing any observable gains in this cognitive domain [38].

Motor skills including simple motor speed, fine motor coordination, and motor precision [13,32,33] have been shown to improve following treatment. However, when comparing change in performance to a group of controls, the gains were no longer statistically significant in one study [30]. As with the findings for some of the executive and attentional measures, this may be secondary to practice effects, but larger cohorts are needed to examine whether there are in fact true practice effects in an NPH sample. Improved methods for determining what constitutes an improvement are also warranted (e.g. reliable change indices).

It is notable that while there is growing evidence that well-selected iNPH patients show improvement across many cognitive domains following successful treatment, cognition does not appear to return to "normal" in most cases. Hellström et al. [47]showed widespread cognitive improvement; however, the performance of the iNPH group remained below the performance of a healthy comparison group, suggesting that the recovery was incomplete.

Differential diagnosis/comorbidities

Variability in the cognitive presentation of iNPH is in part due to the heterogeneity of the disease, but also reflects variability in the latency for a diagnosis to be made. While some patients are identified swiftly via clinical work-up and brain imaging, others do not present to medical attention for months or even years after symptoms begin. In fact, two recent studies examining outcome in iNPH patients both showed that the average duration of symptoms was 24 months (range 12–36 months) [32,33]. Both studies examined whether duration of symptoms was a factor in outcome. One investigation demonstrated that shorter duration was in fact associated with global cognitive improvement and improvement in motor speed [33], whereas the other study did not find a similar association [32]. Despite the uncertainty regarding how duration of symptoms impacts outcome, delays in presentation clearly make differential diagnosis more challenging and the presence of comorbidities further complicates the presentation.

It is not uncommon, especially if diagnosis is delayed, for the neuropsychological test results to suggest involvement of not only frontal systems, but a more widespread cognitive decline that may indicate comorbid AD, vascular cognitive impairment, or another neurodegenerative process. While the existence of cortical deficits such as aphasia, agnosia, and alexia early in the presentation are highly suggestive of an alternate diagnosis, it should be noted that these deficits can be seen in the more advanced stages of iNPH. In some cases they indicate a greater likelihood that a comorbid neurodegenerative disease is also present.

Differential diagnostic considerations

It is important to point out that the presence of a comorbid disorder does not negate the fact that iNPH may contribute to the presentation, and even more importantly, is not necessarily a contraindication for treatment. In our experience, many patients with comorbid neurodegenerative conditions have been successfully treated for iNPH. While the cognitive symptoms typically do not show substantial improvements post-shunt in patients with significant comorbid disease, improvements in gait can be associated with increased independence in activities of daily living and can significantly improve the patient's quality of life as well as making physical management easier for the caregiver.

As described above, there is great variability in the cognitive presentation of patients with iNPH. The profile of deficits typically follows a frontal subcortical pattern, which can often be difficult to distinguish from other disorders that interrupt the integrity of frontal subcortical pathways such as vascular etiologies, parkinsonian syndromes, and even pseudodementia.

Differentiating iNPH from other dementia syndromes is particularly important given that the signs and symptoms can be at least partially reversed with the diversion of CSF through shunt placement. It has been suggested that iNPH may be a contributing factor in to up to 6% of dementia cases [48]. Given the challenge of identifying and differentiating iNPH, this number may be an underestimate. Further, this figure focuses on iNPH cases in which the cognitive presentation has advanced to dementia, yet there are numerous circumstances where mild cognitive dysfunction is a presenting feature and even subtle cognitive changes can impact quality of life and one's ability to function optimally both at home and at work.

Because Alzheimer's disease is so prevalent in the age group at risk for iNPH, distinguishing cognitive symptoms of iNPH from AD is the most frequent differential diagnostic question. There are some data comparing profiles of iNPH and AD groups. While the overlap in cognitive presentation with these disorders may give us clues into the underlying neuropathological mechanisms, additional work is needed in this area to better understand the pathophysiology of iNPH and the mechanisms that are involved both in progression to a dementia that is indistinguishable from AD and the reversibility of certain cognitive features.

Conclusions

Cognitive symptoms of iNPH reflect disturbances in spatially disparate brain networks that mediate executive function, attention, memory, motor sequencing, and visuospatial perception. Cognitive dysfunction in iNPH reflects diverse pathophysiologic processes that are most pronounced in subcortical regions, especially the periventricular white matter of the corona radiata and corpus callosum and subcortical gray structures such as the striatum, thalamus, substantia nigra, and hippocampus. Cognitive disturbances in early stages of iNPH are typically weighted towards frontal systems and are thought to be the product of reversible processes such as interstitial edema and diminished cerebrovascular reserve. Without treatment, iNPH's cognitive symptoms progress and can become irreversible as a result of infarction of white matter and associated metabolic derangements within the brain. With careful selection of shunt candidates as well as management that avoids surgical and postoperative complications, cognitive dysfunction in NPH can be reversed, although only rarely to pre-morbid levels. Common neurodegenerative disorders in the elderly such as AD can coexist with iNPH and diminish the prognosis for long-term recovery of cognitive function after shunt. However, shunt placement can ameliorate symptoms even in cases with coexisting iNPH and neurodegenerative pathology.

Noninvasive methods of studying the structure and function of the human brain and cerebrospinal fluid dynamic are rapidly improving. Ongoing research can be expected to shed further light on the relationship between altered CSF dynamics and neuronal dysfunction leading to cognitive disturbances in iNPH. This should provide new avenues to diagnosis and treatment of iNPH, including the future prospect of improved surgical management and pharmacologic treatment and, ultimately, prevention of the disease.

References

1. Del Bigio MR, Wilson MJ, Enno T. Chronic hydrocephalus in rats and humans: white matter loss and behavior changes. *Ann Neurol* 2003;53:337–46.
2. Roricht S, Meyer BU, Woiciechowsky C, et al. Callosal and corticospinal tract function in patients with hydrocephalus: a morphometric and transcranial magnetic stimulation study. *J Neurol* 1998;245:280–8.
3. Mataro M, Matarin M, Poca MA, et al. Functional and magnetic resonance imaging correlates of corpus callosum in normal pressure hydrocephalus before and after shunting. *J Neurol Neurosurg Psychiatry* 2007;78:395–9.
4. Meier U, Mutze S. Does the ventricle size change after shunt operation of normal-pressure hydrocephalus? *Acta Neurochir Suppl* 2005;95:257–9.
5. Lenfeldt N, Hansson W, Larsson A, et al. Three-day CSF drainage barely reduces ventricular size in normal pressure hydrocephalus. *Neurology* 2012;79(3):237–42.
6. Bradley WG Jr, Scalzo D, Queralt J, et al. Normal-pressure hydrocephalus: evaluation with cerebrospinal fluid flow measurements at MR imaging. *Radiology* 1996;198:523–9.

7. Silverberg GD, Huhn S, Jaffe RA, et al. Downregulation of cerebrospinal fluid production in patients with chronic hydrocephalus. *J Neurosurg* 2002;97(6):1271–5.
8. Kondziella D, Sonnewald U, Tullberg M, Wikkelsø C. Brain metabolism in adult chronic hydrocephalus. *J Neurochem* 2008;106(4):1515–24.
9. Marmarou A, Takagi H, Shulman K. Biomechanics of brain edema and effects on local cerebral blood flow. *Adv Neurol* 1980;28:345–58.
10. Klinge P, Berding G, Brinker T, et al. The role of cerebral blood flow and cerebrovascular reserve capacity in the diagnosis of chronic hydrocephalus – a PET-study on 60 patients. *Acta Neurochir Suppl* 2002;81:39–41.
11. Ziegelitz D, Starck G, Kristiansen D, et al. Cerebral perfusion measured by dynamic susceptibility contrast MRI is reduced in patients with idiopathic normal pressure hydrocephalus. *J Magn Reson Imaging* 2013; doi: 10.1002/jmri.24292.
12. Klinge PM, Brooks DJ, Samii A, et al. Correlates of local cerebral blood flow (CBF) in normal pressure hydrocephalus patients before and after shunting – a retrospective analysis of (15)OH(2)O PET-CBF studies in 65 patients. *Clin Neurol Neurosurg* 2008;110:369–35.
13. Klinge P, Berding G, Brinker T, et al. Regional cerebral blood flow profiles of shunt-responder in idiopathic chronic hydrocephalus: a 15-O-water PET study. *Acta Neurochir Suppl* 2002;81:47–9.
14. Lenfeldt N, Larsson A, Nyberg L, et al. Idiopathic normal pressure hydrocephalus: increased supplementary motor activity accounts for improvement after CSF drainage. *Brain* 2008;131:2904–12.
15. Iddon JL, Pickard JD, Cross JJ, et al. Specific patterns of cognitive impairment in patients with idiopathic normal pressure hydrocephalus and Alzheimer's disease: a pilot study. *J Neurol Neurosurg Psychiatry* 1999;67(6):723–32.
16. Folstein MF, Folstein SE, McHugh PR. "Mini-mental state". A practical method for grading the cognitive state of patients for the clinician. *J Psychiatr Res* 1975;12(3):189–98.
17. Teng EL, Chui HC. The Modified Mini-Mental State (3MS) examination. *J Clin Psychiatry* 1987;48:314–18.
18. Goodglass H, Kaplan E. *The Assessment of Aphasia and Related Disorders*, 2nd edn. Philadelphia, PA: Lea & Febiger; 1987.
19. Spreen O, Benton AL. *Neurosensory Center Comprehension Examination for Aphasia (NCCEA)*. Victoria: University of Victoria; 1969.
20. Benedict RHB, Schretlen D, Groninger L, Brandt J. Hopkins verbal learning test-revised: normative data and analysis of inter-form and test-retest reliability. *Clin Neuropsychol* 1998;12:43–55.
21. Wechsler D. *WAIS-IV Manual*. New York: The Psychological Corporation; 2008.
22. Reitan RM, Wolfson D. *The Halstead-Reitan Neuropsychological Test Battery*. Tucson, AZ: Neuropsychological Press; 1985.
23. Smith A. *Symbol Digit Modalities Test Manual*. Los Angeles, CA: Western Psychological Services; 1973.
24. Klinge P. *A Practical Neuropsychological Battery for Measurement of Cognitive and Motor Function in Patients with Normal-Pressure Hydrocephalus*. Hanover, Germany; 2001.
25. Boon AJ, Tans JT, Delwel EJ, et al. Dutch normal-pressure hydrocephalus study: prediction of outcome after shunting by resistance to outflow of cerebrospinal fluid. *J Neurosurg* 1997;87:687–93.
26. Caltagirone C, Gainotti G, Masullo C, Villa G. Neurophysiological study of normal pressure hydrocephalus *Acta Psychiatr Scand* 1982;65(2):93–100.
27. Merten T. Neuropsychology of normal pressure hydrocephalus *Nervenarzt* 1999;70(6):496–503.
28. Thomsen AM, Børgesen SE, Bruhn P, Gjerris F. Prognosis of dementia in normal-pressure hydrocephalus after a shunt operation. *Ann Neurol* 1986;20(3):304–10.
29. Gallassi R, Morreale A, Montagna P, et al. Binswanger's disease and normal-pressure hydrocephalus. Clinical and neuropsychological comparison. *Arch Neurol* 1991;48(11):1156–9.
30. Katzen H, Ravdin LD, Assuras S, et al. Postshunt cognitive and functional improvement in idiopathic normal pressure hydrocephalus. *Neurosurgery* 2011;68(2):416–19.
31. Scollato A, Gallina P, Gautam B, et al. Changes in aqueductal CSF stroke volume in shunted patients with idiopathic normal-pressure hydrocephalus. *Am J Neuroradiol* 2009;30(8):1580–6.
32. Hellström P, Klinge P, Tans J, Wikkelsø C. The neuropsychology of iNPH: findings and evaluation of tests in the European multicentre study. *Clin Neurol Neurosurg* 2012;114:130–4.
33. Solana E, Sahuquillo J, Junqué C, Quintana M, Poca MA. Cognitive disturbances and neuropsychological changes after surgical treatment in a cohort of 185 patients with idiopathic normal pressure hydrocephalus. *Arch Clin Neuropsychol* 2012;27(3):304–17.
34. Ogino A, Kazui H, Miyoshi N, et al. Cognitive impairment in patients with idiopathic normal pressure hydrocephalus. *Dement Geriatr Cogn Disord* 2006;21(2):113–19.
35. Kanno S, Saito M, Hayashi A, et al. Counting-backward test for executive function in idiopathic

normal pressure hydrocephalus. *Acta Neurol Scand* 2012;126(4):279–86.

36. Ravdin LD, Katzen H. Idiopathic normal pressure hydrocephalus. In: Ravdin LD, Katzen H (Eds.) *Handbook on the Neuropsychology of Aging and Dementia*. New York: Springer Publishing; 2012: 345–54.
37. Thomas G, McGirt MJ, Woodworth GF, et al. Baseline neuropsychological profile and cognitive response to cerebrospinal fluid shunting for idiopathic normal pressure hydrocephalus. *Dement Geriatr Cogn Disord* 2005;20:163–8.
38. Duinkerke A, Williams M, Rigamonti D, Hillis AE. Cognitive recovery in idiopathic normal pressure hydrocephalus after shunt. *Cogn Behav Neurol* 2004;17(3):179–84.
39. Saito M, Nishio Y, Kanno S, et al. Cognitive profile of idiopathic normal pressure hydrocephalus. *Dement Geriatr Cogn Disord* 2011;1:202–11.
40. Otani N, Nawashiro H, Ishihara S, et al. Normal pressure hydrocephalus manifesting as transient prosopagnosia, topographical disorientation, and visual objective agnosia. *J Clin Neurosci* 2004;11(3):313–17.
41. Sasaki H, Ishii K, Kono AK, et al. Cerebral perfusion pattern of idiopathic normal pressure hydrocephalus studied by SPECT and statistical brain mapping. *Ann Nucl Med* 2007;21:39–45.
42. Takaya M, Kazui H, Tokunaga H, et al. Global cerebral hypoperfusion in preclinical stage of idiopathic normal pressure hydrocephalus. *J Neurol Sci* 2010; 298(1):35–41.
43. Klinge P. Updates in diagnostic evaluation and management of normal pressure hydrocephalus. *WFNS Rev Neurosurg* 2012;3(3).
44. Savolainen S, Hurskainen H, Paljärvi L, Alafuzoff I, Vapalahti M. Five-year outcome of normal pressure hydrocephalus with or without a shunt: predictive value of the clinical signs, neuropsychological evaluation and infusion test. *Acta Neurochir* 2002;144(6):515–23.
45. Tsakanikas D, Katzen H, Ravdin LD, Relkin NR. Upper extremity motor measures of tap test response in normal pressure hydrocephalus. *Clin Neurol Neurosurg* 2009;111(9):752–7.
46. Solana E, Poca MA, Sahuquillo J, Benejam B, Junque C, Dronavalli M. Cognitive and motor improvement after retesting in normal-pressure hydrocephalus: a real change or merely a learning effect? *J Neurosurg* 2010;112(2):339–409.
47. Hellström P, Edsbagge M, Blomsterwall E, et al. Neuropsychological effects of shunt treatment in idiopathic normal pressure hydrocephalus. *Neurosurgery* 2008;63(3):527–35.
48. Casmiro M, Benassi G, Cacciatore FM, D'Alessandro R. Frequency of idiopathic normal pressure hydrocephalus. *Arch Neurol* 1989;46:608.

Chapter 8

Incontinence and lower urinary tract symptoms in normal pressure hydrocephalus

Adam P. Klausner and Samuel P. Robinson

Introduction

Since the initial description by Hakim and Adams in 1965 [1], numerous studies have been published on the subject of normal pressure hydrocephalus (NPH). Furthermore, during the nearly five decades since the publication of this landmark paper, significant advancements in the diagnosis and treatment of NPH have been achieved. However, with few exceptions, the majority of studies have focused primarily on only two of the three components of the NPH triad: dementia and gait disturbances. Unfortunately, there have been very few studies that provide a comprehensive characterization of incontinence and lower urinary tract symptoms associated with NPH.

This lack of knowledge may represent a relatively limited state of understanding of the neural circuitry involved in the control of micturition or an unwillingness by patients, families, and providers to consider "incontinence" as a truly important clinical problem. In fact, epidemiologic studies have identified urinary incontinence or overactive bladder as an extremely prevalent problem, affecting nearly 10–20% [2,3] of the worldwide population. However, studies suggest that only a minority of patients with incontinence have ever spoken with a doctor about their condition, and of those who had, a majority were not offered treatment [4]. In this regard, it is important to dispel the myth that incontinence is a *normal* part of aging. In fact, urinary incontinence is always pathologic and almost always can be treated or improved.

For patients with NPH, urinary incontinence is present in roughly 45–90% [5,6] and represents a significant source of bother for both patients and caregivers [7,8]. Therefore, we believe that a thorough evaluation and management of incontinence and other lower urinary tract symptoms should be an integral part of any treatment plan for patients with NPH. This chapter will provide a broad overview of incontinence and lower urinary tract symptoms in NPH and cover areas including dementia and incontinence, differential diagnosis, physiology and pathophysiology, symptoms, evaluation, and treatment. The authors are strong advocates of a multidisciplinary treatment approach involving sub-specialists in neurosurgery, neurology, rehabilitation, psychiatry, nursing, and urology that can work as a team to provide comprehensive care to patients with NPH who have associated incontinence and lower urinary tract symptoms.

Dementia and incontinence

The symptom of urinary incontinence, defined as the involuntary loss of urine, is extremely prevalent in patients with dementia disorders and has been estimated to occur in 53% of these patients [9]. In institutionalized patients with dementia disorders, the prevalence is even higher and has been reported to occur in 83% of nursing home patients with dementia disorders [10,11]. These studies highlight the strong association between dementia and incontinence and also the harsh reality that this combination may be a driving force behind a family's decision to institutionalize a loved one.

However, it is important to recognize that in the setting of dementia, the occurrence and patterns of incontinence may not be uniform. For example, in patients with multi-infarct dementia, incontinence typically occurs *earlier* than in patients with Alzheimer's type dementia and may be preceded by urinary frequency and urgency. In contrast, in patients with post-stroke dementia, incontinence is the rule, occurring in the overwhelming majority. In this regard, understanding the relationship between the onset of incontinence in

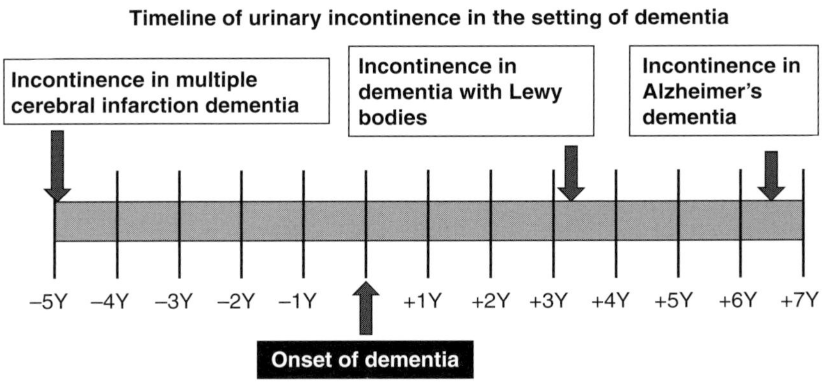

Figure 8.1 In the setting of dementia disorders including multiple cerebral infarct dementia, dementia with Lewy bodies, and Alzheimer's dementia, the onset of urinary incontinence differs. Y = year.

the setting of dementia is important and may help in the diagnosis and treatment of both conditions. In general, it has been observed that incontinence may occur several years prior to the onset of dementia in multiple cerebral infarct dementia. Incontinence occurs about three or more years after the onset of dementia in dementia with Lewy bodies, and six or more years after the onset of dementia in Alzheimer's type dementia [12] (Figure 8.1).

Clearly, an integral component of NPH is the presence of gait disturbances, and this factor may actually be the most bothersome for patients. The relationship between gait disturbances, dementia, and incontinence has profound importance because of the potential heightened risk of falls. Lee and colleagues conducted a cross-sectional study of 159 patients with confirmed dementia which was categorized as mild, moderate, or severe [13]. These investigators found that the overall risk of falls for patients with dementia was 34% with 4-fold higher rates in patients with severe dementia compared to those with mild dementia [13]. In a logistic regression analysis looking at factors of depression, incontinence, nutritional status, poor balance, polypharmacy, dementia severity, and impairment of activities of daily living, the authors found that the only independent factor associated with an increased fall risk was urinary incontinence. This finding highlights the potentially life-threatening nature of incontinence in patients with NPH and other dementia disorders.

Differential diagnosis

One major issue in the evaluation of lower urinary tract symptoms is the lack of consistent and standardized definitions. Specifically, for the diagnosis of urinary incontinence, definitions vary widely with some studies labeling patients as having urinary incontinence if they report "any" episodes of leakage in a 12-month period. Alternatively, other investigations define incontinence as experiencing involuntary loss of urine at least one or more times per week. Incontinence can be objectively measured with the use of *void diaries* in which the time of all voids and incontinence episodes as well as volume of liquids consumed are meticulously recorded for 3, 5, or 7 days [14] and *pad tests* in which patients are told to bring in all the incontinence pads or garments that they have worn in a 24-hour period [15]. The garments are weighed in order to establish an objective measurement of the volume of urinary incontinence. Unfortunately, these tests are extremely labor intensive and inconvenient for patients, and elderly patients with cognitive or physical impairments may not be able to participate.

Furthermore, incontinence may only represent one of many possible lower urinary tract symptoms. Overactive bladder, defined by the International Continence Society as "urinary urgency, with or without urge incontinence, usually with frequency and nocturia" [16], is also highly prevalent and may affect nearly 17% of the worldwide adult population [3,17]. The constellation of symptoms sometimes called "storage" or "irritative" symptoms includes urinary urgency, frequency, nocturia, and urge incontinence. Other lower urinary tract symptoms include straining, hesitancy, intermittent stream, slowed stream, and post-void dribbling. These symptoms, termed "voiding" or "obstructive" symptoms, are also highly prevalent in the geriatric population, and may be related to bladder outlet obstruction induced by benign prostatic hyperplasia [16].

Indeed, a detailed understanding of these subtle differences in terminology and of the extensive differential diagnosis of incontinence and lower urinary tract symptoms in elderly patients is required for the effective treatment of incontinence and lower urinary tract symptoms associated with NPH. Many causes of geriatric lower urinary tract symptoms or incontinence are reversible and can be categorized using the "**DIAPPER**" mnemonic (**D**elirium, **I**nfection, **A**trophic vaginitis, **P**harmaceuticals, **P**sychological disorders, **E**ndocrine disorders, **R**estricted mobility, **S**tool impaction) [18]. For elderly men, benign prostatic hyperplasia is a common condition and can be easily treated with medications or minor surgery. For women, stress urinary incontinence is also common and occurs with exertional activities including coughing, laughing, or getting up from a sitting to standing position.

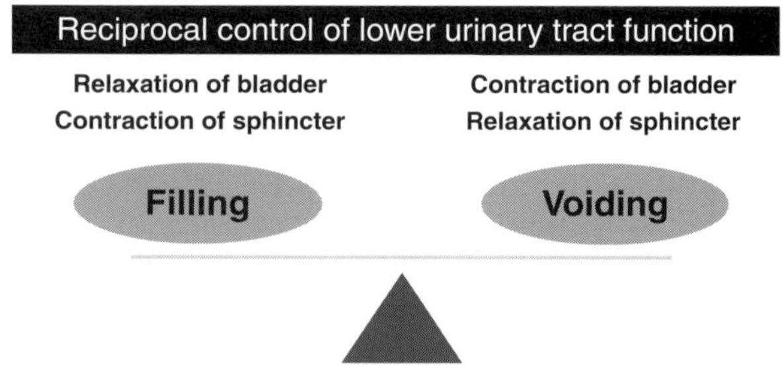

Figure 8.2 The urinary bladder and urethral sphincter are under reciprocal neurologic control. During the filling phase of micturition, the bladder is relaxed and the sphincter is contracted, promoting efficient storage of urine. During the voiding phase, the neurologic switch is reversed, resulting in bladder contraction and sphincter relaxation and promoting efficient emptying of urine.

Pathophysiology of incontinence in NPH

Initially, it was thought that the symptoms of NPH were related to compression and stretching of the major long tracts in the white matter and corpus callosum, which could be at least partially reversed with drainage of cerebrospinal fluid (CSF). Subsequently, a variety of alternative potential pathophysiologic mechanisms have been proposed to explain the NPH clinical triad. Etiologic theories include: decreased ability to reabsorb CSF [19], alterations in cerebral blood flow [20,21], changes in superficial venous compliance [22], presence of occult comorbid conditions [23], changes in the site of CSF reabsorption [24,25], increased CSF pulse pressure [26], and the presence of primary cerebral parenchymal disease [27]. However, the exact pathophysiology of incontinence in the setting of NPH remains unknown.

Normal micturitional physiology

In order to better understand the pathophysiology of NPH-mediated incontinence, a brief review of normal micturitional physiology is required. There are two functional muscular units in the lower urinary tract: the urinary bladder, an organ composed of smooth muscle, and the urinary sphincter, an organ composed of striated muscle surrounding the urethra. In general, these lower urinary tract components are under reciprocal neurologic control (Figure 8.2). In this regard, when the sphincter contracts, the bladder is in a relaxed state, promoting the efficient storage of urine. In the reciprocal state, the urinary sphincter relaxes and the bladder contracts, promoting the efficient emptying of urine.

In the central nervous system, there are two main areas involved in the motor control and reciprocal coordination of lower urinary tract function. At the level of the spinal cord, the motor outflow mediating bladder contraction is parasympathetic and arises in the intermediolateral cell column of the S2–4 spinal cord in the sacral parasympathetic nucleus. At the level of the brainstem, the pontine micturition center is a "point of convergence of pro- and anti-micturition drivers" and is important in the reciprocal control of bladder and urethral function [28]. Areas above the brainstem tend to be inhibitory and mainly function to aid in the voluntary suppression of micturition reflex. Therefore, any neurologic process that occurs at or below the sacral spinal cord (i.e. sacral spinal cord injury, tumor, spinal dysraphism) will result in a lack of motor tone to the bladder and an "acontractile" detrusor. Lesions between the sacral cord and pontine micturition center (i.e. spinal cord injury) will create a lack of inhibitory tone and result in both detrusor overactivity and a lack of bladder and sphincter coordination (detrusor sphincter dyssynergia). Finally, lesions above the pontine micturition center are expected only to cause a lack of inhibitory tone and will result simply in detrusor overactivity with or without incontinence. This pattern is seen with stroke, traumatic brain injury, and tumors [29], and is therefore the expected pattern associated with NPH.

Pathophysiology of incontinence and lower urinary tract symptoms in NPH

Our understanding of lower urinary tract dysfunction in NPH is limited by a lack of detailed knowledge of the supraspinal pathways involved in the control of micturition. The vast majority of neuro-urologic knowledge has been elucidated through the study of specific neurologic lesions and their corresponding clinical presentations. With the use of functional magnetic resonance imaging and positron emission tomography, this anatomic and functional information has been expanded and integrated. At this point, it is clear that supraspinal involvement in storage and micturition is exceedingly complex and requires intact communication between a large number of control centers. A detailed description of these pathways is beyond the scope of this chapter; however, important supraspinal sites identified in control of micturition include: the periaqueductal gray matter, the medial preoptic nucleus of the hypothalamus, the right insula, the dorsal anterior cingulate gyrus, the pontine micturition center, the medial prefrontal cortex, the nucleus retroambiguus, the A11 group of dopaminergic neurons, the "L" region, the paraventricular nucleus, the Köllicke–Fuse nucleus, the locus coeruleus, the A5 group of noradrenergic neurons, the nucleus raphe magnus, the nucleus raphe obscuris, the paraventricular thalamic nucleus, the nucleus raphe pallidus, the medial prefrontal cortex, and the bilateral putamen. Lesions in these areas increase bladder activity presumably through disinhibition [30–33].

A vast network of interconnections exists between these supraspinal structures. The integrity of these connections must be maintained for normal voiding to occur. In addition, it is important to recognize the involvement of many of these areas in emotional control as well as the pathophysiology of depression and anxiety. There is now growing evidence linking functional disorders of the bladder and bowel with common psychiatric conditions [34]. Likewise, in the setting of NPH, it is postulated that the close proximity of some of these micturitional centers and their interconnecting pathways to the ventricular system may result in the urinary symptoms present in NPH. Damage to these areas is presumably mediated through distortion and ischemia [35,36].

Evaluation of urinary symptoms in NPH patients

Terminology

Due to the often vague nature of urinary symptoms, it is important to use standardized terminology as recommended by the International Continence Society (ICS). The ICS uses the term "lower urinary tract symptoms" or "LUTS" and recommends using the terms "storage symptoms" and "voiding symptoms" as broad categorizations [16]. Storage symptoms include urinary frequency, urgency, and nocturia and have been previously described as "irritative." Voiding symptoms include slow stream, intermittency, hesitancy, straining, and terminal dribble and have previously described as "obstructive." Post-void symptoms should be identified as a subcategory of voiding symptoms and documented as a feeling of incomplete emptying and post-micturition dribble [37]. Bladder sensation should be identified as a subcategory of storage symptoms and documented as normal, increased, reduced, or absent [16].

Urologic history

With a good understanding of this complex terminology, the evaluation of patients with NPH should begin with a comprehensive history elicited from the patient, family, and care providers. The history should focus on a detailed characterization of the lower urinary tract symptoms and incontinence, including prior treatments. Special attention should be focused on the *onset* of urinary symptoms and their relationship to other symptoms in the NPH triad. For example, in an elderly woman with idiopathic NPH (iNPH) who complains of longstanding (>10 years) stable urinary incontinence, it is unlikely that the symptoms are NPH-mediated. However, an exacerbation from her baseline level of chronic symptoms would be more typical and revealing. Specific questions should focus on fluid intake, type and timing of medications (specifically diuretics), and any prior history of urologic medical or surgical treatments. Conditions such as recurrent urinary tract infections, benign prostatic hyperplasia, nephrolithiasis, as well as bladder and prostate cancer can present with similar lower urinary tract symptoms and must be differentiated from symptoms that are attributable to NPH.

Validated questionnaires

Subjective information gleaned from patient and family interviews is important and can certainly help guide treatment. However, in terms of lower urinary tract symptoms and incontinence, this type of free-form discussion lacks standardization. Therefore, the use of validated questionnaires to evaluate and characterize the type, severity, and quality-of-life impact of lower urinary tract symptoms has become an accepted means to standardize the assessment of symptoms and to measure outcomes. A wealth of research in this area confirms the utility of validated questionnaires in initial and follow-up patient evaluations [33]. There are a multitude of available questionnaires and choosing the "right" set can be very challenging and can make comparative studies difficult or impossible. To help with this problem, the International Continence Society established an entity called the International Consultation on Incontinence Modular Questionnaires (ICIq) which develops and validates questionnaires evaluating specific domains of lower urinary tract function. It is now recommended that researchers in urinary incontinence use these ICIq instruments in clinical practice and in the performance of research investigations so that outcomes can be more easily compared. Questionnaires are available for free on request at www.iciq.net.

In the evaluation of patients with NPH and urinary symptoms, it has been our standard practice to use instruments that specifically evaluate subdomains of urinary incontinence. For this purpose, we employ the ICIq urinary incontinence short form which asks questions regarding the frequency of incontinence, the volume of each incontinence episode, and the bother associated with incontinence. Based on our experience, we also see patients with typical symptoms of overactive bladder (urgency and frequency) who do not have frank incontinence. Therefore, we also employ the ICIq overactive bladder module which looks at the subdomains of urinary frequency, nocturia, urgency, and urge incontinence. Finally, we administer a detailed quality-of-life instrument (ICIq-LUTSqol) which determines the overall impact of lower urinary tract symptoms on physical, social, and emotional well-being.

Though data are limited, several studies have confirmed the utility of validated questionnaires in NPH patients. Takeuchi and colleagues confirmed an improvement in caregiver satisfaction using the Zarit caregiver burden interview to evaluate caregivers' responses to improvements in gait and urinary symptoms after shunt placement in patients with iNPH [38]. Kuriyama and colleagues used the overactive bladder symptom score developed by Homma et al. to show an association between autonomic dysfunction and urinary symptoms in iNPH patients [39,40]. It is therefore recommended by our group and others to use such questionnaires in the initial assessment of iNPH symptoms [41].

The completion of these questionnaires is a lengthy process and can be stressful for patients and their families. Therefore, it is our policy that all surveys be completed directly by a urologist or a specifically trained designee who is part of the multidisciplinary NPH team. Patients may sometimes protest saying that they "came to see the neurosurgeon and not the urologist" and must be reassured that *all* aspects of the NPH disease require comprehensive evaluation and treatment. Nursing staff can be critically important in helping families understand that the initial evaluation will require visits with multiple providers and may take many long and exhausting hours to complete.

Physical examination

After the initial history, a focused genitourinary physical exam should be performed to rule out treatable causes of incontinence. For example, men may suffer from "phimosis," a condition in which the foreskin cannot be easily retracted, and treatment of this condition can easily improve urinary symptoms. In addition, elderly women frequently suffer from atrophic vaginitis and treatment with topical estrogen cream can readily improve their symptoms.

Diagnostic testing

Diagnostic testing should be individualized in patients with NPH. In our practice, the majority of patients were referred from outside providers and many had their own outside urologists. As a result, we tend to avoid unnecessary repetition of tests. However, in general, it is recommended that the diagnostic evaluation of patients presenting with incontinence or lower urinary tract symptoms include a urinalysis, creatinine, urinary flow rate, and a noninvasive (i.e. bladder scan) measurement of post-void residual volume [42]. Imaging in the form of ultrasound or computed tomography may also be considered in patients who have evidence of hematuria or nephrolithiasis.

Urodynamic testing

Although invasive in nature, urodynamic studies may be the most important investigative procedures performed in patients with significant urinary symptoms and iNPH, as the results will help identify etiologies and guide treatments. The study involves placement of patients on a specialized table or chair and infusing saline through a small urinary catheter. During the study, an additional catheter is placed in the rectum or vagina to allow for the simultaneous measurement of intra-abdominal pressure and intravesical pressures. Electromyography electrodes are placed on the perineum to measure the function of the urethral sphincter mechanism [29].

In our practice, baseline urodynamics (prior to ventriculoperitoneal shunting) was offered to all patients assessed to have moderate to severe urinary symptoms or incontinence, and our research protocol required a follow-up study be performed 3 months after shunting. However, patients are often unwilling to undergo this type of invasive testing as they may not recognize the direct association of lower urinary tract symptoms with NPH. Again, the importance of nursing staff is critical in providing appropriate education and allowing for the mental preparation of our patients and their families. Coordination and scheduling of urodynamic tests can be very challenging as the visit (including preparation and post-test discussion) can easily take 2 hours. Many patients present from great distances and insist that all testing be performed in the fewest possible visits. In this regard, we find that juggling infusion studies, preoperative history and physicals, and anesthesia evaluations presents logistical problems and requires the skill and patience of skilled nurse coordinators.

Characterization of lower urinary tract symptoms in NPH

Since its initial description, incontinence has been included as part of the classic triad in patients with NPH [1]. However, the scope of urinary symptoms in NPH patients is broader than was initially proposed. In patients with secondary NPH, urinary incontinence is variable and is largely dependent upon the severity of the underlying neurologic condition. On the other hand, in patients with iNPH, the presence of urinary incontinence may not be as common and appears to be more of a late finding [36,43]. It has also been suggested, but not well studied, that increased urinary frequency and urgency precede urinary incontinence in NPH patients and are more common presenting symptoms than frank incontinence [5,44,45]. It has also been proposed that the symptoms of urgency and possibly of urge incontinence result from detrusor overactivity, defined urodynamically as the presence of involuntary bladder contractions identified during pressure–flow urodynamic studies. This was first proposed by Ahlberg and colleagues who identified detrusor overactivity in three NPH patients with incontinence [46]. Sakakibara and colleagues confirmed this finding in a separate study and found that 95% of patients with urinary symptoms and iNPH had detrusor overactivity on urodynamic evaluation, and among these patients, the symptoms of urinary urgency and frequency (74%) were more common than actual incontinence (57%) [44]. Despite these findings, controversy still exists given the high correlation between urinary urgency and age-related white matter changes which can occur in combination with or exclusive of iNPH. One study found urinary urgency to be prevalent in 25% of patients with severe age-related white matter changes [47]. Furthermore, some authors still contend that dementia and gait impairment may contribute to the incontinence of NPH through "frontal" release and difficulty with ambulation to the bathroom [36,48,49].

The Virginia Commonwealth University experience

In our own series of 75 patients with new-onset NPH (idiopathic and secondary), patients were not given any incontinence-specific treatments until approximately 3 months post ventriculoperitoneal shunting to determine the degree of incontinence that was potentially NPH-mediated. The mean follow-up from shunt to first urologic follow-up was 158 ± 17 days and baseline responses to the incontinence questionnaire revealed that patients leaked on average less than one time per day with small-to-moderate leakage volume, and only minimal bother (3.6 out of 10) (Figure 8.3). Here, it is important to emphasize that incontinence is a "family" illness and caregivers are often more distressed about the consequences of incontinence than patients, especially in the setting of cognitive impairment. Evaluation of baseline overactive bladder symptoms including urinary frequency, nocturia, urgency, and urge incontinence was performed using a validated overactive bladder instrument. Patients generally reported mild to moderate overactive bladder symptoms with nocturia being the most severe and urge incontinence being the most bothersome (Figure 8.4). Again, evaluating the symptoms in their component parts is extremely helpful in that isolated nocturia (awaking to void during the overnight period) is highly associated with treatable, and unrelated, medical conditions such as congestive heart failure and sleep apnea [50].

At baseline, we were able to perform urodynamic testing on 28 patients who presented with NPH. The results demonstrate that patients had reduced overall bladder capacities (223.6 ± 23.4 ml) with limited warning times and normal detrusor compliance. Involuntary detrusor contractions associated with incontinence were identified in 80%, meeting diagnostic criteria for "neurogenic detrusor overactivity." As expected, nearly 41% (mainly men with benign prostatic hyperplasia) demonstrated evidence of bladder outlet obstruction. However, despite nearly 50% of the patients being women, only 8% of patients displayed urodynamic stress incontinence. Unfortunately, only a handful of patients agreed to have post-shunt follow-up studies, and these were individuals with the most severe and treatment-refractory lower urinary tract symptoms. In addition, many patients with improved cognitive function or improved urinary symptoms refused to undergo the repeat study, stating "why do I need the study if I'm better?" Here again, the importance of education and nursing coordination is critical for the functioning of a multidisciplinary NPH group that includes a dedicated neuro-urologist.

We were able to collect validated questionnaire data from 27 patients with NPH both pre- and post-shunting and found that all incontinence domains improved with significant decreases in score seen for the volume of leakage and the total incontinence score (Figure 8.5). Likewise, all overactive bladder symptoms were significantly improved after shunting with the exception of nocturia (Figure 8.6). This is important because, as discussed above, nocturia may reflect underlying and treatable medical conditions. Improvement for overactive bladder-related bother was not very robust with the exception of urinary urgency.

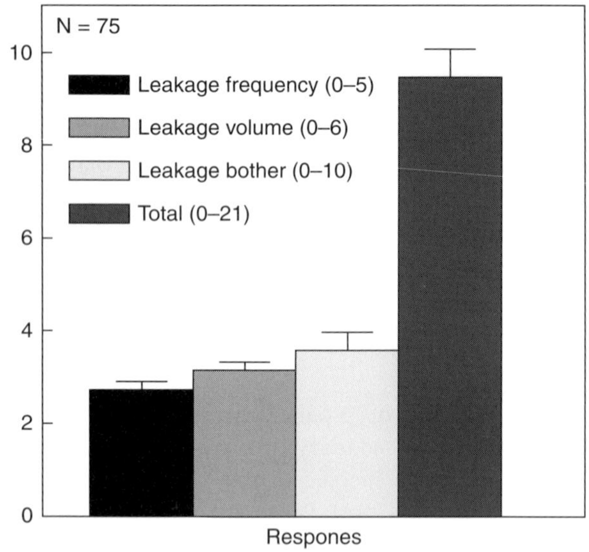

Figure 8.3 In a study of 75 patients at the Virginia Commonwealth University, results from the International Consultation on Incontinence questionnaire (ICIq) module on urinary incontinence demonstrate mild to moderate levels of urinary incontinence.

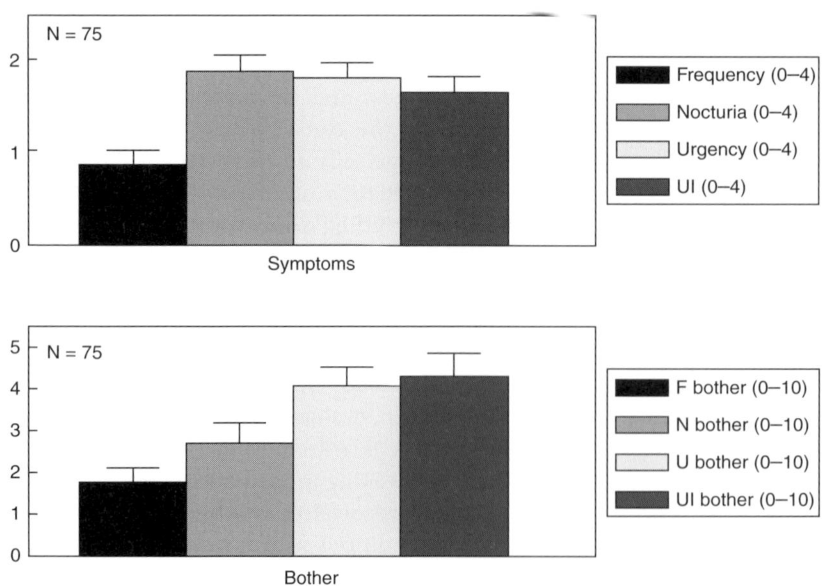

Figure 8.4 In a study of 75 patients at the Virginia Commonwealth University, results from the International Consultation on Incontinence questionnaire (ICIq) module on overactive bladder demonstrate mild to moderate symptoms of urinary frequency (F), nocturia (N), urgency (U), and urge incontinence (UI), with nocturia being the most severe (upper panel). In terms of bother (lower panel), scores revealed mild to moderate bother with the most bothersome symptom being urge incontinence.

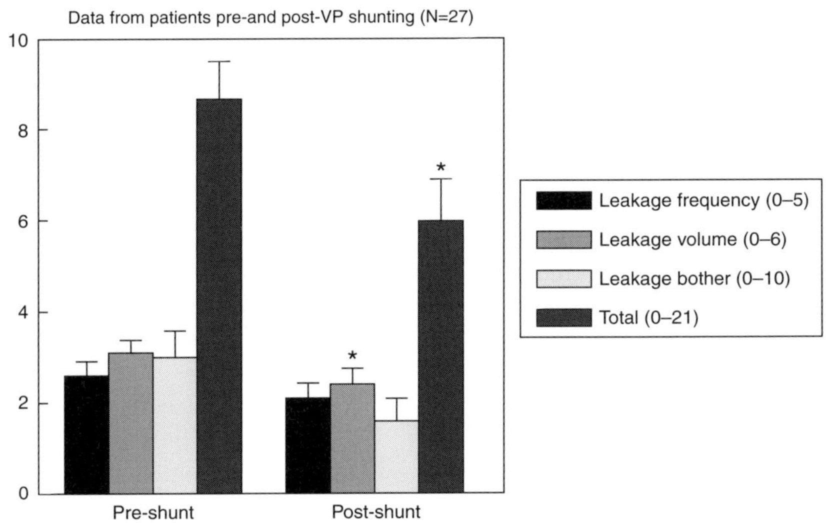

Figure 8.5 In 27 patients who had surveys completed at baseline and again after the placement of a ventriculoperitoneal shunt (VP), results from the International Consultation on Incontinence questionnaire (IClq) module on urinary incontinence demonstrate statistically significant improvements in leakage volume and in total scores. *$p < 0.05$.

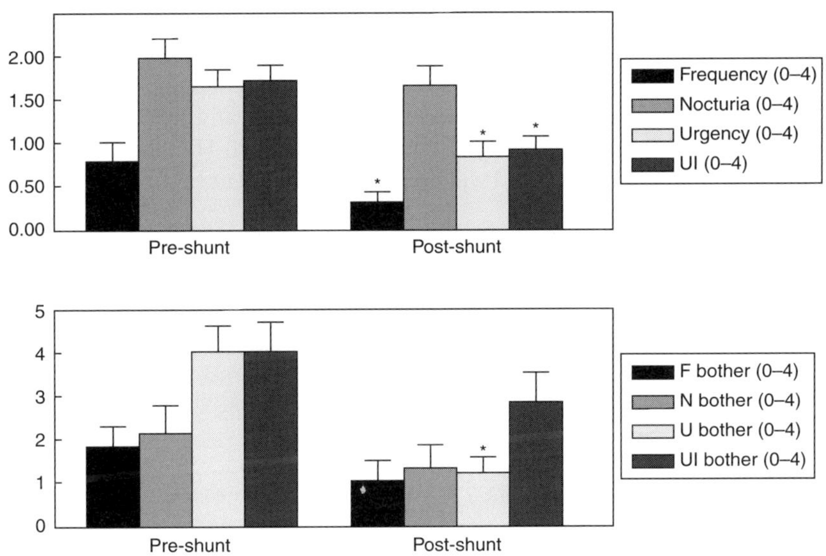

Figure 8.6 In 27 patients who had surveys completed at baseline and again after the placement of a ventriculoperitoneal shunt (VP), results from the International Consultation on Incontinence questionnaire (IClq) module on overactive bladder (OAB) demonstrated significant improvement in the severity of frequency (F), urgency (U), and urge incontinence (UI); however, nocturia did not improve after shunt placement (upper panel). Bother scores related to overactive bladder symptoms (lower panel) showed significant improvement only for urgency. *$p < 0.05$.

Treatment of NPH-mediated incontinence

Given the variability in presentation, it is important to determine the cause of urinary symptoms in patients with presumed NPH prior to the initiation of therapy. If detrusor overactivity has been confirmed with urodynamic testing, then recommended therapy includes antimuscarinic medications and behavioral modification. Patients may be treatment refractory to standard doses or may (with close monitoring) require higher than recommended doses or combination therapies. Nevertheless, in an appropriately selected group of patients, with confirmed diagnosis of iNPH, the mainstay of therapy remains shunt placement.

Short-term results for incontinence after shunt surgery

Controversy exists regarding the most significant preoperative predictor of shunt success. In this regard, a variety of factors have been evaluated and the objective response to external lumbar drainage of cerebrospinal fluid is considered the most significant

[51]. However, even among the most highly selected patients, improvement in gait ataxia consistently outranks improvement in urinary incontinence in the majority of groups surveyed. In an early case series, Ahlberg and colleagues reported 100% improvement in clinical urinary incontinence and found that urodynamic detrusor overactivity improved in three of four patients after shunt placement. They also reported subjective improvement in urinary urgency in the fourth patient [46]. In subsequent studies, the effects of shunting on NPH-mediated incontinence have been more variable. Poca and colleagues reported an 82.4% improvement in urinary incontinence in a group of 236 patients surveyed 6 months after shunt surgery, a more pronounced improvement than observed for both gait (79.3%) and dementia (63.7%) [52].

Long-term results for incontinence after shunt surgery

On the other hand, Cage and colleagues found, using self-reported surveys, that only 55.9% of a cohort of 252 patients showed improvement in incontinence in long-term follow-up, lower than both dementia (64.4%) and gait (81.1%) [53]. In a much smaller series of patients, Savolainen and colleagues reported on long-term outcomes and found that urinary incontinence improved in 58% of the patients with 57% showing improvement in ambulation one year after surgery, with benefits remaining even after 5 years [54]. In a different series, Pujari and colleagues followed patients for 7 years post-shunting with interval evaluations at 3 years after surgery. These investigators found incontinence was the least improved triad symptom with 84% improvement at 3 years and 80% improvement at 7 years [55]. This trend of worsening symptoms over time was not consistent when assessing gait (83% at 3 years and 87% at 7 years) or when assessing dementia (84% at 3 years and 86% at 7 years). However, the most important finding in the Pujari study was the shunt revision rate, which reached 53%, highlighting the importance of appropriate patient selection.

Conclusions

Urinary symptoms are a key component of the NPH triad. Patients typically report overactive bladder symptoms including urinary frequency and urgency and may not experience frank incontinence. The evaluation of urinary symptoms is challenging in geriatric patients and patients with dementia disorders and is best performed by an experienced neurourologist or other provider with expertise in these areas. Understanding the differential diagnoses is also important because many other pathologies can present with urinary symptoms in this age group. The use of validated questionnaires can help standardize the evaluation and management of patients. Furthermore, a multidisciplinary NPH team which includes a dedicated neuro-urologist is critical for the comprehensive management of patients with NPH-mediated urinary symptoms.

Dedication

This work is dedicated to Professor Anthony Marmarou who was recognized internationally as a leading authority and research pioneer in NPH. This current work is made possible by his mentorship and guidance on a project to investigate NPH in geriatric patients funded by the American Geriatrics Society. Professor Marmarou was a consummate gentleman who devoted his life to research, mentorship, and the comfort and well-being of patients with NPH. He passed away in 2010 and will be truly missed but never forgotten.

References

1. Hakim S, Adams RD. The special clinical problem of symptomatic hydrocephalus with normal cerebrospinal fluid pressure. Observations on cerebrospinal fluid hydrodynamics. *J Neurol Sci* 1965;2(4):307–27.
2. Coyne KS, Margolis MK, Kopp ZS, Kaplan SA. Racial differences in the prevalence of overactive bladder in the United States from the epidemiology of LUTS (EpiLUTS) study. *Urology* 2012;79(1):95–101.
3. Irwin DE, Milsom I, Kopp Z, et al. Prevalence, severity, and symptom bother of lower urinary tract symptoms among men in the EPIC study: impact of overactive bladder. *Eur Urol* 2009;56(1):14–20.
4. Milsom I, Abrams P, Cardozo L, et al. How widespread are the symptoms of an overactive bladder and how are they managed? A population-based prevalence study. *BJU Int* 2001;87(9):760–6.
5. Meier U, Zeilinger FS, Kintzel D. Signs, symptoms and course of normal pressure hydrocephalus in comparison with cerebral atrophy. *Acta Neurochir (Wien)* 1999;141(10):1039–48.
6. Hebb AO, Cusimano MD. Idiopathic normal pressure hydrocephalus: a systematic review of diagnosis and outcome. *Neurosurgery* 2001;49(5):1166–84; discussion 84–6.

7. Lim PP, Sahadevan S, Choo GK, Anthony P. Burden of caregiving in mild to moderate dementia: an Asian experience. *Int Psychogeriatr* 1999;11(4):411–20.
8. Toma AK, Tarnaris A, Kitchen ND, Watkins LD. Working towards patient oriented outcome assessment in normal pressure hydrocephalus, what is the most important? *Acta Neurochir (Wien)* 153(1):177–80.
9. Campbell AJ, Reinken J, McCosh L. Incontinence in the elderly: prevalence and prognosis. *Age Ageing* 1985;14(2):65–70.
10. Ouslander JG, Palmer MH, Rovner BW, German PS. Urinary incontinence in nursing homes: incidence, remission and associated factors. *J Am Geriatr Soc* 1993;41(10):1083–9.
11. Palmer MH, German PS, Ouslander JG. Risk factors for urinary incontinence one year after nursing home admission. *Res Nurs Health* 1991;14(6):405–12.
12. Sakakibara R, Uchiyama T, Yamanishi T, Kishi M. Dementia and lower urinary dysfunction: with a reference to anticholinergic use in elderly population. *Int J Urol* 2008;15(9):778–88.
13. Lee CY, Chen LK, Lo YK, et al. Urinary incontinence: an under-recognized risk factor for falls among elderly dementia patients. *Neurourol Urodyn* 2011;30(7):1286–90.
14. Weiss JP, Blaivas JG, Jones M, Wang JT, Guan Z. Age related pathogenesis of nocturia in patients with overactive bladder. *J Urol* 2007;178(2):548–51; discussion 51.
15. Sutherst J, Brown M, Shawer M. Assessing the severity of urinary incontinence in women by weighing perineal pads. *Lancet* 1981;1(8230):1128–30.
16. Abrams P, Cardozo L, Fall M, et al. The standardisation of terminology of lower urinary tract function: report from the Standardisation Sub-committee of the International Continence Society. *Neurourol Urodyn* 2002;21(2):167–78.
17. Coyne KS, Sexton CC, Vats V, et al. National community prevalence of overactive bladder in the United States stratified by sex and age. *Urology* 2011;77(5):1081–7.
18. Resnick NM, Yalla SV. Management of urinary incontinence in the elderly. *N Engl J Med* 1985;313(13):800–5.
19. Børgesen SE, Gjerris F. The predictive value of conductance to outflow of CSF in normal pressure hydrocephalus. *Brain* 1982;105(Pt 1):65–86.
20. Owler BK, Pickard JD. Normal pressure hydrocephalus and cerebral blood flow: a review. *Acta Neurol Scand* 2001;104(6):325–42.
21. Bradley WG. Normal pressure hydrocephalus and deep white matter ischemia: which is the chicken, and which is the egg? *AJNR Am J Neuroradiol* 2001;22(9):1638–40.
22. Bateman GA. The pathophysiology of idiopathic normal pressure hydrocephalus: cerebral ischemia or altered venous hemodynamics? *AJNR Am J Neuroradiol.* 2008;29(1):198–203.
23. Bech-Azeddine R, Hogh P, Juhler M, Gjerris F, Waldemar G. Idiopathic normal-pressure hydrocephalus: clinical comorbidity correlated with cerebral biopsy findings and outcome of cerebrospinal fluid shunting. *J Neurol Neurosurg Psychiatry* 2007;78(2):157–61.
24. Edwards RJ, Dombrowski SM, Luciano MG, Pople IK. Chronic hydrocephalus in adults. *Brain Pathol* 2004;14(3):325–36.
25. Oi S, Di Rocco C. Proposal of "evolution theory in cerebrospinal fluid dynamics" and minor pathway hydrocephalus in developing immature brain. *Childs Nerv Syst* 2006;22(7):662–9.
26. Stephensen H, Tisell M, Wikkelsø C. There is no transmantle pressure gradient in communicating or noncommunicating hydrocephalus. *Neurosurgery* 2002;50(4):763–71; discussion 71–3.
27. Mori K, Mima T. To what extent has the pathophysiology of normal-pressure hydrocephalus been clarified? *Crit Rev Neurosurg* 1998;8(4):232–43.
28. Drake MJ, Fowler CJ, Griffiths D, et al. Neural control of the lower urinary and gastrointestinal tracts: supraspinal CNS mechanisms. *Neurourol Urodyn* 2010;29(1):119–27.
29. Klausner AP, Steers WD. The neurogenic bladder: an update with management strategies for primary care physicians. *Med Clin North Am* 2011;95(1):111–20.
30. Nour S, Svarer C, Kristensen JK, Paulson OB, Law I. Cerebral activation during micturition in normal men. *Brain* 2000;123(Pt 4):781–9.
31. de Groat WC. Anatomy and physiology of the lower urinary tract. *Urol Clin North Am* 1993;20(3):383–401.
32. Griffiths DJ, Tadic SD, Schaefer W, Resnick NM. Cerebral control of the lower urinary tract: how age-related changes might predispose to urge incontinence. *Neuroimage* 2009;47(3):981–6.
33. Abrams P, Cardozo L, Khoury S, Wein A (Eds.) *Incontinence: 2nd International Consultation on Incontinence, Paris*. Health Publications Ltd; 2002.
34. Klausner AP, Ibanez D, King AB, et al. The influence of psychiatric comorbidities and sexual trauma on lower urinary tract symptoms in female veterans. *J Urol* 2009;182(6):2785–90.
35. Vanneste JA. Diagnosis and management of normal-pressure hydrocephalus. *J Neurol* 2000;247(1):5–14.
36. Tsakanikas D, Relkin N. Normal pressure hydrocephalus. *Semin Neurol* 2007;27(1):58–65.

37. Abrams P, Cardozo L, Khoury S, Wein A (Eds.) *Incontinence: 4th International Consultation on Incontinence*. Health Publications Ltd; 2009.
38. Takeuchi T, Goto H, Izaki K, et al. [Postoperative patterns of improvement of symptoms and degrees of satisfaction in families of patients after operations for definite idiopathic normal pressure hydrocephalus: a long-term follow-up study.] (in Japanese) *No Shinkei Geka* 2007;35(8):773–9.
39. Homma Y, Yoshida M, Seki N, et al. Symptom assessment tool for overactive bladder syndrome – overactive bladder symptom score. *Urology* 2006;68(2):318–23.
40. Kuriyama N, Tokuda T, Kondo M, et al. Evaluation of autonomic malfunction in idiopathic normal pressure hydrocephalus. *Clin Auton Res* 2008;18(4):213–20.
41. Shprecher D, Schwalb J, Kurlan R. Normal pressure hydrocephalus: diagnosis and treatment. *Curr Neurol Neurosci Rep* 2008;8(5):371–6.
42. Abrams P, Andersson KE, Birder L, et al. Fourth International Consultation on Incontinence Recommendations of the International Scientific Committee: Evaluation and treatment of urinary incontinence, pelvic organ prolapse, and fecal incontinence. *Neurourol Urodyn* 29(1):213–40.
43. Relkin N, Marmarou A, Klinge P, Bergsneider M, Black PM. Diagnosing idiopathic normal-pressure hydrocephalus. *Neurosurgery* 2005;57(3 Suppl):S4–16; discussion ii–v.
44. Sakakibara R, Kanda T, Sekido T, et al. Mechanism of bladder dysfunction in idiopathic normal pressure hydrocephalus. *Neurourol Urodyn* 2008;27(6):507–10.
45. Sakakibara R, Uchiyama T, Kanda T, et al. [Urinary dysfunction in idiopathic normal pressure hydrocephalus]. *Brain Nerve* 2008;60(3):233–9.
46. Ahlberg J, Norlen L, Blomstrand C, Wikkelsø C. Outcome of shunt operation on urinary incontinence in normal pressure hydrocephalus predicted by lumbar puncture. *J Neurol Neurosurg Psychiatry* 1988;51(1):105–8.
47. Poggesi A, Pracucci G, Chabriat H, et al. Urinary complaints in nondisabled elderly people with age-related white matter changes: the Leukoaraiosis And DISability (LADIS) Study. *J Am Geriatr Soc* 2008;56(9):1638–43.
48. Factora R. When do common symptoms indicate normal pressure hydrocephalus? *Cleve Clin J Med* 2006;73(5):447–50, 52, 55–6 passim.
49. Bejjani GK, Hammer MD. Normal-pressure hydrocephalus: another treatable "dementia": Part 1. *Contemp Neurosurg* 2005;27(16).
50. Tikkinen KA, Auvinen A, Johnson TM, 2nd, et al. A systematic evaluation of factors associated with nocturia – the population-based FINNO study. *Am J Epidemiol* 2009;170(3):361–8.
51. Marmarou A, Young HF, Aygok GA, et al. Diagnosis and management of idiopathic normal-pressure hydrocephalus: a prospective study in 151 patients. *J Neurosurg* 2005;102(6):987–97.
52. Poca MA, Solana E, Martinez-Ricarte FR, et al. Idiopathic normal pressure hydrocephalus: results of a prospective cohort of 236 shunted patients. *Acta Neurochir Suppl* 114:247–53.
53. Cage TA, Auguste KI, Wrensch M, Wu YW, Gupta N. Self-reported functional outcome after surgical intervention in patients with idiopathic normal pressure hydrocephalus. *J Clin Neurosci* 18(5):649–54.
54. Savolainen S, Hurskainen H, Paljarvi L, Alafuzoff I, Vapalahti M. Five-year outcome of normal pressure hydrocephalus with or without a shunt: predictive value of the clinical signs, neuropsychological evaluation and infusion test. *Acta Neurochir (Wien)* 2002;144(6):515–23; discussion 23.
55. Pujari S, Kharkar S, Metellus P, et al. Normal pressure hydrocephalus: long-term outcome after shunt surgery. *J Neurol Neurosurg Psychiatry* 2008;79(11):1282–6.

Chapter 9

Normal pressure hydrocephalus grading scales

Masatsune Ishikawa

Introduction

Hakim and Adams [1] first described a surgically treatable syndrome in patients with symptoms of gait, cognition and urination, ventriculomegaly, and normal cerebrospinal fluid (CSF) pressure. The syndrome is now well known as normal pressure hydrocephalus (NPH). NPH can etiologically be divided into two types: idiopathic and secondary. Secondary NPH (sNPH) can develop within several weeks or months after a subarachnoid hemorrhage or meningitis. In contrast, idiopathic normal pressure hydrocephalus (iNPH) has no identifiable causes. The recent and rapid increase of the elderly population in developed nations has heightened the social importance of precise diagnosis and appropriate treatment for iNPH. An accurate assessment of symptoms and findings on neuroimaging is therefore important in selecting candidates for CSF shunt surgery. In this chapter, we critically review various assessment batteries that have been used in iNPH to date.

Scales

There are many NPH assessing scales, most of which aim to assess (1) level of general activity, (2) severity of respective NPH symptoms, (3) response to interventions such as cerebrospinal fluid (CSF) drainage tests or shunt surgery, and (4) short- and long-term outcome. More recently, the caregiver burden is also being assessed. The requirement of any grading scale should be to clearly define each symptom and be highly reproducible by different observers. They should be able to detect the degree of change in symptoms following interventions such as CSF drainage or CSF shunt surgery. Most assessment scales are qualitative and some are quantitative. The criticism leveled against qualitative assessments is that, although clinically useful, each grade of the scale might not span a similar interval, that the scale itself might exhibit inter-observer difference, and that data are not normalized. In contrast, while quantitative assessments are objective, they may reflect a limited part of NPH symptomatology. It is clear that comparative studies of various grading scales are necessary.

General activity

The well-known NPH scale created by Stein and Langfitt [2] (Table 9.1) assesses a patient's daily activity. This scale is closely related to the modified Rankin Scale [3] (Table 9.2), which is a widely used scale for measuring the degree of disability or dependence in the daily activities of patients with various disorders including NPH. Both scales are useful for assessing the patient's general level of activity; they are not quantitative and they display some indistinctness between the four to seven grades that characterize them.

NPH symptomatology assessment

Qualitative assessment

Gait disturbance, dementia, and urinary incontinence are the cardinal symptoms of NPH. Most NPH grading scales classify the severity of the NPH triad. Black's classification [4] (Table 9.3) has been long used for assessing the NPH triad: each domain of the triad is graded on a 4-point scale. Krauss et al. [5] (Table 9.4) also classified each symptom into four grades. However, because the parameters of each grade are rather ambiguous, this causes inter-observer difference. Furthermore, mild changes following interventions such as CSF drainage or shunting operation are poorly reflected. To overcome these drawbacks, the grading scales increased to five or more grades. Although these grading systems are basically composed of ordinal data, they are often regarded as continuous data and make a total [6] (Table 9.5). This makes it possible to assess relatively mild changes and to compare data before and after the interventions. Kubo et al. [7] confirmed that their five grades in each domain and their total showed high correlation with other qualitative or quantitative measures (Table 9.6). Kiefer et al. [8] added the assessment of headache and dizziness to the NPH triad and graded seven scales in degree. This could be useful for assessment of mild changes in symptoms caused by shunt malfunction or overdrainage during the follow-up period.

Quantitative or semiquantitative assessment

The timed up and go test (TUG) [9] is often used for quantitative assessment of gait in senile patients who are at risk of falls. The TUG measures, in seconds, the time a person takes to stand up from a standard armchair, walk 3 meters, turn, walk back to the chair, and sit down again. A time less than 10 seconds is regarded as normal. A score of more than or equal to 14 seconds has been shown to indicate a high risk of falls. Steps are also measured. TUG requires not only the ability to walk but also the understanding of orders. The ten-meter walk test is commonly used for assessment of gait speed. For older adults, the mean comfortable gait speed at 60 years is 135.9 cm/s for men and 129.6 cm/s for women [10]. These measurements are useful to compare the time or steps before and after the interventions such as the tap test or shunt surgery. Changes of gait can be assessed with video recording. However, there is no consensus for the cut-off level for defining improvement after CSF drainage or shunt surgery.

Dementia is a major symptom of NPH. Various kinds of neuropsychological tests have been used for assessment. For example, Kubo et al. [7] used the mini-mental state examination, frontal assessment battery and Trail Making Test A and B. Thomas et al. [11] used the Wechsler Memory scale, Rey–Osterrieth Complex Figure, Rey Auditory Verbal Learning Test, Line-Tracing test, Stroop Color and Word Test, and some others. Hellström et al. [12] used the Grooved Pegboard, the Rey Auditory Verbal Learning Test, and the Swedish Stroop test. Comparative study of the specificity and sensitivity of these neuropsychological tests is necessary to determine the most reliable test for prediction of shunt surgery.

Urinary incontinence is also a major symptom of NPH. Apart from various NPH grading scales, the international consultation on incontinence questionnaire-short form (ICIQ-SF) is also used [13].

Combination of qualitative and quantitative assessment

Hellström et al. [12] proposed a new NPH scale based on the idea that an iNPH scale should be discriminative,

Table 9.1 Stein–Langfitt classification (used with permission from reference 2)

Grading	Content
0	No neurological deficit, able to work
I	Minimal deficit, able to function independently at home
II	Some supervision required at home
III	Custodial care required in spite of considerable independent function
IV	No practical capacity for independent function

Table 9.2 Modified Rankin Scale (used with permission from reference 3)

Grade	Disability	Content
0	No symptoms	
1	No significant disability	Able to carry out all usual activities, despite some disability
2	Slight	Able to look after own affairs without assistance, but unable to carry out all previous activities
3	Moderate	Requires some help, but able to walk unassisted
4	Moderately severe	Unable to attend to own bodily needs without assistance, and unable to walk unassisted
5	Severe	Requires constant nursing care and attention, bedridden, incontinent
6	Dead	

Table 9.3 Black's classification (used with permission from reference 4)

Grade	Gait difficulty	Memory difficulty	Incontinence
No deficit	Walk with normal steps	No difficulty	Absent
Mild	Walk with small steps	Difficulty demonstrating only on testing	Present
Moderate	Able to walk alone but with a sense of insecurity, a visibly unstable gait, and frequent falls	Noticeable difficulty in daily affairs	Present
Severe	Unable to stand or walk at all or requires constant assistance in walking	Disoriented	Present

Table 9.4 Krauss's classification (used with permission from reference 5)

Grading	Gait disturbance	Cognitive impairment	Urinary disturbance
0	Normal	Normal	Normal
1	Cautious gait or impaired tandem gait	Minimal attentional or memory deficits	Sporadic incontinence or urge phenomena
2	Considerably unstable gait	Considerable attentional or memory deficits but oriented to situational contexts	Frequency incontinence
3	Unaided gait not possible	Not or only marginally oriented to situational context	No or only minimal control of bladder function

Table 9.5 Eide's classification (used with permission from reference 6)

Grading	Gait disturbance	Dementia	Urinary disturbance
5	Normal gait	Normal cognition	No subjective or objective incontinence
4	Gait is abnormal, but walking is possible without support. Imbalance when turning with short steps. Widened base and occasional falling	Memory problems exist that are reported by patient or family	Urinary urgency. Rare incontinence
3	A cane is needed. Independent walking is possible but is unstable or the patient falls	Important memory problems with more or less severe behavior disturbances	Occasional urinary incontinence
2	Support from another person is needed. Ambulation is possible with help	Severe dementia	Continuous urinary incontinence
1	Patient is bedridden or not able to ambulate	Vegetative	Both urinary and fecal incontinence
	Total score = 15.		

that is, it should distinguish well between patients with different levels of symptom severity, but also between iNPH patients and healthy individuals.

The scale consists of the four domains of gait, neuropsychology, balance, and continence (Table 9.7). The former two domains are continuous data and the latter two domains are ordinal data. All scores are calibrated and norm-based using data from an age-matched healthy population. Their NPH scale is well designed with a good statistical basis. However, it is complicated, and its use in clinical practice may be difficult.

Comorbidity

Comorbidity is one of major issues in the management of patients with iNPH.

Kiefer et al. [14] proposed a comorbidity index (Table 9.8). Comorbidity is divided into vascular risk factors, peripheral vascular occlusions, cerebrovascular disease, heart, and others, and each symptom or disease has to be assigned according to the indicated parameter-values (1–3 points). The sum represents the individual comorbidity index.

Further study is necessary to define the clinical significance of each parameter relevant to the clinical outcome.

Caregiver burden scale

In addition to assessing the patient's symptoms or general activity, the change in caregiver burden is a useful measure to assess the patient's ability to cope with daily life. Kazui et al. [15] assessed the change in caregiver burden after shunt surgery. They used the Zarit caregiver burden scale [16] and noted significant improvement in the total score and the personal strain factor one year after surgery, but not in the role strain. The improvement of cognitive impairment was the major factor in reducing caregiver burden.

Table 9.6 Kubo's classification (used with permission from reference 7)

Grading	Gait disturbance	Cognitive disturbance	Urinary disturbance
0	Normal	Normal	Normal
1	Complains of dizziness of drift and dysbasia but no objective gait disturbance	Existence of amnesia or inattention but no objective memory and attentional impairment	Pollakiuria or urinary urgency
2	Unstable but independent gait	Existence of amnesia or inattention but no disorientation of time and place	Occasional urinary incontinence (1–3 or more times per week but less than once per day)
3	Walking with any support	Existence of disorientation of time and place but conversation is possible	Continuous urinary incontinence (1 or more times per day)
4	Walking not possible	Disorientation for the situation or meaningful conversation impossible	Bladder function is almost or completely deficient
	Total score = 12.		

Table 9.7 Hellström's classification (used with permission from reference 12)

Gait

Ordinal rating of gait	Walk 10 min free pace, number of steps	Walk 10 min free pace, seconds
1 = 100	<15.50 = 100	<8.75 = 100
2 = 86	15.50–16.50 = 90	8.75–9.25 = 90
3 = 71	16.75–17.25 = 80	9.50–9.75 = 80
4 = 57	17.50–18.00 = 70	10.00–10.25 = 70
5 = 43	18.25–19.25 = 60	10.50–10.75 = 60
6 = 29	19.50–20.25 = 50	11.00–11.50 = 50
7 = 14	20.50–21.25 = 40	11.75–13.00 = 40
8 = 0	21.50–23.75 = 30	13.25–16.00 = 30
	24.00–27.25 = 20	16.25–19.25 = 20
	27.50–40.00 = 10	19.50–27.00 = 10
	>40 or fail = 0	>27 or fail = 0

The domain score is the mean value of available converted score.

Psychological studies

Grooved Pegboard, fastest trial	Rey, sum	Stroop, color naming	Stroop, interference
<79 = 100	>44 = 100	<68 = 100	<132 = 100
79–87 = 90	38–44 = 90	68–77 = 90	132–160 = 90
88–96 = 80	32–37 = 80	78–81 = 80	161–188 = 80
97–105 = 70	30–31 = 70	82–87 = 70	189–210 = 70
106–114 = 60	28–29 = 60	88–96 = 60	211–239 = 60
115–128 = 50	26–27 = 50	97–106 = 50	240–298 = 50
129–144 = 40	22–25 = 40	107–121 = 40	299–385 = 40
145–173 = 30	19–21 = 30	122–134 = 30	386–600 = 30
174–245 = 20	15–18 = 20	135–171 = 20	>600 = 20
246–600 = 10	11–14 = 10	172–300 = 10	Fail = 10
>600 or fail = 0	<11 or fail = 0	>300 or fail = 0	

The domain score is the mean value of available converted score.

Balance

1.	Able to stand independently for more than 30 s on either lower extremity alone.
2.	Able to stand independently for <30 s on either lower extremity alone.
3.	Able to stand independently with the feet together (at the heels) for more than 30 s.
4.	Able to stand independently with the feet together for <30 s.
5.	Able to stand independently with the feet apart (one foot length) for more than 30 s.
6.	Able to stand independently with the feet apart for <30 s.
7.	Unable to stand without assistance.

The rating is converted into domain scores according to the following: 1 = 100, 2 = 83, 3 = 67, 4 = 50, 5 = 33, 6 = 17 and 7 = 0.

Continence

1.	Normal.
2.	Urgency without incontinence.
3.	Infrequent incontinence without napkin.
4.	Frequent incontinence with napkin.
5.	Bladder incontinence.
6.	Bladder and bowel incontinence.

The rating is based on information of the most trustworthy source available. Patients with reduced awareness may deny incontinence despite its presence.

The results are converted into domain scores according to the following: 1 = 100, 2 = 80, 3 = 60, 4 = 40, 5 = 20 and 6 = 0.

$$\text{NPH Scale} = 2 \times \frac{\text{Gait} + \text{Neuropsychology} + \text{Balance} + \text{Continence}}{\text{5 or number of available domain scores}}$$

Table 9.8 Kiefer's comorbidity index (used with permission from reference 14)

	1 point	2 points	3 points
Vascular risk factors	Hypertension	Diabetes mellitus	
Peripheral vascular occlusions	Aortofemoral bypass Stent ICA stenosis	Peripheral vascular occlusion	
Cerebrovascular disease	Posterior circulation insufficiency	Vascular encephalopathy TIA PRIND	Cerebral infarct
Heart	Arrhythmia Valvular disease Heart failure Stent Aortocoronary bypass Infarction		
Others		Parkinson's disease	

ICA, internal carotid artery; TIA, transient ischemic attack; PRIND, prolonged reversible ischemic neurologic deficit.

Comparison between scales

There are many assessing scales for NPH: the degree of difference between them is not known. This unknown factor might explain, at least in part, the difference between the results of large cooperative studies. For example, the Japanese cooperative study for NPH [17] reported 80% improvement at one year after shunt operation assessed by the grading scale reported by Kubo et al. [7]. In contrast, the European cooperative study [18] reported 92% improvement using the grading scale reported by Hellström et al. [12]. While there appears to be a difference in the improvement rate between the two studies, assessment on the modified Rankin Scale showed 69% improvement in both studies. This discrepancy seems to suggest that the grading scale with more parameters can demonstrate higher improvement rates than that with fewer parameters. To overcome this problem, we need to use the same assessment measures for NPH.

Conclusion

Many grading scales for assessing general activity and symptoms of NPH are readily available from the literature. However, most of them are not validated and normalized. It clearly behooves the medical community to develop standardized measures for NPH assessment without further delay.

References

1. Hakim S, Adams RD. The special clinical problems of symptomatic hydrocephalus with normal cerebrospinal fluid pressure: observations on cerebrospinal fluid dynamics. *J Neurol Sci* 1965;2:302–27.
2. Stein SC, Langfitt TW. Normal-pressure hydrocephalus. Predicting the results of cerebrospinal fluid shunting. *J Neurosurg* 1974;41:463–70.
3. Wilson JL, Hareendran A, Grant M, et al. Improving the assessment of outcomes in stroke: Use of a structured interview to assign grades on the modified Rankin scale. *Stroke* 2002;33:2243–6.
4. Black PM. Idiopathic normal-pressure hydrocephalus Results of shunting in 62 patients. *J Neurosurg* 1980;52:371–7.
5. Krauss JK, Droste DW, Vach W, et al. Cerebrospinal fluid shunting in idiopathic normal-pressure hydrocephalus of the elderly: effect of periventricular and deep white matter lesions. *Neurosurgery* 1996;39:292–9; discussion 299–300.
6. Eide PK. Intracranial pressure parameters in idiopathic normal pressure hydrocephalus patients treated with ventriculo-peritoneal shunts. *Acta Neurochir (Wien)* 2006;148:21–9; discussion 29.
7. Kubo Y, Kazui H, Yoshida T et al. Validation of grading scale for evaluating symptoms of idiopathic normal-pressure hydrocephalus. *Dement Geriatr Cogn Disord* 2008;25:37–45.

8. Kiefer M, Eymann R, Komenda Y, Steudel WI. A grading system for chronic hydrocephalus. *Zentralbl Neurochir* 2003;64:109–15.
9. Podsiadlo D, Richardson S. The timed 'up & go': a test of basic functional mobility for frail elderly persons. *Am Geriatr Soc* 1991;39:142.
10. Bohannon RS. Comfortable and maximum walking speed of adults aged 20–79 years: reference values and detarminants. *Age Ageing* 1997;26:15–19.
11. Thomas G, McGirt M, Woodworth G, et al. Baseline neuropsychological profile and cognitive response to cerebrospinal fluid shunting for idiopathic normal pressure hydrocephalus. *Dement Geriatr Cogn Disord* 2005;20:163–8.
12. Hellström P, Klinge P, Tans J, Wikkelsø C. A new scale for assessment of severity and outcome in iNPH. *Acta Neurol Scand* 2012;126:229–37.
13. Avery K, Donovan J, Abrams P. Validation of a new questionnaire for incontinence: the international consultation on incontinence questionnaire (ICI-Q). *Neurourol Urodyn* 2001;20:510–11.
14. Kiefer M, Eymann R, Steudel WL. Outcome predictors for normal-pressure hydrocephalus. *Acta Neurochir Suppl* 2006;96:364–7.
15. Kazui H, Mori E, Hashimoto M, et al. Effect of shunt operation on idiopathic normal pressure hydrocephalus in reducing caregiver burden: evidence from SINPHONI. *Dement Geriatr Cogn Disord* 2011;31:363–70.
16. Zarit SH, Reever K, Bach-Peterson J. Relatives of the impaired elderly: correlates of feelings of burden. *Gerontologist* 1980;20:649–55.
17. Hashimoto M, Ishikawa M, Mori E, et al. Diagnosis of idiopathic normal pressure hydrocephalus is supported by MRI-based scheme: a prospective cohort study. *CSF Res* 2010;7:18.
18. Klinge P, Hellström P, Tans J, et al. One-year outcome in the European multicenter study on iNPH. *Acta Neurol Scand* 2012;126(3):145–53.

Chapter 10

The differential diagnosis of normal pressure hydrocephalus

Daniele Rigamonti, Marianne Juhler, and Carsten Wikkelsø

Introduction

Hakim and colleagues, in their paper describing the syndrome of normal pressure hydrocephalus (NPH) in three patients, recapitulated the clinical presentation as follows: "a mild impairment of memory, slowness and paucity of thought and action, unsteadiness of gait and unwitting urination" (Hakim's triad) [1]. They also highlighted two important features of the syndrome: "The symptomatology was unobtrusive, having no assignable date of onset, and evolved over a period of weeks and few months ... The most striking feature of the condition was the rapid restitution of the patient's health as the result of lowering of the cerebrospinal-fluid pressure through surgical shunting."

They further stressed that because "the clinical picture corresponds essentially to that of a mild form of dementia," it was obligatory for the treating physician to distinguish such a mild dementia "occurring without obvious cause in a middle-aged person ... from the large number of dementing illnesses of the presenium and the senium." Interestingly, pneumo-encephalography demonstrated, in all three cases described in the original paper by Hakim, an obstruction to the CSF, due to a blockage of the subarachnoid space (SAS) at the cervical-medullary junction in the first two cases and to a colloid cyst in the third [1].

Nowadays, thanks to much improved imaging modalities (CT and MRI) we can quickly recognize ventriculomegaly. However, even in the presence of clinical symptoms, in a significant percentage of cases, in the elderly, no obvious blockage can be detected. NPH in the absence of a definitive cause has been called "idiopathic" NPH (iNPH). The late Professor Marmarou led an effort to better identify this condition from a clinical standpoint. The consensus guidelines published in the USA defined iNPH as probable, possible, and unlikely depending on presence or absence of several elements in the history, neurological examination, imaging, and response to specific diagnostic procedures [2,3]. The guidelines underlined the fact that because iNPH frequently is accompanied by multiple and significant comorbidities, its diagnosis remains challenging. The lack of awareness about NPH on the part of the medical profession further complicates matters [4].

The recently updated Japanese guidelines draw attention to a specific MRI pattern of disproportionately enlarged subarachnoid space hydrocephalus (DESH), believed to be pathognomonic of iNPH [5,6].

This chapter will discuss why establishing the diagnosis of NPH remains a challenge fifty years after its classic description.

The neurological examination of the NPH patient

Hakim and colleagues described the following cognitive elements as characteristic of the syndrome: "lack of spontaneity and initiative, faulty concentration, distractibility, lack of interest, apathy and inertia ... Inner psychic life seemed to be impoverished, and the patient was bereft of thoughts." The findings on the rest of the neurological anamnesis and examination were insignificant: "headache was absent or negligible. Papilledema did not occur. Mild horizontal nystagmus was present in all 3 cases ... Strength of the limbs was maintained; there was no frank cerebellar ataxia. The plantar reflexes were usually flexor or equivocal until a late stage ... The unsteadiness of gait, which was difficult to characterize, was not clearly ascribable to cerebellar deficit. Aphasia, dyspraxia and agnosia were not obvious. The circumference of the cranium was normal" [1].

Adult Hydrocephalus, ed. Daniele Rigamonti. Published by Cambridge University Press.

Younger patients more often have hydrocephalus because of a visible obstruction and in most cases clinical symptoms and signs of elevated intracranial pressure. However, some of these may present later in life with very large ventricles and an "NPH like" clinical picture – an entity that has been described with the acronym LOVA (longstanding overt ventriculomegaly in adults) [7–9].

Elderly patients with presumed iNPH span a continuum from very healthy and functional to very sick and disabled. We have encountered people with impressive ventriculomegaly on MRI and both high IQ and great physical fitness with complaints of subjective difficulties. Given the fact that our tests are based on a control population whose "normal level of function" is at a lower level than the baseline function of these particular individuals (see Cases 1 and 2 at the end of the chapter), we could not detect any deficit.

At the other end of the continuum, we have also many patients with a very complicated medical history and a neurological exam as well (see Cases 3 and 4). This reflects the presence of many comorbidities including hypertension in almost half of the patients, diabetes mellitus in about a fifth, cerebrovascular disease in various degrees in more than half of the patients, and dementia ranging from 15% to 75%, while "pure" cases of iNPH occur in barely a fifth of patients [10–12]. As a consequence, besides gait, cognitive, and urinary symptoms, the careful examiner will find paratonia of lower extremities, increased need of sleep, abnormal Romberg test, and retropulsion, features that are found in more than half of patients, while focal neurological signs, polyneuropathy, and cerebellar signs occur in at least one-fifth of the patients.

The diagnostic work-up of the NPH patient

The original diagnosis of NPH relied upon the presence of mild dementia, gait, and urinary difficulties (Hakim's triad) seen in association with ventriculomegaly on pneumo-encephalogram.

Nowadays the recognition of NPH is complicated by two factors. While the availability of MRI has helped the early recognition of ventriculomegaly, this often precedes the appearance of the full triad. At the other end of the spectrum, in the older population, comorbidities are much more pronounced and might mask the NPH symptomatology especially if it is slow in development [13–15].

Several authors believe that the presence of the full triad most likely represents an advanced stage of the disease and advocate reaching an earlier diagnosis in every case [16]. We were able to document less likelihood of recovery after surgery, as the duration of symptoms increased [10]. Recent data from Sweden confirmed that a delay in intervention after confirmation of the diagnosis, in fact, is accompanied by a measurable deterioration of function and a lesser degree of improvement than in patients who underwent surgery more rapidly [17].

Furthermore, a recent publication claimed a high correlation between presence and severity of all major symptoms in iNPH [18].

Gait dysfunction

The presence of gait difficulties, as the first and prominent symptom, is essential to make the diagnosis of NPH [10].

Gait features that are classically described in iNPH are the wide base, the magnetic or "glued feet," shuffling and slow pace. Gait impairment in NPH, however, ranges from difficulties running, fear of using escalators, difficulties walking on a slope or uneven surfaces or stairs, difficulties getting up from a chair, needing to use an assistive device such as a cane or a walker, to inability to stand and walk. (Please refer to Chapter 6 on pathophysiology of gait for a more detailed discussion of the gait characteristics.)

The 10-meter gait test, the timed up and go (TUG) test, the Tinetti gait and balance test, and the 6 ft walk are widely used, but not always satisfactory and adequate, tools to objectively measure the deficits. Objectively there could be no obvious sign in the patient who cannot run. Conversely, we could assess the patient who takes short steps (less than 1 foot in length), walks at a reduced pace and on a wider base, who has difficulty turning on his/her long axis (more than 4–6 steps to make a 360° turn).

The challenge resides in the fact that gait and balance problems in the elderly can be caused by a plethora of other processes, and it is unrealistic to expect the general practitioner or a family member to recognize the gait of NPH that is quite characteristic to the eyes of the expert. So the lack of awareness of iNPH and the presence of comorbidities frequently confound the general practitioner or the neurologist, leading unfortunately to a harmful delay in diagnosis.

There are several conditions that may deceive the practitioner and prevent the recognition of the causative role of iNPH in the development of gait problems. Parkinsonism (Parkinson's disease and secondary parkinsonism) in its early phase may present a diagnostic challenge because several features are similar: small, shuffling steps, unsteadiness on turning, and a looming posture. However, the narrow-based gait, the loss of the arm swing, and the presence of tremor, hypokinesia, and rigidity are not features of NPH and should not mislead the thoughtful examiner. Lumbar stenosis usually causes low back pain, but weakness and radicular sensory disturbances precipitated by activity might affect the gait and create a source of confusion. Cervical spondylotic myelopathy causing upper motor neuron weakness in the lower extremities, with hyperreflexia and spasticity with or without sensory changes, will affect a person's gait and balance. MRI and CT show the cord compression due to osteophyte formation. Peripheral neuropathy of a metabolic, infectious or other nature, and arthritis of the hip and knees can be aggravating gait problems, too [13–15].

Cognitive deficit

iNPH is responsible only for a small proportion of cognitive difficulties experienced by the elderly; however, because of its reversible nature it must be considered in the differential diagnosis. Because iNPH patients are advanced in age (usually in their seventies or even older), the likelihood of finding Alzheimer's disease (AD) or other forms of dementia in these patients is high.

The mini-mental state examination (MMSE) is useful in broadly assessing the level of dementia (or its absence); a low score in this test is not typical of NPH and should immediately raise the suspicious of a cortical dementia. More sensitive cognitive evaluation of iNPH patients requires specific tests for the assessment of subcortical frontal lobe deficits (executive dysfunction, impaired attention, visuospatial dysfunction, and psychomotor slowing) such as the Rey Auditory Verbal Learning Test, Stroop test, Grooved Pegboard, Trail Making A and B Test, and digit span test.

Aphasia, apraxia, or agnosia should immediately raise suspicion of conditions with cortical pathology (Alzheimer's disease, frontotemporal dementia, and vascular dementia). Depression might mimic dementia and needs to be ruled out. The presence of resting tremor and lead-pipe rigidity with visual hallucinations should raise the suspicion of dementia with Lewy bodies (DLB) [13–15]. (Please refer to Chapter 7 on pathophysiology of the cognitive deficits for a more detailed discussion.)

AD is the most common form of dementia; it usually tends to follow a longer course, with prominent cortical dysfunction like apraxia and language disturbance and prominent memory disorders. Enlarged cortical sulci are seen on MRI. Early AD may resemble depression or pure memory disorders (Korsakoff amnestic syndrome). In AD positron emission tomography (PET) scanning may reveal hypometabolism and hypoperfusion in the temporal and parietal lobes. Cerebrospinal fluid (CSF) levels of Aβ42, tau, and phospho-tau are valuable biomarkers of AD. (Please refer to Chapter 15 on biomarkers for a more detailed discussion.)

Vascular dementia is very common in the elderly; it is often characterized by a long history of hypertension, focal neurological symptoms or signs, stepwise progression and fairly sudden onset of dementia. Pseudobulbar palsy (dysarthria, dysphagia, and emotional instability), focal motor and/or sensory deficit, ataxia, hyperreflexia, and Babinski sign are usually present. MRI shows either multiple cortical infarcts or several smaller infarcts of the deep white matter, basal ganglia, and thalamus (lacunar state). The major challenge to the clinician is subcortical vascular dementia, which can present with symptoms and signs that are more or less identical with those seen in iNPH [13,14].

The presence of a cerebrovascular history and stigmata on MRI should not prevent the recognition of the coexistent ventriculomegaly and reduce the responsibility to investigate if some symptoms might perchance be due to NPH. Recently Tisell et al. showed in a randomized controlled study that patients presented with pronounced white matter changes on MRI and symptoms and signs compatible with iNPH improved significantly after shunting [19].

The European multicenter study on iNPH confirmed that after treatment patients with vascular comorbidity improved to a similar degree as those without, suggesting that patients with vascular comorbidity should not be excluded from being considered for shunt surgery. However, by the same token, it should not be forgotten that severe vascular diseases as determined by a high Kiefer comorbidity score has a very negative prognosis [20–22].

Frontotemporal dementia (FTD) is a heterogeneous group of disorders that produce frontal and temporal lobe degeneration and affect behavior and language. FTD, the third most common cause of dementia after

AD and vascular dementia, affects younger people (before age 60) and presents with behavioral problems or aphasia. MRI shows frontal and temporal lobe atrophy, and PET might show corresponding hypometabolism. Usually the most affected side correlates with the most prominent clinical feature: right-sided in the behavioral variant and left-sided in the language variant. We have occasionally treated patients who were diagnosed with FTD, but also had hydrocephalus: their dementia did not improve, but their gait benefited dramatically from the surgery (Case 3).

Corticobasal degeneration is a tauopathy related to FTD. It involves both cortex and basal ganglia, usually causing unilateral limb clumsiness/sensory loss/apraxia associated with extrapyramidal rigidity, bradykinesia, and postural tremor. In this situation as well, NPH might coexist and an attempt at dealing with it might be considered (Case 4). Progressive supranuclear palsy (PSP) usually is very distinctive in its presentation, with dementia, supranuclear ophthalmoplegia (especially down gaze), pseudobulbar palsy, and dystonia with or without extrapyramidal rigidity being the main features. In Huntington's disease, psychiatric symptoms and chorea usually precede dementia, which is characterized by loss of memory and executive function.

Lewy body disease presents with fluctuating cognitive abilities and visual hallucinations associated with rigidity and bradykinesia typical of parkinsonism. Creutzfeldt–Jakob disease (CJD) is a prion disease causing rapidly progressive dementia that begins either as a mild global cognitive impairment or as a focal cortical disorder (aphasia, agnosia, or apraxia). Psychiatric symptoms and changes in personality can be significant. Myoclonus, extrapyramidal signs, and cerebellar signs are frequently present.

Chronic subdural hematomas (cSDH) usually present with confusion and dementia, and hemiparesis, several weeks or months after a mild trauma in patients with cerebral atrophy, history of alcoholism, or on hemodialysis or anticoagulation. Less common are visual field defects and aphasia. CT and MRI show the frequently bilateral, extra-axial collection of fluid of homogeneous or mixed density, associated with obliteration of the underlying sulci and mass effect on the ventricular system.

A brain tumor, such as an infiltrating glioma, invading the frontal, temporal lobes and the corpus callosum might produce dementia. Apathy, impaired concentration, and slowness are more prominent. In this case too, however, MRI is diagnostic. Radiotherapy and chemotherapy may be aggravating the symptoms.

Leptomeningeal spread of cancer may present with confusion and multiple cranial neuropathies. Cytological study of the CSF will provide the diagnosis if the images do not show meningeal enhancement in the areas where the deficits are caused.

Chronic traumatic encephalopathy following repeated head injuries leads to progressive impairment of concentration and memory, personality changes, rigidity, tremor, and bradykinesia. MRI shows cortical atrophy.

Infectious processes such as HIV, syphilis, and progressive multifocal leukoencephalopathy (PML) due to JC papova virus can produce minor neurocognitive disorders and progress to dementia. The history usually is helpful and appropriate laboratory tests will confirm the diagnosis.

Metabolic diseases such as alcoholism, hypothyroidism, and vitamin B_{12} deficiency should be considered in the differential diagnosis and the appropriate tests ordered if a suspicion occurs.

Organ failures may produce dementia and confound the NPH diagnosis: dialysis dementia, Wilson's disease, and non-wilsonian hepatocerebral degeneration [13,14].

Urinary dysfunction

The bladder symptoms of increased frequency, urgency, and incontinence should be distinguished from other urological conditions. Urinary incontinence could be related to recurrent urinary tract infections and medications, benign prostatic hypertrophy (BPH) in men, and pelvic floor laxity and stress incontinence in women.

Bladder symptoms in NPH result from detrusor hyperactivity. Although several tests can objectively document the dysfunction in these patients, they are rarely used in a consistent fashion. The utilization of a validated questionnaire is a valid surrogate for the assessment and grading of the urinary dysfunction. (Please refer to Chapter 8 on pathophysiology of urologic dysfunction for a more detailed discussion.)

Imaging evaluation

Since Hakim and his colleagues diagnosed NPH on the basis of pneumo-encephalography, imaging has taken gigantic steps. Isotope cisternogram was for a while the gold standard for the diagnosis of NPH and demonstrated NPH secondary to a subarachnoid space blockage when it showed reflux into the ventricular system. But it was the advent of CT first, followed by MRI, that transformed the field. The causes of hydrocephalus, when present, are clearly revealed. Blockage at the foramen of Monro, at the aqueduct, at the outlet of the fourth ventricle, in the basal cisterns, and at the level of the convexity can now be promptly recognized (please refer to Chapter 11 on basic imaging for a more detailed discussion) and the pathophysiology of iNPH is now being actively investigated (please refer to Chapter 12 on advanced imaging for a more detailed discussion).

It is routine these days to use both CT and MRI in the evaluation of NPH patients, although we foresee that this practice might change in the future due to cost or safety concerns.

CT is frequently the initial test and is certainly useful in the diagnosis of hydrocephalus, secondary for example to a subarachnoid hemorrhage (SAH). A CT scan could immediately give information on the degree of ventriculomegaly, the presence of periventricular edema, and the tightness of the cortical SAS.

MRI provides a superior anatomical and physiological definition of the ventricular system and the SAS. There is evidence that MRI could help discriminate between NPH and AD by studying the degree of dilatation of the perihippocampal fissures (PHFs), which are much more dilated inAD [23].

Several sequences are used, some of which should be considered "core" images and others "advanced" images. Core sequences provide information that is essential to the management of the patient; advanced imaging sequences provide images that are critical in furthering the understanding of the mechanism of the disease. (Please refer to Chapters 11 and 12 on basic and advanced imaging for more details.)

Invasive evaluation of CSF physiology

This diagnostic test provides information about CSF dynamics and predicts outcome. It consists in either removal of CSF accompanied by pre- and post-functional evaluation, or an infusion (bolus or continuous) test.

Spinal tap test (STT)

STT consists of the removal of more than 30 ml of CSF from the patient. Opening pressure should be measured at the beginning. CSF should be sent for routine and special examinations. Routine examinations include cytology, microbiology, and chemistry. (For special testing please refer to Chapter 15.)

An unequivocal improvement in the functioning of the patient after the STT has a very strong positive predictive value (PPV) for a beneficial effect of shunting. Different authors have different criteria that rely on either percentage improvement or improvement beyond 1 standard deviation (SD) in either gait or cognitive testing.

Continuous spinal or ventricular drainage

The test requires the insertion of an indwelling spinal or ventricular catheter for a few days and an hourly drainage of 5–10 ml of CSF. The CSF is analyzed in the same fashion as with the STT. This test has the advantage of demonstrating an improvement in some patients who do not respond to the STT.

Infusion test

There are several infusion methods available: bolus, the continuous and the pressure controlled.

In spite of some data suggesting the contrary, several series reporting the results of intrathecal infusion technique with constant flow suggest that outflow resistance (R_{out}) is pathologically elevated in patients with NPH, while it is normal in patients with cerebral atrophy; the compliance (C_p) is normal (see Chapters 13 and 14 for more details).

Intracranial pressure (ICP) measurements

We have not found ICP monitoring helpful in our experience at Johns Hopkins. The problem might reside in the fact that measurements have been performed in patients with symptoms suggestive of a CSF circulation disorder and patients with "low" pressures have been presumed to be normal. Thus "normal values" have been extrapolated from a symptomatic population. If truly normal values were found to be lower than so far assumed, then NPH could be a disorder of moderately, chronically elevated ICP. Data from the department at the University of Copenhagen are suggestive of normal ICP around 0 mmHg in supine position and −10 mmHg or below in standing position.

According to the recently concluded European iNPH multicenter study, CSF tap test and R_{out} can be used for selecting patients for shunt surgery, given their high positive predictive value (PPV >90%), but they cannot be used for excluding patients for surgery, given the very low negative predictive value (NPV <20%) [24].

iNPH grading scales

Over the years several authors have attempted to grade the clinical severity of NPH patients and assess their outcome after treatment. These tools have helped us enormously to improve preoperative assessment of patients and assessment of outcome. (Please refer to Chapter 9 for more details on grading scales.)

Outcome

Considering that surgery produces long-term improvement in about 70% of cases and that improvement might affect all three elements of the triad, we lament the fact that in the medical community at large there is not enough interest in trying to recognize this reversible form of dementia, offering patients a chance of even partial recovery [10,25]. A reason for this lack of enthusiasm could reside in a negative attitude about aggressively managing what some neurologists believe to be a nonexistent condition. More sadly, the lack of interest could be the result of sheer ignorance as documented by Conn [4]. For whatever reason the patient goes undiagnosed, the delay leads to further progression of the deficits and a diminished recovery after a delayed surgery. Several authors have commented on the negative correlation between diagnostic delay and postsurgical recovery [10, 16]. The presence of coexisting AD (31.3%) might provide yet another reason for poor long-term outcomes after shunting [26]. (Please refer to Chapter 20 on outcome for a more detailed discussion of this topic.)

Final thoughts

A study from Japan demonstrated a prevalence of iNPH of 0.51% in people aged 61 years or older, while asymptomatic ventriculomegaly with iNPH features on MRI (AVIM) occurred in 1.01% of this elderly population [27]. A population study from Norway showed a prevalence of probable iNPH of 21.9/100 000 and an incidence of 5.5/100 000/year; the age-related prevalence climbed to 181.7/100 000 above age 70 [28]. The total incidence of surgery for hydrocephalus in Norway over a 5-year period was 1.09/100 000/year (ranging between 0.84 and 1.47/100 000/year) [29]. In Sweden the annual incidence of surgery for every type of hydrocephalus was 3.4/100 000; surgery for iNPH was the most common (47%) [30]. (Please refer to Chapter 5 on epidemiology for a more detailed discussion of this topic.)

These data suggest that only 18–31% of patients with iNPH were offered surgery in the Scandinavian countries, where the condition is better known than in the USA. This clearly suggests a failure of recognition of the disease.

The medical profession clearly does not think enough about NPH, and the reasons are unclear. We think that we should stop overwhelming the medical community with a complicated classification and an even more complicated explanation of the pathogenesis. We believe that focusing on "ventriculomegaly" would be much more beneficial in raising the awareness of the condition.

The patient with ventriculomegaly should be referred to a neurological or neurosurgical center, where an appropriate evaluation would place him/her into the appropriate category based on the degree of symptomatology:

(1) Asymptomatic patients or patients with minimal symptoms of NPH.
(2) Patients with clear symptoms of NPH, no obvious comorbidities and clear response to diagnostic tests.
(3) Patients with advanced symptoms of NPH and significant associated pathology.

Patients with minimal or no symptoms should be carefully monitored, evaluated with a detailed neurocognitive and motor examination their status, and encouraged to undergo a spinal tap at some point to determine if their perceived sense of well-being is masking an insidiously developing deficit.

Patients with clear symptoms and clear response to CSF challenge that can be unequivocally measured are easier to manage. There is, however, fairly powerful evidence from the European hydrocephalus study that the tap test and the infusion tests have a poor NPV [24]. It is then prudent in patients in whom the symptoms and the images are characteristic of NPH to discuss the possibility of surgery even in the absence of a positive response to a CSF challenge test.

Patients with advanced symptoms of NPH and associated pathology represent a major challenge. In these patients the task is to determine if by eliminating the contribution of NPH to the disability a significant improvement in the quality of life could be obtained. Given some recent evidence obtained by the group of Wikkelsø and our own personal experience, it seems wise to at least consider surgery in this group as well.

In all groups undergoing surgery we recommend paying close attention to the long-term function of the shunt and intervening at the first sign of malfunction.

Case 1 A 53-year-old executive underwent a work-up for thyroid problems that included an MRI. He walks for 40 minutes every day with his wife. His neurological exam is completely within normal limits. His timed up and go (TUG) test time is 6 seconds, his Tinetti gait and balance score is 28/28. He can stand on one leg for 1 minute and 46 seconds with no problem. MRI showed ventriculomegaly, crowding on the convexity, bowing of the corpus callosum, dilatation of the third ventricle with bulging outward of the wall and aqueductal pathology. (See Figure 10.1.)

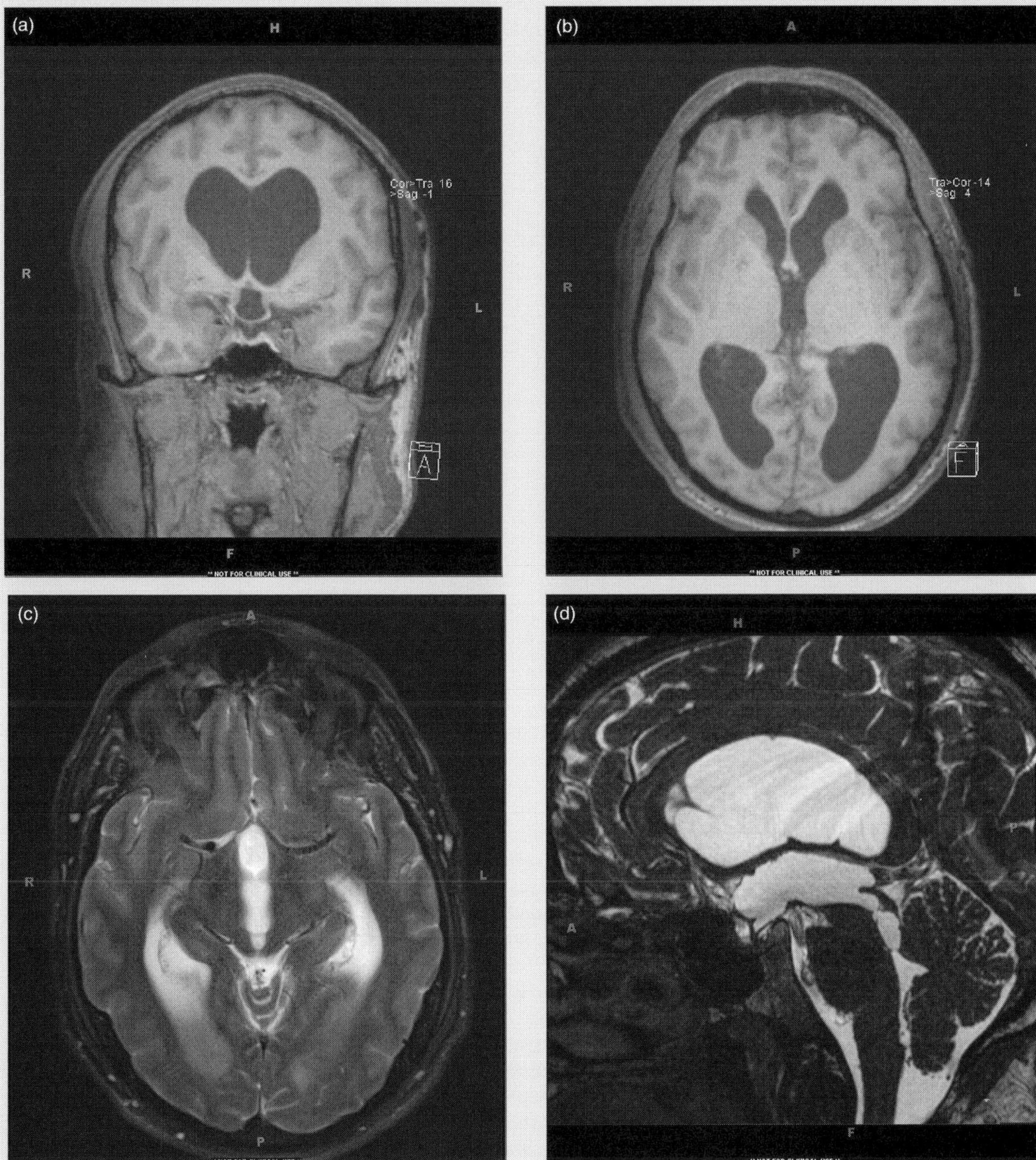

Figure 10.1 (a and b) Coronal and axial T1 demonstrate tight subarachnoid space (SAS) associated with ventriculomegaly. (c and d) Axial and sagittal T2 show a cyst in the posterior portion of the aqueduct.

Case 2 A 58-year-old professor slipped on ice in February 2010 while jogging and landed on her head. Afterward she felt dizzy when putting on make-up, washing hair, and working in the yard. A marathoner, she became unable to run. She noted occasional difficulty remembering a word during a lecture and irritability. She had urinary urgency, and frequency. Her neurological exam was normal, her Tinetti was 28/28 and her TUG was 7 s, 7 s, and 6 s.

MRI showed ventriculomegaly without an obvious obstruction. She underwent a lumbar puncture on June 24, 2011 and for several days afterward she could run and her thoughts were "streaming" better. Her friends noted that her language was more fluent. She insisted on having surgery and underwent ventriculoperitoneal shunting on August 19, 2011. At follow-up 18 months later, she felt the best: her energy was back, she was training for a marathon, and doing heavy yard work. (See Figure 10.2.)

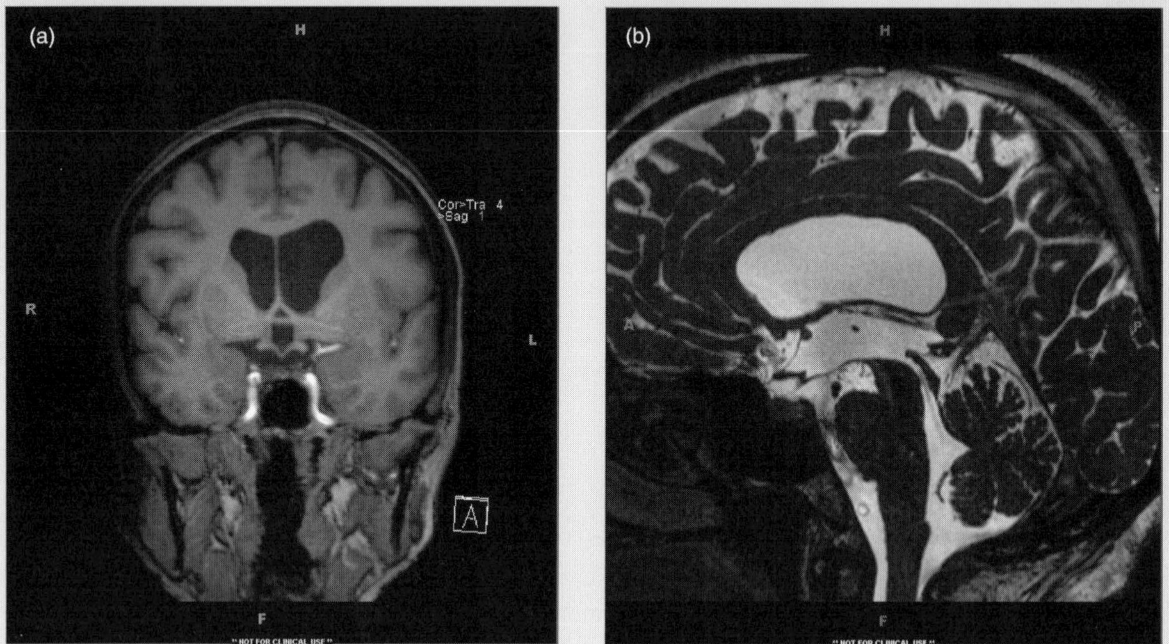

Figure 10.2 (a) Coronal T1 shows ventricular dilatation, the SAS is less tight. (b) Sagittal T2 shows that the floor of the third ventricle is bulging, suggesting a gradient of pressure.

Case 3 A 64-year-old woman began having urgency and incontinence in 2009. A year later, she developed short-term memory loss, and needed assistance with activities of daily living. A neurocognitive evaluation suggested possible frontotemporal dementia. At the same time she developed a shuffling, slow, wide-based gait and tendency to fall. She rapidly went from walking normally, to using a walker first, then a wheelchair. Sinemet, Aricept, and Namenda did not help.

At the time of her visit in March 2011, she was unable to do any chores around the house or bathe herself. Her MMSE was 24/30 (missed orientation answers, forgot one item, was unable to copy two pentagons). Her Tinetti was 5/28 (with maximal support). Her TUG was 1 min 36 s, 1 min 22 s with maximal support. MRI showed a significant amount of atrophy and some periventricular edema and no evidence of obstruction. She improved after a large volume spinal tap and underwent shunting on April 6, 2011 and revision on January 6, 2012. On follow-up visit on January 23, 2013 she was walking independently. Her MMSE was 28/30 (missing date and unable to draw intersecting pentagons): a dramatic improvement up from 24/30. Her Tinetti was 19/28: also a dramatic improvement up from 5/28. Her TUG decreased to a good 22 s, 22 s, 20 s down from 1 min 36 s, 1 min 22 s. (See Figure 10.3.)

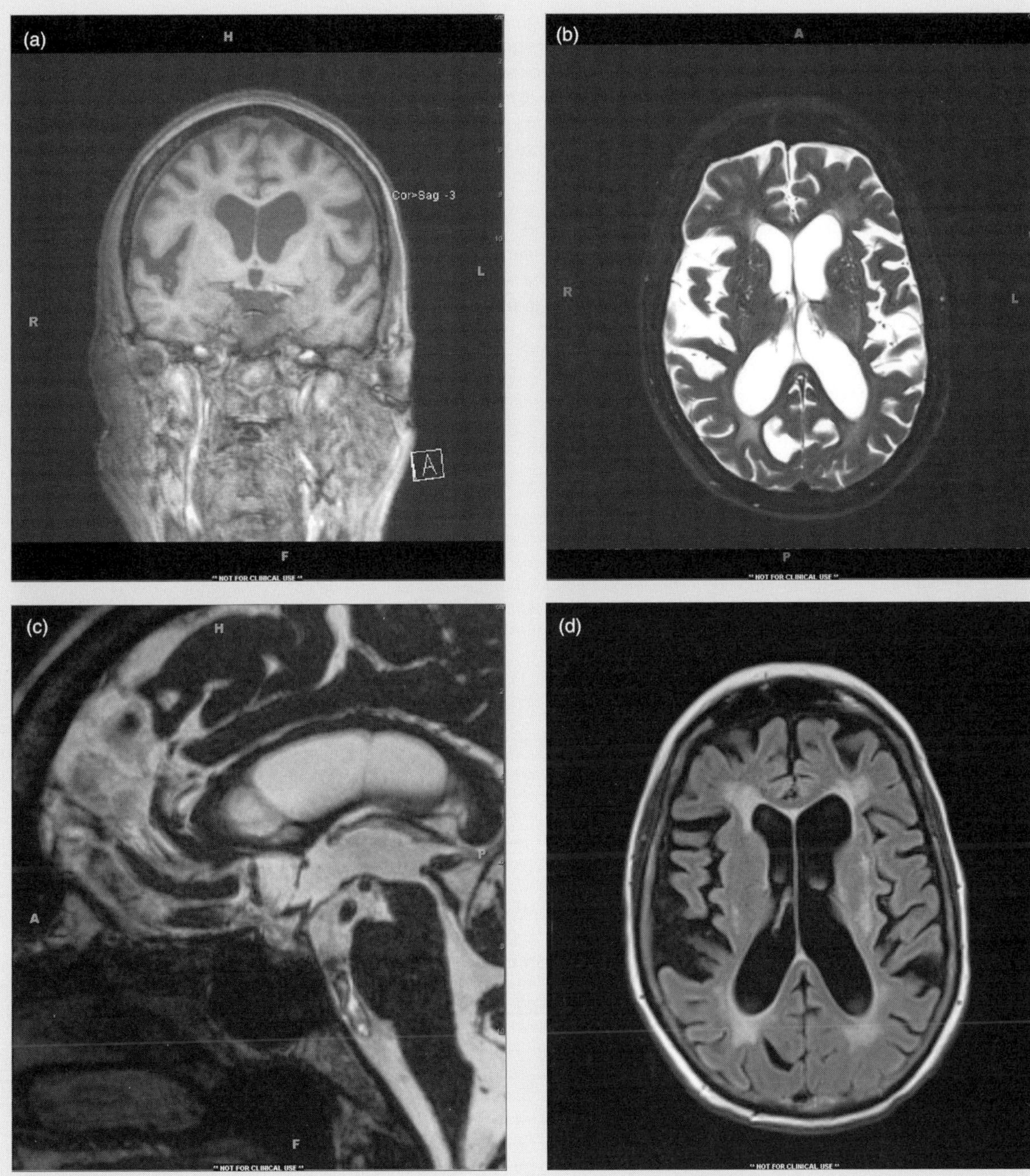

Figure 10.3 (a) Coronal T1 shows dilated ventricles and dilated SAS. (b) Axial T2 shows a severe degree of atrophy. (c) Sagittal T2 shows normal appearance of the third ventricle walls. (d) Axial FLAIR shows atrophy, white matter changes.

Case 4 A 70-year-old woman had problems with cognition and memory for several years ago. She had been a competitive softball and basketball player until 30–31 years of age (she did not remember why she stopped). MRI obtained because of severe headache at age 50 (1993) showed hydrocephalus. At the time, she was fully functional. In September 2008, after hip surgery her memory deteriorated. In fall of 2011, there was a rapid decline: she slowed down in her walking and began to have frequent falls, she developed urinary incontinence, and slept about 12 hours a night as well as napping during the day. She needed assistance to walk into the clinic. Her MMSE score was 7/30. Formal neurocognitive tests suggested dementia, and PET showed hypometabolism in temporal regions. Tinetti was 9/28; TUG was 18 s, 18 s, and 17 s.

MRI showed significant ventriculomegaly with Evans index of 0.42 and aqueductal stenosis.

Endoscopic third ventriculostomy and brain biopsy were performed on September 5, 2012. Biopsy indicated a moderate level of AD-related pathology and a non-Alzheimer tauopathy. On November 9, 2012 her follow-up exam showed MMSE of 9/30, up from 7/30. Tinetti was 26/28, up from 9/28. TUG times were 11 s and 12 s, down from 18 s, 18 s, and 17 s.

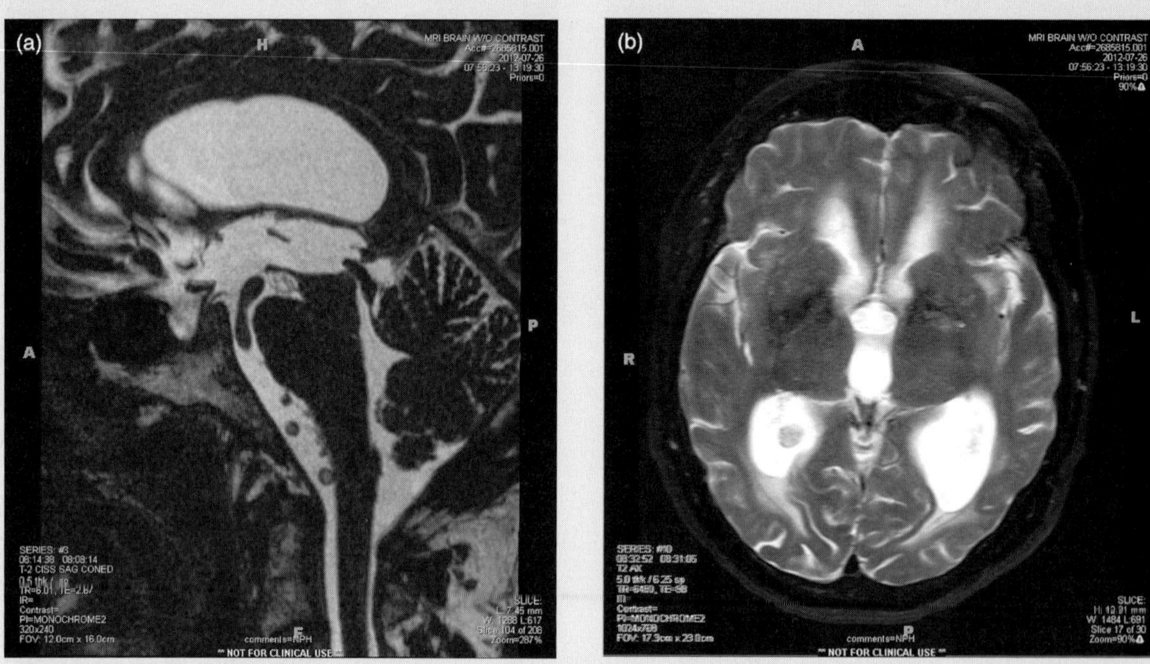

Figure 10.4 (a) Sagittal T2 shows aqueductal obstruction, bulging floor of the third ventricle. (b) Axial T2 shows massive dilatation with relatively tight SAS.

References

1. Adams RD, Fisher CM, Hakim S, Ojemann RG, Sweet WH. Symptomatic occult hydrocephalus with 'normal' cerebrospinal-fluid pressure. A treatable syndrome. *N Engl J Med* 1965;273(3):117–26.
2. Marmarou A, Bergsneider M, Relkin N, Klinge P, Black PM. Development of guidelines for idiopathic normal-pressure hydrocephalus: introduction. *Neurosurgery* 2005;57(3 Suppl):S1–3.
3. Relkin N, Marmarou A, Klinge P, Bergsneider M, Black PM. Diagnosing idiopathic normal-pressure hydrocephalus. *Neurosurgery* 2005;57(3 Suppl):S4–16.
4. Conn H. Normal pressure hydrocephalus: a case report by a physician who is the patient. *Clin Med* 2007;7:296–9.
5. Kitagaki H, Mori E, Ishii K, et al. CSF spaces in idiopathic normal pressure hydrocephalus: morphology and volumetry. *Neuro Radiol* 1998;19:1277–84.
6. Mori, E, Ishikawa M, Ishii K, et al. Guidelines for management of idiopathic normal pressure hydrocephalus: second edition. *Neurol Med Chir (Tokyo)* 2012;52:775–809.

7. Al-Jumaily M, Jones B, Jenkinson C, et al. Long-term neuropsychological outcome and management of 'decompensated' longstanding overt ventriculomegaly in adults. *Br J Neurosurg* 2012;5:717–21.
8. Kiefer M, Eymann R, Steudel WI, Strowitzki M. Gravitational shunt management of long-standing overt ventriculomegaly in adult (LOVA) hydrocephalus. *J Clin Neurosci* 2005;12(1):21–6.
9. Oi S, Shimoda M, Shibata M, et al. Pathophysiology of long-standing overt ventriculomegaly in adults. *J Neurosurg* 2000;12(1):933–40.
10. McGirt M, Woodworth G, Coon A, et al. Diagnosis, treatment, and analysis of long-term outcomes in idiopathic normal pressure hydrocephalus. *Neurosurgery* 2005;57:699–705.
11. Bech-Azzedine R, Hogh P, Juhler M, Gjerris F, Waldemar G. Idiopathic normal-pressure hydrocephalus: clinical comorbidity correlated with cerebral biopsy findings and outcome of cerebrospinal fluid shunting. *J Neurol Neurosurg Psychiatry* 2007;78:157–61.
12. Golomb J, Wisoff J, Miller DC, et al. Alzheimer's disease comorbidity in normal pressure hydrocephalus: prevalence and shunt response. *J Neurol Neurosurg Psychiatry* 2000;68:778–81.
13. Greenberg DA, Aminoff MJ., Simon RP. *Clinical Neurology*, 8th edn. New York: McGraw-Hill Medical; 2012: 122–3.
14. Shprecher D, Schwalb J, Kurlan R. Normal pressure hydrocephalus: diagnosis and treatment. *Curr Neurol Neurosci Rep* 2008;8(5):371–6.
15. Gallia G, Rigamonti D, Williams MA. The diagnosis and treatment of idiopathic normal pressure hydrocephalus. *Nat Clin Pract Neurol* 2008;8(5):371–6.
16. Meir U, Zelinger FS, Kintzel D. Signs, symptoms and course of normal pressure hydrocephalus in comparison with cerebral atrophy. *Acta Neurochir* 1999;141:1039–48.
17. Wikkelsø C. *First Brazilian Symposium on Hydrocephalus*. Porto Alegre, March 8 and 9, 2013.
18. Hellström P, Klinge P, Tans J, Wikkelsø C. A new scale for assessment of severity and outcome in iNPH. *Acta Neurol Scand* 2012;126(4):229–37.
19. Tisell M, Tullberg M, Hellström P, et al. Shunt surgery in patients with hydrocephalus and white matter changes. *Neurosurgery* 2011;114:1432–8.
20. Kiefer M, Eymann R, Steudel WI. Outcome predictors for normal-pressure hydrocephalus. *Acta Neurochir Suppl* 2006;96:364–7.
21. Meier U, Lemcke J. Co-morbidity as a predictor of outcome in patients with idiopathic normal-pressure hydrocephalus. *Acta Neurochir Suppl.* 2010;106:127–30.
22. Kiefer M, Utenberg A. The differential diagnosis and treatment of normal-pressure hydrocephalus. *Dtsch Arztebl Int* 2012;106(1–2):15–26.
23. Holodny AI, Waxman R, George AE, et al. MR differential diagnosis of normal-pressure hydrocephalus and Alzheimer disease: significance of perihippocampal fissures. *AJNR Am J Neuroradiol* 1998;19(5):813–19.
24. Wikkelsø C, Hellström P, Klinge P, Tans JT. The European iNPH Multicentre Study on the predictive values of resistance to CSF outflow and the CSF Tap Test in patients with idiopathic normal pressure hydrocephalus. *J Neurol Neurosurg Psychiatry* 2013;84(5):562–8.
25. Pujari S, Kharkar S, Metellus P, et al. Normal pressure hydrocephalus: long-term outcome after shunt surgery. *J Neurol Neurosurg Psychiatry* 2008;70(11):1282–6.
26. Savolainen S, Paljarvi L, Vaparanti M. Prevalence of Alzheimer's disease in patients investigated for presumed normal pressure hydrocephalus: a clinical and neuropathological study. *Acta Neurochir* 1999;141:849–53.
27. Iseki C, Kawanami T, Kato T, et al. Asymptomatic ventriculomegaly with features of idiopathic normal pressure hydrocephalus on MRI (AVIM) in the elderly: a prospective study in a Japanese population. *Neurol Sci* 2009;277:54–7.
28. Brean A, Eide PK. Prevalence of probable idiopathic normal pressure hydrocephalus in a Norwegian population. *Acta Neurol Scand* 2008;118:48–53.
29. Brean A, Fredo HL, Sollid S, et al. Five-year incidence of surgery for idiopathic normal pressure hydrocephalus in Norway. *Acta Neurol Scand* 2009;120:314–16.
30. Tisell M, Höglund M, Wikkelsø C. National and regional incidence of surgery for adult hydrocephalus in Sweden. *Acta Neurol Scand* 2005;112:72–5.

Chapter 11

Core imaging in adult hydrocephalus

Benjamin D. Elder, Patrick Bankah, Ari M. Blitz, C. Rory Goodwin, Thomas A. Kosztowski, Ignacio Jusué-Torres, and Daniele Rigamonti

Introduction

Advances in neuroimaging have greatly improved the management of hydrocephalus. The various imaging modalities are useful in confirming the diagnosis, determining the etiology of hydrocephalus, providing intraoperative guidance, and improving the follow-up of patients who have undergone treatment including cerebrospinal fluid (CSF) shunting or endoscopic third ventriculostomy (ETV). The various imaging modalities that are utilized include:

- conventional X-rays;
- ultrasonography;
- computerized axial tomography (CT);
- magnetic resonance imaging (MRI);
- radionuclide shunt patency imaging.

As systematically as possible, we will list for each modality their use in the preoperative, perioperative, and postoperative period.

Conventional X-rays

Conventional X-rays often are used to evaluate shunted patients as the entire shunt hardware can be visualized to assess the continuity of the shunt. However, as the majority of shunt malfunctions are unrelated to mechanical discontinuity, the majority of images obtained will demonstrate intact tubing; Lehnert et al. [1] found only 4% of shunt surveys to be abnormal in a series of 296 patients in the emergency room. Similarly, Griffey et al. [2] assessed the utility of shunt surveys in diagnosing shunt malfunctions in the emergency room in adult hydrocephalus patients and found a sensitivity of only 0.11 but a specificity of 0.98. A similar study in the pediatric population demonstrated a slightly higher sensitivity of 0.31 [3]. Conventional X-rays are also utilized to verify the shunt setting, because programmable shunt valves generally have radiopaque markers.

In addition to the use of plain films for diagnosing shunt discontinuities, we routinely obtain plain-film shunt surveys immediately postoperatively as a baseline and to verify shunt continuity. For pleural or atrial distal catheters, we also obtain a chest X-ray (often as part of the shunt survey) to verify the location of the distal catheter and to confirm that there is no pneumothorax (Figure 11.1). For peritoneal distal catheters, we perform an abdominal X-ray 12–24 hours after the shunt survey to confirm movement of the distal catheter as evidence that it is not pre-peritoneal or in a loculated cavity (Figures 11.2 and 11.3).

Ultrasonography

The use of duplex ultrasound of the internal jugular vein is often helpful in preoperative planning for ventriculoatrial shunt placement to confirm patency of the vein; it is being used intraoperatively to guide the percutaneous insertion of the distal catheter (Figure 11.4) and even to navigate around venous obstructions [4].

Ultrasonography is useful in the assessment of possible fluid collections around the distal shunt tubing in peritoneal, pleural, and atrial (Figure 11.5) catheters that may be suggestive of shunt malfunction or infection. However, a CT scan of the chest or abdomen is required if more detailed imaging is needed to better assess the fluid collection.

CT imaging

Diagnosis of hydrocephalus

CT scans are often the first-line imaging in hydrocephalus due to wide availability, ease with which they are performed, minimal contraindications, and low expense relative to MRIs. Generally, in the presence of hydrocephalus, the temporal horns, which are normally barely visible, look dilated. The appearance of the

Adult Hydrocephalus, ed. Daniele Rigamonti. Published by Cambridge University Press.

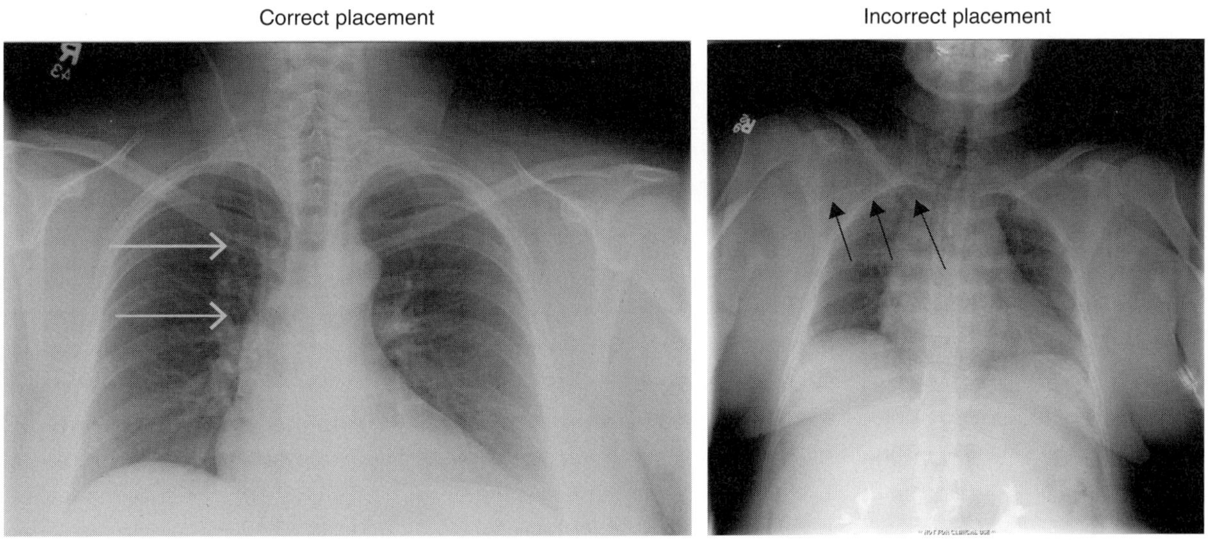

Figure 11.1 A postoperative chest radiogram shows correct and incorrect placement of the distal tip of the ventriculoatrial catheter.

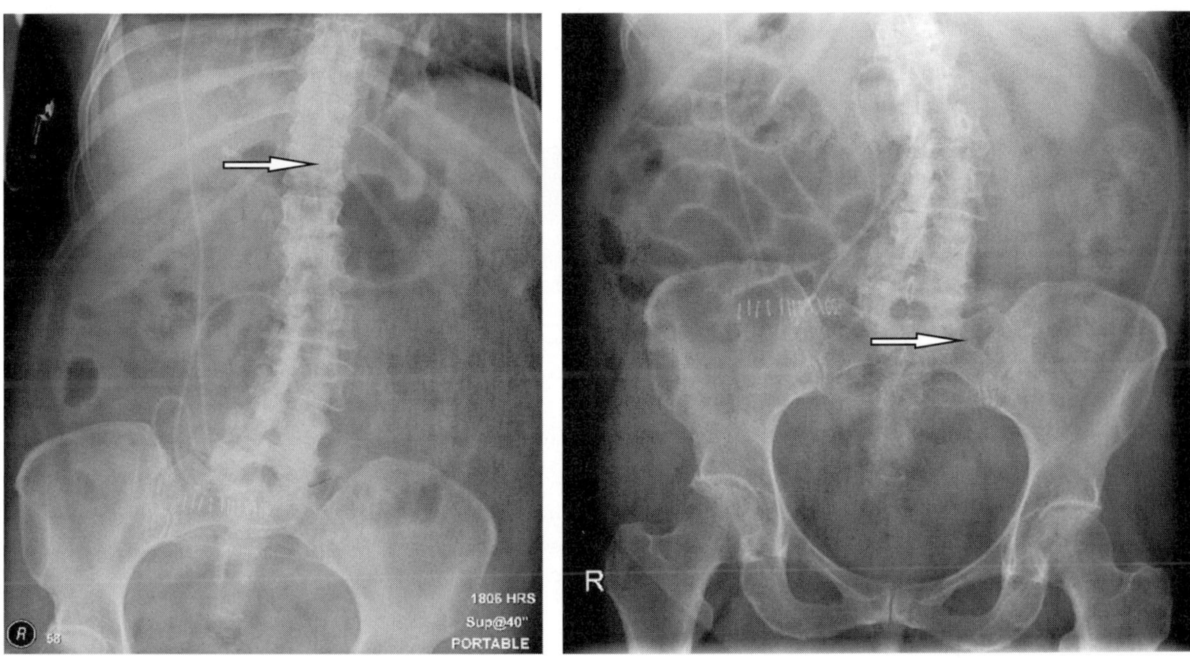

Figure 11.2 A postoperative abdominal radiogram shows that the tip of the catheter is moving in the course of several hours because of the peristalsis, confirming intra-abdominal placement.

sylvian fissure, interhemispheric fissure, and cerebral sulci depends on the type of hydrocephalus. They are barely visible in the case of obstructive hydrocephalus and clearly visible in idiopathic normal pressure hydrocephalus (iNPH). An Evans ratio (defined as the ratio of the frontal horn to the maximal biparietal distance measured in the same CT slice) greater than 0.3 is generally considered a reliable sign of hydrocephalus (Figure 11.6) [5]. The Japanese guidelines for iNPH also describe this measurement [6], although some groups advocate the use of volumetric ventricular measurements in the diagnosis of iNPH now that high resolution CT scans are widely available; one recent study proposed a ventricular volume greater than 77

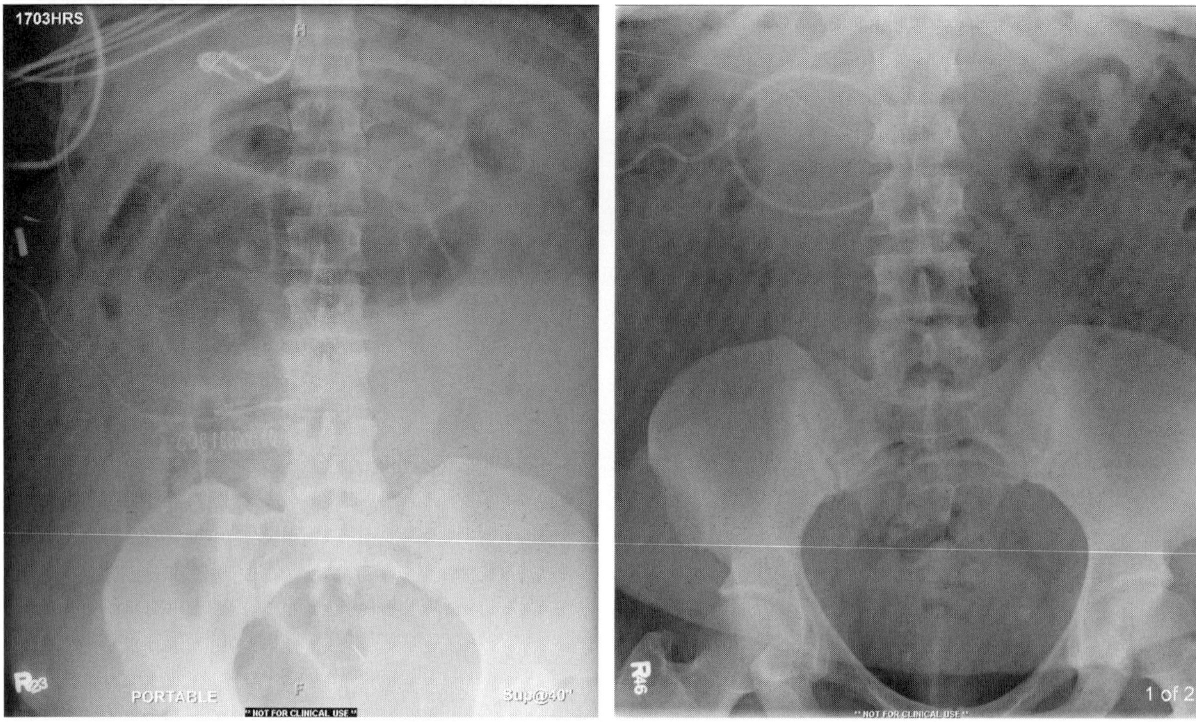

Figure 11.3 A postoperative abdominal radiogram and a later one show that the tip of the catheter, initially in the abdomen, migrated to an extraperitoneal subcutaneous location.

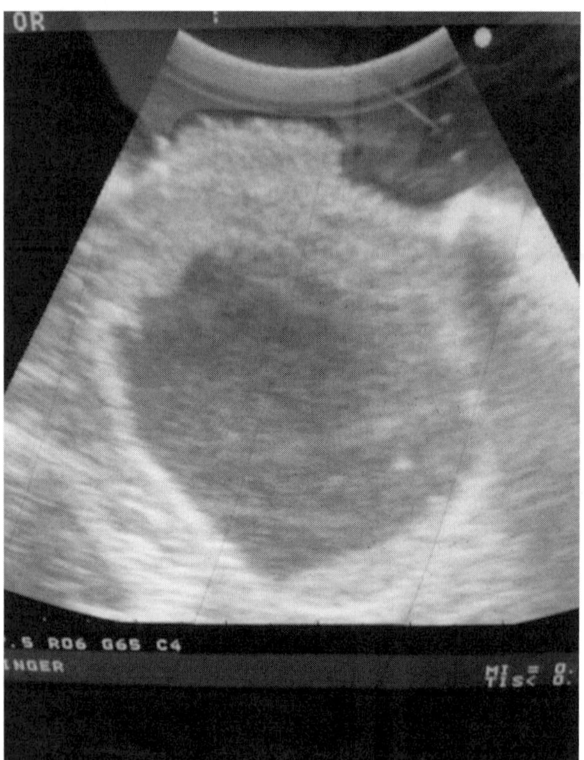

Figure 11.4 Ultrasound visualizes a pocket of CSF surrounding a proximal lumbar catheter that migrated from the spinal canal to the subcutaneous location.

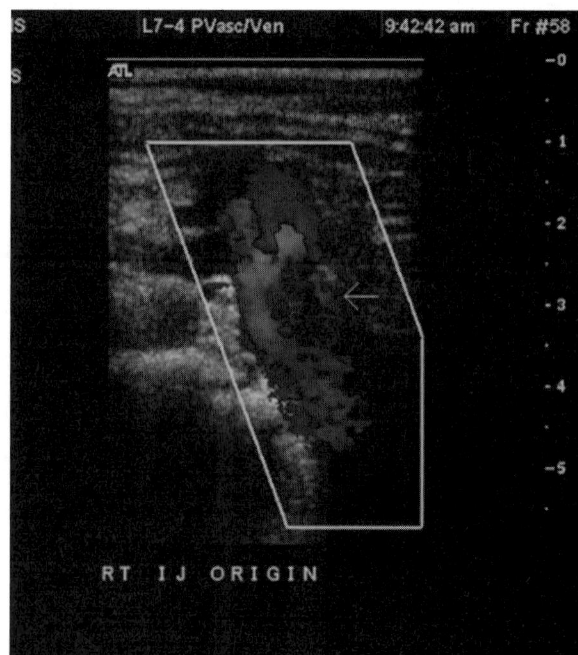

Figure 11.5 Thoracic ultrasound visualizes a small thrombus at the distal tip of a ventriculoatrial shunt. A full-color version is included in the color plate section.

ml as suggestive of iNPH [7]. Hydrocephalus is also suggested on imaging when the size of both temporal horns (TH) exceeds 2 mm in width. Additionally, a ratio of the FH/ID exceeding 0.5 is suggestive, where FH is the largest width of the frontal horns and ID is the internal diameter from inner table to inner table at the same level. Other generally accepted evidence of hydrocephalus includes ballooning of the frontal horns of the lateral ventricle ("Mickey Mouse" ventricles), or transependymal flow suggestive of acute hydrocephalus.

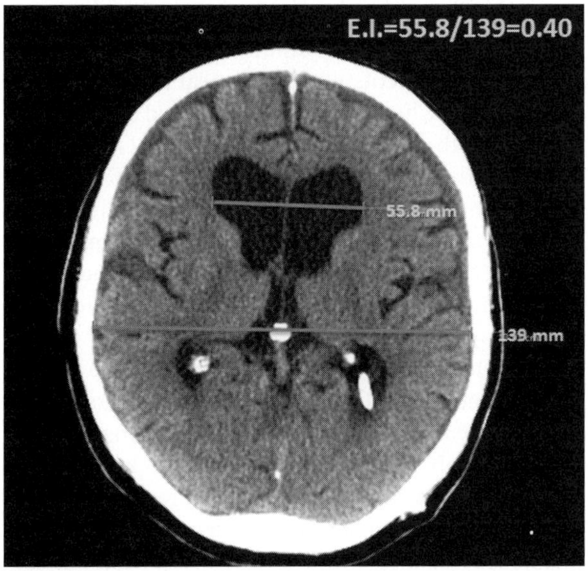

Figure 11.6 Different from the original description based on coronal pneumo-encephalography, we routinely measure the Evans index as the ratio between the maximum frontal horn span, measured in front of the caudate nucleus, and the maximum biparietal inner skull diameter in the same section.

Volumetric analysis (VA) by CT or MRI of the CSF spaces

VA is an interesting tool to assess the size of the ventricles, the size of the subarachnoid space (SAS), their relationship, and changes in the size of the ventricles or SAS after shunting [8]. Although it seemed to hold great promise, the tool is presently considered still experimental and its clinical use is limited (Figure 11.7).

Postoperative management: shunt malfunction

CT scans are performed to obtain a baseline image postoperatively to demonstrate the location of the proximal catheter in the ventricular system, the baseline size of the ventricles, and any postoperative intraventricular hemorrhage (Figure 11.8). CTs are helpful in diagnosing shunt malfunctions in younger patients: a CT image should ideally be compared to a prior baseline image obtained when the patient was doing well clinically; however, this is not always possible, particularly in the emergency room setting, though every

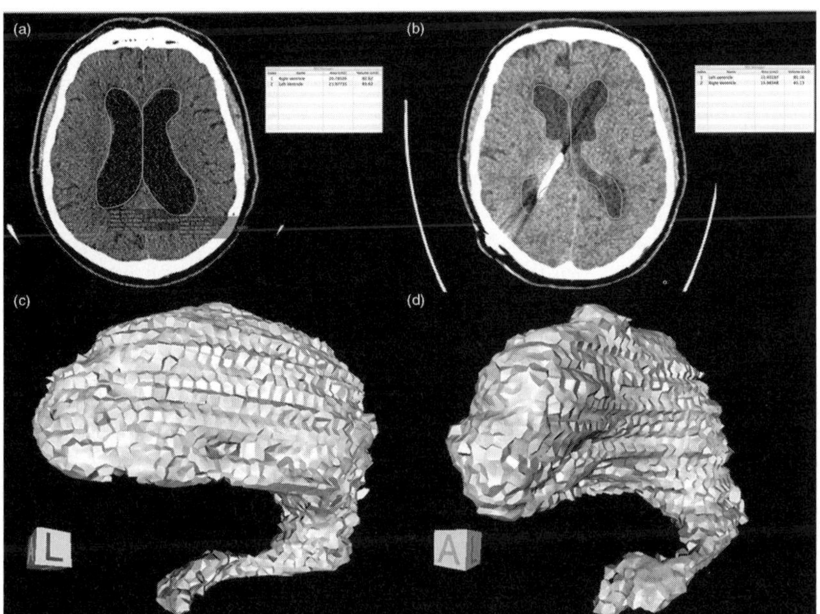

Figure 11.7 The preoperative and postoperative ventricle volumes are measured using non-enhanced 1.5–3 mm CT sections. The sum of areas from all axial sections is used to compute ventricle volume using MIPAV software in a semi-automated fashion (OsiriX, Los Angeles, CA Center for Information Technology, National Institutes of Health, Bethesda, MD).

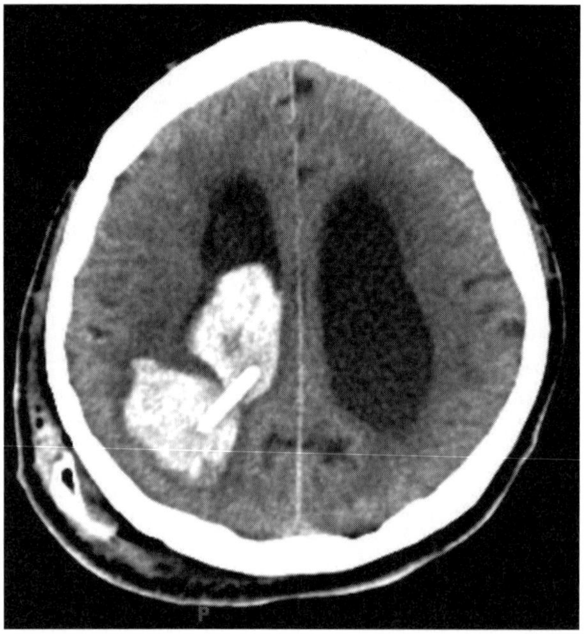

Figure 11.8 Early postoperative CT shows the new intracerebral hemorrhage (ICH) secondary to the insertion of a ventriculoperitoneal shunt.

attempt should be made to obtain prior imaging with which to compare. In general, an increase in ventricular caliber may be indicative of a shunt malfunction, or may be an expected outcome if a programmable shunt was recently changed to a higher setting. Likewise, a decrease in ventricular caliber may be due to a recent programmable valve change to a lower setting or recent shunt revision due to malfunction, but can be a sign of overdrainage.

A recent retrospective study examined the utility of head CT scans in a series of 296 patients who presented to the emergency room, and found that 18% of the scans were positive and that there was a significant association between abnormal head CT and surgical revision [1]. Another study demonstrated the importance of obtaining prior imaging for comparison as having increased ventricular size since a prior CT scan had a sensitivity of 48% for shunt malfunction, but enlarged ventricular size without a prior comparison CT only had a sensitivity of 28% for shunt malfunction [9]. Finally, particularly with bone windows, CT images can verify the continuity of the tubing and valve connection in the cranial region. However, in adult patients shunt malfunction is less likely to be diagnosed on the basis of CT, because in these situations there may be minimal change in ventricular size. Patients with iNPH [10] or pseudotumor cerebri, or patients with the slit ventricle syndrome or decreased compliance [11], may not demonstrate a change in ventricular size on CT imaging. CT imaging is also ideal to rule out subdural hematoma or hygroma formation in the setting of overdrainage (Figure 11.9).

In addition to its use in diagnosing shunt malfunction with cranial imaging, CT scanning is very helpful in diagnosing abdominal shunt-related complications in patients with peritoneal distal catheters. For example, Chung et al. [12] examined a series of 70 patients with ventriculoperitoneal shunts who presented with abdominal complaints and found that almost 23% of the patients had evidence of abdominal shunt-related complications including shunt migration (Figure 11.10), infection, CSF pseudocyst, abdominal abscess, infected fluid collection, or rarely bowel or bladder perforation (Figure 11.11).

Despite its widespread use in hydrocephalus diagnosis and treatment, CT scanning is not without its risks, as the patient is exposed to a large dose of ionizing radiation with each scan. This is especially a drawback in the pediatric population. For instance, a recent review estimated a 1% lifetime risk of head and neck malignancies from diagnostic radiation exposure in children with ventriculoperitoneal shunts [13]. To mitigate this risk, many centers have developed lower-dose head CT protocols for both the adult [14] and pediatric [15] populations.

MRI

MRI is considered the gold standard imaging modality in the evaluation of hydrocephalus in adults. In addition to providing much of the same diagnostic evidence and measurements as can be obtained on CT imaging, MRI can provide substantially more anatomic detail. It provides excellent multiplanar anatomic definition of the ventricular system, subarachnoid spaces, and brain parenchyma. It is the preferred examination for the diagnosis of iNPH, especially with T2-weighted images. T2 steady-state free precession (SSFP) images (e.g. CISS or FIESTA) are extremely valuable in outlining the fine anatomy of the aqueduct, third ventricle, foramen of Monro, fourth ventricle, and the subarachnoid space. This sequence can confirm the patency of the aqueduct prior to a large volume lumbar puncture or lumbar drainage (Figure 11.12a and b). The sequence can outline an obstruction due to a web (Figure 11.12c) or tumor at the level of the aqueduct or of the foramen of Monro. In the presence of an obstruction, the walls of the third ventricle are characteristically bulging

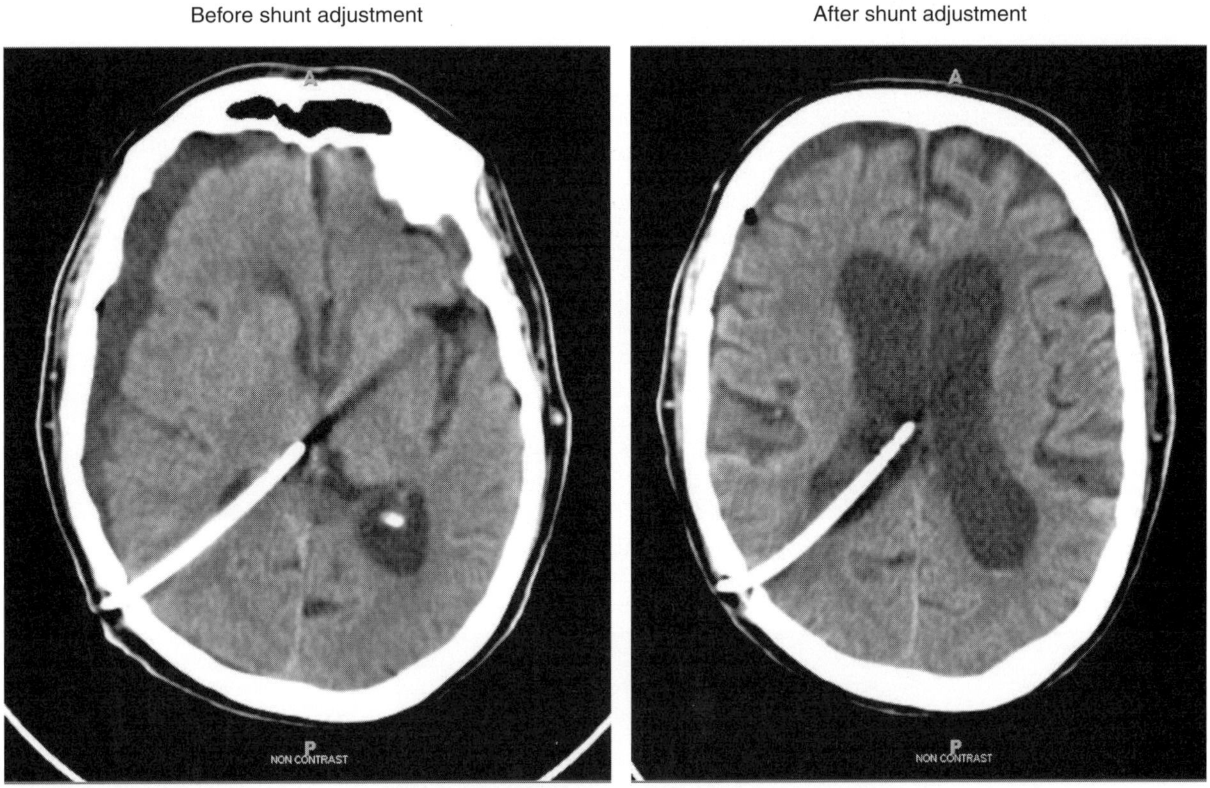

Figure 11.9 CT shows a left subdural hygroma and its disappearance after adjusting the valve to a higher setting.

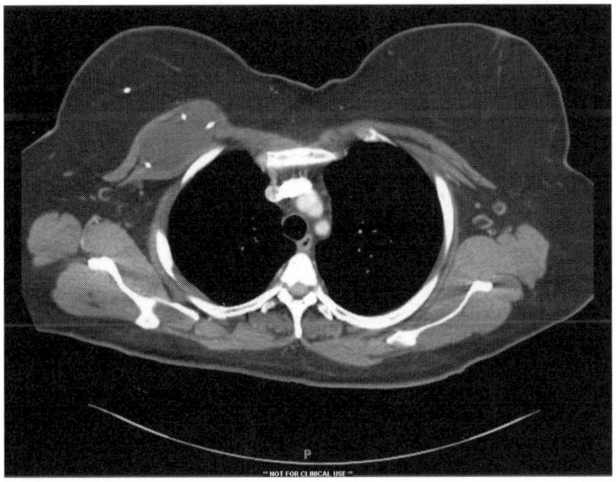

Figure 11.10 Chest CT confirms the migration into a subcutaneous location of a ventriculopleural shunt.

outward (Figure 11.12c). The same sequence is used to document the patency of a third ventriculostomy after ETV (Figure 11.12d). Coronal MRI sequences may demonstrate a disproportionately enlarged subarachnoid space hydrocephalus (DESH) pattern that the Japanese authors consider pathognomonic of idiopathic NPH (Figure 11.13) [6]. Finally, transependymal CSF flow suggestive of acute hydrocephalus may be seen on T2 or FLAIR imaging (Figure 11.14).

MRI does not require ionizing radiation, making it ideal for use in the pediatric population or when a patient requires serial imaging. However, some drawbacks to MRI use include the time length of the scan, need for sedation or anesthesia in patients with claustrophobia or pediatric patients, multiple contraindications due to metal implants, difficulty performing scans in patients with pacemakers or implanted defibrillators, as well as the significant expense relative to CT scans. It should also be noted that patients with older programmable shunts must have the valve reset following the MRI as the older valves can have their setting changed by the magnetic field during the scan.

Phase-contrast MRI

Phase-contrast or "cine" MR imaging was originally applied to CSF imaging by Levy and Di Chiro [16] in order to demonstrate pulsatile CSF flow, and the process

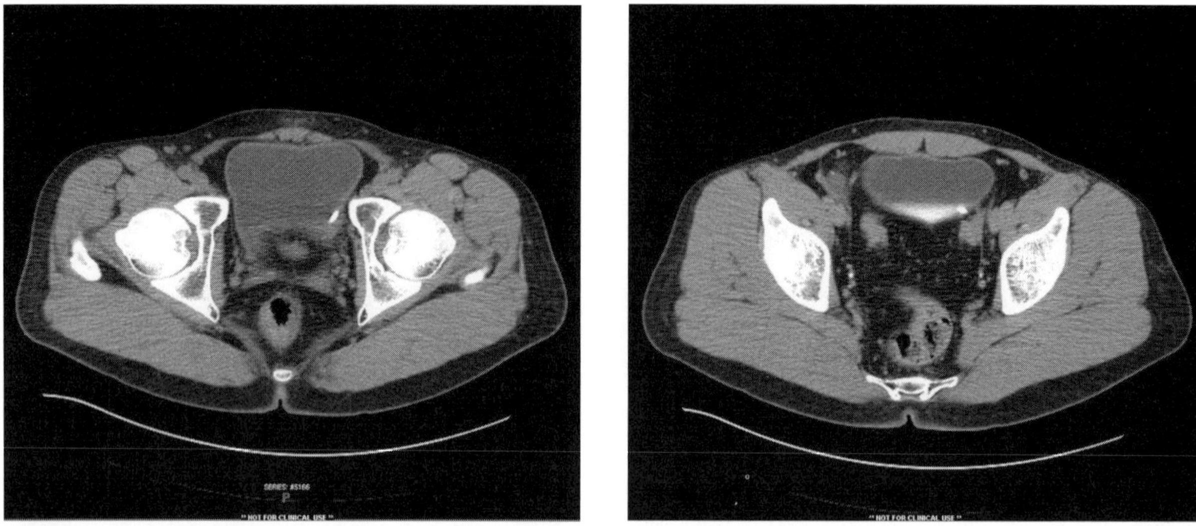

Figure 11.11 Abdominal CT confirms the perforation into the bladder of a ventriculoperitoneal shunt.

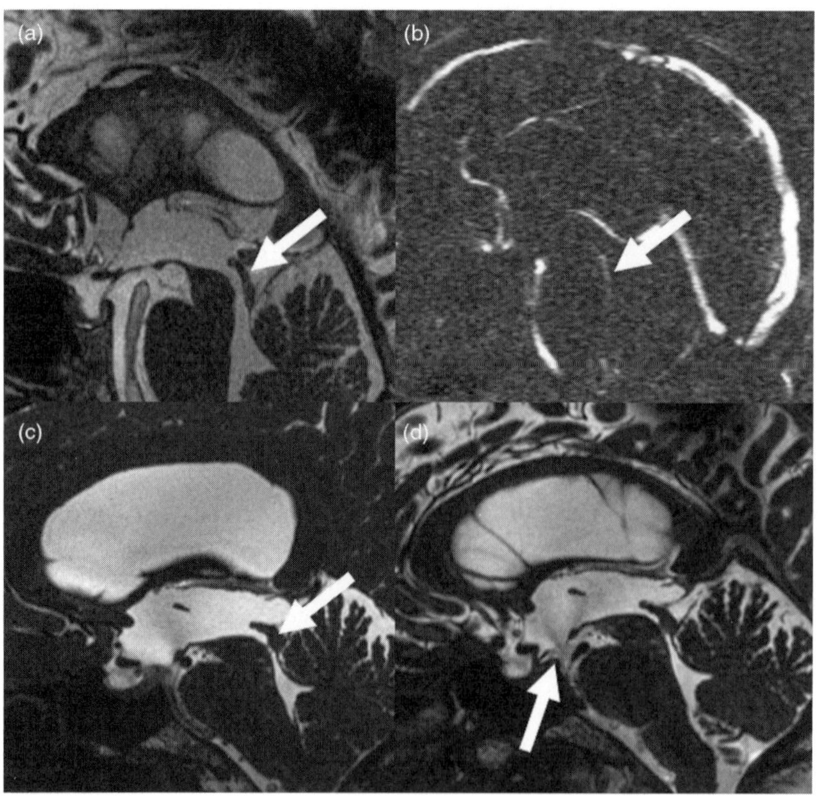

Figure 11.12 (a) Sagittal midline CISS image demonstrates anatomic patency of the cerebral aqueduct (arrow). (b) Aqueductal patency is confirmed with the use of cardiac gated phase-contrast imaging. Hyperintensity on the magnitude of phase images demonstrates the presence of CSF flow in the cerebral aqueduct (arrow). (c) Sagittal midline CISS images in another patient demonstrate obstruction of the caudal aspect of the cerebral aqueduct due to two thin webs (arrow). CSF flow could not be demonstrated through the region of the cerebral aqueduct on cardiac gated phase-contrast images (not shown). (d) The patient underwent endoscopic third ventriculostomy, the patency of which is confirmed by an anatomic defect in the floor of the third ventricle on CISS images through which a flow void extends (arrow). Cardiac gated phase-contrast images confirmed the presence of CSF flow (not shown).

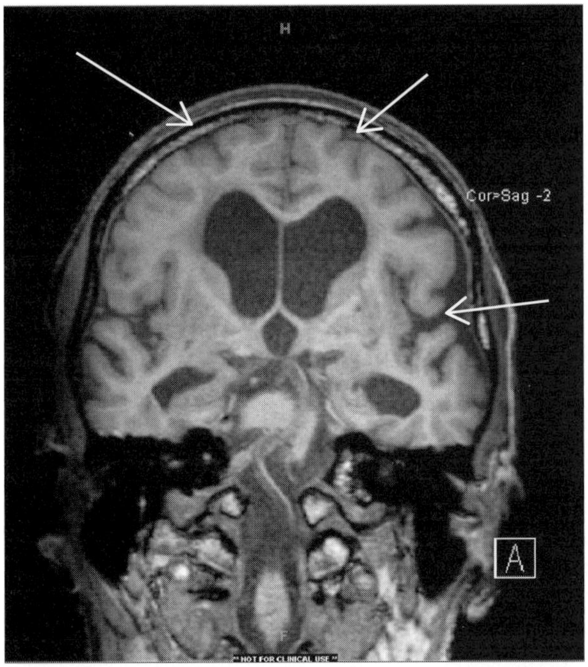

Figure 11.13 A coronal T1-weighted MRI demonstrates crowding of the sulci over the convexity and the enlarged subarachnoid space of the sylvian fissure that produce the characteristic DESH pattern described by the Japanese authors [6].

was later refined to better quantify CSF flow rates [17]. It has been most useful in the diagnosis of aqueductal stenosis [18] and CSF obstruction, as described above, and has been shown to be more sensitive than conventional MR imaging (Figure 11.12b). For instance, in a retrospective study, 17/17 patients were found to have altered flow with aqueductal obstruction on phase-contrast imaging whereas only 10/17 were found to have aqueductal stenosis on conventional MR imaging [19]. It can also be used to determine the patency of a prior ETV [20]. Phase-contrast imaging also has some utility in identifying proximal shunt flow to assess for proximal malfunction. Although it has proven beneficial in the diagnosis of aqueductal stenosis and proximal shunt flow, a prior study demonstrated that it was not beneficial in predicting which iNPH patients will respond to shunting [21], though research is still ongoing in this area.

MRI with gadolinium enhancement

The administration of gadolinium allows the visualization of vascular structures. The appearance of a thickened dural layer suggests the presence of intracranial hypotension secondary to overdrainage of CSF by the shunt (Figure 11.15).

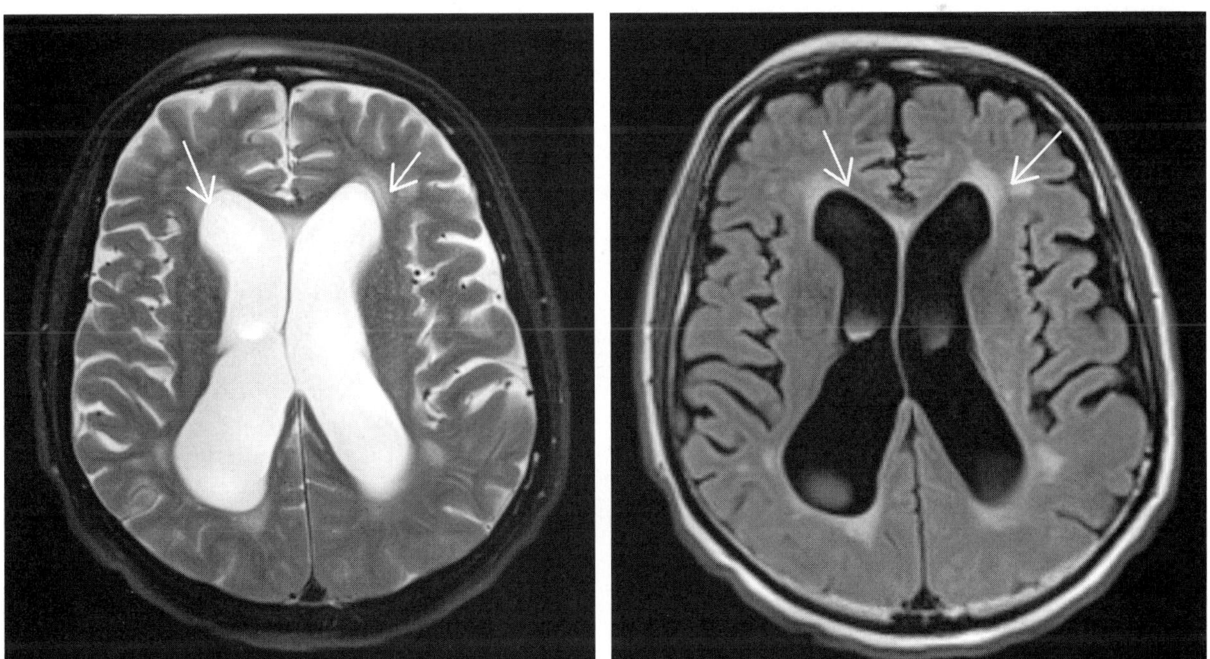

Figure 11.14 T2-weighted and FLAIR MR images show the characteristic "capping" of the frontal horns secondary to presumed retrograde CSF reabsorption into the parenchyma.

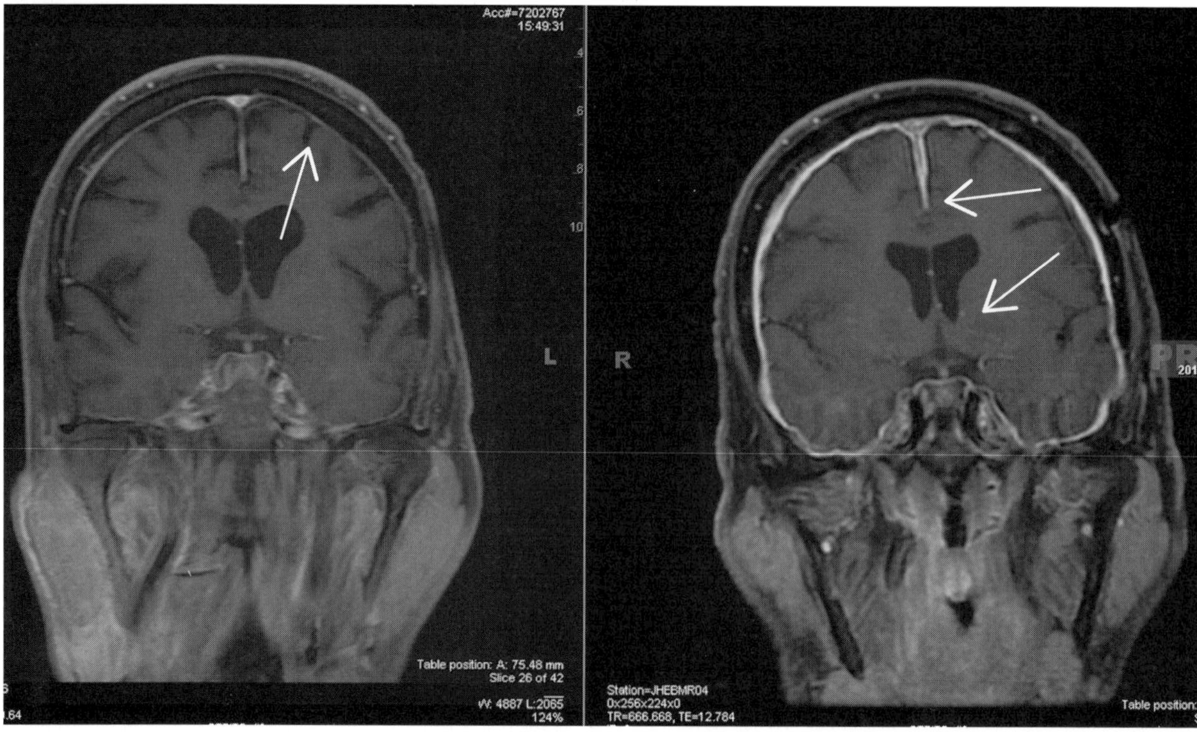

Figure 11.15 On gadolinium-enhanced T1-weighted images the appearance of diffuse pachymeningeal enhancement, even in the absence of brainstem sagging, is suggestive of intracranial hypotension.

Radionuclide shunt patency test

It is not always easy to diagnose shunt obstruction. The presence of enlarging ventricles, compared to historical baseline, on standard imaging modalities such as CT or MRI is usually sufficient proof. However, even with enlarging ventricles on cranial imaging, it is difficult to assess if malfunction is at the level of the proximal catheter, valve, or distal catheter. The problem is compounded in iNPH as shunting results in a minimal change in ventricle size [22], and there is a similarly minor change in ventricle size with shunt malfunction. A similar diagnostic dilemma can be encountered when assessing possible shunt malfunction in children with slit ventricle syndrome or pseudotumor cerebri patients.

We have employed the use of radionuclide shunt patency (SP) studies in the work-up of shunt malfunctions in these groups. This procedure was developed in 1966 by Di Chiro and Grove [23], and has been modified by other groups with water-soluble contrast medium [24], termed a "shuntogram." The radionuclide SP study was recently studied and validated in the iNPH population by our own group [25].

The SP study allows for the assessment of four variables in the diagnosis of shunt malfunction which also isolate the region of the shunt that has malfunctioned. These include ventricular entry, opening pressure, $T_{1/2}$ time, and peritoneal distribution. Using all four variables, the positive predictive value of the SP study was 80% [25]. Ventricular entry of radiotracer helps rule out proximal malfunction. Elevated opening pressure with brisk flow of CSF indicates malfunction of the valve or distal catheter, or demonstrates an inappropriate shunt setting in a programmable system. The peritoneal distribution of radionuclide is classified as diffuse, loculated, or none, and indicates potential failure of the distal shunt tubing.

The $T_{1/2}$ time is calculated as the time for radioactivity counts in the shunt bulb to decrease to half of the starting value (Figure 11.16). In iNPH patients, a $T_{1/2}$ >8.7 min is suggestive of shunt malfunction, with a positive predictive value of 87.5% [25]. However, the $T_{1/2}$ is less accurate in patients with low CSF pressures (<5 cmH_2O), as there may be no spontaneous CSF flow during the SP study in the supine position, when the $T_{1/2}$ is calculated.

In addition to helping to diagnose shunt malfunction in the iNPH population, a major benefit of its use

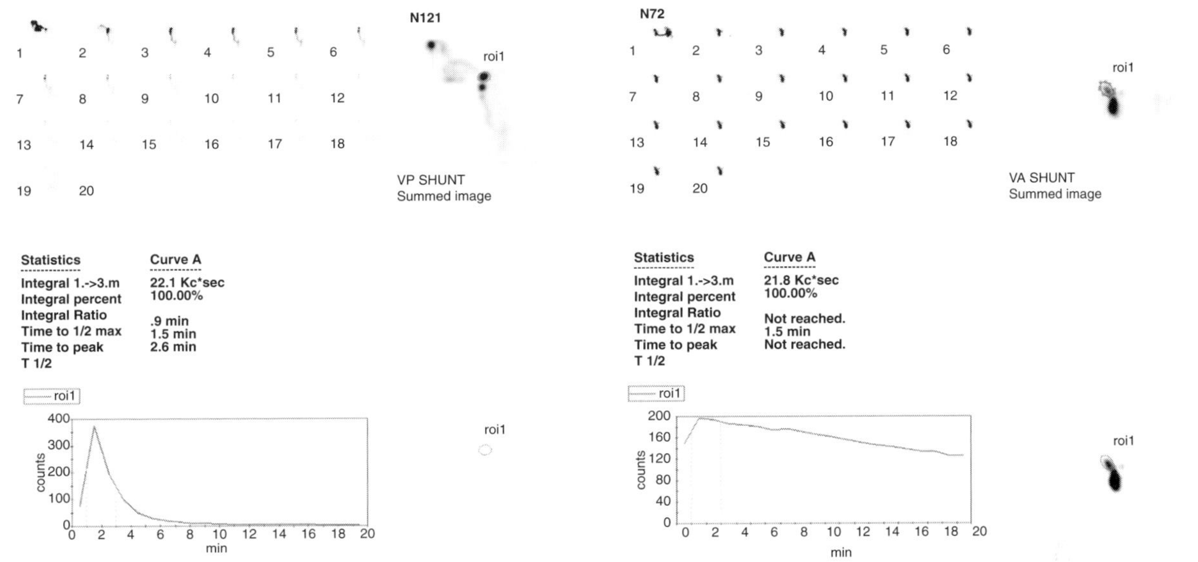

Figure 11.16 Shunt patency tests show the different appearance of the clearance curve when the shunt is patent (on the left) and when the shunt is obstructed (on the right). The $T_{1/2}$ time is normal on the left and prolonged on the right.

is helping to isolate the exact site of malfunction. This allows surgical revision to be targeted to the region of obstruction, which in iNPH patients is almost always in the distal peritoneal catheter [25]. Furthermore, as the distal catheter is often the site of obstruction in iNPH patients, the traditional method of assessing rapid refill of the shunt bulb following manual compression is less useful as this just assesses proximal catheter function, and will not diagnose a valve or distal tubing malfunction.

In conclusion, the SP study is a valuable tool in the diagnosis of shunt malfunction particularly in the iNPH patient population. It requires the same invasiveness as the traditional shunt tap, yet yields significantly more information with confirmation of shunt patency and flow or isolation of the site of malfunction.

References

1. Lehnert BE, Rahbar H, Relyea-Chew A, et al. Detection of ventricular shunt malfunction in the ED: relative utility of radiography, CT, and nuclear imaging. *Emerg Radiol* 2011;18(4):299–305.
2. Griffey RT, Ledbetter S, Khorasani R. Yield and utility of radiographic "shunt series" in the evaluation of ventriculo-peritoneal shunt malfunction in adult emergency patients. *Emerg Radiol* 2007;13(6):307–11.
3. Desai KR, Babb JS, Amodio JB. The utility of the plain radiograph "shunt series" in the evaluation of suspected ventriculoperitoneal shunt failure in pediatric patients. *Pediatr Radiol* 2007;37(5):452–6.
4. Momin EN, Recinos PF, Coon AL, Rigamonti D. Use of intraoperative venography to guide the distal portion of a ventriculoatrial shunt past an obstruction in the central veins: technical case report. *Neurosurgery* 2010;66(6 Suppl Operative):370–1; discussion 371.
5. Synek V, Reuben JR, Du Boulay GH. Comparing Evans' index and computerized axial tomography in assessing relationship of ventricular size to brain size. *Neurology* 1976;26(3):231–3.
6. Mori E, Ishikawa M, Kato T, et al. Guidelines for management of idiopathic normal pressure hydrocephalus: second edition. *Neurol Med Chir (Tokyo)* 2012;52(11):775–809.
7. Ambarki K, Israelsson H, Wåhlin A, Birgander R, Eklund A, Malm J. Brain ventricular size in healthy elderly: comparison between Evans index and volume measurement. *Neurosurgery* 2010; 67(1): 94–9.
8. Kitagaki H, Mori E, Ishii K, et al. CSF spaces in idiopathic normal pressure hydrocephalus: morphology and volumetry. *AJNR Am J Neuroradiol* 1998;19(7):1277–84.
9. Zorc JJ, Krugman SD, Ogborn J, Benson J. Radiographic evaluation for suspected cerebrospinal fluid shunt obstruction. *Pediatr Emerg Care* 2002;18(5):337–40.
10. Lenfeldt N, Hansson W, Larsson A, et al. Three-day CSF drainage barely reduces ventricular size in normal pressure hydrocephalus. *Neurology* 2012;79(3):237–42.

11. McNatt SA, Kim A, Hohuan D, Krieger M, McComb JG. Pediatric shunt malfunction without ventricular dilatation. *Pediatr Neurosurg* 2008;44(2):128–32.

12. Chung JJ, Yu JS, Kim JH, Nam SJ, Kim MJ. Intraabdominal complications secondary to ventriculoperitoneal shunts: CT findings and review of the literature. *AJR Am J Roentgenol* 2009;193(5):1311–17.

13. Smyth MD, Narayan P, Tubbs RS, et al. Cumulative diagnostic radiation exposure in children with ventriculoperitoneal shunts: a review. *Childs Nerv Syst* 2008;24(4):493–7.

14. Mullins ME, Lev MH, Bove P, et al. Comparison of image quality between conventional and low-dose nonenhanced head CT. *AJNR Am J Neuroradiol* 2004;25(4):533–8.

15. Udayasankar UK, Braithwaite K, Arvaniti M, et al. Low-dose nonenhanced head CT protocol for follow-up evaluation of children with ventriculoperitoneal shunt: reduction of radiation and effect on image quality. *AJNR Am J Neuroradiol* 2008;29(4):802–6.

16. Levy LM, Di Chiro G. MR phase imaging and cerebrospinal fluid flow in the head and spine. *Neuroradiology* 1990;32(5):399–406.

17. Enzmann DR, Pelc NJ. Cerebrospinal fluid flow measured by phase-contrast cine MR. *AJNR Am J Neuroradiol* 1993;14(6):1301–7; discussion 1309–10.

18. Kadowaki C, Hara M, Numoto M, Takeuchi K, Saito I. Cine magnetic resonance imaging of aqueductal stenosis. *Childs Nerv Syst* 1995;11(2):107–11.

19. Stoquart-El Sankari S, Lehmann P, Gondry-Jouet C, et al. Phase-contrast MR imaging support for the diagnosis of aqueductal stenosis. *AJNR Am J Neuroradiol* 2009;30(1):209–14.

20. Bargallo N, Olondo L, Garcia AI, et al. Functional analysis of third ventriculostomy patency by quantification of CSF stroke volume by using cine phase-contrast MR imaging. *AJNR Am J Neuroradiol* 2005;26(10):2514–21.

21. Dixon GR, Friedman JA, Luetmer PH, et al. Use of cerebrospinal fluid flow rates measured by phase-contrast MR to predict outcome of ventriculoperitoneal shunting for idiopathic normal-pressure hydrocephalus. *Mayo Clin Proc* 2002;77(6):509–14.

22. McConnell KA, Zou KH, Chabrerie AV, Bailey NO, Black PM. Decreases in ventricular volume correlate with decreases in ventricular pressure in idiopathic normal pressure hydrocephalus patients who experienced clinical improvement after implantation with adjustable valve shunts. *Neurosurgery* 2004;55(3):582–92; discussion 592–3.

23. Di Chiro G, Grove AS, Jr. Evaluation of surgical and spontaneous cerebrospinal fluid shunts by isotope scanning. *J Neurosurg* 1966;24(4):743–8.

24. Savoiardo M, Solero CL, Passerini A, Migliavacca F. Determination of cerebrospinal fluid shunt function with water-soluble contrast medium. *J Neurosurg* 1978;49(3):398–407.

25. Kharkar S, Shuck J, Kapoor S, et al. Radionuclide shunt patency study for evaluation of suspected ventriculoperitoneal shunt malfunction in adults with normal pressure hydrocephalus. *Neurosurgery* 2009;64(5):909–16; discussion 916–18.

Chapter 12

Imaging of the cerebrospinal fluid circulation

Olivier Balédent

Imaging of flows

Magnetic resonance imaging (MRI) is the preferred medical technique for brain and central nervous system investigations. This technique is sensitive to the motion of hydrogen atoms that represent the main component of biological fluids. These displacements of protons are the source of prevalent artifacts in morphological MR imaging: depending on the motion velocity of the fluid elements present in the considered slice, phenomena known as inflow and outflow artifacts modulate the intensity of the impacted voxels. The example of the fast CSF flow induced artifact in the aqueduct of Sylvius (flow void), well known by radiologists as evidence of a permeable aqueduct on T2-weighted images, can also be used to qualitatively point out the hyperdynamic aspect of specific hydrocephalus pathologies.

The understanding and exploitation of this type of artifact allowed the development of time-of-flight MR angiography. These sequences are particularly sensitive to the signal enhancement induced by the uninterrupted inflow in the slice of "fresh" blood that did not undergo earlier magnetization flip and presents a full magnetization at the origin of the observed enhanced signal.

However, morphological imaging methods do not allow quantitative studies of blood flow.

The phase-contrast MRI (PC-MRI) technique, based on the classical gradient echo sequence allowing fast imaging, is very sensitive to the motion of biological structures. It can be useful to quantify liquid flow rates in order to detect slow or absent flows. This method detects the magnetization's phase-shift of spins moving through magnetic field gradients (or alignment of individual spins relative to one another) with respect to static spins. Measurement of these phase-shift effects makes it possible to reconstruct images composed of flow sensitive pixels, where the pixel intensity reflects the local velocity [1].

The quality of PC-MRI acquisitions is dependent upon magnetic field inhomogeneities and local susceptibility artifacts. In order to cancel out the effects of external sources of spin dephasing, two gradients with the same magnitude but opposite direction are applied (bipolar gradient). Each of the gradients will shift the phase of spins within the tissues. In stationary tissues, the effects of the second pulse will exactly reverse those of the first. Conversely, fluid particles moving through the acquisition plane (vascular or CSF) will experience a net phase-shift proportional to its velocity.

Usually, the acquisition plane is selected perpendicular to the assumed flow direction axis. The reconstruction process then gathers the data in two-dimensional phase images, in which each pixel intensity is related to the local flow velocity. Depending on the manufacturers of MR scanners, this intensity can directly correspond to the velocity value or have to be calculated using specific vendors' information. In addition to the velocity maps covering the acquisition slice, phase-contrast MRI generally simultaneously acquires sets of T2-weighted amplitude images depicting the anatomy.

This technique was initially developed to image the beating heart and quantify flow velocities through cardiac valves and shunts. As heart motion is periodic, cardiac triggering or gating must be linked to the bipolar gradient echo pulse sequence [2,3].

The cardiac pulse can be recorded by using either the electrocardiogram (ECG) or the plethysmograph signal. The ECG signal is the most widely used in cardiac gating techniques because systole identification is very accurate using this method. The detection of the R-wave on the ECG signal serves as reference for automatic acquisition. Nevertheless, this technique is tedious and may require repeated electrode repositioning.

Adult Hydrocephalus, ed. Daniele Rigamonti. Published by Cambridge University Press.

In addition, as the ECG signal is sensitive to the magnetic field gradients, ECG-gated acquisition may induce a significant increase in the sequence duration. In contrast, the plethysmography method using a peripheral transducer, less prone to magnetic field gradients influence, can be easily handled.

MRI cardiac gating can be retrospective or prospective:

- Prospective gating technique sets the number of temporal phases splitting the cardiac cycle (CC) according to the lowest estimated CC length, which may induce misrepresentation of the diastolic phase.
- Retrospective gating technique is preferred because the number of temporal frames is initially set, reducing signal discrepancies between the first and final phases of the CC. In clinical practice, 32 images per cycle is a good compromise between temporal resolution and acquisition time. The number of temporal frames covering the CC depends on echo time (TE), repetition time (TR), and flip angle. By using gradient refocused echo sequence, short TR, and low flip angles, the temporal resolution can be significantly increased and the duration of the sequence reduced [4].

Depending on the MR apparatus manufacturers, PC-MRI sequence can be associated with acceleration methods such as parallel imaging, partial field of view reconstruction, or view sharing techniques (e.g. number of views per segment). Nevertheless, these techniques reduce the accuracy and signal to noise ratio of images.

The main parameters that can potentially influence the quality and the accuracy of flow imaging are briefly recalled below.

Phase encoding is related to the velocity of spins within the limits of ±180°. If the absolute phase-shift is higher than 180°, phase wrapping will occur and the measured velocity will be underestimated. It is thus necessary to fit the velocity scale to the probable maximum flow velocity in the vessel. This scale factor is the velocity encoding parameter (V_{enc}), which would correspond to a phase-shift of 180°. The V_{enc} parameter sets the range of measurable velocities ($-V_{enc}$, $+V_{enc}$) without phase wrapping. The previous estimation of the extreme values of the detected velocities can therefore increase the measurement accuracy.

If V_{enc} is lower than the actual flow velocity, aliasing artifacts due to phase wrapping will be encountered in the studied vessel; they visually correspond to areas where discontinuities in pixel intensities appear. The more V_{enc} is small, the more aliasing areas will affect the velocity map. If V_{enc} is higher than the expected maximum flow velocity, the signal to noise ratio decreases concomitantly with the measurement's accuracy. Then, V_{enc} must be adjusted depending on the studied flows and anatomical levels. For example, blood velocities are different in internal carotid and in small epidural veins; in the same way CSF oscillations in the narrow aqueduct of Sylvius can be hyperdynamic compared to CSF oscillations in the large pontine cistern.

A grayscale is used to represent PC-MRI measured velocities. Static tissues, corresponding to null flows, will be represented with gray pixels. Hyper- or hypointense pixels correspond to areas where circulation occurs at a velocity close to V_{enc} absolute value.

The slice can be positioned so as to be parallel to the direction of flow; in this case, results are not quantitative but rather give a qualitative overview of the anatomical regions where fluid motion occurs (see Figure 12.7b, c). In order to record quantitative flow data, the acquisition slice must be perpendicular to the presumed direction of the flow (see (Figure 12.3).

If the plane is oblique with respect to the flow axis, each pixel velocity will be underestimated. Nevertheless, as the vessel section area is then proportionally overestimated, the flow rate (Flow = Velocity × Area) is theoretically preserved but spatial resolution limits generate a significant decrease in accuracy.

Main PC-MRI parameters usually encountered in cerebral acquisitions:

TE	Minimum
TR	Minimum
Flip angle	20° to 45°
Field of view	10 × 10 to 24 × 24 cm²
Matrix	256 × 128 to 512 × 512
Slice thickness	2–7 mm
View per segment	1 to 4
Number of images per CC	16 to 40 (32 currently used)
Acquisition flow direction	*Slice* for quantitative acquisition
	All directions for qualitative acquisition
V_{enc}	2–20 cm/s (CSF)
	60–150 cm/s (main arteries)
	10–60 cm/s (main veins)

Signal to noise ratio can be improved by increasing the number of excitations (or averaging) at the expense of the duration of the acquisition. The spatial resolution and the subject's cardiac frequency also influence the temporal length of the PC-MRI exam; this duration can vary from less than a minute to more than 10 minutes.

The best possible protocol results from a compromise between reasonable time acquisition for clinical exam and reasonable accuracy to suit specific "flow questions": PC-MRI protocol could be different if the question is simply "*Are there hyperdynamic CSF oscillations in this large aqueduct?*" or precisely "*What is the accurate value of CSF net flow in this very narrow aqueduct?*"

Pelc et al. studied the cine PC-MRI sequence in terms of blood flow quantization within deep vessels (portal trunk) in dogs. The values measured using MRI were compared to an invasive Doppler echography technique (the Doppler probe was directly inserted in the studied vessel) [5]. This comparison exhibited a strong correlation between the two methods. The authors concluded that MRI would probably be able to quantify blood flow circulation in deep vessels in humans.

Buonocore and Bogren established the factors influencing the measurement accuracy of the PC-MRI sequence. According to their results, the slice thickness, the encoding velocity, and the temporal resolution as well as the choice of TR, TE, and flip angle, were parameters in which suitable settings were paramount in order to reach an acceptable measurement accuracy [6].

Greil et al. studied, in vitro, the different acquisition parameters and their potential effect on the velocity measurement accuracy. They concluded that the key factor was the spatial resolution of the image modulated by the field of view and the matrix [7].

During an in vitro study using an MRI phantom, McCauley et al. validated the PC-MRI sequence for velocity measurements in unsteady flows. After comparison of MRI to standard Doppler velocimetry, they showed that the second technique was significantly less accurate [8].

Enzmann et al. and Wahlin et al. showed the good reproducibility of the PC-MRI technique for quantization of weak liquid oscillations such as those encountered at the aqueduct level [9,10].

For all PC-MRI flow measurements, one must take into account the effects of eddy currents in all vendors' scanners as they introduce a significant velocity phase offset. Sequence and protocol optimization is required to reduce this intrinsic source of errors [6,9,11,12].

As PC-MRI is a functional imaging method, the post-processing step is crucial. PC-MRI was at first mainly used for vascular flow quantization and many software packages were developed by MR vendors to measure blood flows in vessels. As blood flows are mainly unidirectional and vessels' boundaries present simple geometrical shapes, several automatic algorithms were developed, allowing quick, reproducible, and accurate blood vessel segmentation [13]. CSF flow oscillations arise in complex anatomical regions such as subarachnoid spaces. Thus CSF flow studies require a specific CSF segmentation algorithm, which may explain why CSF flow investigations have not been widespread in clinical practice.

Balédent et al. and Alperin and Lee developed home-made flow software based on the analysis of CSF and blood velocity changes during CC. Using this tool, dedicated to both blood vessels and subarachnoid space (SAS) segmentation, the authors showed that one could extract velocimetric data of blood and CSF flows in a reproducible way (inter- and intra-observer), allowing an accurate, reproducible, and automatic segmentation of blood vessel and SAS lumens [14,15].

In this chapter, CSF and blood flow values were calculated using the PC-MRI post-processing software developed by Balédent et al. (software can be freely downloaded at: www.tidam.fr [14]). The methodology of this pixel-based software is focused on several robust frameworks that provide reliable results. The main ideas underlying the algorithm are described below.

In order to correct for possible phase offset, the average apparent velocity of a neighboring region of interest was first subtracted from the phase velocity [11,16]. The segmentation algorithm consisted of two successive steps: the creation of a new parametric image, obtained for all time frames, followed by the application of a threshold. In this new image, each pixel intensity depended on the magnitude of the fundamental frequency, i.e. the subject's cardiac frequency. The magnitude of this spectral component was assessed using a fast Fourier transformation (FFT) for each pixel signal during CC. Regions exhibiting cardiac periodicity, such as CSF areas, were highlighted on the new image where pixel intensities were characterized by their dependence of flow on heart rate. A threshold was applied to the parametric image so as to extract all the pixels with a velocity signal at the cardiac frequency

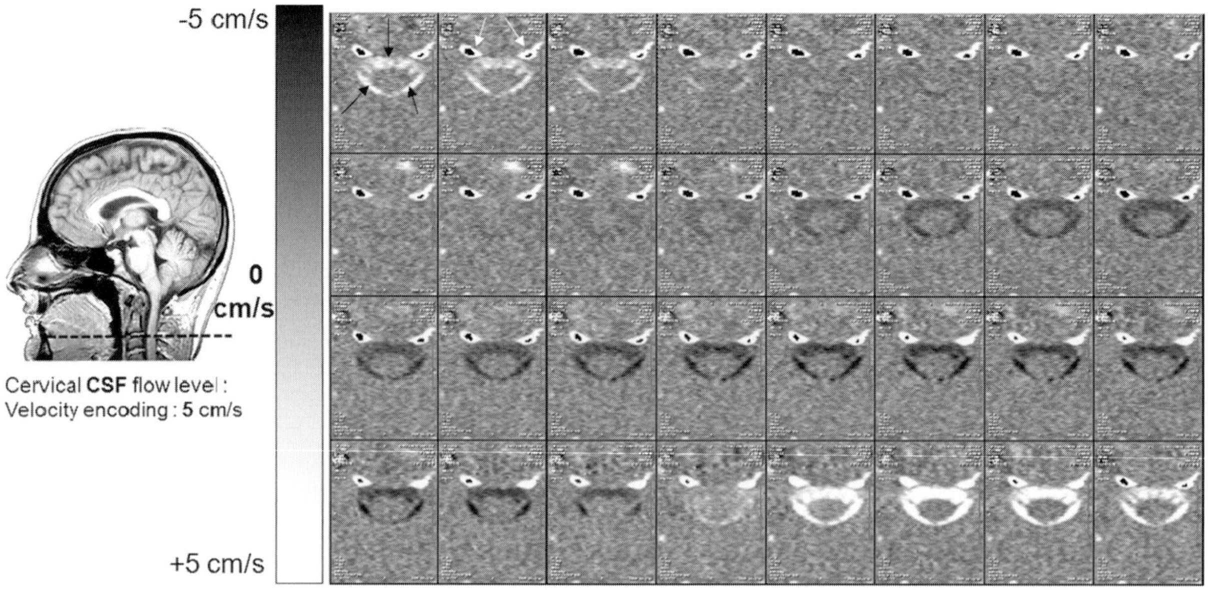

Figure 12.1 Cervical CSF flow intensity changes during the cardiac cycle.

above a visually selected threshold. This threshold usually made it possible to differentiate tissue with low fundamental component magnitude and identify CSF pulsating motion, which has a large fundamental component magnitude (see Figure 12.2). If CSF and non-CSF regions were adjoining, a phase threshold was then applied to identify actual CSF pixels.

Temporal normalization

All the temporal data were expressed as percentage of CC and the time of internal carotid systolic peak flow of an individual was used as time reference. This time shift was applied to all the velocity curves for each subject.

Aliasing correction

Aliasing pixels are characterized by their high velocity in the opposite direction to the average velocity of the segmented area. Corrected velocity values for such pixels were recalculated as $V_{corrected} = (2 * V_{enc} - |V_{error}|) * (-|V_{error}|/V_{error})$.

CSF flow parameters

The flow rate through a region of interest (ROI) is estimated as the product of the averaged velocity of the pixels within the ROI and the area of the given ROI. Stroke volume (SV expressed in μl/CC) corresponds to the mean of the two oppositely directed displaced volumes during the CC. This is the most prevalent parameter, often applied in the aqueduct of Sylvius to characterize CSF flow [16,17].

In Figure 12.1, a series of 32 phase images resulting from PC-MRI is depicted. Images were zoomed to clearly visualize CSF intensity changes during a whole cardiac cycle. The slice being studied was positioned perpendicularly to the spine at the C2–C3 level. In the first images, white pixels represent the flush of CSF in the subarachnoid spaces around the spine and black arrows show the main CSF compartments separated by spinal nerves.

During CC, CSF pixel intensities gradually decrease toward gray color where the liquid velocities reach a null value. Then, the color progressively darkens toward black, which corresponds to the moment when CSF fills the cranium. Periods of CSF flushing/filling alternate, paced by the heart beat.

In these images, white arrows point at two regions showing the blood flow in the epidural veins, which are close the subarachnoid spaces. In this example, as epidural blood flow exhibits velocities up to 5 cm/s, the aliasing phenomenon (dark areas) arises in the vessel.

Available processing software, using automatic segmentation, makes it possible to quickly obtain a reproducible time evolution curve during the CC. After background correction using a manually drawn area, flow parameters such as CSF stroke volume are directly calculated (Figure 12.2).

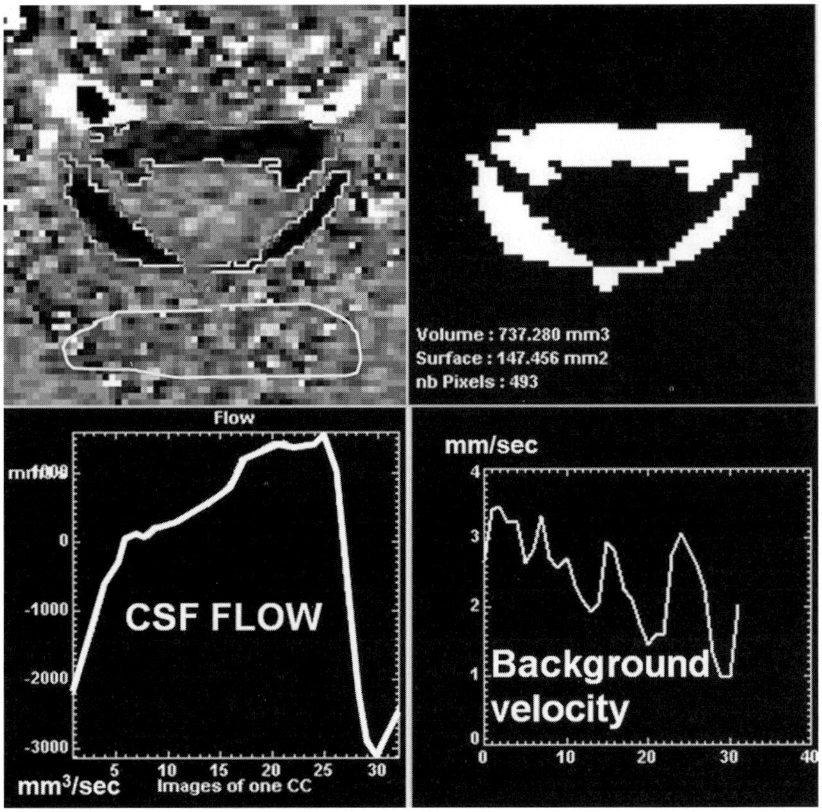

Figure 12.2 PC-MRI post-processing. PC-MRI image of CSF flow at cervical level (C2–C3). The software extracts the outline of regions of interest (ROIs) and calculates flow curve. To correct for the phase offset due to eddy currents, the average apparent velocity of a static neighboring region throughout the cardiac cycle was subtracted from the phase velocity of the ROIs. This background region is manually drawn (white line) in a static anatomical region. Vascular vessels and CSF flows from other anatomical levels are measured in the same way.

CSF and blood flow interaction

As CSF is an incompressible fluid, Pascal's law indicates that, from a static point of view, any pressure variation in an elementary volume of the CSF compartment would thus be integrally transmitted at any point in the whole CSF volume.

The compliance of a compartment can be defined as the ratio of volume change to the corresponding pressure change. This parameter is an indicator of the distensibility of the compartment and corresponds to the ability to bear a pressure increase, resulting from volume fluctuation, without disruption of the structure function. When compliance is known, it should be possible to assess the magnitude of the CSF pressure required to bring the CSF compartment back to its initial volume after a volume change in one of the other intracranial compartments (blood or brain).

The cranio-rachidian skeleton and the meningeal dura mater can be considered to constitute a rigid undeformable structure in adulthood. In children, fibrous and elastic cranial sutures and fontanelles provide the cranial box with the flexibility necessary for nervous growth and development; these fontanelles usually close progressively from birth until the end of the second year in infancy. CSF and blood flow also change during this growing period [18].

In this rigid closed "box," three compartments interact: the nearly incompressible vascular (arterial, capillary, and venous) and CSF compartments and brain parenchyma. Blood and CSF compartments are incompressible. Although the glial cells constitute a soft flexible embedding, the cerebral parenchyma is also usually supposed to be incompressible and needs the extracranial compliance distributed in the spinal canal and the dural sac.

The interactions between these various compartments consist of periodical liquid volume displacements and exchanges. Actually, the cranial box deals continuously with two imperatives. The first obvious requirement is an intracranial inflow of arterial blood at each cardiac cycle (CC), which is necessary to supply the brain with essential nutrients for regular cerebral functioning. The second requirement is to regulate the outgoing venous and CSF flows in order to maintain a stable pressure in the cranial box, as a significant increase in intracranial pressure might be harmful for the brain, hindering normal cerebral functioning.

In this context, PC-MRI is a valuable tool to investigate and quantify these CSF and blood flow interactions throughout the cardiac cycle. In the following parts of this chapter, normal adult hydro- and hemodynamics will be described. Then these results will be used as references to better detect cerebral flow alterations of hydrocephalus patients.

In healthy adults, MRI flow studies showed that the CSF flush venting from the intracranial SAS into the cervical spinal SAS, which had a high magnitude and elapsed very quickly, was the main lever control in instantaneous regulation of ICP. In contrast, the ventricular CSF flow represented less than 6% of the intracranial blood variation, and occurred at almost 20–25% of the CC duration. Therefore, it appeared that, in healthy subjects, the ventricular system plays a minor role in the dampening of the general systolic expansion [14], while the "CSF mobile compliance" [19] of the intracranial cavity depends mainly on the SAS. Additionally, the temporal analysis of flow curves tended to confirm previous theories about the relation between brain expansion and the ventricular pulsations. We [14] hypothesized that the early CSF flush through the fourth ventricle reflects the early infratentorial expansion, while the delayed CSF flush through the aqueduct, the third ventricle, and the foramina of Monro rather reflects the delayed supratentorial expansion. Finally, a close correlation between CSF aqueductal stroke volume and time point of jugular peak flow was found, which indicated a direct quantitative relation between brain expansion and ventricular pulsation. Based on these findings, we suggested a global modeling of both CSF and blood flow relationships throughout the different phases of the cardiac cycle. The description and understanding of these successive phenomena in healthy subjects would enable detailed and extensive volumetric analysis in clinical practice, in order to access pathological changes and to detect the perturbations of CSF dynamic patterns in several neurological disorders.

PC-MRI is a powerful tool to investigate CSF and blood circulation but its use in clinical practice requires careful selection of the anatomical part for investigation. Figure 12.3 displays an example of the four main regions explored in an efficient CSF flow protocol. In less than 10 minutes a global overview of the hydro- and hemodynamics of the craniospinal system is made possible.

By applying this protocol in healthy adults, we observed that CSF and vascular curves presented comparable and reproducible oscillations even if amplitude variations in vascular and CSF flow due to age, anatomy, or physiology were present [20]. These variations are moderate compared with important alterations in CSF and blood flows induced by cerebral pathologies such as hydrocephalus, syringomyelia, and cerebral hemorrhage [17,21,22].

Figure 12.4 displays an example of normal CSF and blood flow curves during the CC in a 30-year-old woman. These curves are representative of flows measured in the healthy young adult population described in Table 12.1.

The knowledge of individual arterial flow curves makes it possible to calculate the cerebral blood inflow, Figure 12.4a, which is the sum of left and right internal carotid flows with the vertebral artery flow. Mean cerebral arterial blood flow was close to 700 ml/min in adults.

The cerebral venous outflow resulted from the sum of left and right internal jugular flows and epidural veins flow. In order to take into account unmeasured small veins, the amplitude of the measured cerebral venous waveform was corrected, so that the average of the corrected cerebral venous flow rate was equal to the previously measured average arterial inflow (Figure 12.4b). Cerebral venous flow is not steady during the cardiac cycle but presents noteworthy oscillations resulting from arterial pulsations, intracranial pressure, and probably also from heart suction. It is interesting to note that arterial and venous flows exhibit an equivalent amplitude during the diastole period (x-axis: 9–12) and just prior to the systolic peak flow (x-axis: 24–26). The equilibrium period (called "brain equilibrium pressure") when arterial inflow and venous outflow are almost balanced corresponds to the moment when CSF reverses its flow at the cervical level, as displayed in Figure 12.4c.

Indeed, the curve depicted within this figure represents the intracranial arterio-venous flow difference (subtraction of venous flow from arterial flow) throughout the CC: a positive systolic peak flow (arterial flow > venous flow) and two diastolic negative bumps (venous flow > arterial flow) are shown. The positive values of this calculated curve represent an increase in blood volume whereas negative values are related to a decrease in blood volume. The integration of the positive part

Table 12.1 Blood and CSF flow in healthy subjects, hydrocephalus stenosis patients before and after endoscopic third ventriculostomy (ETV), and normal pressure hydrocephalus (NPH) patients

Population	N	Age	CBF (ml/min)	Cervical CSF (μl/CC)	Ventricular CSF (μl/CC)
Healthy young	19	27 ± 4	688 ± 115	575 ± 124	48 ± 23
Healthy aging	12	71 ± 9	509 ± 103	457 ± 147	34 ± 16
Hydrocephalus stenosis	11	63 ± 10	555 ± 123	594 ± 250	0
Post ETV			670 ± 105	496 ± 149	210 ± 100
NPH	12	49 ± 23	525 ± 206	467 ± 260	196 ± 100

N, number of subjects; CBF, mean cerebral blood flow; cervical CSF, CSF stroke volume at C2–C3; ventricular CSF, CSF stroke volume in the aqueduct or in the aperture of the third ventricle for patients who underwent ETV.

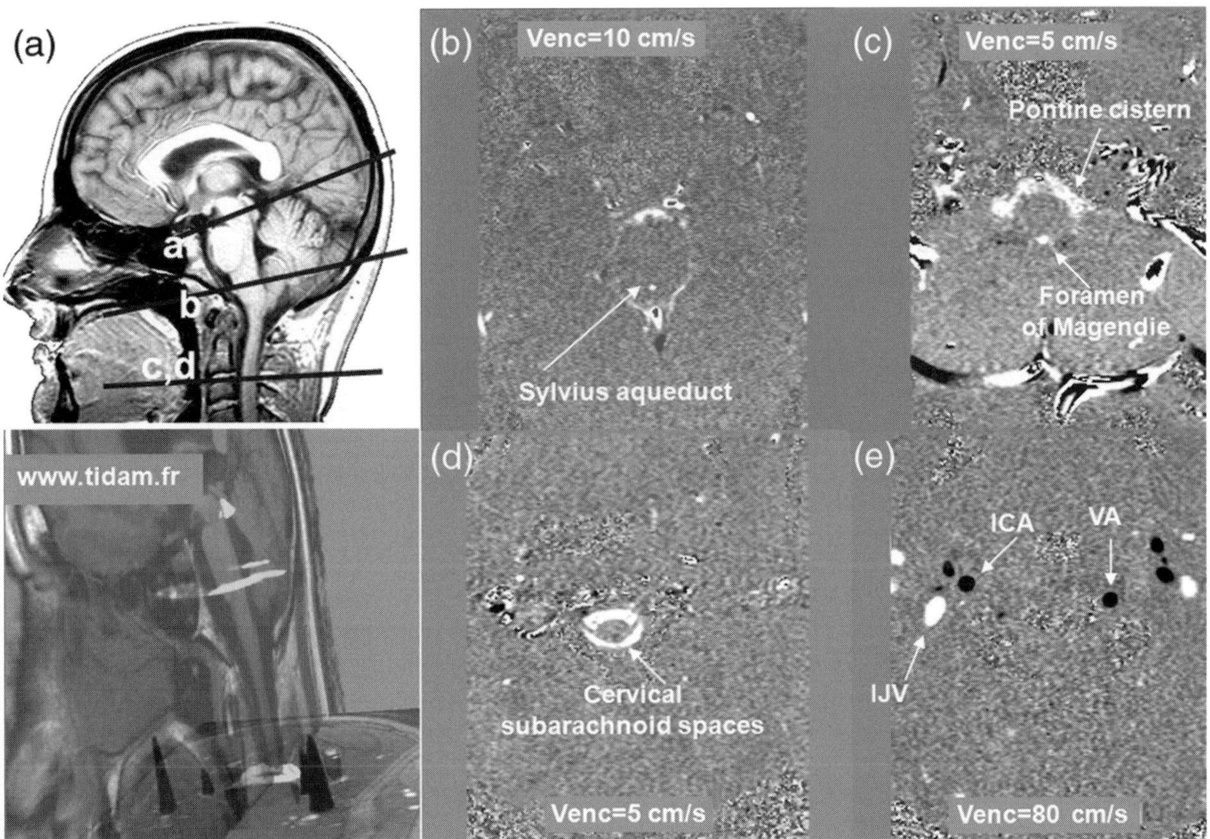

Figure 12.3 Data acquisition. Sagittal scout view sequences were used as localizer to select the anatomical levels for flow quantification (a). The acquisition planes were selected perpendicular to the presumed direction of the flows. Sections through the aqueduct of Sylvius (b), pontine cistern and foramen of Magendie (c), and C2–C3 subarachnoid spaces level (d), were used for CSF flow measurement. By varying the velocity encoding (V_{enc}), the same cervical section level (e) was used to measure vascular flows in left and right internal carotids (ICA), vertebral arteries (VA), and internal jugular veins (IJV). Black pixels represent the flows entering the slice, white pixels represent flows directed out of the slice, and gray pixels correspond to immobile tissues. A full-color version is included in the color plate section.

of the curve represents the intracranial blood volume change during the CC. The arterio-venous curve, reflecting the pulsatility of the brain during the cardiac cycle, is the main source of intracranial pressure (ICP) fluctuation during the CC. Actually, ICP amplitude is also dependent on CSF volume changes in the cranium as well as intracranial compliance.

As can be observed in Figure 12.4c, arterio-venous difference and CSF flow measured at the cervical level are oscillating in opposite phase with similar

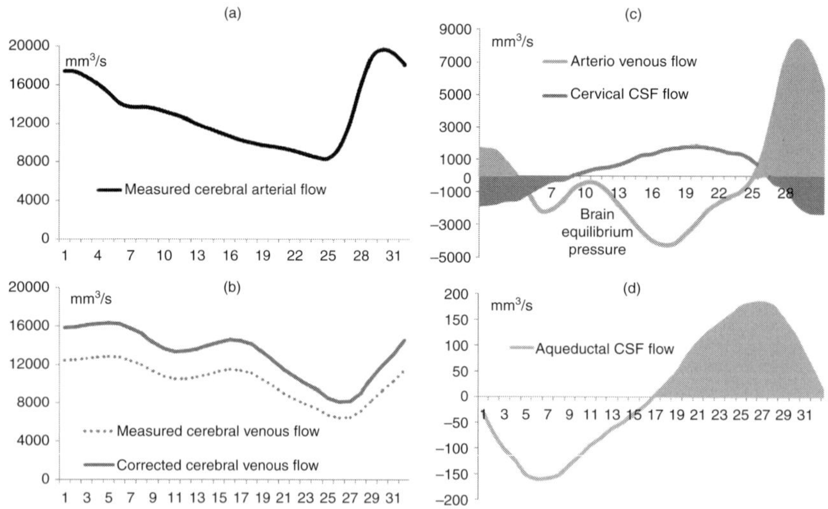

Figure 12.4 CSF and cerebral blood flow during the cardiac cycle in healthy adults (see text for full explanation). A full-color version is included in the color plate section.

amplitudes: positive flow values correspond to CSF flushing through the spinal canal and negative values correspond to CSF filling the cranium. CSF seems to balance the vascular expansion so as to minimize the potential increase in ICP during the systolic phase because arterial inflow is not instantaneously drained by the venous system.

In the same way, summation of CSF and vascular flow curves are calculated to obtain the intracranial volume change (IVC) during a CC [23]. As a function of the craniospinal compliance, IVC generates pressure changes in the equilibrium ICP. The pressure fluctuations due to volume variations were determined by Marmarou's monoexponential function [24]:

$$P(t) = P_0.\exp^{(k.\mathrm{IVC}(t))}$$

where P is the instantaneous intraventricular pressure, P_0 is the resting equilibrium pressure, and k is the elastance (inverse of compliance) factor. This highlights the major role of CSF in the control of ICP during the CC.

The intracranial compartment can be assimilated to a "black box" that converts the arterial input signal into venous and CSF output signals. The ICP temporal evolution controls the cerebral blood perfusion. Then, monitoring of ICP during the CC is a key parameter for understanding and diagnosis of diseases related to CSF flow alterations.

The PC-MRI CSF–blood approach may help to estimate the ICP waveform but a missing link still remains. Although Alperin [25] proposed, through various assumptions, a PC-MRI method to assess intracranial elastance and ICP in six baboons, no paper in the literature has demonstrated or corroborated this finding in large human populations or in specific phantom models. In the future, this scientific void may be filled using specific phantom models of the craniospinal system [26].

Figure 12.4d displays the CSF oscillation in the aqueduct during CC; the green area represents the aqueductal CSF stroke volume. In comparison with the cervical level, the amplitude of aqueductal CSF oscillation is nearly 10 times smaller and presents a significant phase-shift [14]. The volume of CSF in intracranial SAS is around the value of CSF ventricular volume. Nevertheless, as the long and narrow tubular aqueduct of Sylvius imposes a substantial resistance to flow, the impact of ventricular CSF flow in ICP amplitude change during CC is then very low in healthy subjects. It highlights the major influence of CSF at the intracranial SAS level (pontine, cerebellar cisterns), which oscillates between the cranium and the spinal canal.

From the CSF and blood flow curves measured in a healthy population, a chronological sequence of events has been generated. Figure 12.5 shows how the fast systolic blood inflow impacts on the volume exchanges between the compartments. A more global and synthetic depiction is displayed in Figure 12.6.

As CSF is mainly produced in the ventricular choroid plexus, we can rationally hypothesize that a residual net flow directed toward the fourth ventricle arises. Theoretically, the PC-MRI method could measure or approach this secretion [27] but many constraints such as spatial and temporal resolution, eddy currents [12], intermittent CSF secretion, or variable heart rate limit the chance to meet this challenge. New MRI sequences based on spin labeling technique seem more relevant to

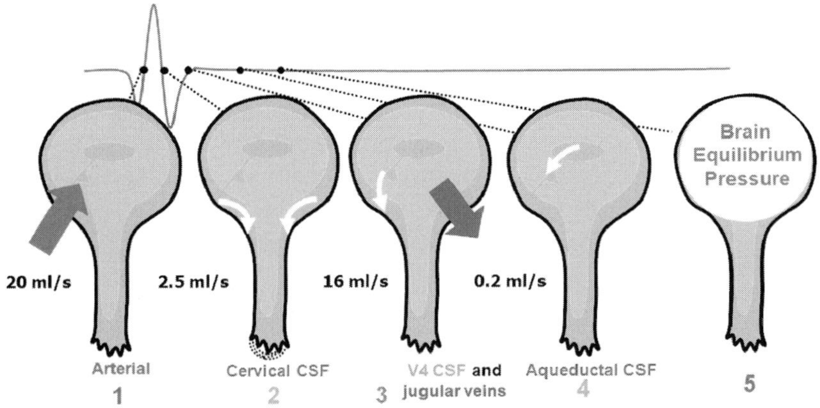

Figure 12.5 Chronological sequence of cerebral blood and CSF peak flows during early phase of the cardiac cycle. The cardiac systole can be divided into five phases according to the CSF or blood peak flows; the time of appearance of these peaks and their magnitude (in ml/s) are depicted. During the first phase, the cerebral blood volume instantaneously increases because of the vertebral and internal carotid systolic peak flows. The quickest way to absorb this and to regulate brain volume expansion is to flush extracerebral CSF into the spinal SAS (second phase), thanks to the spinal and dural sac compliance. During the third phase, a significant jugular output flow occurs and CSF progressively flushes out of V4; later (fourth phase), aqueduct, V3, and Monro flushes appear, with a very small contribution to the volume regulation. During the fifth phase, after a transient equilibrium state, brain CSF filling occurs and the reverse sequence begins. A full-color version is included in the color plate section.

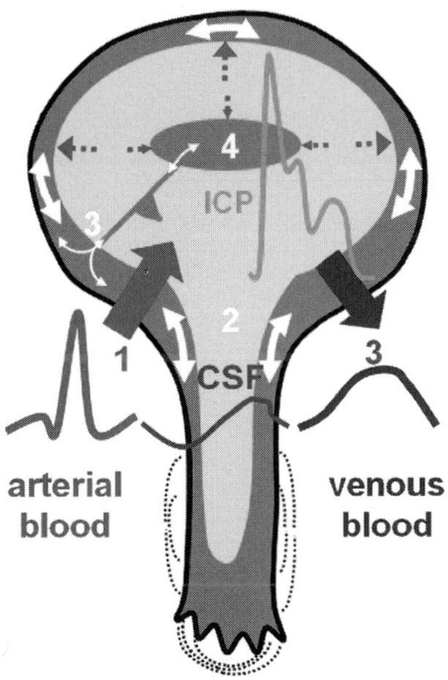

Figure 12.6 Diagram of CSF and blood flow. The large and rapid amplitude change in cerebral arterial input flow [1] increases the brain volume over the intracranial subarachnoid spaces (large red arrows). In these areas, resistance to flow is low and as CSF viscosity is low, CSF is quickly displaced out of the cranium toward the compliant spinal canal [2]; ICP increase is therefore limited. Nevertheless, this first CSF response is scanty and has to be supplemented with the cerebral blood venous outflow [3]. Due to blood viscosity, this venous contribution is slower but brings a greater displaced volume. Finally, the pressure decreases at the brain periphery induce a CSF ventricular flow, out of the fourth ventricle and through the aqueduct of Sylvius, resulting in a small inner displacement of the brain directed toward the ventricles (small red arrows). After this series of flow events during the systolic phase of CC, arterial inflow equals venous outflow and cervical CSF flush stops. After this brief equilibrium pressure moment, venous heart aspiration increases the cerebral venous outflow, decreases ICP, and reverses the cervical CSF flow to fill the cranium and prepare the next cycle. A full-color version is included in the color plate section.

observe and measure the CSF net flow in the aqueduct [28]. The choroid plexus may also play a role in CSF absorption and is not the sole source of CSF production [27,29,30].

Imaging of CSF disorders

In clinical practice, the most commonly encountered CSF disorders observed using radiological images are *hydrocephalus* in the brain and *syringomyelia* in the spine. These two pathologies have a characteristic in common: CSF volume increases in the center of the nervous system, generating compression of the surrounding tissues.

The aim of the following section is to show how PC-MRI of CSF can help clinicians to diagnose and understand these disorders as well as how it can help neurosurgeons to guide treatment.

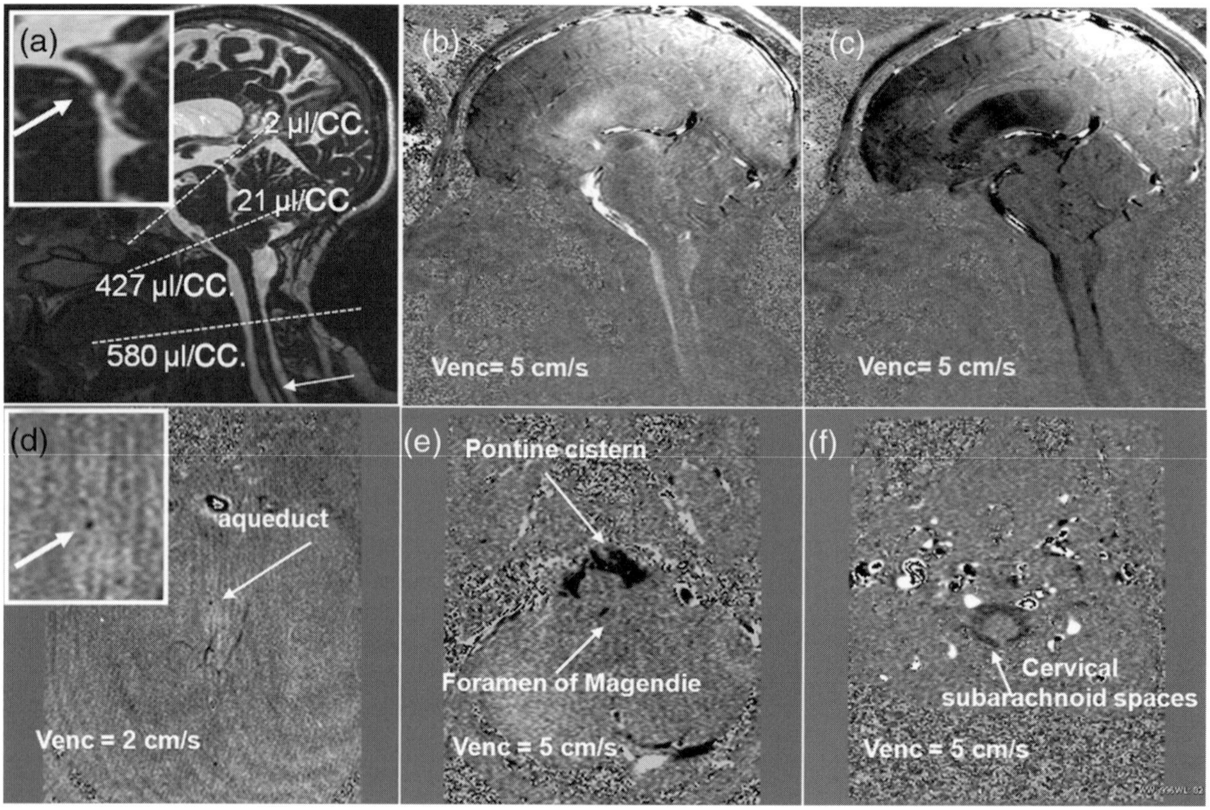

Figure 12.7 Incomplete stenosis of the aqueduct of Sylvius. CSF MRI investigations in a 42-year-old woman presenting with hydrocephalus and syringomyelia. Control 3 months after foramen magnum surgery. (a) 3D-FIESTA image highlights CSF splitting and hyposignal in the aqueduct probably due to aqueductal stenosis. At the bottom of the image, hypersignal inside the spine indicates the beginning of a syringomyelia cavity. (b, c) Sagittal PC-MRI view with velocity sensitivity selected in the up–down direction. Image (b) corresponds to systolic phase with CSF flushing towards the spinal canal, CSF appears in white around the spine and in the subarachnoid spaces but not clearly in the aqueduct and the foramen of Magendie. Aliasing inside the pontine cistern corresponds to the blood flow in the basilar artery whose velocities are much greater than 5 cm/s. Image (c) corresponds to the diastolic phase with CSF filling the cranium. These sagittal images (b, c) cannot be used for quantitative investigation of CSF flow but allow a global qualitative view of the CSF circulation during the cardiac cycle. (d) Quantitative PC-MRI exam has been carried out at the aqueduct of Sylvius level with very low velocity encoding (V_{enc}) to depict very small but real oscillations. When V_{enc} was adjusted to 10 cm/s, no flow was detected. (e) PC-MRI shows also the functional pontine cistern, foramen of Magendie, and cervical subarachnoid spaces in the cervical canal (f). The stroke volumes of CSF during the cardiac cycle were calculated after post-processing and are written on image (a) at their respective levels. Results show that, though surgery established a normal CSF circulation between the cranium and the spinal canal, communication between the ventricles and the subarachnoid spaces remained abnormal.

Hydrocephalus can be seen as an alteration of the CSF circulation between its production and absorption sites but also, in light of the previous section, as an alteration of its displacements between the various CSF compartments of the craniospinal system. Aqueductal stenosis, one of the common origins of hydrocephalus, can be induced by tumor compression detected using standard morphological MR imaging. Absence of flow void in T2-weighted images can be a good indicator of stenosis and 3D-SSFP (three-dimensional balanced steady-state free precession) sequence is available to investigate a wide range of CSF pathologies when traditional MRI sequences do not provide the desired anatomic information (Siemens TrueFISP, General Electrics FIESTA, and Philips balanced TFE) [31].

During our clinical experience, according to the morphological images, we have observed patients with suspected aqueductal stenosis showing CSF oscillations in the aqueduct and patients without evidence of stenosis demonstrating null flow in the aqueduct on PC-MRI images [32].

As a consequence of this observation, the PC-MRI protocol is performed in all cases of suspected aqueductal stenosis in our hospital. Low V_{enc} (5 or 2 cm/s) is required to confirm the absence of CSF flow in the aqueduct (Figure 12.7).

Table 12.1 shows that hydrocephalus patients with aqueductal stenosis have an increase in CSF oscillations in the spinal canal probably due to the associated ICP increase.

Endoscopic third ventriculostomy (ETV) is an interesting surgical treatment for aqueductal stenosis pathologies. Nevertheless, the aperture made in the third ventricle (V3) is not characterized by the same hydrodynamic characteristics as the functional aqueduct. Indeed, CSF flow rate can be calculated by the ratio of pressure difference between the third ventricle and subarachnoid spaces to the resistance of the relevant channel (aqueduct or V3 aperture). These resistances, related to the radius and length of the fluid passage, are obviously not of the same order of magnitude in the geometrically different aqueduct and V3 aperture. It is then interesting to quantify CSF oscillations through the V3 aperture and to evaluate the impact of ETV on hydro- and hemodynamics.

After ETV, cervical CSF oscillations significantly decreased in aqueduct stenosis patients (Table 12.1). This decrease is probably associated with the decrease in ICP [33].

As was done in the aqueduct, the functionality of the third ventricle aperture has also been quantified using PC-MRI by computation of temporal flow curves in order to extract the associated stroke volume (Figure 12.8). Through this aperture, CSF presented oscillations with a temporal evolution similar to the one observed in volunteers' aqueducts but amplitudes were greatly increased. No significant correlation was found between the V3 CSF oscillation and the aperture area, the cervical CSF oscillation, or the arterial flow amplitude.

As noted for the aqueduct analysis, it is important to carefully position the PC-MRI slice; at the V3 level, it must be close to the roof and perpendicular to presumed direction of CSF flow. In the case of huge flow through the aperture, the presence of flow void in T2-weighted images can help in choosing the best slice location.

Another potential issue is the proximity of the basilar artery as blood can generate aliasing artifacts which can be difficult to differentiate from CSF flow.

The V_{enc} factor used for the V3 acquisition varies from 5 to 15 cm/s, depending on the size of the aperture and the pressure distribution.

Quantization of CSF oscillations through the V3 aperture is very useful to control its permeability and to check the efficiency of the treatment. This could be useful also in understanding the physiological aspects of the surgery and may, in the future, help to select patients who finally need a shunt because other CSF flow alterations still persist.

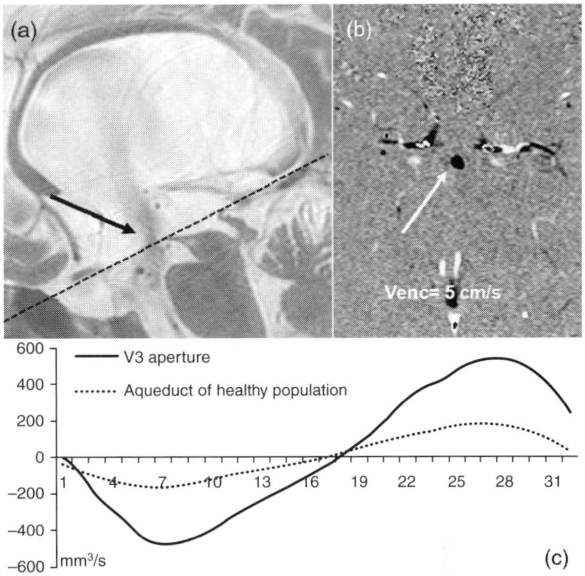

Figure 12.8 CSF flow in the V3 aperture after ETV. (a) Sagittal T2-weighted image showing flow void (black arrow) in the aqueduct characterizing flow blockage. (b) CSF flow through the aperture performed by the neurosurgeon re-established CSF communication between the third ventricle and the subarachnoid spaces. (c) CSF oscillation through the aperture compared to aqueduct CSF oscillation calculated in a healthy population.

Since its first description in 1965 [34,35], the syndrome of normal pressure hydrocephalus (NPH) has remained a diagnostic and therapeutic challenge. Paradoxically, despite the name of this syndrome, the ICP pulse waveform of chronic adult hydrocephalus patients is not so normal [36] and NPH can be a confusing name [37].

In 2005, an independent study group was assembled and addressed evidence-based guidelines for the management of NPH patients [38]. A part of this assessment examined the value of supplemental tests in the diagnosis of NPH and prediction of which patients would benefit from placement of a shunt. Among all of these tools (cisternography, ICP monitoring, tap test, external lumbar drainage, CSF resistive outflow R_{out}), PC-MRI seemed to be of potential interest through the evaluation of aqueductal stroke volume, but neither CSF flow void sign nor quantitative CSF flow velocity seemed to have significant diagnostic value. Greitz et al.

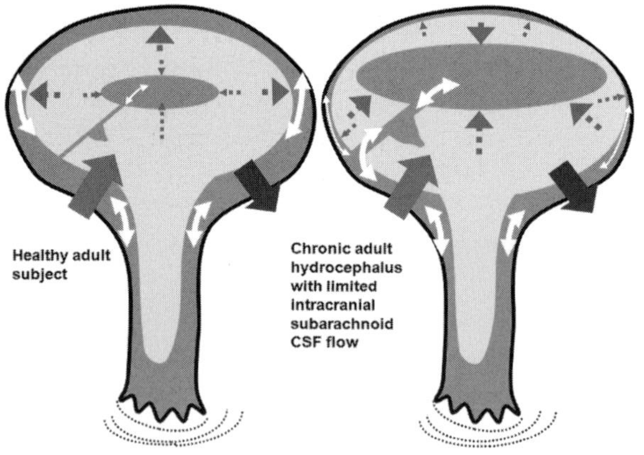

Figure 12.9 Schematic representation of CSF circulation in a healthy subject and chronic adult hydrocephalus. Red arrow represents arterial flow. Blue arrow represents venous outflow. White arrows represent CSF oscillation during cardiac cycle. In this model restricted CSF oscillations in the intracranial subarachnoid compartment increase CSF oscillations in the ventricle to maintain cervical CSF oscillations, then balance vascular expansion and preserve a large increase in ICP during the cardiac cycle. A full-color version is included in the color plate section.

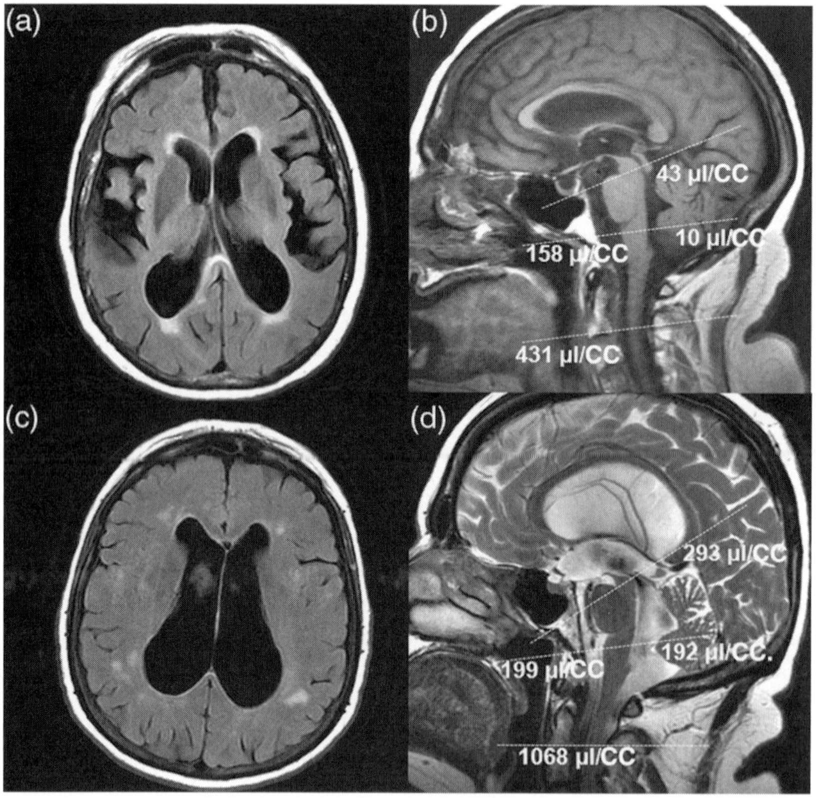

Figure 12.10 CSF flow in two patients with suspected NPH. (a, b) Morphological MRI of a 72-year-old woman with slowly progressive dementia, Parkinson syndrome, and a significant gait disturbance. (a) Her ventricles were dilated with hypersignal signs of transependymal resorption of CSF with significant atrophy. (b) The CSF stroke volumes from PC-MRI acquisition at the level of the aqueduct, the pontine cistern, the foramen of Magendie, and in the spinal canal at the C2–C3 level are displayed. Cerebral arterial inflow was 492 ml/min. A tap test was done and resulted in a negative response and post lumbar puncture headache. No surgical treatment was undertaken. (c, d) Morphological MRI of a 56-year-old woman with isolated gait disturbance. (c) T2 axial FLAIR image showing dilation of the ventricles without important signs of transependymal resorption. (d) CSF stroke volume is presented in sagittal T2-weighted MRI: flow void is important inside the aqueduct in accordance with the very large calculated stroke volume. Cerebral arterial inflow was 566 ml/min. Tap test response was positive, then the patient was shunted and a few days after surgery her walking had improved. CSF dynamics of the first patient (a, b) was in the range of normal values (Table 12.1) whereas the second (c, d) had greatly increased oscillations.

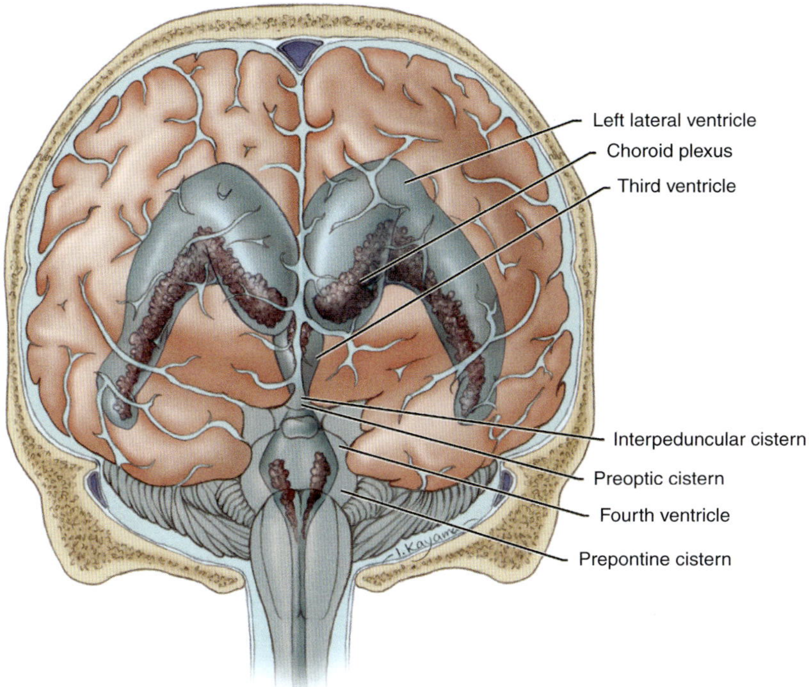

Figure 1.1 Overview of the ventricular system and cisterns. CSF is produced and flows from the lateral ventricles into the third and then fourth ventricles. From the fourth ventricle, CSF empties into the cisterns of the skull base, which will then flow into CSF cisterns of the cerebral convexities.

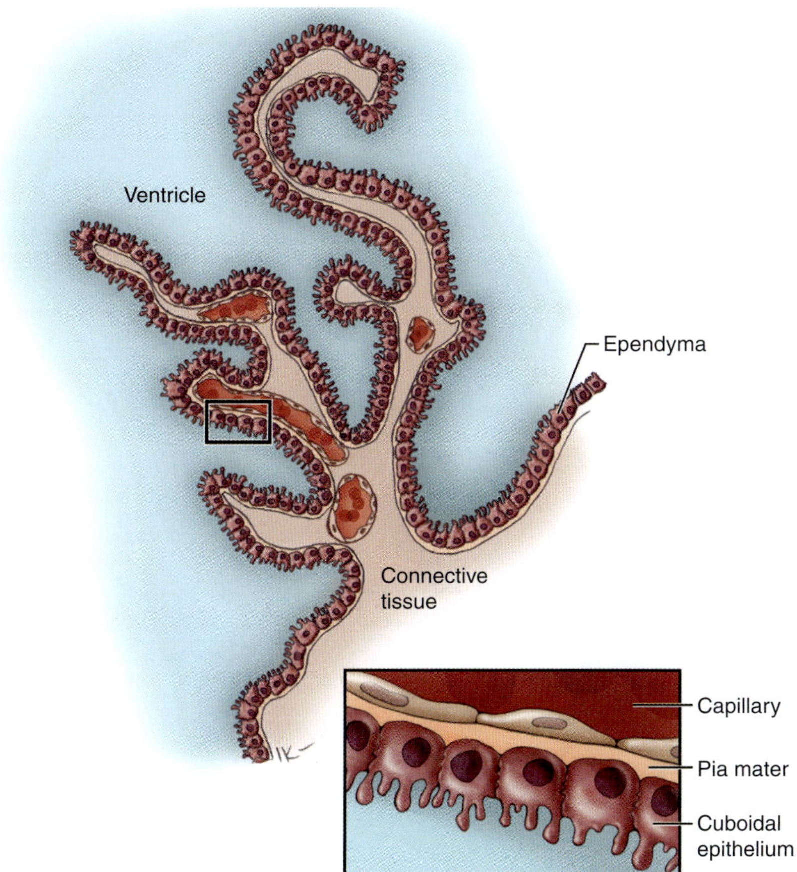

Figure 1.2 The choroid plexus has a "hobnail" appearance. It consists of a layer of cuboidal epithelial cells that surround an inner core comprised of connective tissue, pia mater, and capillaries.

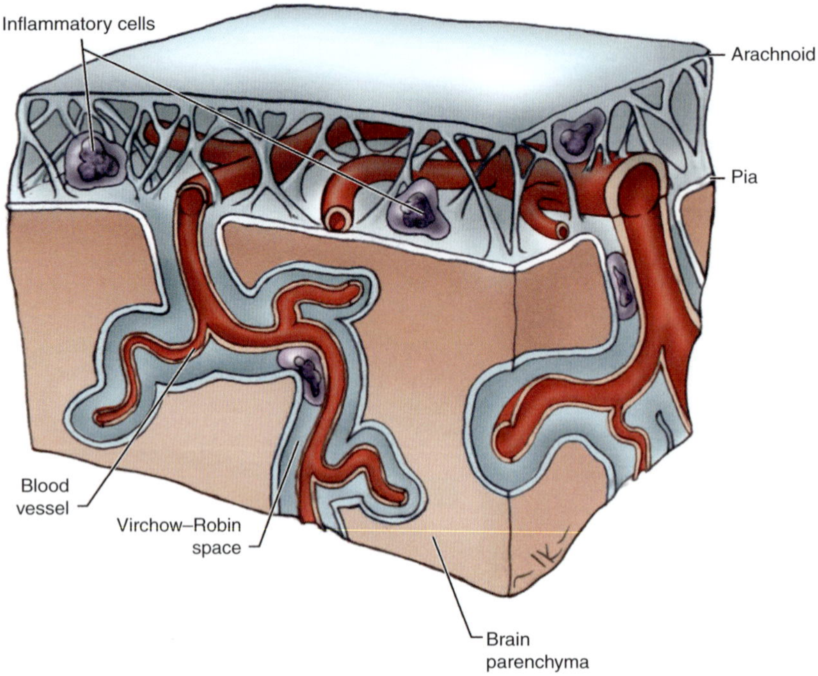

Figure 1.3 Virchow–Robin spaces are fluid-filled spaces surrounding perforating arteries and veins coming into and out of the brain parenchyma, respectively. They are found in the subarachnoid and subpial spaces.

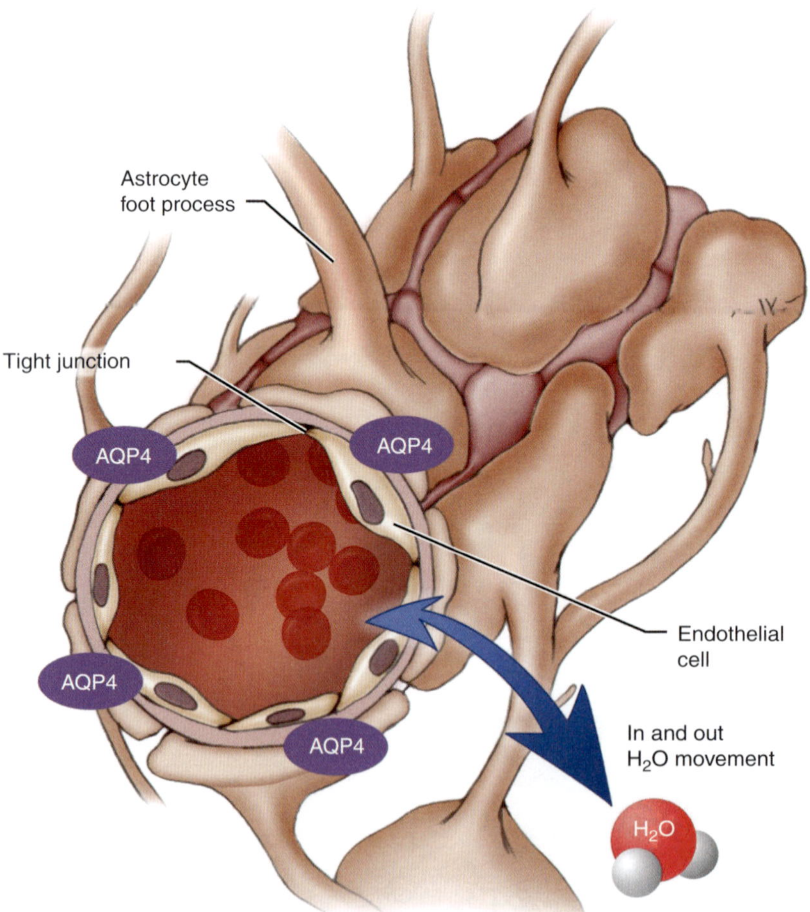

Figure 1.4 AQP4 can be identified at the astrocytic endfeet, at the level of the blood–brain-barrier and plays a significant role in the movement of water into and out of the brain.

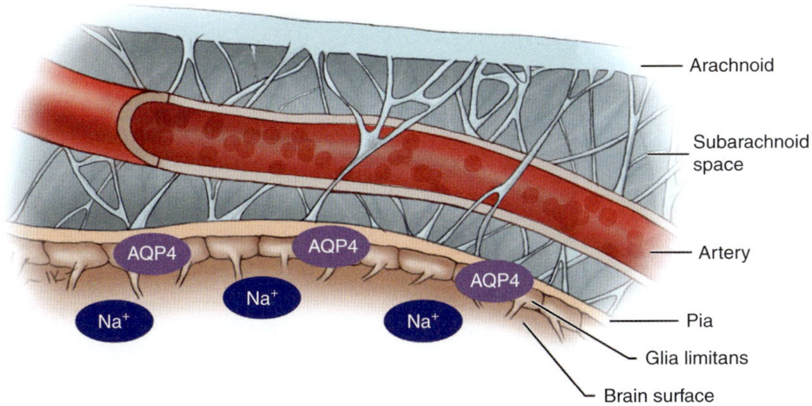

Figure 1.5 AQP4 is found mainly at the brain cortical surface, at the glia limitans layer just below the pia matter.

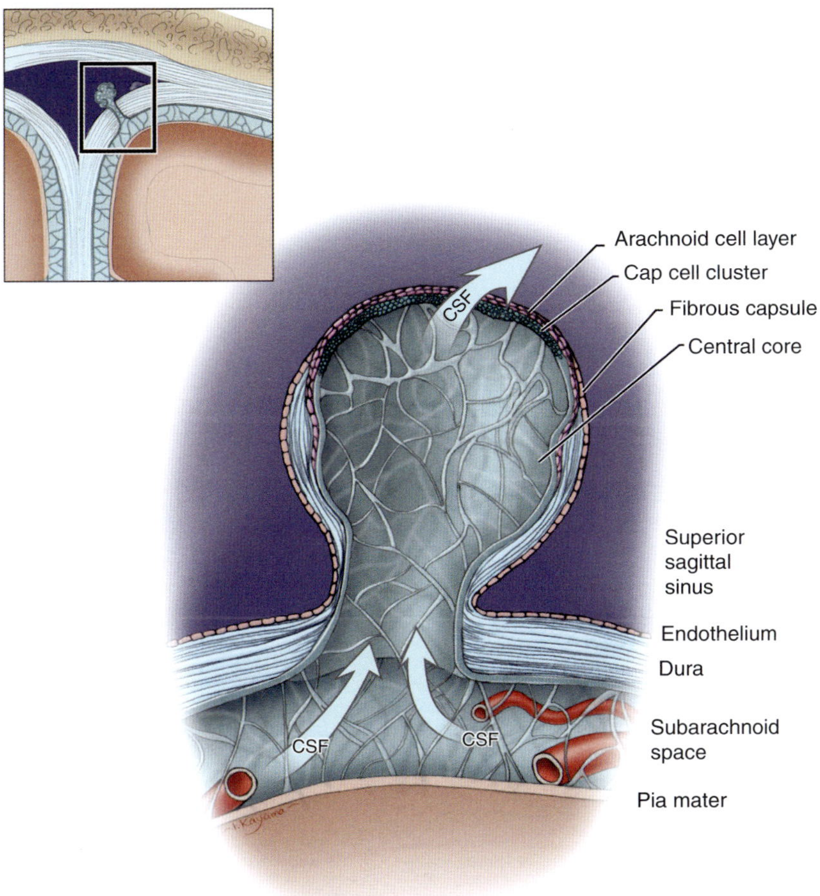

Figure 1.6 Arachnoid granulations consist of invaginations of arachnoid into the venous space. CSF from the subarachnoid space drains into the arachnoid villi and ultimately into the venous sinus.

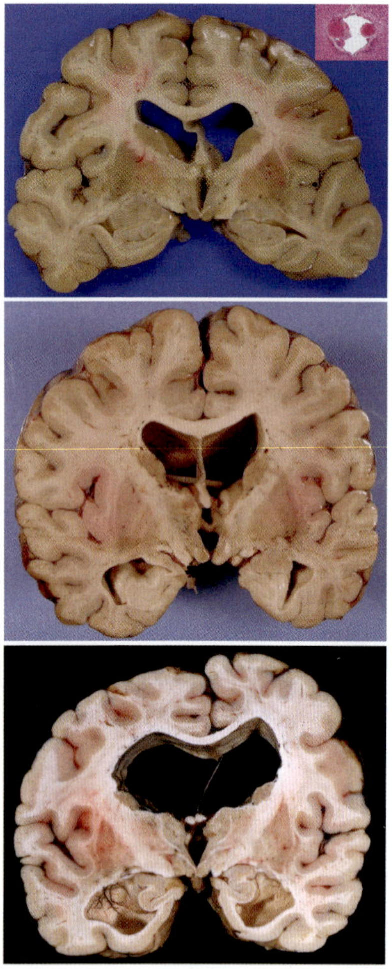

Figure 2.2 Photographs of coronal slices of hydrocephalic brains at the frontotemporal level highlighting the unpredictability of functional impairment. The upper slice is from a patient with clinical diagnosis of idiopathic NPH (case A5 in Table 2.2). The inset shows the cerebral aqueduct partially obstructed by granular extrusions, likely the consequence of an irritating process (possibly mild ventriculitis) many years earlier. The middle slice is from a patient with clinical diagnosis of secondary NPH (case B3 in Table 2.2). The shunt (piercing the septum pellucidum) was no longer functional and the symptoms had recurred. The lower slice is from an individual whose ventricles had enlarged considerably over the preceding 9 years but was asymptomatic (case C13 in Table 2.2). The septum pellucidum is destroyed and the corpus callosum thinned.

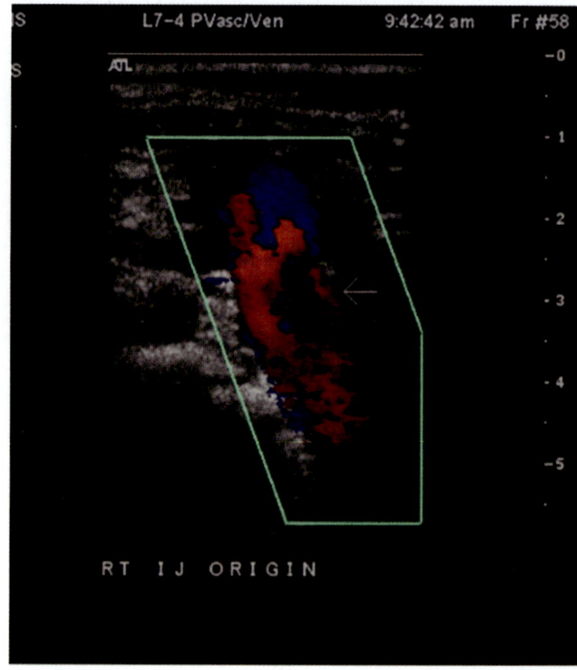

Figure 11.5 Thoracic ultrasound visualizes a small thrombus at the distal tip of a ventriculoatrial shunt.

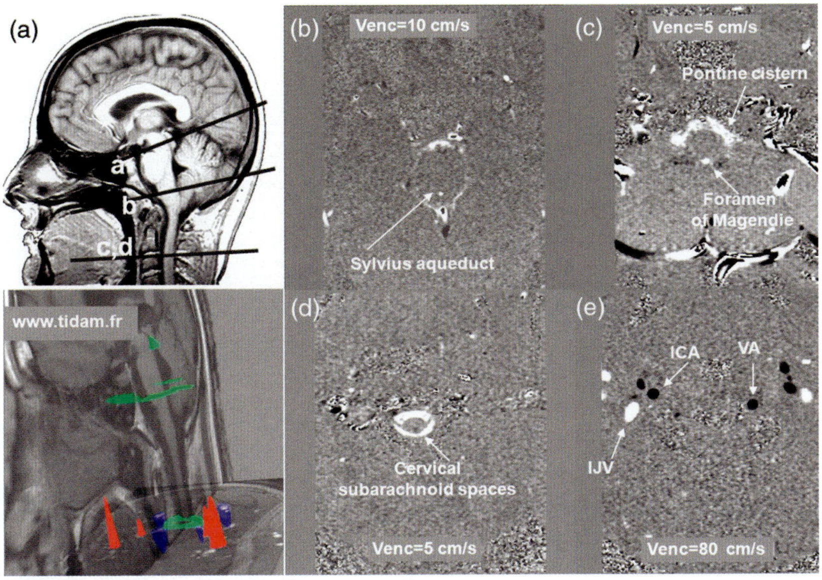

Figure 12.3 Data acquisition. Sagittal scout view sequences were used as localizer to select the anatomical levels for flow quantification (a). The acquisition planes were selected perpendicular to the presumed direction of the flows. Sections through the aqueduct of Sylvius (b), pontine cistern and foramen of Magendie (c), and C2–C3 subarachnoid spaces level (d), were used for CSF flow measurement. By varying the velocity encoding (V_{enc}), the same cervical section level (e) was used to measure vascular flows in left and right internal carotids (ICA), vertebral arteries (VA), and internal jugular veins (IJV). Black pixels represent the flows entering the slice, white pixels represent flows directed out of the slice, and gray pixels correspond to immobile tissues.

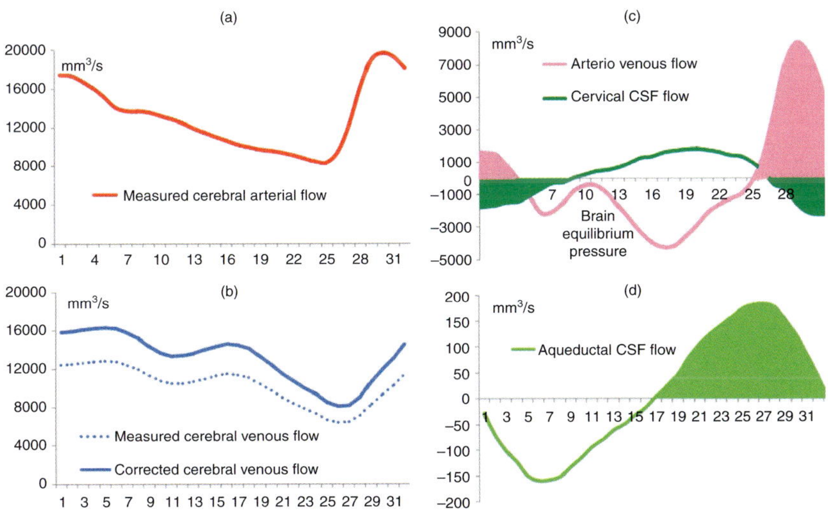

Figure 12.4 CSF and cerebral blood flow during the cardiac cycle in healthy adults (see text for full explanation).

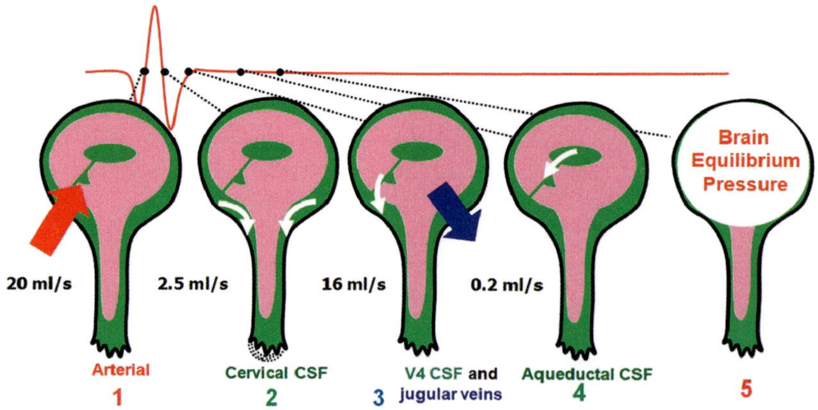

Figure 12.5 Chronological sequence of cerebral blood and CSF peak flows during early phase of the cardiac cycle. The cardiac systole can be divided into five phases according to the CSF or blood peak flows; the time of appearance of these peaks and their magnitude (in ml/s) are depicted. During the first phase, the cerebral blood volume instantaneously increases because of the vertebral and internal carotid systolic peak flows. The quickest way to absorb this and to regulate brain volume expansion is to flush extracerebral CSF into the spinal SAS (second phase), thanks to the spinal and dural sac compliance. During the third phase, a significant jugular output flow occurs and CSF progressively flushes out of V4; later (fourth phase), aqueduct, V3, and Monro flushes appear, with a very small contribution to the volume regulation. During the fifth phase, after a transient equilibrium state, brain CSF filling occurs and the reverse sequence begins.

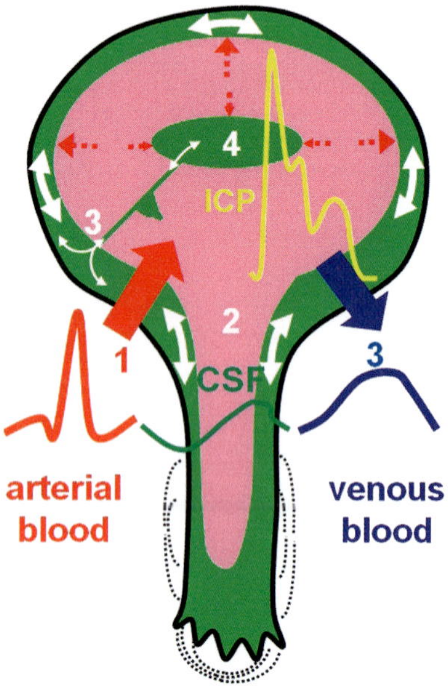

Figure 12.6 Diagram of CSF and blood flow. The large and rapid amplitude change in cerebral arterial input flow [1] increases the brain volume over the intracranial subarachnoid spaces (large red arrows). In these areas, resistance to flow is low and as CSF viscosity is low, CSF is quickly displaced out of the cranium toward the compliant spinal canal [2]; ICP increase is therefore limited. Nevertheless, this first CSF response is scanty and has to be supplemented with the cerebral blood venous outflow [3]. Due to blood viscosity, this venous contribution is slower but brings a greater displaced volume. Finally, the pressure decreases at the brain periphery induce a CSF ventricular flow, out of the fourth ventricle and through the aqueduct of Sylvius, resulting in a small inner displacement of the brain directed toward the ventricles (small red arrows). After this series of flow events during the systolic phase of CC, arterial inflow equals venous outflow and cervical CSF flush stops. After this brief equilibrium pressure moment, venous heart aspiration increases the cerebral venous outflow, decreases ICP, and reverses the cervical CSF flow to fill the cranium and prepare the next cycle.

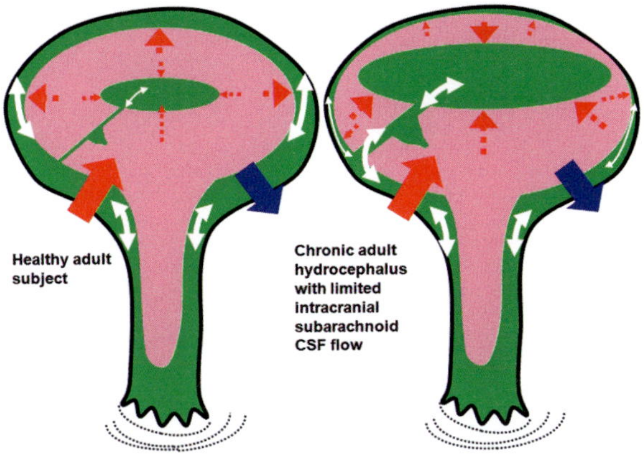

Figure 12.9 Schematic representation of CSF circulation in a healthy subject and chronic adult hydrocephalus. Red arrow represents arterial flow. Blue arrow represents venous outflow. White arrows represent CSF oscillation during cardiac cycle. In this model restricted CSF oscillations in the intracranial subarachnoid compartment increase CSF oscillations in the ventricle to maintain cervical CSF oscillations, then balance vascular expansion and preserve a large increase in ICP during the cardiac cycle.

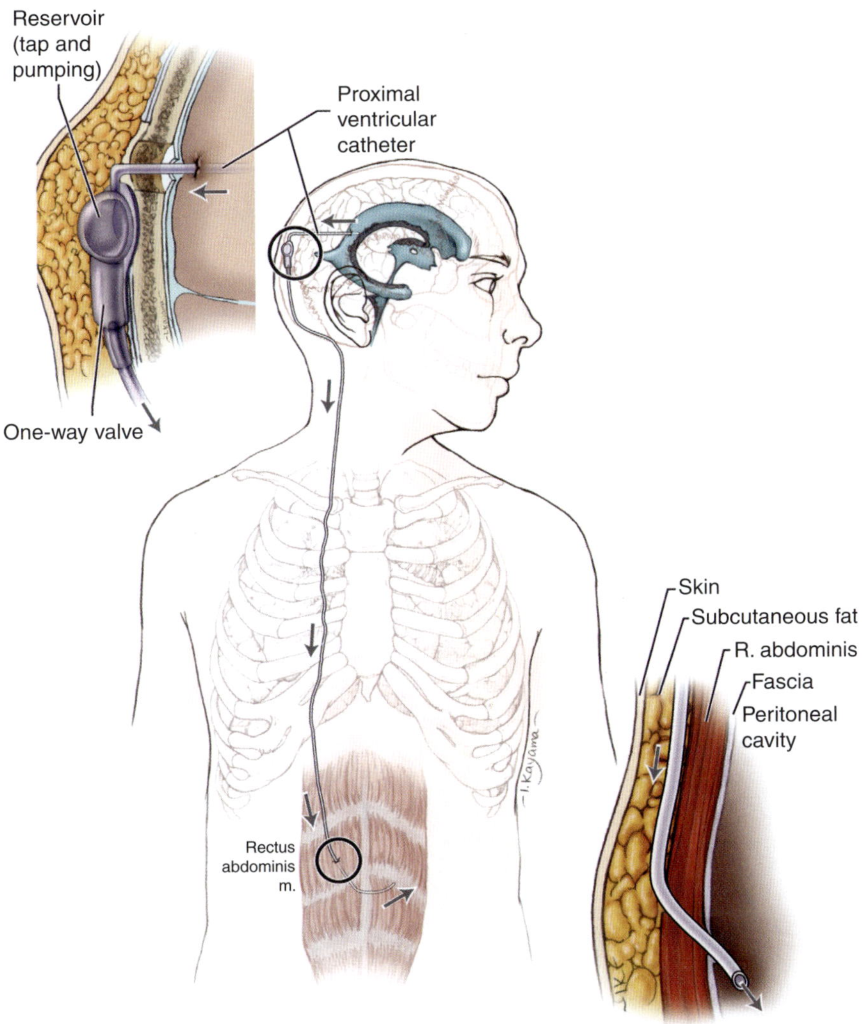

Figure 16.1 Ventriculoperitoneal shunt insertion. The distal catheter generally is inserted off midline, through the rectus abdominis muscle and fascia, although many other techniques can be used.

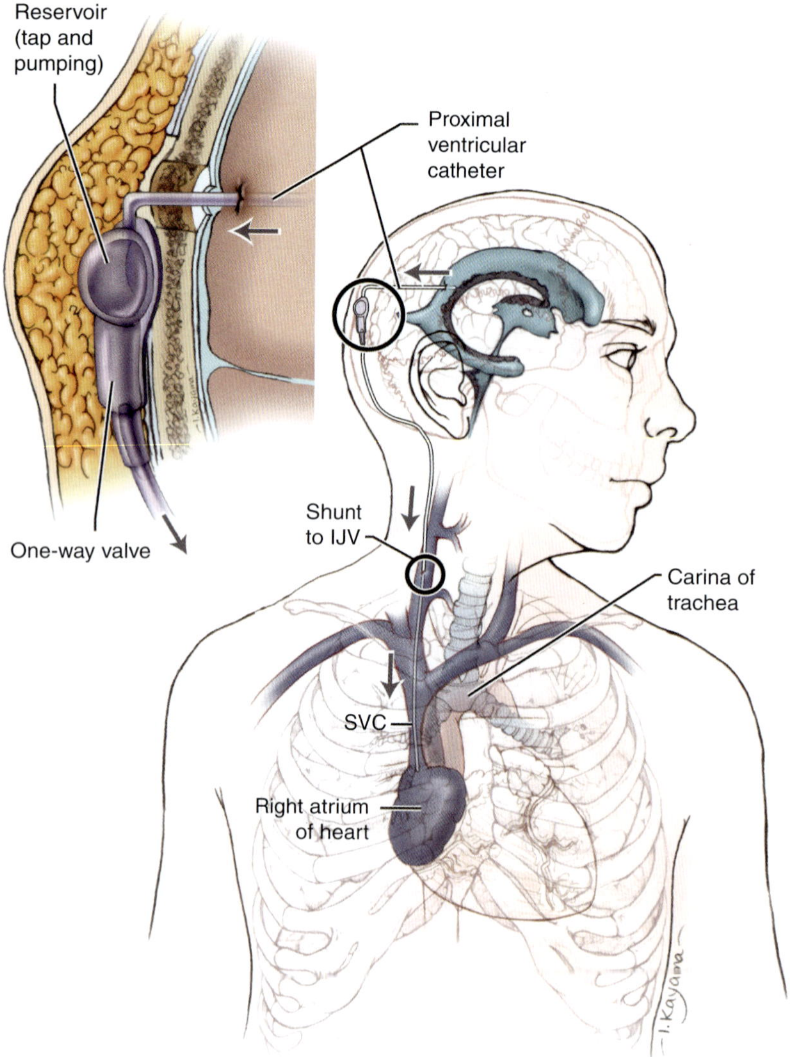

Figure 16.2 Ventriculoatrial shunt insertion. The distal catheter is introduced through the internal jugular vein (IJV), with a goal termination at the cavoatrial junction. SVC, superior vena cava.

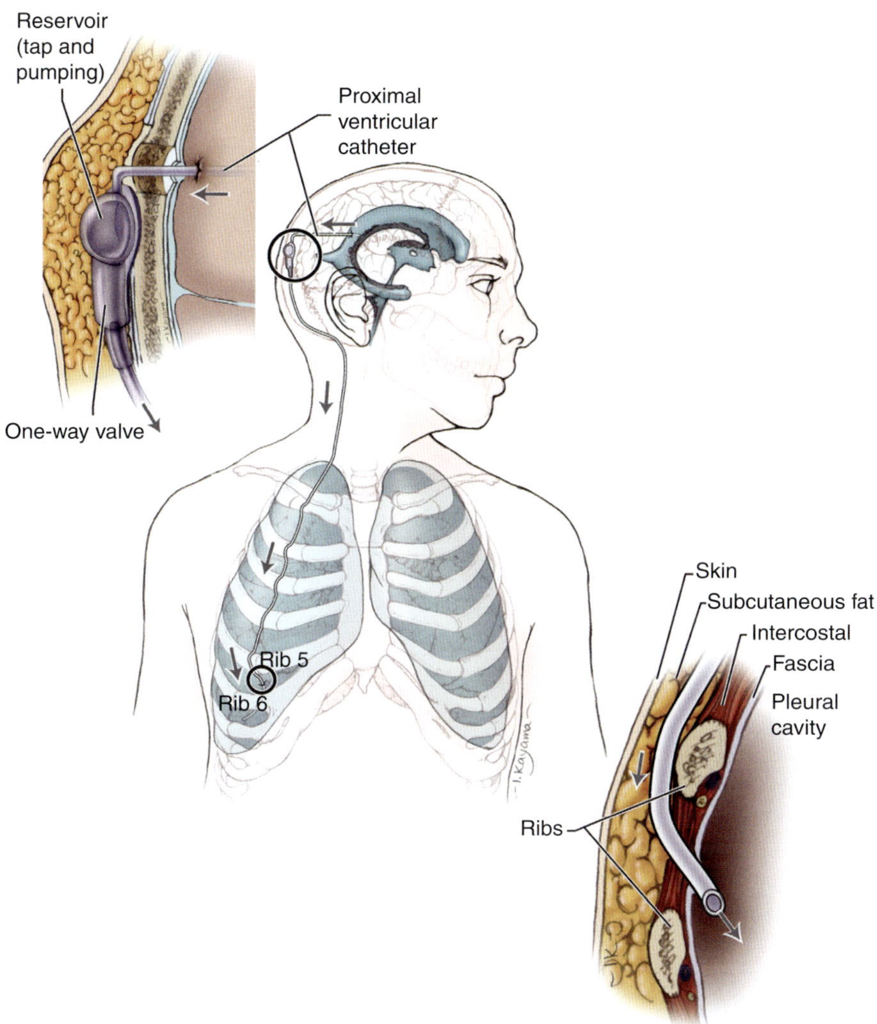

Figure 16.3 Ventriculopleural shunt insertion. The distal catheter is introduced above the sixth rib in order to avoid the intercostal vessels and nerve.

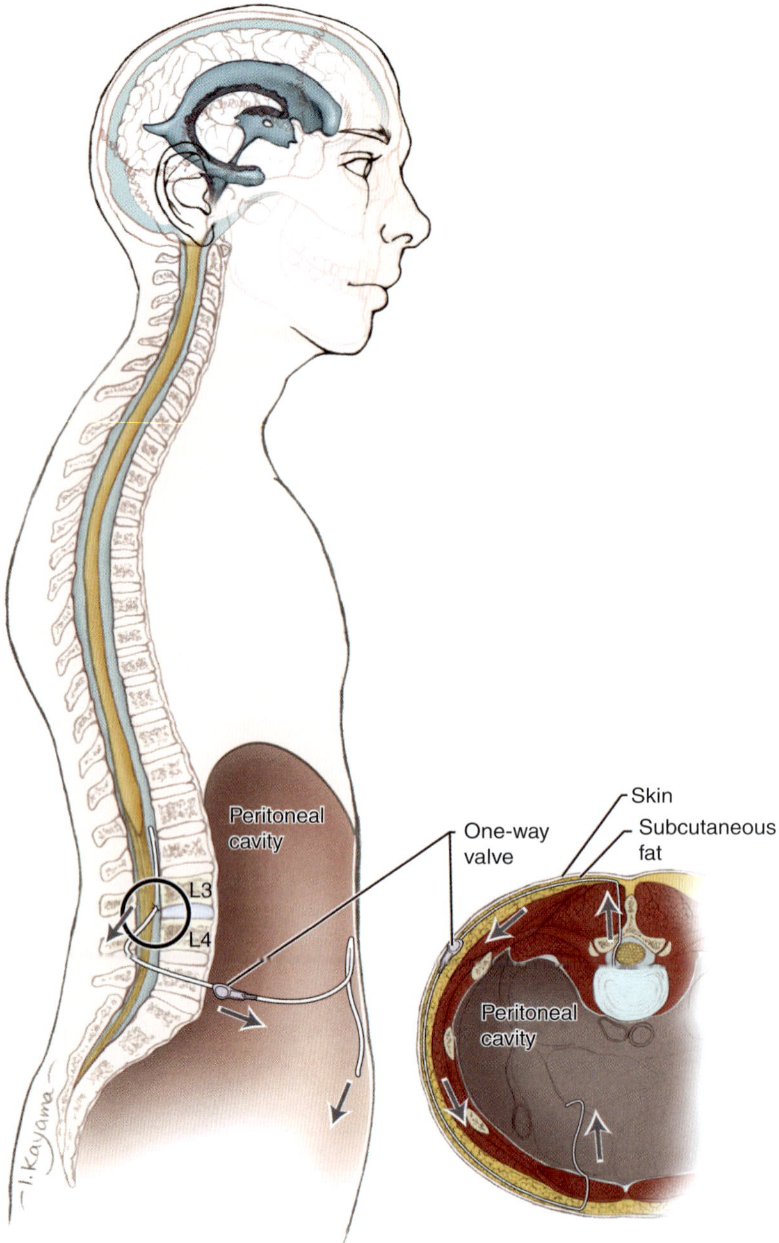

Figure 16.4 Lumboperitoneal shunt insertion. The proximal catheter is often introduced at the L3–4 level, although adjacent levels are also used commonly.

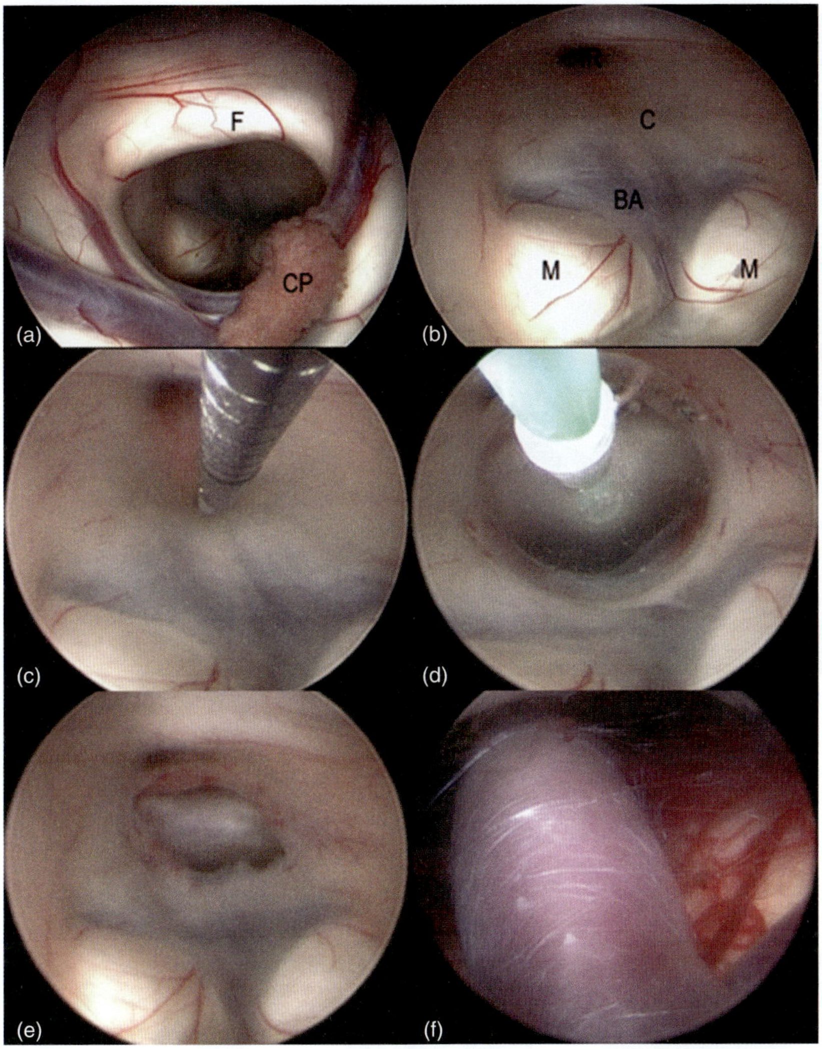

Figure 19.3 Endoscopic third ventriculostomy. (a) View through the foramen of Monro (CP, choroid plexus; F, fornix). (b) Floor of the third ventricle (BA, basilar artery; M, mammillary bodies; C, clivus; IR, infundibular recess). (c) Blunt perforation of the floor of the third ventricle with the Decq forceps. (d) Dilation of the stoma by inflating the balloon of the Fogarty catheter. (e) Sufficient open stoma after ETV. (f) Inspection of the prepontine cistern showing the basilar artery.

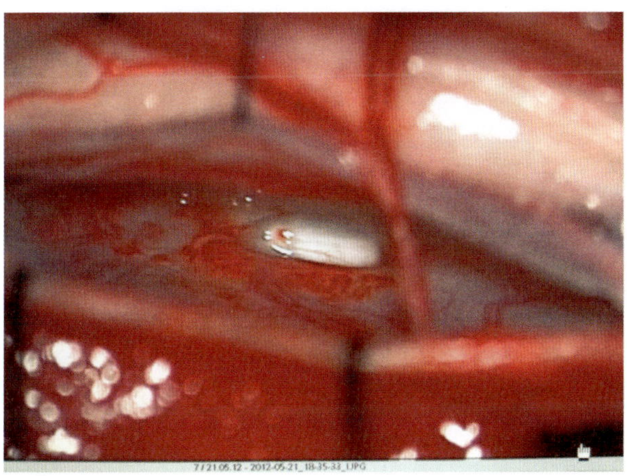

Figure 22.3 Intraoperative picture of a ventral dural tear in a patient with spontaneous intracranial hypotension.

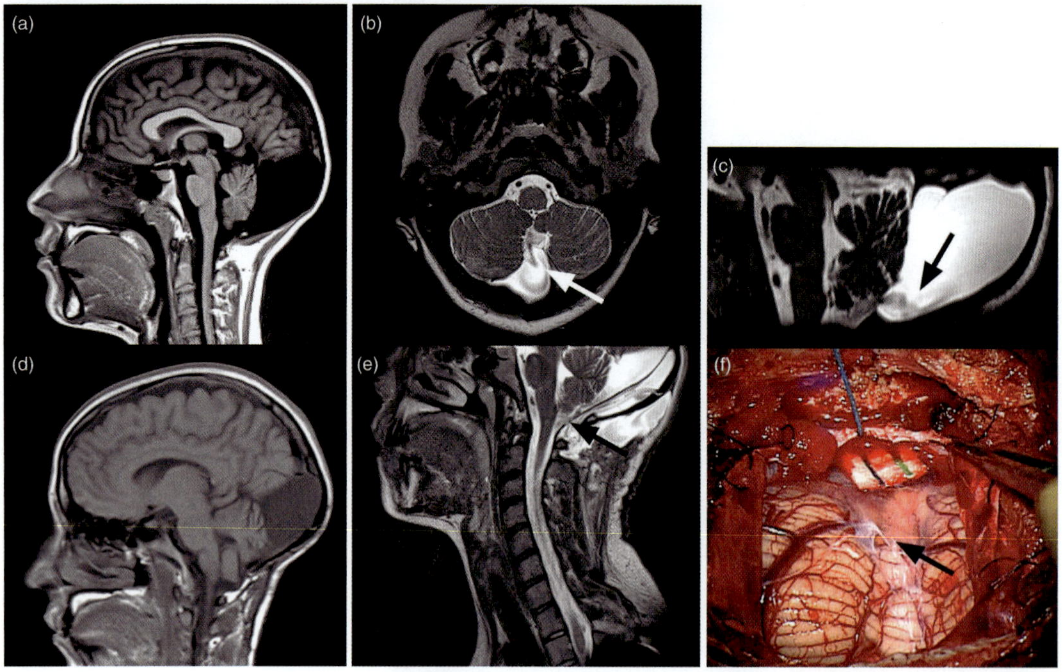

Figure 24.2 Posterior fossa cyst without hydrocephalus. (a–c) Preoperative MRI findings showing a retrocerebellar cystic lesion with some mass effect on the cerebellum as indicated in a midline sagittal T1-weighted image (a). The axial T2-weighted image (b) shows a flow void signal in the cisterna magna suggestive of CSF turbulences (white arrow), which was supported by a sagittal CISS sequence focusing on that area that indicated a focal communication inferiorly, inferior to the fourth ventricle, suggestive of a "ball-valve" mechanism causing the cyst to expand (c, black arrow). (d–e) Postoperative MRI shows reduction of the cyst and expansion of the cerebellum in a sagittal T1-weighted image as well as restored CSF flow at the level of the foramen magnum as indicated by physiological flow void signals at the foramen of Magendie, and between the cisterna magna and the cervical spinal CSF compartment (e, black arrow). The intraoperative microscopic view during microsurgical fenestration of the cyst supports the finding of an arachnoid cyst with a pre-existing focal opening (black arrow) to support the "ball-valve" mechanism as suggested by the radiographic findings (f).

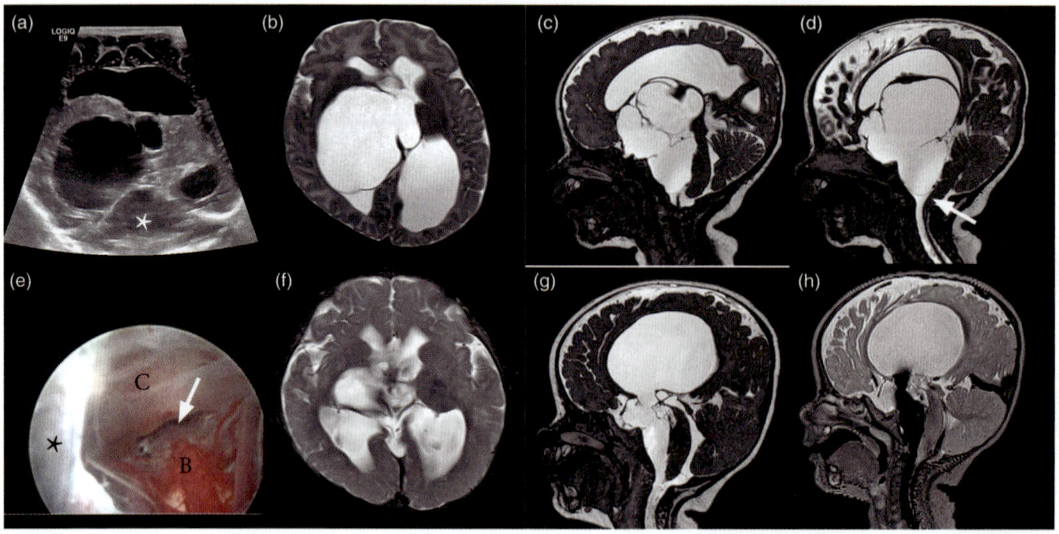

Figure 24.6 Hydrocephalus associated with a giant suprasellar arachnoid cyst diagnosed in a fetus. (a–d) Preoperative findings of a fetal ultrasound showing hydrocephalus and infratentorial pathology, suggestive of a posterior fossa cyst or Dandy–Walker malformation (a, white asterisk). T2-weighted axial MRI (B) and sagittal CISS sequences (c, d) at day 3 post-partum show a giant arachnoid cyst extending into the supra- and infratentorial compartment with multiple septi; however, the CISS sequences suggest one compartment cyst of suprasellar origin, and endoscopic fenestration into the spinal canal and opening of the caudal cyst membrane (d, white arrow) was attempted. A left frontal transventricular endoscopic approach was performed and fenestration of the cyst into the spinal compartment was accomplished as seen by the intraoperative endoscopic view (e; C = clivus, B = brainstem basilar artery, asterisk = cyst membrane, white arrow = spinal subdural space). (f–h) Postoperative corresponding MRI findings show significant reduction of cyst size and improved hydrocephalus in both axial and sagittal T2-weighted and CISS sequences (f, g) as well as CSF flow signal suggestive of communication of the lateral ventricles with the spinal compartment shown by T2 CSF space imaging (h).

[39] observed that aqueductal flows in NPH patients were 10 times greater than those in normal subjects. Luetmer et al. found the average flow rate in patients with NPH to be significantly higher than the flow rate in normal age-matched controls or in patients with Alzheimer's disease [40].

Actually, the value of ventricular CSF was first suggested by the exaggerated aqueductal flow void on axial MRI scans. Jack et al. [41] noted that the increase in CSF flow dynamics at the level of the aqueduct and the fourth ventricle was correlated with NPH patients' response to shunting. In contrast, although Krauss et al. [42] found a significant increase in the extension of the flow void in the aqueduct and the third and fourth ventricles in the NPH group, they did not find any correlation with the postoperative outcome.

The usefulness of stroke volume in the evaluation of postoperative prognosis was first suggested by Bradley et al. [17], but this was not replicated in the study of Dixon et al. [43] which found no significant correlation between increased aqueductal CSF flow and outcome following shunt. However, Dixon et al. as well as El Sankari et al. observed an increase in mean aqueductal CSF flow in patients who improved after shunting although they had a negative tap test [40,44].

Wagshul et al. [45] suggested a stroke volume ratio as a measure of hyperdynamic flows in NPH, reflecting a readjusted distribution of flows between the subarachnoid and the ventricular spaces as previously proposed by Balédent et al. [46]. They observed that cervical CSF flow was similar in NPH patients and healthy volunteers whereas ventricular flow was greater in the control group. Ventricular CSF represented 11% of the cervical CSF stroke volume in healthy volunteers, compared to 42% in NPH patients. Therefore, intracranial subarachnoid flow was dramatically reduced in NPH subjects. These results are in accordance with the findings of Kitagaki et al. [47], who observed that CSF volume in patients with idiopathic normal pressure hydrocephalus was significantly decreased in the subarachnoid spaces.

In healthy subjects, intracranial CSF mobile compliance depends predominantly on intracranial subarachnoid CSF pulsations. Conversely, in NPH patients, the ventricular pulsations play a major role in cerebral pressure damping during vascular brain expansion; ventricular dilation seems to be an adaptive response to the alterations of subarachnoid intracranial CSF pulsations (Figure 12.9). An increase in CSF flow is linked to a pressure difference increase as Czosnyka et al. observed an ICP amplitude increase during invasive pressure monitoring in NPH patients [36].

In NPH, ventricular dilation may be related to ventricular wall modifications induced by an increase in the pressure difference between ventricular and extraventricular CSF, whereas in atrophic brain, ventricles are dilated because tissue is missing. When reliable diagnosis is difficult, CSF oscillation studies could be helpful to differentiate one state from the other.

As an example, Figure 12.10 demonstrates how PC-MRI can be used in patients presenting with ventricular dilation and clinical signs of NPH. PC-MRI results were compared to the reference values summarized in Table 12.1. Patient 1 (a, b) presented with normal CSF circulation indicating that the pressure differences which generate CSF flows were not altered: the observed ventricular dilation was probably due to atrophy rather than NPH. Patient 2 (c, d) presented with hyper-oscillations between all of the CSF compartments. CSF oscillations in the spinal canal were twice the normal value, indicating a probable increase in ICP amplitude and normal functionality of spinal spaces. Aqueductal CSF oscillations were six times the normal value and represented 30% of cervical CSF oscillations versus only 10% in the healthy subject. In this case, ventricular dilation was probably due to an increase in the amplitude of pressure difference between the CSF compartments during CC.

From a previous study on achondroplasia [48] and the observation of patients undergoing hydrocephalus associated with craniostenosis, Sainte-Rose et al. [49] concluded that an increase in the superior sagittal sinus venous pressure could be the cause of enlarged ventricles.

PC-MRI is also a good tool to investigate cerebral venous flows [50,51]. Bateman [52] explored the pulsatility of venous flows, showing that NPH patients exhibited a significant increase in pulsatility inside the straight sinus. Such a patient with hydrocephalus associated with jugular stenosis invites the question: "*which is the chicken and which is the egg*?" (Figure 12.11).

Coupling of the cardiovascular and cerebrospinal fluid (CSF) system is considered to be important in understanding the pathophysiology of cerebrovascular and craniospinal disease. A coupled cardiovascular and CSF system model was designed to examine the relation of spinal cord blood flow and CSF pulsations along the spinal subarachnoid space [53].

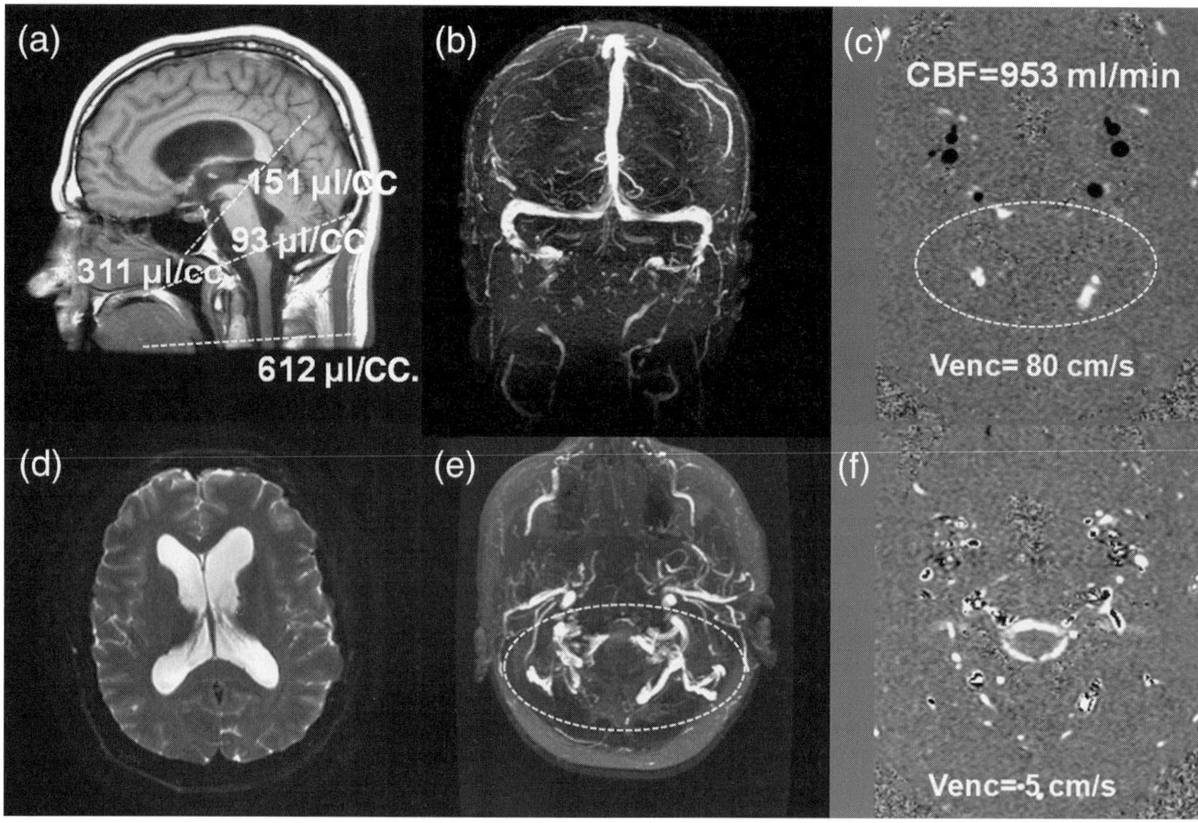

Figure 12.11 CSF and cerebral venous blood flow alterations in a hydrocephalus patient. MRI of a 32-year-old hydrocephalus patient suffering from severe headache and presenting with ventricular dilation (a, d). CSF stroke volumes in the aqueduct, foramen of Magendie, pontine cistern, and spinal spaces are displayed. (b,e) Venous angiography showed that cerebral venous outflow was restricted in jugular veins and predominantly in the posterior part (white ellipse). Axial vascular (c) and CSF (f) flow investigation confirmed the results. Cerebral arterial flow was 953 ml/s. The PC-MRI report pointed to a possible venous origin of hydrocephalus in this patient.

As hydrocephalus mainly results from a brain compression initiated by CSF flows, it seems logical to associate this flow-induced stress mechanism with pathologies affecting the spine such as Chiari malformation or syringomyelia.

Figures 12.12 and 12.13 present the case of two patients where PC-MRI could quantify CSF flow alterations in the spinal canal. However, these examples do not aim to explain these complex pathologies which, according to previous experience, present large variabilities.

Although numerous studies have been conducted to assess PC-MRI as sensitive and specific diagnosis, evidence-based recommendations are still lacking because of heterogeneities in evaluation protocols, measured parameters, measurement techniques, and often because of small isolated and heterogeneous populations. PC-MRI applications in the management of CSF disorders and the understanding of its pathogenesis would benefit from multicenter standardized study research protocols. Nevertheless, PC-MRI is a powerful tool to explore the fluid biomechanics inside the cranium [54], to point out CSF flow disorders [55], and to help the neurosurgeon.

Brain and spine are altered when CSF is submitted to chronic abnormal pressure. We can also hypothesize that small hydrodynamic instability or disorganization of inflow–outflow in the different CSF compartments during the cardiac cycle could be the origin of CSF disorders such as hydrocephalus.

In order to work in this way, the PC-MRI technique gives us some original keys and the recently developed 3D PC-MRI sequence will increase the potentiality of CSF flow imaging [56,57].

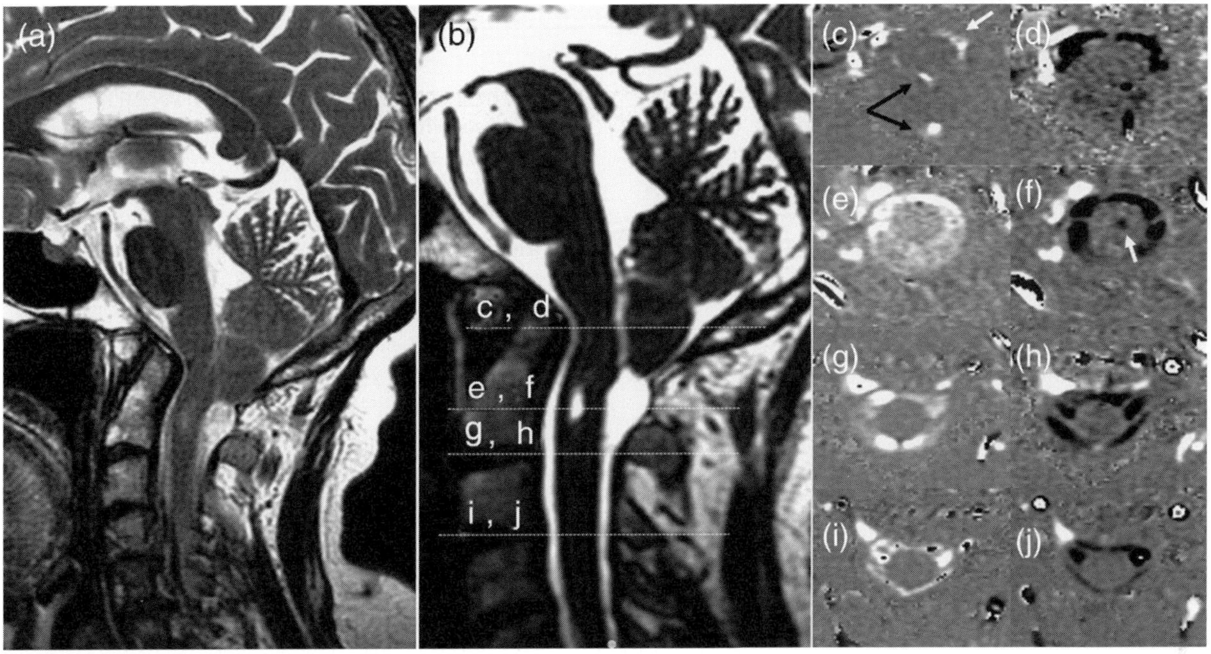

Figure 12.12 CSF flow in Chiari malformation. MRI of Chiari malformation in a 62-year-old woman. Sagittal T2-weighted image (a) and sagittal FIESTA acquisition (b) showed hypersignal in the middle of the spine at the C2 level and accumulation of CSF in the posterior subarachnoid spaces below the cerebellum. PC-MRI data were acquired at different levels along the spine: foramen magnum (c, d), C1 (e, f), C2–C3 (g, h) and C3–C4 (i–j). The respective CSF flow images, during systole (white intensities) when intracranial CSF is quickly flushing to the spinal canal and diastole (black intensities) when CSF is filling the cranium, are displayed. Image (c) demonstrates restricted CSF flow in the anterior subarachnoid spaces (white arrow) and two jet flows from the foramen of Magendie and from the compressed cerebellum cistern (black arrows). Image (f) shows normal CSF flows in the subarachnoid spaces and a little flow inside the cavity (white arrow). Image (g) shows CSF flows in the predominant channels whereas images (h–j) present homogeneous distribution of CSF flows. Paradoxically, CSF stroke volumes (mean of 550 μl/CC) were subnormal from foramen magnum to C3–C4. V_{enc} was set to 5 cm/s for all PC-MRI acquisitions and aliasing was corrected post-acquisition. In this example of Chiari malformation, CSF communication between the cranium and the spinal canal was not decreased. But CSF flow was concentrated in small areas, inducing an increase in the fluid kinetic energy that stressed the epidural canal of the spine, which could eventually result in the development of a cavity.

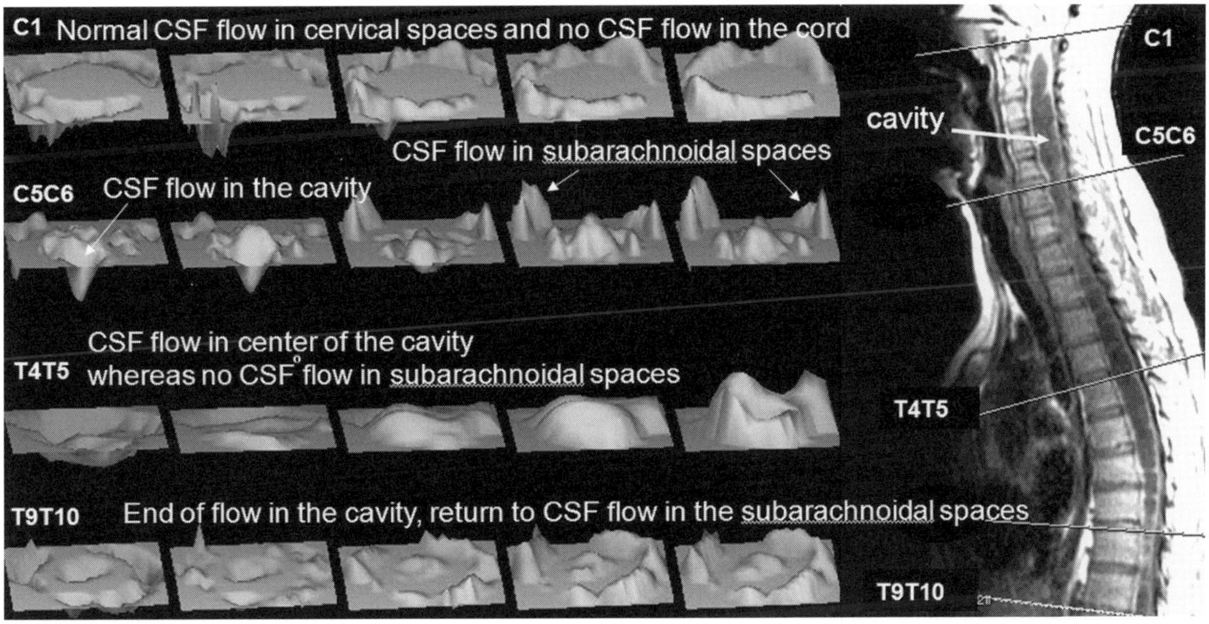

Figure 12.13 CSF flow in a syringomyelia cavity in a 25-year-old woman. PC-MRI velocity profiles were displayed in three dimensions to observe the CSF flow around the spine, before and inside the large cavity which appears in the sagittal T1-weighted image from C1 to T10. Addition of stroke volumes of CSF flow inside and outside the cavity was normal at each level.

References

1. Feinberg DA, Mark AS. Human brain motion and cerebrospinal fluid circulation demonstrated with MR velocity imaging. *Radiology* 1987;163(3):793–9.
2. Nayler GL, Firmin DN, Longmore DB. Blood flow imaging by cine magnetic resonance. *J Comput Assist Tomogr* 1986;10(5):715–22.
3. Pelc NJ, Herfkens RJ, Shimakawa A, Enzmann DR. Phase contrast cine magnetic resonance imaging. *Magn Reson Q* 1991;7(4):229–54.
4. Sechtem U, Pflugfelder P, Higgins CB. Quantification of cardiac function by conventional and cine magnetic resonance imaging. *Cardiovasc Intervent Radiol* 1987;10(6):365–73.
5. Pelc LR, Pelc NJ, Rayhill SC, et al. Arterial and venous blood flow: noninvasive quantitation with MR imaging. *Radiology* 1992;185(3):809–12.
6. Buonocore MH, Bogren H. Factors influencing the accuracy and precision of velocity-encoded phase imaging. *Magn Reson Med* 1992;26(1):141–54.
7. Greil G, Geva T, Maier SE, Powell AJ. Effect of acquisition parameters on the accuracy of velocity encoded cine magnetic resonance imaging blood flow measurements. *J Magn Reson Imaging* 2002;15(1):47–54.
8. McCauley TR, Pena CS, Holland CK, Price TB, Gore JC. Validation of volume flow measurements with cine phase-contrast MR imaging for peripheral arterial waveforms. *J Magn Reson Imaging* 1995;5(6):663–8.
9. Enzmann DR, Pelc NJ. Normal flow patterns of intracranial and spinal cerebrospinal fluid defined with phase-contrast cine MR imaging. *Radiology* 1991;178(2):467–74.
10. Wahlin A, Ambarki K, Hauksson J, et al. Phase contrast MRI quantification of pulsatile volumes of brain arteries, veins, and cerebrospinal fluids compartments: repeatability and physiological interactions. *J Magn Reson Imaging* 2012;35(5):1055–62.
11. Pelc NJ, Sommer FG, Li KC, et al. Quantitative magnetic resonance flow imaging. *Magn Reson Q* 1994;10(3):125–47.
12. Wentland AL, Wieben O, Korosec FR, Haughton VM. Accuracy and reproducibility of phase-contrast MR imaging measurements for CSF flow. *AJNR Am J Neuroradiol* 31(7):1331–6.
13. Burkart DJ, Felmlee JP, Johnson CD, et al. Cine phase-contrast MR flow measurements: improved precision using an automated method of vessel detection. *J Comput Assist Tomogr* 1994;18(3):469–75.
14. Balédent O, Henry-Feugeas MC, Idy-Peretti I. Cerebrospinal fluid dynamics and relation with blood flow: a magnetic resonance study with semiautomated cerebrospinal fluid segmentation. *Invest Radiol* 2001;36(7):368–77.
15. Alperin N, Lee SH. PUBS: pulsatility-based segmentation of lumens conducting non-steady flow. *Magn Reson Med* 2003;49(5):934–44.
16. Enzmann DR, Pelc NJ. Cerebrospinal fluid flow measured by phase-contrast cine MR. *AJNR Am J Neuroradiol* 1993;14(6):1301–7; discussion 9–10.
17. Bradley WG, Jr., Scalzo D, Queralt J, et al. Normal-pressure hydrocephalus: evaluation with cerebrospinal fluid flow measurements at MR imaging. *Radiology* 1996;198(2):523–9.
18. Capel C, Gondry-Jouet C, Krejpowicz B, et al., eds. Intracranial compliance study by phase contrast magnetic resonance imaging in newborns and children. *International Society for Magnetic Resonance in Medicine*; 2012; Melbourne, Australia.
19. Bateman GA. Vascular compliance in normal pressure hydrocephalus. *AJNR Am J Neuroradiol* 2000;21(9):1574–85.
20. Stoquart-ElSankari S, Balédent O, Gondry-Jouet C, et al. Aging effects on cerebral blood and cerebrospinal fluid flows. *J Cereb Blood Flow Metab* 2007;27(9):1563–72.
21. Brugieres P, Idy-Peretti I, Iffenecker C, et al. CSF flow measurement in syringomyelia. *AJNR Am J Neuroradiol* 2000;21(10):1785–92.
22. Saliou G, Paradot G, Gondry C, et al. A phase-contrast MRI study of acute and chronic hydrodynamic alterations after hydrocephalus induced by subarachnoid hemorrhage. *J Neuroimaging* 2012;22(4):343–50.
23. Balédent O, Fin L, Khuoy L, et al. Brain hydrodynamics study by phase-contrast magnetic resonance imaging and transcranial color doppler. *J Magn Reson Imaging* 2006;24(5):995–1004.
24. Marmarou A, Shulman K, Rosende RM. A nonlinear analysis of the cerebrospinal fluid system and intracranial pressure dynamics. *J Neurosurg* 1978;48(3):332–44.
25. Alperin NJ, Lee SH, Loth F, Raksin PB, Lichtor T. MR-Intracranial pressure (ICP): a method to measure intracranial elastance and pressure noninvasively by means of MR imaging: baboon and human study. *Radiology* 2000;217(3):877–85.
26. Bouzerar R, Czosnyka M, Czosnyka Z, Balédent O. Physical phantom of craniospinal hydrodynamics. *Acta Neurochir Suppl* 2012;113:65–9.

27. Gideon P, Stahlberg F, Thomsen C, et al. Cerebrospinal fluid flow and production in patients with normal pressure hydrocephalus studied by MRI. *Neuroradiology* 1994;36(3):210–15.

28. Yamada S, Miyazaki M, Kanazawa H, et al. Visualization of cerebrospinal fluid movement with spin labeling at MR imaging: preliminary results in normal and pathophysiologic conditions. *Radiology* 2008;249(2):644–52.

29. Bulat M, Klarica M. Recent insights into a new hydrodynamics of the cerebrospinal fluid. *Brain Res Rev* 2011;65(2):99–112.

30. Johanson CE, Duncan JA, 3rd, Klinge PM, et al. Multiplicity of cerebrospinal fluid functions: new challenges in health and disease. *Cerebrospinal Fluid Res* 2008;5:10.

31. Hingwala D, Chatterjee S, Kesavadas C, Thomas B, Kapilamoorthy TR. Applications of 3D CISS sequence for problem solving in neuroimaging. *Indian J Radiol Imaging* 2011;21(2):90–7.

32. Stoquart-El Sankari S, Lehmann P, Gondry-Jouet C, et al. Phase-contrast MR imaging support for the diagnosis of aqueductal stenosis. *AJNR Am J Neuroradiol* 2009;30(1):209–14.

33. Oi S, Shimoda M, Shibata M, et al. Pathophysiology of long-standing overt ventriculomegaly in adults. *J Neurosurg* 2000;92(6):933–40.

34. Adams RD, Fisher CM, Hakim S, Ojemann RG, Sweet WH. Symptomatic occult hydrocephalus with "normal" cerebrospinal-fluid pressure. A treatable syndrome. *N Engl J Med* 1965;273:117–26.

35. Hakim S, Adams RD. The special clinical problem of symptomatic hydrocephalus with normal cerebrospinal fluid pressure. Observations on cerebrospinal fluid hydrodynamics. *J Neurol Sci* 1965;2(4):307–27.

36. Czosnyka M, Czosnyka Z, Keong N, et al. Pulse pressure waveform in hydrocephalus: what it is and what it isn't. *Neurosurg Focus* 2007;22(4):E2.

37. Bret P, Guyotat J, Chazal J. Is normal pressure hydrocephalus a valid concept in 2002? A reappraisal in five questions and proposal for a new designation of the syndrome as "chronic hydrocephalus". *J Neurol Neurosurg Psychiatry* 2002;73(1):9–12.

38. Marmarou A, Bergsneider M, Relkin N, Klinge P, Black PM. Development of guidelines for idiopathic normal-pressure hydrocephalus: introduction. *Neurosurgery* 2005;57(3 Suppl):S1–3; discussion ii–v.

39. Greitz D, Hannerz J, Rahn T, Bolander H, Ericsson A. MR imaging of cerebrospinal fluid dynamics in health and disease. On the vascular pathogenesis of communicating hydrocephalus and benign intracranial hypertension. *Acta Radiol* 1994;35(3):204–11.

40. Luetmer PH, Huston J, Friedman JA, et al. Measurement of cerebrospinal fluid flow at the cerebral aqueduct by use of phase-contrast magnetic resonance imaging: technique validation and utility in diagnosing idiopathic normal pressure hydrocephalus. *Neurosurgery* 2002;50(3):534–43; discussion 43–4.

41. Jack CR, Jr., Mokri B, Laws ER, Jr., et al. MR findings in normal-pressure hydrocephalus: significance and comparison with other forms of dementia. *J Comput Assist Tomogr* 1987;11(6):923–31.

42. Krauss JK, Regel JP, Vach W, et al. Flow void of cerebrospinal fluid in idiopathic normal pressure hydrocephalus of the elderly: can it predict outcome after shunting? *Neurosurgery* 1997;40(1):67–73; discussion 73–4.

43. Dixon GR, Friedman JA, Luetmer PH, et al. Use of cerebrospinal fluid flow rates measured by phase-contrast MR to predict outcome of ventriculoperitoneal shunting for idiopathic normal-pressure hydrocephalus. *Mayo Clin Proc* 2002;77(6):509–14.

44. El Sankari S, Fichten A, Gondry-Jouet C, et al. Correlation between tap test and CSF aqueductal stroke volume in idiopathic normal pressure hydrocephalus. *Acta Neurochir Suppl* 2012;113:43–6.

45. Wagshul ME, Chen JJ, Egnor MR, McCormack EJ, Roche PE. Amplitude and phase of cerebrospinal fluid pulsations: experimental studies and review of the literature. *J Neurosurg* 2006;104(5):810–19.

46. Balédent O, Gondry-Jouet C, Meyer ME, et al. Relationship between cerebrospinal fluid and blood dynamics in healthy volunteers and patients with communicating hydrocephalus. *Invest Radiol* 2004;39(1):45–55.

47. Kitagaki H, Mori E, Ishii K, et al. CSF spaces in idiopathic normal pressure hydrocephalus: morphology and volumetry. *AJNR Am J Neuroradiol* 1998;19(7):1277–84.

48. Pierre-Kahn A, Hirsch JF, Renier D, Metzger J, Maroteaux P. Hydrocephalus and achondroplasia. A study of 25 observations. *Childs Brain* 1980;7(4):205–19.

49. Sainte-Rose C, LaCombe J, Pierre-Kahn A, Renier D, Hirsch JF. Intracranial venous sinus hypertension: cause or consequence of hydrocephalus in infants? *J Neurosurg* 1984;60(4):727–36.

50. Bhadelia RA, Bogdan AR, Wolpert SM. Cerebrospinal fluid flow waveforms: effect of altered cranial venous outflow. A phase-contrast MR flow imaging study. *Neuroradiology* 1998;40(5):283–92.

51. Stoquart-Elsankari S, Lehmann P, Villette A, et al. A phase-contrast MRI study of physiologic cerebral venous flow. *J Cereb Blood Flow Metab* 2009;29(6):1208–15.
52. Bateman GA. The pathophysiology of idiopathic normal pressure hydrocephalus: cerebral ischemia or altered venous hemodynamics? *AJNR Am J Neuroradiol* 2008;29(1):198–203.
53. Martin BA, Reymond P, Novy J, Balédent O, Stergiopulos N. A coupled hydrodynamic model of the cardiovascular and cerebrospinal fluid system. *Am J Physiol Heart Circ Physiol* 302(7):H1492–509.
54. Miller K, ed. *Biomechanics of the Brain*. New York, Dordrecht, Heidelberg, London: Springer Science+Business Media; 2011.
55. Mallucci C, Sgouros S, eds. *Cerebrospinal Fluid Disorders*. New York, London: Informa Healthcare; 2010.
56. Bunck AC, Kroeger JR, Juettner A, et al. Magnetic resonance 4D flow analysis of cerebrospinal fluid dynamics in Chiari I malformation with and without syringomyelia. *Eur Radiol* 2012;22(9):1860–70.
57. Stadlbauer A, Salomonowitz E, Brenneis C, et al. Magnetic resonance velocity mapping of 3D cerebrospinal fluid flow dynamics in hydrocephalus: preliminary results. *Eur Radiol* 2012;22(1):232–42.

Chapter 13

Cerebrospinal fluid dynamics and infusion techniques

Cemil Kayis and Gunes A. Aygok

Introduction

Normal pressure hydrocephalus (NPH) is a pathopsychological condition that has potentially reversible symptoms of gait apraxia, dementia, and urinary incontinence [1,2]. Therefore, proper diagnosis is extremely crucial for the timely treatment and subsequent quality of a patient's life. Since NPH is defined as excessive accumulation of cerebrospinal fluid (CSF) in and around the ventricles with no signs of significant pressure elevation, the hydrodynamics of CSF is one of the key phenomena in diagnosis and management of NPH. The treatment is usually shunting the patients who are responsive to the diagnostic tests such as external lumbar drainage (ELD) and transient monitoring of CSF dynamics [3]. CSF pressure is considered as the main variable monitored from an invasively conducted test and conceptually can be defined as the pressure that must be exerted against a needle placed in the CSF space to just prevent the escape of fluid. It is also proposed that the outflow resistance (R) of CSF and the pulsing characteristics of CSF pressure may be a good candidate to analyze and derive diagnostic conclusions through the same test; however, there is still so much that is unknown. In this chapter, we will briefly describe the CSF dynamics and how fluid inside the central nervous system (CNS) is generated, stored, and absorbed within the context of a mathematical model developed by Marmarou [4,5]. Then, we proceed to explain the main infusion techniques in theory and their practical applications by various clinics. Finally, we will present a comparative analysis of clinically accepted methods followed by a brief discussion and conclusion.

CSF dynamics

The CSF is secreted through the choroid plexus in the ventricles [6]. The rate of formation was reported to be on average constant and about 0.35 ml/min [7]. After being secreted mainly in the lateral and third ventricles, the CSF follows a path to the fourth ventricle through the aqueduct of Sylvius. Then, it flows into the subarachnoid space through the foramina of Luschka and the foramen of Magendie, where most of it is absorbed by the superior sagittal sinus through the arachnoid villi. Some absorption of CSF also takes place in the spinal subarachnoid space [8].

Marmarou [4] developed a model analogous to an electric circuit with some key parameters which are beneficial in diagnosis of NPH. According to Marmarou's theory [4], the CSF formation is balanced by its storage and absorption in equilibrium condition:

$$I_f = I_s + I_e \qquad (13.1)$$

where I_f, I_s, and I_a are formation, storage, and absorption rates, respectively, in the units of ml/min. A general equation governing time-dependent pressure dynamics was derived in terms of the following parameters: The quantized intracranial compliance, i.e. pressure–volume index (PVI), dural sinus pressure (P_d), resistance to absorption (R), and an external input rate of fluid summed up with the intrinsic CSF formation rate.

Compliance means the elasticity or compensatory mechanism of brain parenchyma in response to nonequilibrium conditions such as an external volume addition to CSF space and/or internal pressure fluctuations. It is formulated as volume change per unit pressure difference, $\Delta V/\Delta P$. However, Figure 13.1a shows that the compliance curve has an exponential trend and it varies moving along the curve. Thus, plotting the same data on a semilog scale exhibits a linear behavior and yields a unique constant value as obtained from

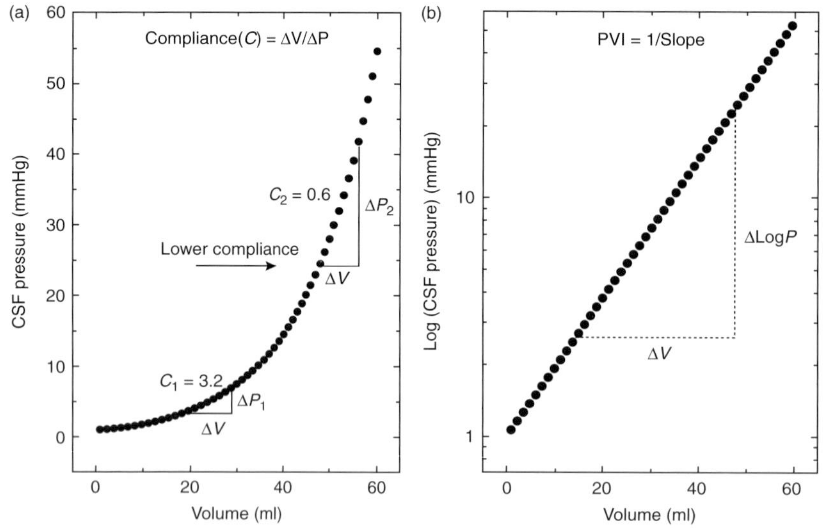

Figure 13.1 (a) A representative simulation of pressure–volume (P-V) curve, which is a characteristic property for each brain. The P-V relationship was shown to be exponential [4]. (b) PVI is the inverse slope obtained from a semilog plot of the P-V curve.

the slope of the line (Figure 13.1b). The inverse slope is called PVI (measured in ml), which is defined as the extra fluid volume necessary to increase the CSF pressure 10-fold.

Absorption rate (I_a) is defined as the gradient of pressure between CSF space (P) and the venous system of the dural sinus (P_d) divided by the resistance to absorption (R):

$$I_a = \frac{(P - P_d)}{R} \tag{13.2}$$

Storage rate is by definition the rate of change of CSF volume stored:

$$I_s = \frac{dV}{dt} \tag{13.3}$$

In addition, compliance (C) can be expressed differentially as:

$$C = \frac{dV}{dP} \tag{13.4}$$

Due to the exponential feature of the compliance curve, C can be expressed as follows:

$$C = \frac{1}{KP} \tag{13.5}$$

where K is a constant determining the steepness of compliance curve. Combining equations (13.4) and (13.5) and differentiating with respect to time yields the form:

$$\frac{dP}{dt} = KP\frac{dV}{dt} = KPI_s \tag{13.6a}$$

and

$$I_s = \frac{1}{KP}\frac{dP}{dt} \tag{13.6b}$$

Thus, a first order nonlinear differential equation can be obtained by substituting the new terms for I_s (13.6b) and I_a (13.2) in (13.1):

$$I_f = \frac{1}{KP}\frac{dP}{dt} + \frac{P - P_d}{R} \tag{13.7}$$

A simplification by rearranging the terms yields the standard differential equation form below:

$$\frac{dP}{dt} + \frac{K}{R}P^2 - K\left(I_f + \frac{P_d}{R}\right)P = 0 \tag{13.8}$$

The general analytical time-dependent solution of (13.8) for pressure is achieved by a specific mathematical transformation and the result is as follows:

$$P(t) = \frac{\psi(t)}{\left[\frac{1}{P_0} + \left(\frac{K}{R}\right)\int_0^t \psi(\tau)d\tau\right]} \tag{13.9}$$

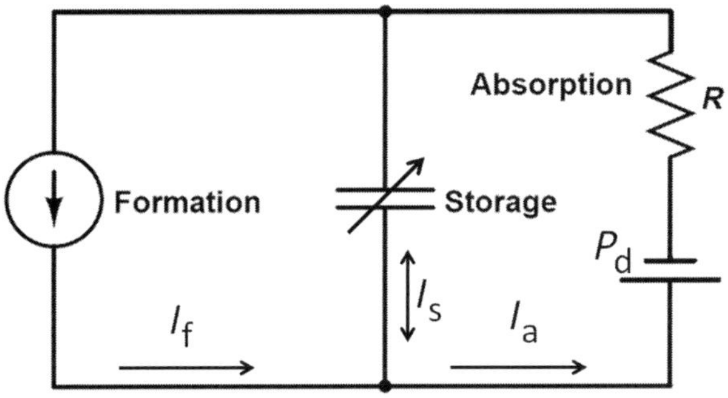

Figure 13.2 The CSF system was modeled by analogy to an electrical circuit and the equations were derived using the rules of circuit operation. Formation and storage are represented by a current source and a nonlinear capacitance, respectively. In addition, absorption branch is represented by a potential difference and a resistance element, which are for dural sinus pressure, P_d and resistance to outflow, *R*, respectively.

where $\psi(t) = e^{K\int_0^t I(\tau)d\tau}$ is the integration factor. Details may be found in the appendix of reference 4.

In addition, the model invokes two physiological constraints: the venous drainage is linear, i.e., drainage is linearly proportional to the pressure gradient between CSF pressure on the granulation side (*P*) and pressure on the dural sinus side (P_d) as verified for adult cats by Marmarou et al. [4]. In addition, CSF pressure must be greater than dural sinus pressure, i.e., $P > P_d$, to have actual drainage. It is also assumed that the dural sinus pressure is constant under normal physiological circumstances.

Once the governing CSF model has been developed, it can be solved for both steady-state and transient conditions. At steady-state condition as imposed by the model, CSF pressure is governed by the dural sinus pressure and the product of constant formation rate and resistance to absorption:

$$P = P_d + I_f R \tag{13.10}$$

Note that there is no storage term involving the compliance component at equilibrium condition. This is analogous to the capacitor model acting as open circuit under direct current operating conditions in an electrical circuit. In fact, Marmarou [4] proposed his model using an electrical circuit analogy to the CSF circulation as seen schematically in Figure 13.2. Meanwhile, Eq. (13.10) suggests that the slope gives the outflow resistance and an increase in formation rate will reflect as an increase in the CSF pressure under the assumption of *R* and P_d held constant. In addition, at zero formation rate, CSF pressure is pinned to the dural sinus pressure for which there is no absorption expected.

Lumbar infusion techniques

The infusion of fluid to the CSF space was clinically introduced by Katzman and Hussey [9,10] and since then it has been effectively implemented as a useful diagnostic tool for hydrocephalus and in vivo patency tests of malfunctioning shunts as well as for research conducted on animals [4,8]. In principle, the infusion test is done by introducing a sufficient amount of fluid (saline or artificial CSF) to the CSF space. Marmarou used the above-mentioned mathematical model (Eq. 13.9) for three different types of external inputs which are for bolus injection, volume removal, and constant infusion methods. Current clinical applications are mainly based on those with slight modifications comprising the specifics for a particular method. The solution depicts the transient effects as a response to the specific input types summed up with the constant formation rate. The mathematical equivalent of a selected physical external input, i.e., $I(\tau)$, must be inserted in Eq. (13.9) for the corresponding desired solution (Table 13.1, columns B and C). Ideally a positive/negative square-pulse function represents a rapid injection/removal as in the case of the bolus method. For example, the external input rate for bolus injection is 1 ml/s for a few seconds. In contrast, constant infusion is simply a summation of two constant-rate inputs, which are the intrinsic formation rate and constant infusion rate. The ideal mathematical representation for this type of physical input is a step function, for which the starting moment for the infusion process corresponds to the location of the step-like feature (Table 13.1, bottom row, column B).

The solutions and output responses for time-dependent pressure, *P*(*t*), have specific results with respect to the constraints imposed as well as the infusion type, as summarized in Table 13.1. After collecting the output response data, one can subsequently solve for desired quantities (*R*, I_f, *C*, PVI, etc.) by using the expression for *P*(*t*) at any time. The main parameters of interest are resistance to outflow and the pressure–volume index.

Bolus injection

The bolus injection method is defined as a small amount of volume (≈4 ml) introduced to the CSF system in a short amount of time, usually within about 4–5 s. The

Table 13.1 Three different infusion methods (rows) were evaluated using the Marmarou model for CSF dynamics [4]. Column (A) is the volume added to the CSF system as a function of time; (B) external input rate summed up with constant intrinsic production rate; (C) the mathematical equivalent of the added/removed volume; (D) the solution of the model for pressure as a function of time with respect to the given inputs; (E) the output response of the respective solutions for each infusion method

(A) Type of input	(B) Total input	(C) Math form of input	(D) Solution for pressure, $P(t)$	(E) Output response
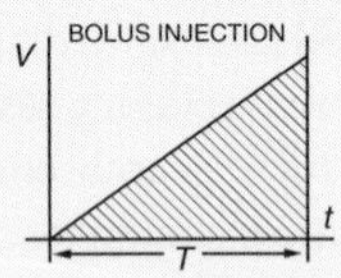	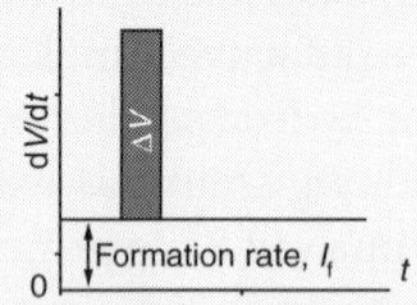	$I_f + V\delta(t)$	$P(t)=\dfrac{P_o e^{KV+\frac{KtP_o}{R}}}{1+e^{KV}\left[e^{\frac{KtP_o}{R}}-1\right]},\ t<t_c$	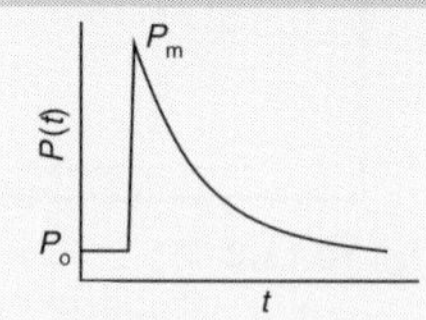
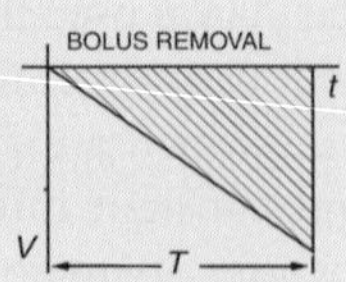	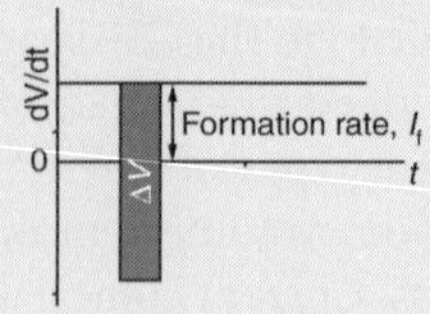	$I_f - V\delta(t)$	$P(t)=P_o e^{KI(I_f t-V)},\ t<t_c$ $P(t)=\dfrac{P_o e^{-KV+\frac{KtP_o}{R}}}{1+e^{-KV}\left[e^{\frac{KtP_o}{R}}-1\right]},\ t\geq t_c$	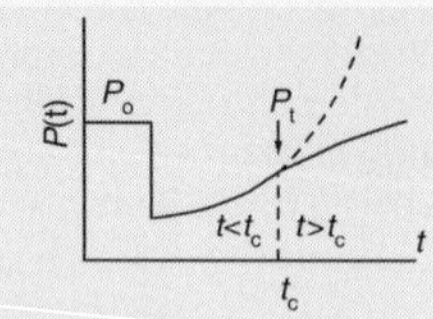
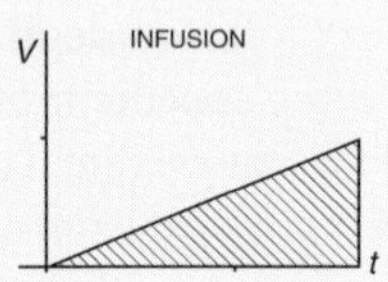	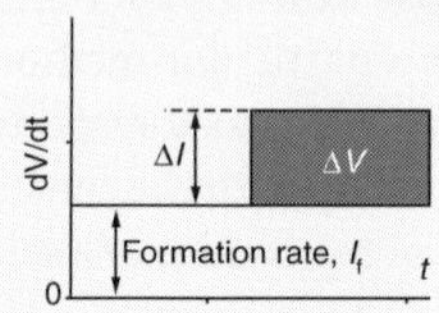	$I_f + \Delta I$	$P(t)=\dfrac{P_o[P_o+R\Delta I]}{P_o+R\Delta I\left[e^{\frac{Kt(P_o+R\Delta I)}{R}}\right]}$	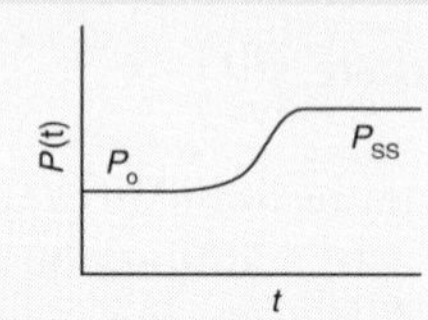

amount of liquid must be small but significant enough to create an observable transient as invasively monitored from the CSF pressure. The injected amount is mathematically formulated using a delta function keeping the formation rate as a constant background. The pressure profile exhibits an abrupt increase from its equilibrium state reaching a maximum value immediately after introduction of the injected amount. Then, pressure starts to decrease as a function of the compliance parameter, K, and resistance to outflow, R. Finally, the CSF system is expected to restore itself ideally at opening pressure, P_o.

The general solution for R is shown below as derived from the time-dependent pressure result (Table 13.1, top row, column D):

$$R=\frac{tP_0}{(\mathrm{PVI})\log\left[\left(\frac{P_t}{P_p}\right)\left(\frac{P_p-P_o}{P_t-P_o}\right)\right]} \tag{13.11}$$

where t is time, P_o is the resting (base) pressure, P_p is peak pressure immediately after injection, and P_t is the pressure value recorded at a selected time after injection.

Similarly, PVI is calculated using the data obtained from bolus method through the following expression:

$$\mathrm{PVI}=\frac{\Delta V}{\log\left(\frac{P_p}{P_o}\right)} \tag{13.12}$$

where ΔV is the total volume injected. Equation (13.12) can be derived from the definition of PVI and using Figure 13.1b.

Bolus infusion measurement can be performed in an outpatient clinic. The procedure conducted at the Medical College of Virginia (Virginia Commonwealth University, Richmond, USA) can be described as follows. After surgical preparation of the site and application of a local analgesic, a 25-gauge needle is used to access percutaneously into the lumbar intrathecal space. After reaching CSF space, the needle, sterile saline syringe, and strain-gauge type pressure

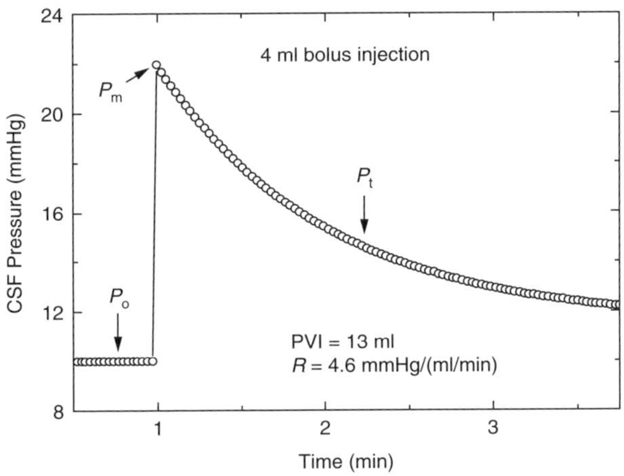

Figure 13.3 An example of bolus injection data obtained from a patient. PVI and *R* can be calculated by picking the values of the relevant parameter from the patient data collected. Data were processed to smooth the ripples.

transducer are interconnected through a tube and three-way stopcock. An auxiliary setup consisting of a tube and stopcock is also used to get air-free tubing filled with saline. Then, the output of the transducer is connected to a bedside monitor (Philips Intellivue MP5), which provides a pressure waveform on the screen. Similarly, the output of the bedside monitor is connected to a computer to store and analyze the pressure data. Finally, the transducer reading must be zeroed to atmosphere, and a careful check of the fluid lines is needed to ensure that they are continuously filled with fluid with no air bubbles. Following these steps, the operator may inject 4 ml of fluid at a rate of 1 ml/s and monitor and record the time course of pressure for data analyses. The number of necessary bolus injections is three or four for each patient and the total test duration is approximately 20 to 30 minutes including preparation.

Figure 13.3 shows an example of bolus injection data obtained from a patient. The outflow resistance can be calculated by picking the values of relevant parameters and plugging in Eq. 13.11. The normal range for *R* lies within 4–6 mmHg/(ml/min) from the clinical studies conducted at the Medical College of Virginia NPH clinic [3]. Below this range is considered to be still normal yielding even better conductance (*G*), where conductance is defined as the reciprocal of resistance ($G = 1/R$). In contrast, values above 6 mmHg/(ml/min) are regarded as a diagnostic indication of possible NPH, i.e. positive shunt responder. Additionally, an approximate value of 25 ml is considered to be a normal PVI value for a healthy person, whereas a PVI below 15 ml is an indication of low compliance, which implies a "tight brain." PVI values higher than 25 ml may be caused by some anomalies such as an atrophic brain.

Volume removal

Volume removal is defined as the opposite of bolus injection and is also called bolus withdrawal. In this scenario one must take into account that another condition emerges by removal of CSF as follows: The model suggests that absorption of CSF is only possible when the gradient between the CSF pressure and dural sinus pressure is positive, i.e., $P > P_d$. However, CSF pressure may drop below the dural venous sinus pressure immediately after bolus removal. Thus the time evolution after bolus removal must be separated into two regimes where the resistance to absorption is effectively infinite for the first part. The second regime starts at the threshold point where CSF pressure becomes greater than or equal to the dural venous pressure, which builds up by constant formation of CSF. The time-dependent CSF pressure can be formulated by considering these two pre- and post-threshold regions. Before the threshold point, CSF pressure recovers as a function of formation rate and compliance coefficient, whereas when absorption starts to take place after threshold, CSF pressure evolves as a function of absorption resistance and compliance coefficient until it reaches the equilibrium pressure as in the case of bolus injection.

Volume removal technique also enables calculation of PVI. In addition, the formation rate can be calculated using the region right after volume removal until the threshold point through the equation below:

$$I_f = \frac{PVI}{t}\log\frac{P}{P_m} \tag{13.13}$$

where *P* and *t* must be picked at a point before the threshold level, i.e., $t < t_c$ (Table 13.1, center row, column D).

In 1934, Masserman [11] reported an average CSF formation rate of 0.32 ml/min by relatively rapid removal of 20–35 ml of CSF and observing spontaneous recovery of pressure up to its resting value. Although Masserman's prediction turned out to be pretty close to the recently accepted rate of 0.35 ml/min, his method has been criticized due to the assumption of constant absorption rate during the pressure restoration and not allowing for the vascular compensation of the initial pressure drop. In addition, Ekstedt [12] measured formation rate through a modified method by continuous lumbar drainage of CSF. The value reported was 0.4 ml/min, which is also within range of the commonly accepted rate. The bolus removal method also relies on the assumption that no absorption takes place before the CSF pressure surpasses the dural sinus pressure following a rapid withdrawal of fluid, for which pressure drops below the threshold value.

Gradual infusion methods

The bolus technique introduces a relatively sudden perturbation to the CSF system. Monitoring of the subsequent relaxation to the equilibrium state allows acquisition of the data necessary to calculate R and PVI. In contrast, gradual infusion methods suggest adding fluid in a controlled manner and simultaneously monitoring the time course of CSF pressure. Here we cover two main types of gradual infusion techniques, which are constant flow infusion and constant pressure infusion methods.

Constant flow infusion

As a third method, the constant flow infusion technique comprises a continuous infusion of fluid at a constant rate on top of the intrinsic formation rate [9,10,13]. The model suggested a solution for time-dependent pressure $P(t)$ which results in a rapid increase in time and then slowly levels off. Finally, it forms a plateau, where the CSF system attains its new equilibrium with a steady-state pressure of P_{ss} caused by spontaneous balancing of external infusion through an increased absorption rate. The outflow resistance R can be calculated from the dynamic pressure expression given in Table 13.1 (bottom row, column D) as a response to an applied external input. Other relevant parameters such as the resting pressure (P_o), compliance constant (K), and pressure (P) must be determined from a curve fitting to experimental data. It is also possible to solve for R using the static approach by simply dividing the difference between steady-state pressure (P_{ss}) and resting pressure (P_o) by the infusion rate (ΔI) as follows:

$$R = \frac{P_{ss} - P_o}{\Delta I} \tag{13.14}$$

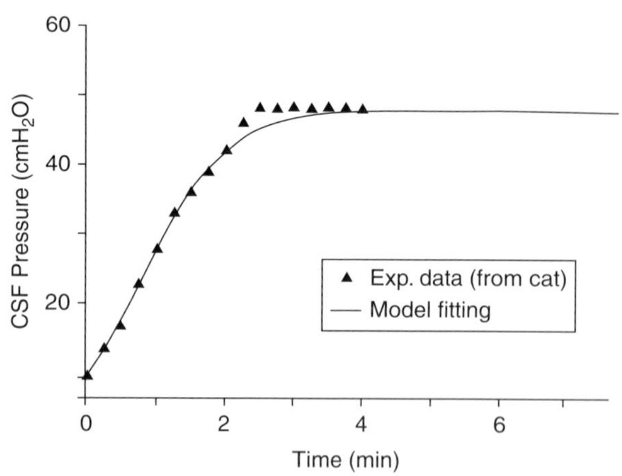

Figure 13.4 Model compared with experimental CSF pressure responses. Fluid was infused into the cisterna magna at a constant rate of 0.35 ml/min [4].

After Katzman and Hussey [9,10] clinically introduced the constant rate infusion technique in 1970, it was adopted and modified by several others [14–20]. In particular, Marmarou tested his model on adult cats by comparing the data monitored during an infusion into the cisterna magna at a constant rate of 0.35 ml/min. His original work published in 1978 exhibited a good agreement between theory and experiment, confirming that the model successfully governs the time course of CSF pressure for constant and bolus infusion methods. Figure 13.4 shows a selected dataset comparing the model with the data obtained from the constant infusion method. However, he picked the transient method (bolus infusion) to assess outflow resistance for clinical practice mainly due to the fact that the bolus method is faster than other methods, which is especially beneficial for patient comfort and low complication rates. Also, the transient method was expected to yield more novel data due to the impulsive nature of the technique compared with the constant flow rate method.

In contrast, Børgesen et al. [21] applied a modified version of lumbo-ventricular constant flow method called the "constant pressure constant infusion rate technique." They used the software developed by Czosnyka et al. [22] to capture the time course of pressure and faster assessment of outflow resistance using the Davson equation [23]. In particular, Juniewicz et al. [24] measured an elevation in resting pressure of about 3 mmHg following a constant infusion test. Figure 13.5 displays a typical recording of constant flow infusion at a rate of 1 ml/min [24]. The time evolution of pressure response exhibited an expected increase and plateau formation during the infusion and subsequent exponential pressure decay, resting at a higher value than the opening pressure. The possible suggestions to explain

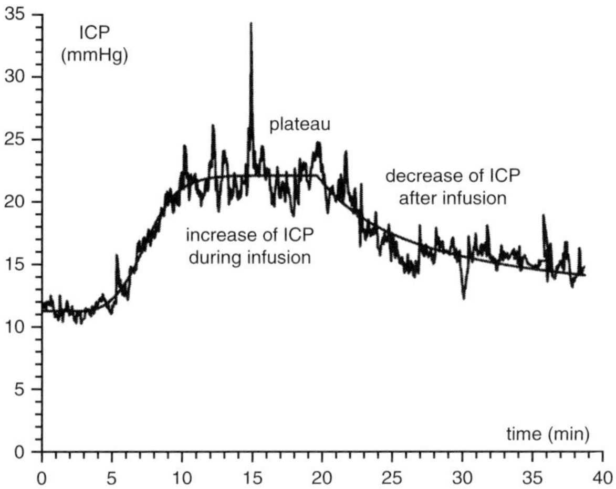

Figure 13.5 Typical clinical data monitored using constant infusion method at a rate of 1 ml/min [24].

this hysteresis effect were either through transient volume change caused by excessive CSF diffusion into parenchyma [25] or by increase in the vascular component of intracranial pressure after infusion [26].

Constant pressure infusion

The constant pressure method was suggested by Ekstedt in 1977 [27]. Principally, the technique is based on keeping the pressure at a constant level during the flow of sustaining artificial CSF. A peristaltic infusion pump and a computer-based regulating feedback system are utilized to achieve this for several pressure steps. For each level, flow rate and CSF pressure must be recorded. Then, R can be calculated based on steady-state solution for the model using Eq. (13.14).

In this method, two needles must be used, one assigned for infusion and the other for pressure measurement. The patient needs to rest in the supine position for about 20 min followed by about 5 min of resting pressure (P_o) monitoring. The step height for each consecutive pressure level is kept about 4 mmHg and each step is sustained at a stable level for 5–8 min. The overall procedure may take 1–1.5 h [28].

Figure 13.6a displays typical data collected for constant pressure infusion [28]. Six different pressure steps are clearly achieved by regulating the flow rate. In addition, the pressure level goes back to the resting pressure after the infusion process has halted. In principle, the constant pressure method is based on the dynamics of constant flow infusion. The basic modification is as follows: instead of monitoring the data several times under the same pressure–flow conditions

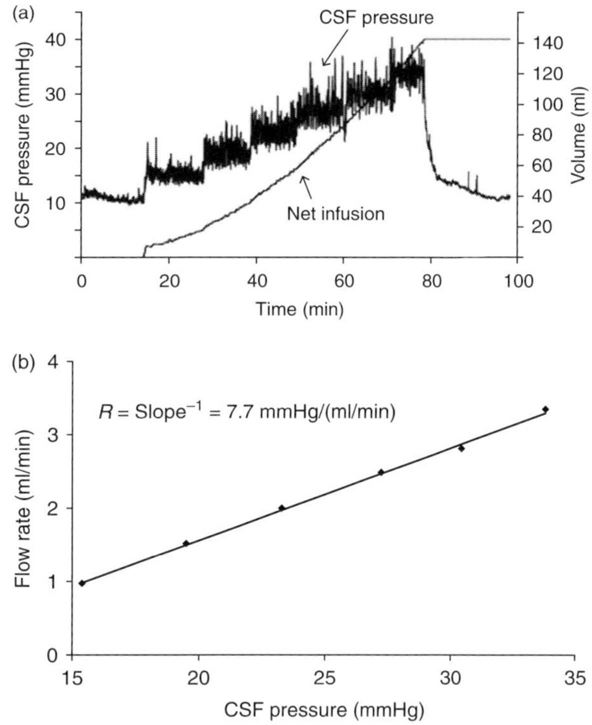

Figure 13.6 (a) Clear observation of pressure levels by regulating the flow rate [28]. (b) Linear fit on the data collected by recording flow rate corresponding to each pressure level. The inverse slope yields outflow resistance [28].

and averaging them all, the constant pressure method suggests monitoring CSF pressure with the increments of small offset values. This would allow plotting flow as a function of pressure or vice versa. The linear relationship between pressure and flow is shown in Figure 13.6b as Marmarou assumed in his circuit model and confirmed experimentally on cats [4]. The linearity also implies that resistance to outflow is constant as long as one does not exceed the compensatory system of the brain, i.e., by staying within a reasonable compliance range.

External lumbar drainage and tap test

External lumbar drainage (ELD) is an excellent prognostic tool for which the accuracy of prediction rate can be more than 90% [3]. The test is based on the idea of simulating the shunt operation in real life by withdrawing CSF for relatively long time durations at drainage rates roughly comparable to regular shunt drainage. The standard application of the method usually requires 48–72 hours at an inpatient setting. The drainage rate may change depending on the patient's condition such as age and brain atrophy. For the patients below

75 years and having a relatively "tight" brain, the rate is kept at around 10 ml/h. However, for patients older than 75 years or having an atrophic brain, the rate must be reduced and watched carefully. ELD yields the most accurate prognostic indications since it simulates the shunt for an extended time duration, which also helps to exclude some placebo effects. However, the long-term hospitalization may cause high complication rates and very uncomfortable conditions for elderly patients. Therefore, the possible elimination of ELD by replacing it with a combination of other tools is favored.

The tap test can be considered as a method for partial replacement of ELD; it involves the removal of one-shot large-volume CSF, i.e. withdrawal of about 40–50 ml within 15–30 min. It is possible to conduct the tap test in an outpatient clinic usually following an infusion test. Patients may leave the clinic after resting for an hour. The outcome can be evaluated by comparing the symptoms of gait impairment and cognitive findings before and after the CSF removal, supported by imaging and infusion test results. The symptoms may also alleviate after the patient goes home and rests overnight. Therefore good patient communication and follow-up is necessary.

Discussion

Infusion tests are mainly used as an auxiliary diagnostic tool for patients with NPH symptoms along with other clinical diagnostic methods such as the tap test or ELD [3,29–32]. In addition, outflow resistance is beneficial for testing in vivo shunt patency, which is effectively utilized to determine suspected malfunctioning shunt valves and antisiphon devices [33–36]. Moreover, coupling between vascular pulsing effect and CSF pressure also draws attention and is still being extensively studied after the advent of continuous computerized monitoring of intracranial pressures. Hence, monitoring of CSF pulse pressure amplitude during the lumbar infusion test was proposed for further understanding of CSF dynamics as well as for predicting outcome after NPH treatment [37–39]. The parameters of CSF dynamics extracted from an infusion test may also be beneficial for differential diagnostics such as distinguishing atrophic brain from hydrocephalus [40].

Technically, clinical prognostic applications of infusion methods can be classified into two groups: transient and steady-state. The bolus method is a means of monitoring transient behavior of CSF pressure after a rapid injection, whereas gradual infusion methods simply use the steady-state conditions by regulating the infusion process. The underlying basic principle of both methods is the linearity of the pressure–flow relationship within safe compensatory limits of the central nervous system. The pressure–flow linearity intrinsically holds the concept of constant R. However, clinical studies designed for shunt outcome prediction showed that there is no consensus on the magnitude of R calculated from the data collected using both methods. The threshold of resistance to outflow for the bolus method was determined as 4 mmHg/(ml/min) from a clinical study on 151 patients [3]. In contrast, centers using steady-state methods suggest significantly higher threshold values scattered in the range of 8–18 mmHg/(ml/min) [29,41–46]. Both methods offer positive predictive values (PPV) above 70%. However, negative predictive values (NPV) are not as high as PPVs, especially for constant infusion methods [29]. Thus, the use of other complementary diagnostic tools such as imaging, evaluation of the triad of symptoms, and CSF removal via tap test or ELD is imperative for the purpose of accurate outcome prediction. The gold standard process for predicting shunt responders is ELD, for which the accuracy rate is 92% [3]. However, the procedure requires an inpatient setting, and patients undergoing the ELD test may suffer from various complications. Moreover, 48- to 72-hour hospitalization may not be suitable for many elderly patients. Therefore, an infusion test with the aforementioned complementary diagnostic tools may increase outcome prediction accuracy comparable to the ELD prediction level and possibly eliminate hospitalization.

Clinically, there is no clear evidence to judge that the transient method is superior to the steady-state method or vice versa in terms of prognostic impact. The two methods are based on different physical standpoints yielding two different threshold outflow resistances for steady-state and transient solutions, even though the model suggests unique outflow resistance for both. The underlying cause of the difference is not known yet, possibly due to a missing parameter or a scaling factor which may unify the results. Therefore, each method should be treated separately and self consistently. For comparison in terms of application, the bolus method takes much less time, requiring a maximum of 30 min for each patient. In addition, it does not require complex equipment such as infusion pumps and regulatory systems and only one needle is necessary for lumbar puncture. The total amount of injected fluid is also much less than the amount necessary for constant pressure infusion, which is about 12 ml for three consecutive injections. In contrast, it demands more experience and better understanding of CSF dynamics while handling the process.

Since NPH is considered to occur at a late age, generally over 60, a large number of patients have atrophic brains of varying severities. The response of atrophic brain to bolus injection may skew the results for the first infusion. Hence, a second injection is necessary to compensate for the "pseudo-compliance" induced by atrophic brain. Injections that are applied following the first one exhibit similar *R* and PVI values, confirming the reliability of data. Imaging may be highly beneficial to assess dilation of sylvian fissures, which was reported as an indication of NPH [47,48]. Assessment of PVI together with imaging may also be useful to evaluate any atrophic brain and observations can be incorporated for interpretation of outflow resistance.

CSF pulse pressure is another aspect of CSF dynamics. CNS consists of three major components: brain parenchyma, CSF, and cerebral blood. Pressures exerted by the active compartments (CSF and cerebral blood) are in communication with each other and arterial/venous pressure components are scaled with a lever arm factor, i.e. the compensatory reserve of the aforementioned three components. The arterial blood pressure is roughly scaled down by more than an order of magnitude, where peak-to-peak CSF pulse amplitudes may vary in a range of 3–10 mmHg. The infusion technique is an integral part of probing the pulsed feature of CSF pressure for which the compliance response can be deduced and used for prediction of prognosis in NPH [39]. However, there are no theoretical and practical certainties and well-established clinical thresholds to date. Nevertheless, periodic pulse amplitude measurements should continue to support and enrich the interpretation of findings obtained from an infusion test. The periodic pulse feature superimposed on top of CSF pressure acts like an AC signal (with some distortion factor) straddled on a DC signal. Addition of this concept to the Marmarou circuit model and solving it quantitatively may lead to a better understanding of CSF dynamics, filling the gaps between theory and acquired data and in turn improving the overall results obtained from an infusion test.

Conclusions

Infusion tests enable direct probing of cerebrospinal fluid dynamics yielding independent data to compare with the results obtained from other assessments and beneficial for diagnosis and treatment of hydrocephalus. The main physical parameters are pressure–volume index and resistance to CSF outflow as extracted from a model developed analogous to an electrical circuit. However, full benefit could not be harnessed due to the complex structure of the central nervous system in regard to its neural structure and hydrodynamic function. NPH in elderly patients is mostly an idiopathic disease possibly caused by imbalance of the latter. Comorbidity is also a major cofounder in this patient population. These challenges greatly impede efforts to resolve the real etiology of NPH. The link between the hydrodynamic imbalance, its hypothetical damage in the periventricular region, and the presence of the clinical symptoms has not been clarified yet. Hence, improving the current infusion models by understanding the correlation between the key parameters of CSF infusion techniques, incorporating novel relevant parameters such as the pulsed feature of CSF pressure, and supporting these with the findings from other disciplines is imperative and may pave the way to resolving underlying etiology. Nevertheless, both bolus and constant infusion methods are excellent tools for detecting a shunt failure in many cases since functioning shunts act as a parallel route for CSF flow and decrease the resistance to outflow substantially.

References

1. Hakim S, Adams RD. The special clinical problem of symptomatic hydrocephalus with normal cerebrospinal fluid pressure. Observations on cerebrospinal fluid hydrodynamics. *J Neurol Sci* 1965;2:307–27.
2. Adams RD, Fisher CM, Hakim S. Symptomatic occult hydrocephalus with "normal" cerebrospinal fluid pressure. A treatable syndrome. *N Engl J Med* 1966;273:117–26.
3. Marmarou A, Young HF, Aygok GA, et al. Diagnosis and management of idiopathic normal-pressure hydrocephalus: a prospective study in 151 patients. *J Neurosurg* 2005;102:987–97.
4. Marmarou A, Shulman K, Rosende RM. A nonlinear analysis of the cerebrospinal fluid system and intracranial pressure dynamics. *J Neurosurg* 1978;48:332–44.
5. Marmarou A. A theoretical model and experimental evaluation of the cerebrospinal fluid system. PhD thesis, Drexel University, Philadelphia, PA; 1973.

6. Cushing HW. Studies on the cerebrospinal fluid. *J Med Res* 1914;8:406–9.
7. Ekstedt J. CSF hydrodynamic studies in man. Normal hydrodynamic variables related to CSF pressure and flow. *J Neurol Neurosurg Psychiatry* 1978;41:345–53.
8. Marmarou A, Shulman K, Lamorgese J. Compartmental analysis of compliance and outflow resistance of the cerebrospinal fluid system. *J Neurosurg* 1975;43:523–34.
9. Katzman R, Hussey F. A simple constant-infusion manometric test for measurement of CSF absorption. I. Rationale and method. *Neurology* 1970;20:534–44.
10. Hussey F, Schanzer B, Katzman R. A simple constant-infusion manometric test for measurement of CSF absorption. II. Clinical studies. *Neurology* 1970;20:665–80.
11. Masserman JH. Cerebrospinal hydrodynamics: IV. Clinical experimental studies. *Arch Neurol Psychiatry* 1934;32:523–53.
12. Ekstedt J. CSF hydrodynamic studies in man. Normal hydrodynamic variables related to CSF pressure and flow. *J Neurol Neurosurg Psychiatry* 1978;41:345–53.
13. Foldes FF, Arrowood JG. Changes in cerebrospinal fluid under the influence of continuous subarachnoidal infusion of normal saline. *J Clin Invest* 1948;27:346–51.
14. Nelson JR, Goodman SJ. An evaluation of the cerebrospinal fluid infusion test for hydrocephalus. *Neurology (Minneap)* 1971;21:1038–53.
15. Martins AN, Kobine AI, Larsen DF. Pressure in the sagittal sinus during intracranial hypertension in man. *J Neurosurg* 1974;40:603–8.
16. Di Rocco C, Maira G, Rossi GF, Vignati A. Cerebrospinal fluid pressure studies in normal pressure hydrocephalus and cerebral atrophy. *Eur Neurol* 1976;14:119–28.
17. Trotter JL, Luzecky M, Siegel BA, Gado M. Cerebrospinal fluid infusion test. Identification of artifacts and correlation with cisternography and pneumoencephalography. *Neurology (Minneap)* 1974;24:181–6.
18. Czosnyka M, Batorski L, Laniewski P, et al. A computer system for the identification of the cerebrospinal compensatory model. *Acta Neurochir* 1990;105:112–16.
19. Kosteljanetz M. Resistance to outflow of cerebrospinal fluid determined by bolus injection technique and constant rate steady state infusion in humans. *Neurosurgery* 1985;16:336–40.
20. Børgesen SE, Gjerris F, Sørensen SC. The conductance to outflow of cerebrospinal fluid absorption in normal pressure hydrocephalus. *Acta Neurol Scand* 1978;57:88–96.
21. Børgesen SE, Albeck MJ, Gjerris F, Czosnyka M, Laniewski P. Computerized infusion test compared to steady pressure constant infusion test in measurement of resistance to CSF outflow. *Acta Neurochir (Wien)* 1992;119:12–16.
22. Czosnyka M, Wollk-Laniewski D, Darwaj P. Software for neurointensive care. In: Hoff JT, et al. (Eds.) *Intracranial Pressure VIII*. Berlin, Heidelberg, New York: Springer; 1989: 84–7.
23. Davson H, Hollingsworth G, Segal MB. The mechanism of drainage of the cerebrospinal fluid. *Brain* 1970;93:665–78.
24. Juniewicz H, Kasprowicz M, Czosnyka M, et al. Analysis of intracranial pressure during and after the infusion test in patients with communicating hydrocephalus. *Physiol Meas* 2005;26:1039–48.
25. Kasprowicz M, Czosnyka M, Czosnyka Z, et al. Hysteresis of the cerebrospinal pressure–volume curve test in hydrocephalus. *Acta Neurochir Suppl* 2003;86:529–32.
26. Czosnyka M, Richards HK, Czosnyka Z, Piechnik S, Pickard JD. Vascular components of cerebrospinal fluid compensation. *J Neurosurg* 1999; 90:752–9.
27. Ekstedt J. CSF hydrodynamic studies in man 1. Method of constant pressure CSF infusion. *J Neurol Neurosurg Psychiatry* 1977;40:105–19.
28. Andersson N, Malm J, Backlund T, Eklund A. Assessment of cerebrospinal fluid outflow conductance using constant pressure infusion – a method with real time estimation of reliability. *Physiol Meas* 2005;26:1137–48.
29. Boon AJ, Tans JT, Delwel EJ, et al. Dutch normal-pressure hydrocephalus study: prediction of outcome after shunting by resistance to outflow of cerebrospinal fluid. *J Neurosurg* 1997;87:687–93.
30. Kahlon B, Sundbärg G, Rehncrona S. Comparison between the lumbar infusion and CSF tap tests to predict outcome after shunt surgery in suspected normal pressure hydrocephalus. *J Neurol Neurosurg Psychiatry* 2002;73:721–6.
31. Albeck MJ, Skak C, Nielsen PR, et al. Age dependency of resistance to cerebrospinal fluid outflow. *J Neurosurg* 1998; 89:275–8.
32. Meier U, Miethke C. Predictors of outcome in patients with normal-pressure hydrocephalus. *J Clin Neurosci* 2003;10(4):453–9.
33. Woodford J, Saunders RL, Sachs, Jr. E. Shunt system patency testing by lumbar infusion. *J. Neurosurg* 1976;45:60–5.
34. Czosnyka ZH, Czosnyka M, Pickard JD. Shunt testing in-vivo: a method based on the data from the UK

shunt evaluation laboratory. *Acta Neurochir Suppl* 2002;81:27–30.

35. Lundkvist B, Koskinen L-OD, Birgander R, Eklund A, Malm J. Cerebrospinal fluid dynamics and long-term survival of the Strata valve in idiopathic normal pressure hydrocephalus. *Acta Neurol Scand* 2011;124:115–21.

36. Eklund A, Koskinen L-OD, Williams MA, et al. Hydrodynamics of the Certas™ programmable valve for the treatment of hydrocephalus. *Fluids Barriers CNS* 2012;9:12.

37. Czosnyka M, Wollk-Laniewski P, Batorski L, Zaworski W. Analysis of intracranial pressure waveform during infusion test. *Acta Neurochir* 1988;93:140–5.

38. Kim D-J, Carrera E, Czosnyka M, et al. Cerebrospinal compensation of pulsating cerebral blood volume in hydrocephalus. *Neurol Res* 2010;32(6):587–92.

39. Eide PK, Brean A. Cerebrospinal fluid pulse pressure amplitude during lumbar infusion in idiopathic normal pressure hydrocephalus can predict response to shunting. *Cerebrospinal Fluid Res* 2010;7:5.

40. Eklund A, Lundkvist B, Koskinen L-OD, Malm J. Infusion technique can be used to distinguish between dysfunction of a hydrocephalus shunt system and a progressive dementia. *Med Biol Eng Comput* 2004;42:644–9.

41. Børgesen SE, Gjerris F. The predictive value of conductance to outflow of CSF in normal pressure hydrocephalus. *Brain* 1982;105:65–86.

42. Ekstedt J. CSF hydrodynamic studies in man. 2. Normal hydrodynamic variables related to CSF pressure and flow. *J Neurol Neurosurg Psychiatry* 1978;41:345–53.

43. Delwel EJ, de Jong DA, Avezaat CJJ, et al. CSF dynamics in patients with suspected normal pressure hydrocephalus. In: Hoff JT, Betz AL (Eds.) *Intracranial Pressure VII*. Heidelberg: Springer-Verlag; 1989: 379–82.

44. Lundar T, Nones H. Determination of ventricular fluid outflow resistance in patients with ventriculomegaly. *J Neurol Neurosurg Psychiatry* 1990;53:896–8.

45. Price DJ. Attempts to predict the probability of clinical improvement following shunting of patients with presumed normal pressure hydrocephalus. In: Hoff JT, Betz AL (Eds.) *Intracranial Pressure VII*. Heidelberg: Springer-Verlag; 1989: 390–3.

46. Tans JTJ, Poortvliet DCJ. Reduction of ventricular size after shunting for normal pressure hydrocephalus related to CSF dynamics before shunting. *J Neurol Neurosurg Psychiatry* 1988;51:521–5.

47. Ishikawa M, Hashimoto M, Kuwana N, et al. Guidelines for management of idiopathic normal pressure hydrocephalus. *Neurol Med Chir (Tokyo)* 2008;48(Suppl.):S1–S23.

48. Mori E, Ishikawa M, Kato T, et al. Guidelines for management of idiopathic normal pressure hydrocephalus: second edition. *Neurol Med Chir (Tokyo)* 2012;52(11):775–809.

Chapter 14

Monitoring of intracranial pressure and assessment of cerebrospinal fluid dynamics

Marek Czosnyka, Martin U. Schuhmann, Stefano Signoretti, Zofia Czosnyka, and John D. Pickard

Quantitative assessment of cerebrospinal fluid (CSF) dynamics may support clinical intuition with a description of CSF circulatory and compensatory dysfunction, particularly when both clinical and imaging evidence is subtle and ambiguous. For normal pressure hydrocephalus (NPH) the consensus regarding the use of physiological parameters in conjunction with clinical and imaging information is still uncertain, despite guidelines for the management of NPH [1] published some time ago. The main problem is that they have never been based on sufficiently hard clinical and experimental evidence.

The current range of clinical applications for CSF dynamics testing includes hydrocephalus, idiopathic intracranial hypertension, craniosynostosis, and traumatic brain injury – in the latter case useful for differentiating post-traumatic hydrocephalus from atrophy and assessing CSF pathways following decompressive craniectomy.

Main mechanisms and models of CSF circulation and pressure–volume compensation

Generally, CSF dynamics depends on interaction between four components: CSF production, flow, absorption, and pulsations.

CSF production occurs by active secretion at a relatively constant rate but dependent upon brain metabolic rate and reducing with age. The role of free, unobstructed flow of CSF is 3-fold: (1) it provides a shock absorptive function for the brain and spinal cord, important in trauma; (2) it allows clearance of brain metabolites; (3) it allows for an even distribution of pressure throughout the intracranial vault, reducing any pressure gradients and preventing brain shifts or herniation. The last point explains why a very high intracranial pressure (ICP; >40 mmHg) can be tolerated relatively asymptomatically in communicating hydrocephalus (e.g. during CSF infusion tests). In contrast, when CSF pathways are obstructed, as in cerebral edema after traumatic brain injury, marked clinical deterioration is seen at ICP exceeding 20–25 mmHg.

CSF absorption occurs, according to the traditional view proposed by Weed in 1916 [2], in a pressure-dependent fashion via the arachnoid granulations at the superior sagittal sinus, also called the major pathway, mathematically described by Davson [3]. Dandy and Blackfan, following animal experiments and human observations, concluded that CSF reabsorption could not be refined to the arachnoid granulations but occurs diffusely from the subarachnoid space throughout the CNS [4]. Since microscopic arachnoid villi appear just around birth and arachnoid granulations are not detectable before the age of about 7 years, several alternative CSF absorption mechanisms have been proposed by various authors and have also been summarized as the “minor pathway” as opposed to the major pathway [5]. Alternative outflow of CSF may probably occur via periventricular leakage into the brain parenchyma, as suggested in NPH.

CSF circulates not only in a constant way with a rate equivalent to CSF production, but also in pulsations. CSF pulsatile flow is observed in the cerebral aqueduct (approx. 40 microliters in stroke volume in normal subjects) and in the cervical region of the subarachnoid space (approx. 500 microliters stroke volume) [6]. For a half of the cardiac cycle, CSF flows down into the spinal subarachnoid space and for the other half, upward into cranial compartments. The role of pulsatile CSF flow and pressure pulsations is still unclear, but is becoming more frequently studied in hydrocephalus and other diseases manifesting with abnormal CSF dynamics.

Adult Hydrocephalus, ed. Daniele Rigamonti. Published by Cambridge University Press.

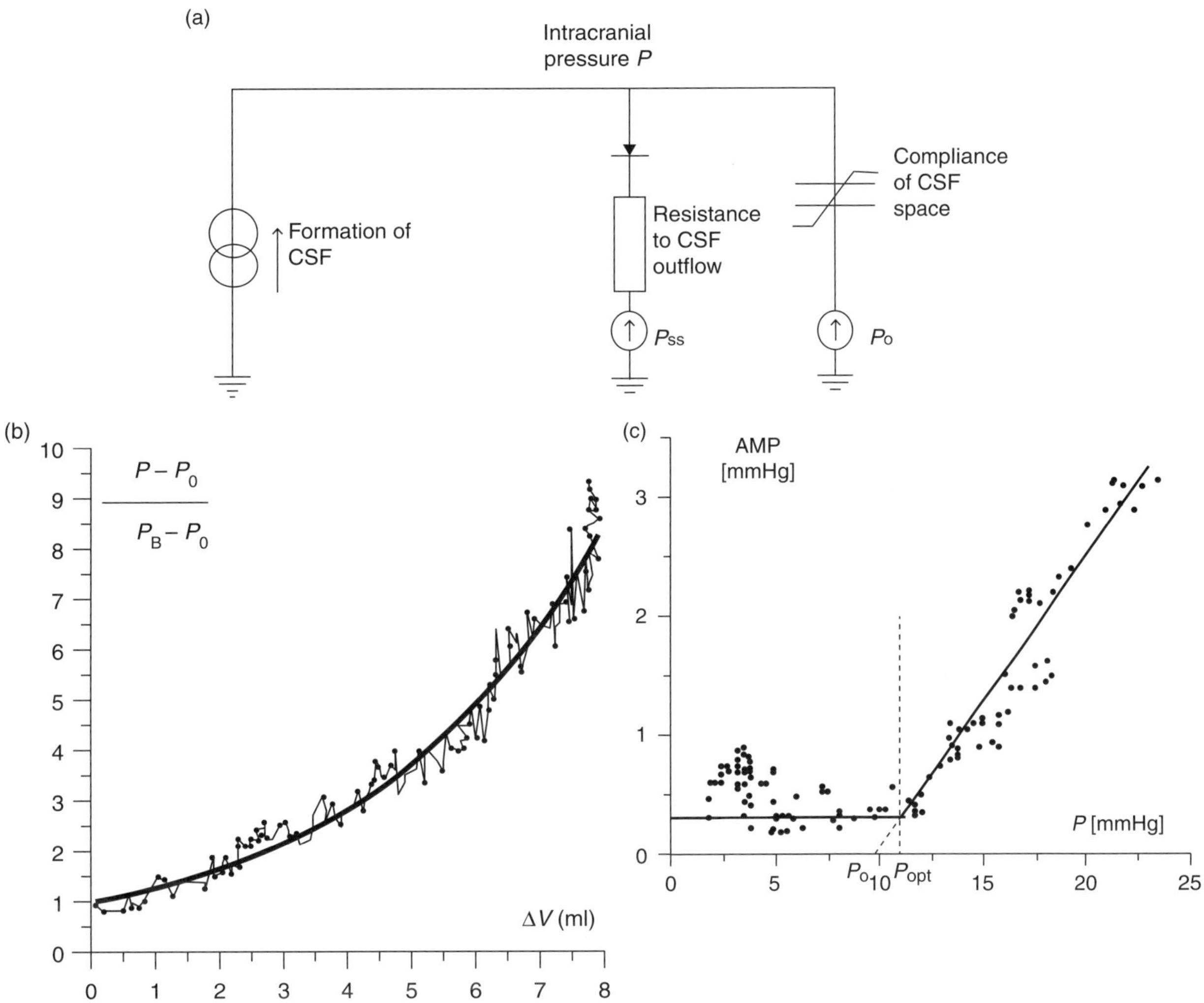

Figure 14.1 (a) Electrical model of CSF circulation adapted from Marmarou, 1978 [7]. The current source reflects formation of CSF; resistor with diode – unilateral absorption of CSF into the sagittal sinuses; capacitor and voltage source – nonlinear compliance of CSF space. (b) Exponential relationship between added volume and relative rise in ICP. (c) Linear relationship between pulse amplitude of ICP and mean ICP. Below a certain ICP level (P_{opt}), amplitude stabilizes and is no longer rising proportionally to mean ICP. Accordingly, below P_{opt} the pressure–volume curve becomes linear.

The mathematical model of CSF pressure–volume compensation, introduced by Marmarou [7] and modified in later studies [8], provides a theoretical basis for the differential diagnosis in hydrocephalus. Components of this model have been identified in many clinical scenarios and are in use in clinical diagnostic procedures. The most popular version of the model is commonly depicted as an electronic circuit (Figure 14.1a).

Under normal conditions production of CSF is balanced by its storage and reabsorption to the venous blood:

$$\text{Production of CSF} = \text{Storing of CSF} + \text{Reabsorption of CSF} \quad (14.1)$$

Production of CSF is almost constant. Reabsorption is proportional to the gradient between CSF pressure (P) and pressure in the sagittal sinus (P_{ss}):

$$\text{Reabsorption} = \frac{P - P_{ss}}{R} \quad (14.2)$$

P_{ss} is considered to be determined mainly by central venous pressure. However, it is obvious that interaction between changes in CSF pressure and P_{ss} exists in patients with idiopathic intracranial hypertension, where P_{ss} is frequently elevated due to stenosis of "collapsible" lateral sinuses.

The coefficient R (symbol R_{out} is also used) is termed the resistance to CSF outflow (units: mmHg/[ml/min]).

Storage of CSF is proportional to the cerebrospinal compliance C (units: ml/mmHg):

$$\text{Storage} = C \times \frac{dP}{dt} \quad (14.3)$$

The compliance of the cerebrospinal space is inversely proportional to the gradient of CSF pressure P and the reference pressure P_o (14.4):

$$C = \frac{1}{E \times (P - P_o)} \quad (14.4)$$

Some authors suggest that the relationship (14.4) is valid only above a certain pressure level called the "optimal pressure"; however, this is still a point of some dispute. The coefficient E is termed the cerebral elasticity (or elastance coefficient; units: ml^{-1}). Elevated elasticity (>0.18 ml^{-1}) signifies a poor pressure–volume compensatory reserve [8].

The reference pressure P_o is a parameter of uncertain significance. Some authors suggest that it is the pressure in the most distal part of the cerebral venous compartment and may be equal to P_{ss}. Others assume that this variable can be neglected [7].

The relationship (14.4) expresses a fundamental law of the cerebrospinal dynamic compensation: when the CSF pressure increases, the compliance of the brain decreases.

Combination of (14.1) with (14.2) and (14.4) gives a final equation (14.5):

$$\frac{1}{E \times (P - P_o)} \times \frac{dp}{dt} + \frac{P - P_b}{R} = I(t) \quad (14.5)$$

where $I(t)$ is the rate of external volume addition and P_b is a baseline pressure.

Solution of this equation provides important mathematical relationships describing the physics of CSF compensation. The first describes the shape of the relationship between the effective volume increase ΔV and the CSF pressure, called the pressure–volume curve or V as exponential (Figure 14.1b):

$$P = (P_b - P_o) \times e^{E\Delta V} + P_o \quad (14.6)$$

Secondly, the equation (14.6) can be helpful in the theoretical evaluation of the relationship between the pulse wave amplitude of ICP and the mean CSF pressure. If we presume that the rise in the blood volume after a heart contraction is equivalent to a rapid bolus addition of CSF fluid at the baseline pressure P_b, the peak-to-peak pulse amplitude (AMP_{pp}) can be expressed as:

$$AMP_{pp} = P_p - P_b = (P_b - P_o) \times (e^{E\Delta V} - 1) \quad (14.7)$$

In almost all cases, when CSF pressure is increased by an external volume addition, the pulse amplitude rises – see Figure 14.1c. The gradient of the regression line between AMP and P (so-called AMP/P line) is proportional to the exponent of elasticity. The intercept point, theoretically, marks the reference pressure P_o.

In all pressure–volume testing techniques, parameters of model (14.5) are estimated using various algorithms and various volume-adding techniques. However, the presented model has limited scope: it cannot interpret dynamic interactions between the rising CSF pressure, expanding ventricles, and cerebral blood volume. More complex models have been formulated but none of them has yet become established in clinical practice.

ICP monitoring

Monitoring of ICP over a longer period can be performed safely using intraparenchymal probes. Less reliably and with more infection risks, the same can be achieved by lumbar puncture or a needle inserted in a preimplanted reservoir. Continuous, real-time analysis of the data, using a pressure monitor connected to a computerized system, is helpful. To obtain the most reliable results overnight monitoring is required; however, when this is impossible, a minimum of one hour monitoring with the patient resting in a horizontal position is necessary. In contrast, it is well established that a single manometric lumbar CSF pressure measurement may be misleading.

Furthermore, ICP recording made overnight or at baseline before the infusion test allows the observation of various cyclical or random dynamic changes in ICP of vasogenic origin (i.e. forced by endogenous change in cerebral blood volume or fluctuations of arterial and venous pressure). These include pulse, respiratory, or slow vasogenic waves (Figure 14.2).

Pulse waveform

Our own experience indicates that pulse amplitude helps in interpretation of recordings in cases of disturbed CSF compensation, shunt blockage, or slit ventricles. It also helps in distinguishing postural

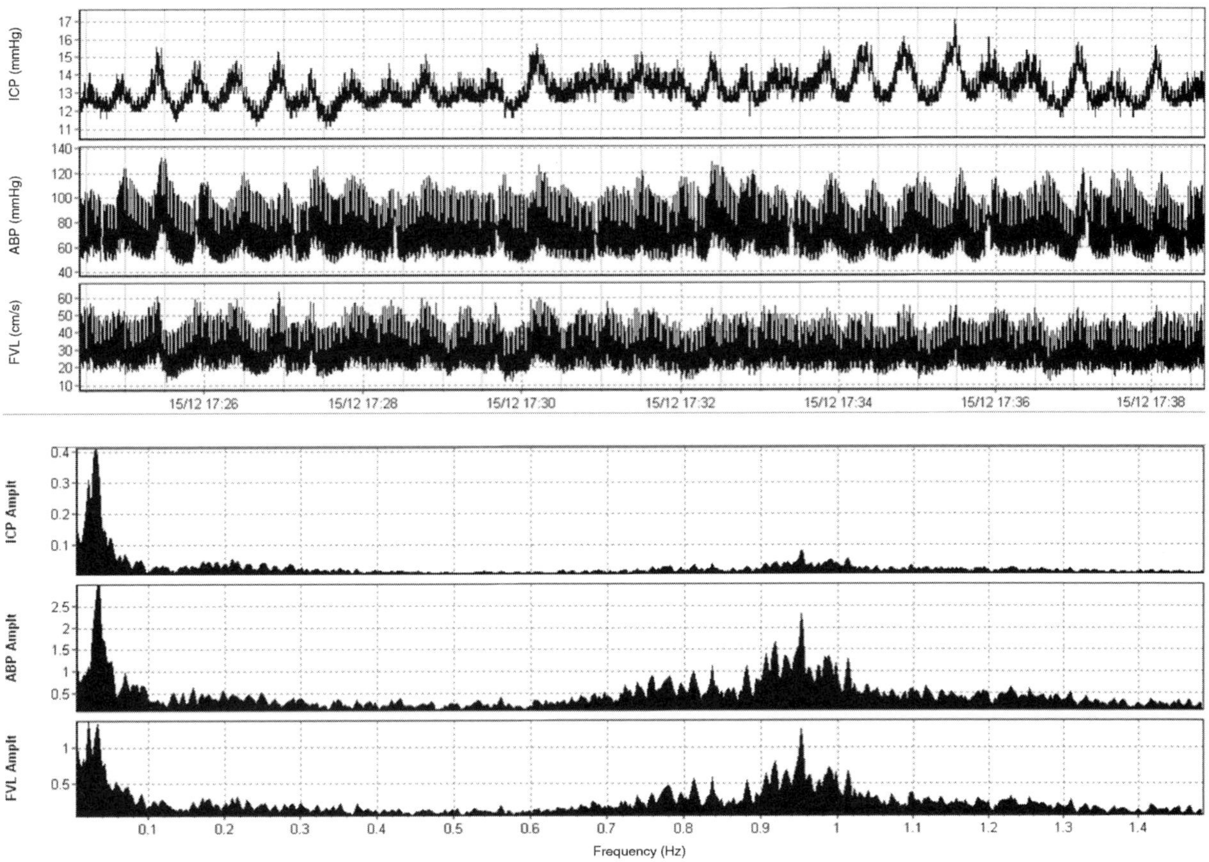

Figure 14.2 Components of simultaneously recorded ICP, arterial blood pressure (ABP), and TCD blood flow velocity on the left side (FVL): pulse, respiratory and slow waves. In time (top panel) and frequency domain (bottom panel).

changes and vasogenic ICP elevations during overnight monitoring.

We do not interpret pulse amplitude alone as a single parameter influencing management. It is interpreted in conjunction with the clinical picture, neuroimaging evidence, neuropsychological tests, etc.

Detection of pulse amplitude proves that the ICP waveform is properly transmitted to the transducer. Lack of amplitude may implicate invalid pressure recording.

Pulse amplitude of ICP is synchronized with pulse amplitude of arterial pressure and the pulse amplitude of blood flow velocity in the middle cerebral artery (Figure 14.2).

Pulse amplitude increases proportionally to mean CSF pressure during the infusion study [8]. All slow vasogenic waves of ICP produce correlated variations in amplitude. In contrast, in patients with predominant brain atrophy, the rise in AMP is very sluggish and vasogenic variations are absent.

The slope of the AMP/*P* line in our group analysis does not correlate with magnitude or frequency of B waves, contrary to results suggested previously [9].

Similarly, in our experience, the slope of the AMP/*P* line may correlate with outcome after shunting for NPH, according to recent reports [10].

Correlation of pulse amplitude with the brain elastance coefficient is insignificant.

In our own experience, pulse amplitude is not a strong predictor of outcome after shunting; however, other authors advocate such a relationship [11].

The interesting theory that an increase in pulse amplitude may reflect insufficient cerebral "Windkessel" seems to need more convincing experimental and clinical evidence. Increased pulse amplitude of ICP has been previously reported to be responsible for dilatation of the ventricles [12]. However, in idiopathic NPH there is no evidence of any association between pulse amplitude and size of the ventricles.

The cerebral "Windkessel effect" helps in damping of arterial blood pulse pressure over the cardiac cycle and assists in the maintenance of brain perfusion during diastole when cardiac ejection ceases. In brain, arterial pulsations are then progressively dissipated to render the capillary circulation smooth, almost pulseless. The Windkessel effect becomes diminished with age as the elastic arteries become less compliant. Breakdown of this phenomenon increases pulsation in the subarachnoid space and this causes an increase of pulsation in the choroidal artery and plexus, thus increasing the CSF ventricular pulsation amplitude. The new increased amplitude of ventricular CSF pressure exceeds the amplitude of pulsation of CSF in the subarachnoid space. This causes a pulsating transmantle pressure gradient, possibly explaining ventricular dilation [13]. Moreover, it is likely that the loss of the Windkessel effect results in an increased pressure in the subarachnoid capillary circulation causing narrowing or reversal of the CSF/venous gradient, responsible for CSF malabsorption. Some scientists suggest that the elevation of capillary and venous pulse pressure that occurs as a consequence of redistribution of pulsation may diminish the hydrostatic gradient necessary for CSF absorption.

In conclusion, "Windkessel theory" says that communicating hydrocephalus may be a disorder of intracranial cerebral blood flow (CBF) pulsation – but it still requires more comprehensive evidence.

On the other hand, it is also likely that CSF and brain pulsations are not only influenced by compliance of arterial walls and the brain "Windkessel" mechanism, but more importantly, by the subarachnoid space patency to compensate for the effects of brain expansion as a CSF pulsatile movement as seen using phase-coded MRI [6]. Only if CSF can move freely in basal cisterns and get out from there, can Windkessel dampening of the arterial pulse work properly.

Injection of kaolin into the basal cisterns and subarachnoid hemorrhage in the basal cisterns following aneurysmal rupture both create hydrocephalus by blocking this CSF pulse movement by clogging up basal subarachnoid spaces.

Correlation of pulse amplitude with R_{out} is positive and significant although weak (correlation coefficient in a range from 0.2 to 0.3). There is no difference in amplitude between males and females. Pulse amplitude increases slightly with age but does not show any correlation with duration of symptoms of NPH or their severity (measured using NPH scale). Pulse amplitude is much lower in idiopathic NPH (iNPH) patients without any evidence of coexisting cerebrovascular disease than in those patients with clear evidence of vascular problems. After shunting, pulse amplitude decreases.

While mean ICP potently reacts to a change of posture (usually becomes negative in an upright body position), the pulse amplitude usually does not follow postural ICP variations.

In analysis of pulse waveform, peak-to-peak pulse values [8,11] or first harmonic of pulse waveform are usually taken into account. This is probably an oversimplification. Morphological analysis of pulse amplitude usually indicates several peaks: P1, P2, and often P3. Peak P1 is usually attributed to passive transmitting of the arterial pulse wave through arterial walls (percussion peak). Peak P2 is associated with transport of arterial blood volume along arteries, which produces a pressure–volume response. Peak P2 increases when compliance of the brain is reduced; therefore, the so-called P2/P1 ratio was historically interpreted as a dimensionless index of brain compliance. Automatic detection of the separate peaks is complex [14], but their continuous descriptors seem to be promising in interpretation of pulse waveform of ICP.

Finally, pulse amplitude in ICP recording may be weak and noisy. Proper computer detection is helpful in most cases.

Assessment of B waves

According to classical standards [15], when so-called "B waves" were present for more than 80% of the duration of ICP monitoring, shunting was recommended. However, using computer detection, B waves (slow waves of ICP of periods from 20 seconds to 2 minutes) are almost universally present, probably even in healthy volunteers. There are no data derived from normal subjects, as a measurement of ICP is invasive. A variable has been proposed, being an amplitude of sine wave bearing the same energy as B waves, calculated using spectral analysis. This amplitude has to remain greater than 1 mmHg for a duration longer than 15 minutes to qualify as a sign of pathological level of "B waves" [16]. However, in an original paper by Børgesen and Gjerris [15], recordings were classified for the "presence" of B waves when they reached a much larger amplitude (5–10 mmHg).

B waves are coherent with fluctuations of cerebral blood flow velocity (see Figure 14.2) and near infrared spectroscopy. The average energy of slow waves did not correlate well with R_{out} in those patients in whom both overnight monitoring and infusion test were performed (our own study). This result is quite disturbing: it may be explained that the survey was conducted in a limited group of "difficult" patients, for whom the results of infusion study indicated a "borderline" state of CSF compensation or the picture was dramatically divergent from the clinical or radiological findings. The utility of B waves in prognostication in hydrocephalus should be readdressed, preferably by multicenter trial.

Cerebrospinal pressure–volume compensatory reserve – RAP index

Conventionally, pressure–volume compensatory reserve is assessed using intracranial volume addition [7]. Changes in ICP in response to a known volume change allow such parameters as the pressure–volume index (PVI) to be derived from bolus volume addition or *E* (which characterizes the shape of the pressure–volume curve over its exponential region) using constant rate infusion. However, under certain assumptions, external volume addition is not necessary as it is possible to assess pressure–volume compensation by taking into account the change in pressure with every heart beat, where a volume of arterial blood is added to the cerebrospinal space in a pulsatile manner. Although the added volume is not known and may be variable, the pressure response is recorded continuously in the form of the pulse waveform of the ICP recording. The RAP index (correlation coefficient [*R*] between the pulse amplitude [*A*] and the mean intracranial pressure [*P*]) is derived by linear correlation between 30 consecutive, time-averaged datapoints of pulse amplitude of ICP (AMP) and mean ICP acquired within a 10 second-wide time-window. RAP describes the degree of correlation between AMP and mean ICP over short periods of time (5 minutes). Theoretically, the RAP coefficient indicates the relationship between ICP and changes in intracerebral volume – the "pressure–volume" curve. A RAP coefficient close to 0 indicates a good pressure–volume compensatory reserve at low ICP, i.e. the situation when the "working point" is still below the exponential region of the curve. When the pressure–volume curve starts to increase exponentially, AMP co-varies directly with mean ICP and consequently RAP rises to +1. This indicates a low compensatory reserve [17].

Cerebrovascular pressure reactivity (PRx)

Another useful ICP-derived variable is the pressure reactivity index (PRx), which is based on the concept of assessment of cerebrovascular pressure reactivity by observing the response of ICP to spontaneous fluctuations of ABP. Using computational methods similar to the calculation of the RAP index, PRx is the correlation coefficient between 30 consecutive, time-averaged datapoints of ICP and ABP. A positive PRx signifies a positive gradient of the regression line between the slow components of ABP and ICP, which has been shown to be associated with passive behavior of a non-reactive vascular bed. A negative value of PRx reflects normal reactive cerebral vessels, as ABP waves provoke inversely correlated waves in ICP. This index correlates well with indices of autoregulation based on transcranial Doppler ultrasonography (see below).

Example of clinical use of ICP monitoring: pediatric hydrocephalus

Pediatric hydrocephalus is quite different in most aspects from adult hydrocephalus, especially NPH. Most cases of pediatric hydrocephalus have a clear obstructive component regarding etiology (Chiari malformation, post-hemorrhagic, post meningitis, aqueductal stenosis, fourth ventricular outflow obstruction), even if obstruction can often only be detected using high resolution MRI techniques [18]. Despite the fact that obstruction is classically associated with pressure active hydrocephalus presenting typical signs and symptoms of raised intracranial pressure, children also exhibit pressure compensated hydrocephalus. They also might undergo shunt dysfunction or ETV failure without becoming symptomatic in the sense of the above-mentioned classical signs and symptoms of raised ICP. In these cases of compensated hydrocephalus or occult treatment dysfunction, ICP overnight monitoring and shunt infusion studies have been shown to be very helpful. Figure 14.3 shows a typical example of elevated baseline ICP, exaggerated nocturnal ICP dynamics during REM sleep, increase of RAP during these episodes indicating exhaustion of cerebrospinal reserve capacity, and elevated baseline AMP in a totally asymptomatic child with known ETV re-closure.

CSF dynamics: infusion test

The computerized infusion test [19] is a modification of the traditional constant rate infusion as described by Katzman and Hussey [20]. The method requires fluid infusion to be made into any

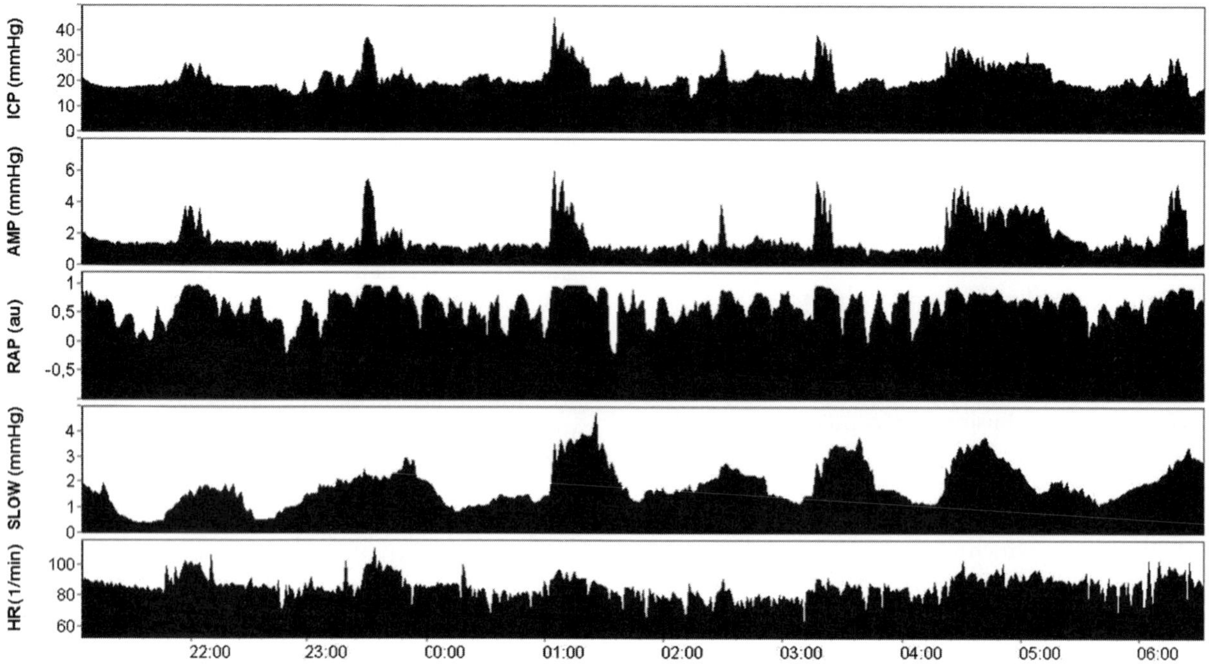

Figure 14.3 Example of ICP overnight monitoring during sleep of a 5-year-old boy with known Blake's pouch (outflow obstruction of the fourth ventricle) and large ventricles, who was found to have complete shunt obstruction despite being totally asymptomatic. Because of very large ventricles he received ETV as an alternative treatment instead of shunt revision which was found to be re-closed after 6 months. He was evaluated regarding shunt-independent ventriculomegaly. His baseline ICP was elevated at 20 mmHg; during REM sleep induced vasogenic wave periods he encountered overshooting peak ICP values (minute average values) of almost 40 mmHg. RAP rose during these episodes almost to 1 indicating exhaustion of reserve capacity. Baseline AMP was slightly increased at about 1.5 mmHg and rose during vasogenic wave periods to values of about 5 mmHg. In summary highly abnormal values were recorded and a shunt was reinserted. Ventricle size thereafter decreased considerably.

accessible CSF compartment. Lumbar infusion, even if it has understandable limitations, is less invasive than intraventricular.

The alternative is an infusion into a subcutaneously positioned reservoir, connected to an intraventricular catheter or shunt antechamber. In such cases two hypodermic needles (gauge 25) are used: one for the pressure measurement and the second for the infusion.

During the infusion, the computer calculates and graphically presents mean pressure and pulse amplitude over time (Figure 14.4). The resistance to CSF outflow can be calculated using simple arithmetic as the difference between the value of the plateau pressure during infusion and the baseline pressure, divided by the infusion rate. However, the precise measurement of the final plateau pressure is not possible when strong vasogenic waves arise or an excessive elevation of the pressure above the safe limit of 40 mmHg is recorded. Computerized analysis produces results even in difficult cases when the infusion is terminated prematurely. The pressure–volume curve is additionally investigated (see Figure 14.1). The algorithm utilizes time-series analysis for volume–pressure curve retrieval, the least-mean-square model fitting, and an examination of the relationship between the pulse amplitude and the mean CSF pressure.

R_{out} and baseline CSF pressure

Infusion study (constant rate [20], or any other variation of controlled but variable rate [21]) allows indices describing the state of CSF compensatory reserve to be estimated. Briefly, there are two types of infusion methods: the steady-state studies (constant pressure infusion [21] and constant flow infusion [20]), and the "dynamic study" (bolus infusion [7]). Although each examination has its advantages and drawbacks, they are all based on the same theoretical background inspired by the mathematical model developed by Marmarou et al. [7]. Traditionally, the two most important parameters are resistance to CSF outflow (R_{out}) and baseline CSF pressure. Elevated R_{out} (>13 mmHg/[ml/min] [15] or >18 mmHg/[ml/min] [22]) denotes disturbed CSF

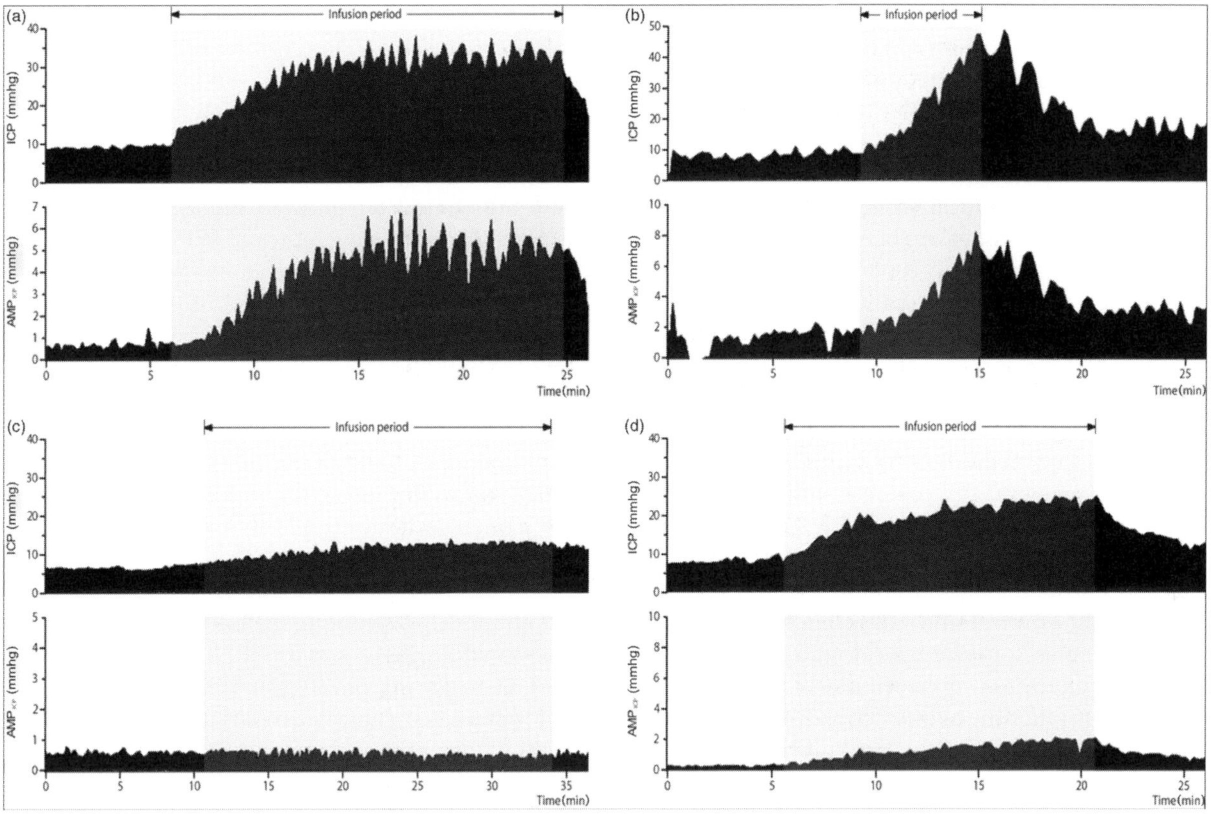

Figure 14.4 Examples of constant rate infusion test. ICP: mean ICP (10 second average) and AMP: pulse amplitude of ICP. The gray section is the duration of infusion of Hartman solution at a rate of 1 or 1.5 ml/min. (a) Normal pressure hydrocephalus (NPH): although the baseline pressure is normal, the resistance to CSF outflow increased, there are lots of strong vasogenic waves, and changes in pulse amplitude are fairly well correlated with changes in mean ICP. (b) Acute hydrocephalus post-subarachnoid hemorrhage (SAH): the normal baseline pressure was measured, but the resistance to CSF outflow is high. Good response of shunt surgery was expected. (c) Cerebral brain atrophy: the baseline pressure is low, and the resistance to CSF outflow is low. No vasogenic waves were recorded and pulse amplitude does not respond. (d) Normal: the baseline pressure, the resistance to CSF outflow, and other parameters are normal and, thus, the result demonstrates the normal CSF circulation.

circulation. Elevated baseline pressure (>18 mmHg) may signify an uncompensated cerebrospinal volume-expanding process.

However, there is still controversy about the value of R_{out} for predicting improvement after shunting, which shows an interesting timeline. In 1992 Børgesen et al. [19] indicated 100% both positive and negative predictive power for an R_{out} threshold of 13 mmHg/(ml/min). A Dutch study in 1997 [22] showed 97% positive predictive power for R_{out} >18 mmHg/(ml/min) but only 36% negative predictive power. In the 2005 "NPH guidelines" Marmarou and coworkers [1] recognized sensitivity/specificity of R_{out} above 80% (this was done on a meta-analysis of sizable published studies). However, in 2012 the so-called "European Trial" [23] indicated no association of R_{out} and improvement after shunting. The trial was not very large (around 100 patients), conducted in divergent centers, and directly sponsored by one big shunt manufacturer. Nevertheless, the results were spectacularly different from historical data. Are we managing different patients than in the 1980s and 1990s? Or do we tend to estimate R_{out} with greater variation?

A further difficulty when trying to determine the predictability of R_{out} arises from the fact that different centers use different infusion methods to calculate it, and this can lead to interpreting in the same manner cut-off levels that are not necessarily the same. It has been stated that for unknown reasons [1], physiologic R_{out} as calculated by using the bolus infusion, results in systematically and significantly lower values (<4 mmHg/ml/min) than those determined by steady-state infusion methods. Interestingly, a recent paper from Sundström et al. [24] that aimed to compare values of

R_{out} determined from the bolus, the constant-flow, and the constant-pressure infusion methods demonstrated that in experimental conditions, with well-known characteristics, R_{out} values showed good concordance among all methods. These findings confirm the robust theory of the mathematical model. Notwithstanding, when shifting to a clinical setting R_{out} shows clear and significantly different values between steady-state and bolus methods, as already reported in previous studies [25]. The key to understanding such differences lies in the presence of physiological pressure variations introduced when applying this model in humans (e.g. breathing, cardiac variation, and so on). The first big difference with the bolus infusion when compared to the steady-state methods is the magnitude of the created "peak pressure" that together with the volume of injected fluid permits calculation of the PVI (pressure–volume index). The bolus itself allows a wide range of increase in baseline pressure, while constant-pressure and constant-flow infusions cause much less variation. Moreover, bolus R_{out} values are calculated using the PVI together with the new pressure selected on the return curve at different time points. Then PVI and momentary chosen pressure on the pressure trace decaying after bolus back to baseline values determine the final R_{out} value. Any error in the estimation of PVI will affect the R_{out} estimation. At the same time, especially when resistance to outflow is high, the pressure differences on the return curve are much smaller, limiting the signal processing options for extracting R_{out}-related data from the curve and therefore making the method more susceptible to physiological variations. Finally, the R_{out} values obtained from each of these time points is averaged to yield one R_{out} value for each bolus. The bolus injection is then repeated at least three times and the R_{out} values for all three injections are averaged to yield the final R_{out} value for the patient. All these considerations could explain the difference in R_{out} between methods.

The "dynamic" response of the bolus method should be seen as an advantage, since potentially we measure a more "physiological" R_{out}; however, this test might require an operator with extensive experience, while the better repeatability of the steady-state methods makes them the recommended approach for estimating R_{out}, at least in iNPH.

A different situation, where a more dynamic physiological response might be needed, could be represented by the extremely heterogeneous population suffering from secondary forms of hydrocephalus (post-traumatic, post-hemorrhagic, post-infectious hydrocephalus, etc.). Here, determining opening pressure, brain compliance (PVI), and R_{out} in a relative short time might represent a true clinical advantage to distinguish between atrophy and hydrocephalus as the two possible causes of "secondary" ventriculomegaly. Here are some examples: an elevated baseline ICP (>15 mmHg) with slow return of ICP to baseline after the bolus injection indicates an elevated CSF outflow resistance (bolus R_{out} >5 mmHg/[ml/min]) in patients who should be promptly shunted. A normal baseline ICP with the bolus injection causing a relatively smaller increase in ICP, indicating an enhanced PVI, might reveal true brain atrophy. On the other hand, when the bolus injection causes a relatively larger increase in an initially normal baseline ICP, with rapid return to baseline, it might indicate exquisitely low brain compliance, and the need for a "low pressure" shunt. If the same peak pressure after the bolus returns to the baseline ICP at a much slower rate than normal, this suggests an elevated R_{out} (as occurs in iNPH) and most likely the need for an adjustable valve, since in this case there are more parameters subjected to variation after shunt that might require several changes of the valve setting.

Elastance coefficient (or elasticity)

The exact clinical significance and interpretation of the elastance coefficient (*E*) is not yet fully documented, though theoretically it describes brain stiffness. Tans and Poortvliet [26] showed that *E* weakly correlated with the resistance to CSF outflow, although no further studies exploring this concept have followed. Tisell et al. [27] demonstrated that *E* correlated positively with the result of third ventriculostomy: those with a stiffer brain (higher *E*) have a better chance of improving after surgery.

Analysis of slow waves, compensatory reserve, and pressure reactivity during infusion study

Parameters describing vascular effects and pressure–volume compensation can also be evaluated during the infusion study. The study usually starts with 10–15 minutes of baseline assessment, which can be easily extended. Consequently, the same parameters as during an overnight ICP monitoring can be calculated.

Of all the CSF compensatory parameters derived from the infusion test, the resistance to CSF outflow demonstrates significant associations with cerebrovascular reactivity (PRx): patients with lower R_{out} tend to have more frequently disturbed cerebrovascular reactivity.

Also the results of correlation analyses between R_{out} and pulse amplitude of ICP, energy of slow waves, and respiratory wave at baseline demonstrate significant associations. Increases in all vasogenic components during infusion as compared to the baseline values are commonly observed [28]. Practically these indices are used as an additional descriptor of CSF dynamics and help in understanding CSF circulatory disorders.

Who needs a shunt: CSF dynamics perspective

Our practice indicates that not a single parameter, but all above described variables and indices characterizing CSF dynamics, are useful for prognostication of hydrocephalus management.

CSF dynamics in normal pressure hydrocephalus is characterized by a normal baseline pressure during sleep in a strictly horizontal position without head elevation (ICP <15 mmHg). The resistance to CSF outflow is increased (>13 mmHg/[ml/min]). B waves recorded during infusion are elevated and regular. Pulse amplitude is well correlated with mean ICP and may be slightly elevated. Compensatory reserve at baseline is sometimes found to be elevated (RAP index above 0.6) and usually elastance coefficient is slightly increased ($E > 0.2\ ml^{-1}$) (see Figure 14.4a).

Patients suffering predominantly from brain atrophy have normal CSF circulation. Typically, opening pressure, resistance to CSF outflow, and pulse amplitude are low (ICP <12 mmHg, R_{out} <10 mmHg/[ml/min], amplitude <1 mmHg). The compensatory reserve at baseline is good (RAP <0.5), reflecting low elasticity of the atrophic brain ($E < 0.2\ ml^{-1}$). Vasogenic waves are rather limited during recording. The mean ICP increases smoothly during the infusion and decreases in a similar fashion following infusion, comparable to the inflation and deflation of a balloon (Figure 14.4c).

Lumbar infusion is not recommended in non-communicating hydrocephalus because of the risk of brain herniation in the event of uncontrolled CSF leak. However, this type of hydrocephalus may not always be easy to detect with a brain scan. In those few instances of non-communicating hydrocephalus when lumbar infusion is performed, the resistance to CSF outflow is normal because the lumbar infusion is not able to detect the proximal narrowing in CSF circulatory pathways. In acute hydrocephalus R_{out} is elevated, the resting pressure and pulse amplitude are elevated, and paradoxically elastance is relatively low (ICP >15 mmHg, pulse amplitude >4 mmHg, $E < 0.20\ ml^{-1}$).

Active obstructive hydrocephalus can be safely assessed using ventricular infusion (via a reservoir). This demonstrates high intracranial resting pressure and high resistance to CSF outflow (ICP >15 mmHg, R_{out} >13 mmHg/[ml/min]). The elasticity is high (>0.20 ml^{-1}), RAP is elevated above 0.6, and the pulse amplitude is high (>4 mmHg) indicating poor compensatory reserve.

Acute communicating hydrocephalus (such as post subarachnoid hemorrhage) presents with a similar pattern of parameters, with frequent deep vasogenic waves (including plateau waves) (Figure 14.4b).

Finally, normal CSF circulation is characterized by low baseline pressure (<15 mmHg), normal resistance to CSF outflow (<10 mmHg/[ml/min]), low magnitude of slow waves at baseline (<1.5 mmHg), good compensatory reserve ($E < 0.18\ ml^{-1}$), low RAP index at baseline (RAP <0.6), and limited pulse amplitude of ICP (<1 mmHg) (Figure 14.4d).

Vascular components of CSF circulation

The tone of cerebral vessels has been reported to influence CSF compensatory reserve as described by brain compliance, brain stiffness, or CSF pulse amplitude [8].

No significant change in the elastance coefficient during arterial hypotension has been reported [29]. In contrast, during hypercapnia the elastance coefficient increases, signifying an increase in brain stiffness. The most intriguing finding in this study is a change in the resistance to CSF outflow, observed during different cerebral vasodilatatory maneuvers. The R_{out} decreased with hypotension but increased with hypercapnia. Changes of R_{out} with deep hypotension (reduction in ABP by 50%) are restricted (30% change in R_{out}).

Transcranial Doppler-derived pressure autoregulation

Some studies have indicated that cerebral blood flow may be compromised in areas around the ventricles in patients presenting with a degree of ventricular dilatation and clinical symptoms of NPH. A relationship between the resistance to CSF outflow and cerebral autoregulation in patients diagnosed with NPH has been reported [30]. An index of autoregulation was calculated in 40 patients during infusion study using transcranial Doppler ultrasonography. It was significantly correlated with the resistance to CSF outflow, indicating better autoregulation in those patients with higher R_{out}. Patients presenting with ventricular dilatation may have either low (atrophy?) or increased (NPH?) resistance to CSF outflow. Increased resistance correlates with preserved autoregulation. Those with a low resistance, suggestive of brain atrophy, have severely disturbed autoregulation in the middle cerebral artery territory.

CO_2 reactivity

CO_2 reactivity testing is commonly used in patients with increased risk of stroke. Whether this test can reveal underlying vascular disease in patients suffering from hydrocephalus still remains to be demonstrated [31].

The test is noninvasive: bilateral transcranial Doppler (TCD) probes are placed over the temporal bone windows to enable middle cerebral artery insonation at a depth of approximately 50 mm. The probes are secured to the scalp with a headband. Arterial blood pressure can be measured noninvasively using a cuff placed around the middle finger of the left hand. A mixture of 5% CO_2 in air is administered via a facemask. End-tidal CO_2 ($EtCO_2$) concentration is monitored. Signals are studied over 10 minutes breathing normally for baseline recordings (normocapnia). Then patients breathe air containing 5% CO_2 to achieve a steady increase in $EtCO_2$ (usually greater than 1 kPa) for 10 minutes.

The traditional cerebrovascular reactivity (CR) has been calculated as a percentage rise of mean flow velocity per 1 kPa change in $PaCO_2$.

When deep changes in arterial pressure are observed, CR should be corrected accordingly. The normal values of CR are still controversial, but by consensus we chose the threshold of 12%/kPa as the lower limit under which CR should be considered as altered.

Cerebral blood flow studies

In NPH, global mean CBF has generally been demonstrated to be lower than in normal controls and a postoperative increase of CBF has often been demonstrated after successful shunting [32,33]. A CBF increase has also often been evidenced after CSF withdrawal by lumbar puncture in patients ultimately responding to shunting [34]. The reduction in baseline CBF is often more pronounced in the frontal region and appears to predominate in the white matter (WM) [36] and, in some cases, although the mean global CBF was within the normal range, the regional CBF pattern was abnormal compared to normal controls with a slightly reduced rCBF in the central WM. Therefore, a possible primary dysfunction of the axons in the WM rather than a primary dysfunction of the gray matter might have a dominating role in the generation of the clinical syndrome.

In a PET/MRI study [36] the distribution of the regional periventricular WM CBF using $H_2{}^{15}O$ positron emission tomography (PET) co-registered on MRI anatomy was assessed. Also the relationship between WM CBF response to a controlled rise of ICP (and hence a fall of cerebral perfusion pressure) induced by an infusion of CSF has been studied. Ten patients with idiopathic NPH (mean age 69 years) underwent a CSF infusion study via a previously implanted right frontal ventricular catheter connected to a subcutaneous reservoir. CBF was measured by $H_2{}^{15}O$ PET at baseline and then during the steady-state plateau of raised ICP. The PET images were co-registered to 3D structural T1-weighted MR images (voxel 1 mm^3). In 10 healthy normal volunteers image acquisition and reconstruction were accomplished in the same manner, except that only a baseline CBF determination was performed. Distributions of the baseline WM CBF and of the percent change of WM CBF as a function of the normalized distance from the ventricles (0: WM adjacent to the ventricle; 1: outermost subcortical WM) were plotted.

The profile of baseline regional WM CBF in NPH patients showed a logarithmic increasing relationship with distance from the ventricles, whereas in controls no relationship was apparent. The profile of the percent changes of regional WM CBF in patients during raised ICP showed a "U" shape function of the distance.

The increasing profile of WM baseline CBF might suggest that a potential mechanism for CBF reduction in NPH is the collapse of the microcirculation induced by a parenchymal interstitial pressure gradient during infusion study. The maximal WM CBF reduction occurred at 0.3 of normalized distance, which corresponds to a mean distance of 9 mm. This falls into the boundary zone vascular territory between the deep and superficial territories of the middle cerebral artery, which suggests that NPH may promote watershed ischemia (Figure 14.5).

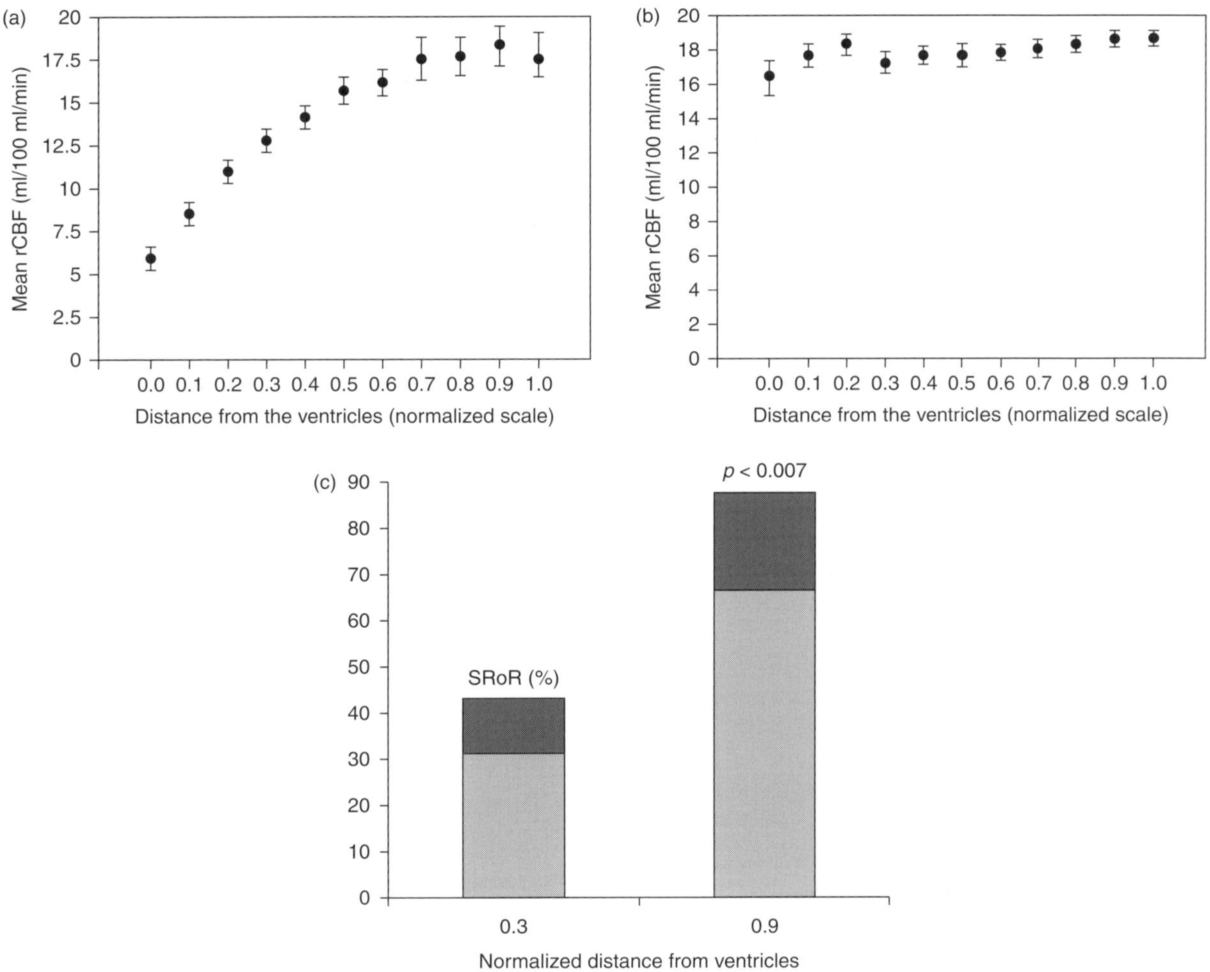

Figure 14.5 Baseline white matter CBF in patients suffering from NPH (a) and in control subjects (b) (ref), as a function of normalized distance from walls of ventricles (0) to gray matter border (1). (c) Difference in static rate of autoregulation (SRoR) at 30% of distance from walls of ventricles and 90%.

New trends in studies devoted to cerebrovascular–CSF coupling in hydrocephalus are emerging as we type this chapter. It is worthwhile emphasizing "pulsatile theory" in hydrocephalus [37], all novel MRI-based techniques for tracing CSF flow and its pulsations [38], tissue oxygenation [39], and cerebral microdialysis [40].

Conclusion

Studies of CSF dynamics including ICP and CBF monitoring are undoubtedly useful although they do not always offer straightforward answers about the likelihood of improvement after shunting or ETV. This is because hydrocephalus is predominantly a multifactorial disease and the link between its complex pathophysiology and clinical improvement is difficult to establish. Nevertheless, knowing and understanding failures in CSF dynamics helps to understand the nature of the problems that need to be corrected. Methods of assessment of CSF dynamics also help to review and correct cases of shunt or ETV failure; this point will be highlighted in the chapter on hydrocephalus shunts (Chapter 17).

Acknowledgments

The authors would like to credit the great intellectual input of many colleagues participating in the "hydrocephalus project" in Cambridge 1991–2012: Mrs. Nicole Keong, Mrs. Helen Whitehouse, Dr. Jo Iddon, Professor Barbara Sahakian, Dr. Alonso Pena, Mr.

Ruwan Weerakkody; PhD students/visiting scholars: Mr. Eric Schmidt (Toulouse), Mr. Brian Owler (Sidney), Mr. Shahan Momjian (Geneva), Dr. Gianpaolo Petrella (Rome), Dr. Olivier Balédent (Amiens); and clinical staff at the Hydrocephalus Clinic (run by Professor J. D. Pickard) in Addenbrooke's Hospital, Cambridge, UK.

References

1. Marmarou A, Bergsneider M, Klinge P, Relkin N, Black PM. The value of supplemental prognostic tests for the preoperative assessment of idiopathic normal-pressure hydrocephalus. *Neurosurgery* 2005;57(3 Suppl):S17–28.
2. Weed LH. The establishment of the circulation of cerebro-spinal fluid. *Anat Rec* 1916;10:256–8.
3. Davson H, Hollingsworth G, Segal MB. The mechanism of drainage of the cerebrospinal fluid. *Brain* 1970;93:665.
4. Dandy WE, Blackfan KD. An experimental and clinical study of internal hydrocephalus, *JAMA* 1913;25:2216–17.
5. Oi S, Di Rocco C. Proposal of "evolution theory in cerebrospinal fluid dynamics" and minor pathway hydrocephalus in developing immature brain. *Childs Nerv Sys* 2006;22(7):662–9.
6. Balédent O, Gondry-Jouet C, Stoquart-Elsankari S, et al. Value of phase contrast magnetic resonance imaging for investigation of cerebral hydrodynamics. *J Neuroradiol* 2006;33(5):292–303.
7. Marmarou A, Shulman K, Rosende RM. A nonlinear analysis of the cerebrospinal fluid system and intracranial pressure dynamics. *J Neurosurg* 1978;48:332.
8. Avezaat CJJ, Eijndhoven JHM. Cerebrospinal fluid pulse pressure and craniospinal dynamics. A theoretical, clinical and experimental study. Thesis, Jongbloed, The Hague; 1984.
9. Lenfeldt N, Andersson N, Agren-Wilsson A, et al. Cerebrospinal fluid pulse pressure method: a possible substitute for the examination of B waves. *J Neurosurg* 2004;101(6):944–50.
10. Anile C, De Bonis P, Albanese A, et al. Selection of patients with idiopathic normal-pressure hydrocephalus for shunt placement: a single-institution experience. *J Neurosurg* 2010;113(1):64–73.
11. Eide PK, Brean A. Intracranial pulse pressure amplitude levels determined during preoperative assessment of subjects with possible idiopathic normal pressure hydrocephalus. *Acta Neurochir (Wien)* 2006;148(11):1151–6.
12. Di Rocco C, Pettorossi VE, Caldarelli M, Mancinelli R, Velardi F. Experimental hydrocephalus following mechanical increment of intraventricular pulse pressure. *Experientia* 1977;33(11):1470–2.
13. Lee HS, Yoon SH. Hypothesis for lateral ventricular dilatation in communicating hydrocephalus: new understanding of the Monro-Kellie hypothesis in the aspect of cardiac energy through arterial blood flow. *Med Hypotheses* 2009;72(2):174–7.
14. Hu X, Xu P, Scalzo F, Vespa P, Bergsneider M. Morphological clustering and analysis of continuous intracranial pressure. *IEEE Trans Biomed Eng* 2009;56:696–705.
15. Børgesen SE, Gjerris F. The predictive value of conductance to outflow of CSF in normal pressure hydrocephalus. *Brain* 1982;105:65–86.
16. Stephensen H, Andersson N, Eklund A, et al. Objective B wave analysis in 55 patients with non-communicating and communicating hydrocephalus. *J Neurol Neurosurg Psychiatry* 2005;76(7):965–70.
17. Kim DJ, Czosnyka Z, Keong N, et al. Index of cerebrospinal compensatory reserve in hydrocephalus. *Neurosurgery* 2009;64(3):494–501.
18. Dincer A, Kohan S, Ozek MM. Is all "communicating" hydrocephalus really communicating? Prospective study on the value of 3D-constructive interference in steady state sequence at 3T. *AJNR Am J Neuroradiol* 2009;30(10):1898–906.
19. Børgesen SE, Albeck MJ, Gjerris F, Czosnyka M, Laniewski P. Computerized infusion test compared to steady pressure constant infusion test in measurement of resistance to CSF outflow. *Acta Neurochir* 1992;119:12–16.
20. Katzman R, Hussey F. A simple constant infusion manometric test for measurement of CSF absorption. *Neurology (Minneap)* 1970;20:534–44.
21. Frieden H, Ekstedt J. Instrumentation for cerebrospinal fluid hydrodynamic studies in man. *Med Biol Eng Comput* 1982;20:167–80.
22. Boon AJ, Tans JT, Delwel EJ, et al. Dutch normal-pressure hydrocephalus study: prediction of outcome after shunting by resistance to outflow of cerebrospinal fluid. *J Neurosurg* 1997;87(5):687–93.
23. Wikkelsø C, Hellström P, Klinge PM, Tans JT; European iNPH Multicentre Study Group. The European iNPH Multicentre Study on the predictive values of resistance to CSF outflow and the CSF Tap Test in patients with idiopathic normal pressure hydrocephalus. *J Neurol Neurosurg Psychiatry*. 2013;84(5):562–8.
24. Sundström N, Andersson K, Marmarou A, Malm J, Eklund A. Comparison between 3 infusion methods to measure cerebrospinal fluid outflow conductance. *J Neurosurg* 2010;113(6):1294–303.
25. Kosteljanetz M: Resistance to outflow of cerebrospinal fluid determined by bolus injection technique

and constant rate steady state infusion in humans. *Neurosurgery* 1985;16:336–40.

26. Tans JT, Poortvliet DC. Relationship between compliance and resistance to outflow of CSF in adult hydrocephalus. *J Neurosurg* 1989;71(1):59–62.
27. Tisell M, Edsbagge M, Stephensen H, Czosnyka M, Wikkelsø C. Elastance correlates with outcome after endoscopic third ventriculostomy in adults with hydrocephalus caused by primary aqueductal stenosis. *Neurosurgery* 2002;50:70–6.
28. Momjian S, Czosnyka Z, Czosnyka M, Pickard JD. Link between vasogenic waves of intracranial pressure and cerebrospinal fluid outflow resistance in normal pressure hydrocephalus. *Br J Neurosurg* 2004;18(1):56–61.
29. Czosnyka M, Richards HK, Czosnyka Z, Piechnik S, Pickard JD. Vascular components of cerebrospinal fluid compensation. *J Neurosurg* 1999;90:752–9.
30. Czosnyka Z, Czosnyka M, Whitfield PC, Donovan T, Pickard JD. Cerebral autoregulation among patients with symptoms of hydrocephalus. *Neurosurgery* 2002;50(3):526–32.
31. Lee EJ, Hung YC, Chang CH, Pai MC, Chen HH. Cerebral blood flow velocity and vasomotor reactivity before and after shunting surgery in patients with normal pressure hydrocephalus. *Acta Neurochir (Wien)* 1998;140:599–604.
32. Mamo HL, Meric PC, Ponsin JC, et al. Cerebral blood flow in normal pressure hydrocephalus. *Stroke* 1987;18:1074–80.
33. Klinge PM, Berding G, Brinker T, Knapp WH, Samii M. A positron emission tomography study of cerebrovascular reserve before and after shunt surgery in patients with idiopathic chronic hydrocephalus. *J Neurosurg* 1999;91:605–9.
34. Mori K, Maeda M, Asegawa S, Iwata J. Quantitative local cerebral blood flow change after cerebrospinal fluid removal in patients with normal pressure hydrocephalus measured by a double injection method with N-isopropyl-p-[123I] iodoamphetamine. *Acta Neurochir (Wien)* 2002;144(3):255–63.
35. Owler BK, Pickard JD. Normal pressure hydrocephalus and cerebral blood flow: a review. *Acta Neurol Scand* 2001;104(6):325–42.
36. Momjian S, Owler BK, Czosnyka Z, et al. Pattern of white matter regional cerebral blood flow and autoregulation in normal pressure hydrocephalus. *Brain* 2004;127:965–72.
37. Egnor M, Zheng L, Rosiello A, et al. A model of pulsations in communicating hydrocephalus. *Pediatr Neurosurg* 2002;36(6):281–303.
38. Yamada S, Miyazaki M, Kanazawa H, et al. Visualization of cerebrospinal fluid movement with spin labeling at MR imaging: preliminary results in normal and pathophysiologic conditions. *Radiology* 2008;249(2):644–52.
39. Weerakkody RA, Czosnyka M, Zweifel C, et al. Near infrared spectroscopy as possible non-invasive monitor of slow vasogenic ICP waves. *Acta Neurochir Suppl* 2012;114:181–5.
40. Eide PK, Stanisic M. Cerebral microdialysis and intracranial pressure monitoring in patients with idiopathic normal-pressure hydrocephalus: association with clinical response to extended lumbar drainage and shunt surgery. *J Neurosurg* 2010;112(2):414–24.

Chapter 15

Cerebrospinal fluid biomarkers in idiopathic normal pressure hydrocephalus

Andrew A. Tarnaris

History of setting up biomarkers in idiopathic normal pressure hydrocephalus

Biological markers have been traditionally used in clinical practice to support a diagnosis, or monitor the progression of a disease by surveying levels longitudinally.

The definition as given by the Biomarkers Definition Working Group was "*A characteristic that is objectively measured and evaluated as an indicator of normal biological, pathogenic processes or pharmacological responses to a therapeutic intervention*" [1]. Biomarkers can aid us in this task as they provide an insight to the changes in the milieu associated with a condition.

To establish their use in routine clinical practice they should display high sensitivity and specificity. As in other medical specialties, in neurosciences there is a currently a tendency to develop disease-specific biomarkers.

Biomarkers have been proposed as an aid in the diagnosis of several neurodegenerative disorders. "*The ideal biomarker for Alzheimer's disease (AD) should detect a fundamental feature of neuropathology and be validated in neuropathologically-confirmed cases; it should have a sensitivity of 80% for detecting AD and a specificity of 80% for distinguishing other dementias; it should be reliable, reproducible, non-invasive, simple to perform, and inexpensive. Recommended steps to find out a biomarker include confirmation by at least two independent studies conducted by qualified investigators with the results published in peer-reviewed journals.*" This definition given by the Consensus Report of the Working Group on Molecular and Biochemical Markers of Alzheimer's Disease (Ronald and Nancy Reagan Research Institute and the NIA Working Group-1998) [2] highlights adequately the problems any attempts to find biomarkers for idiopathic normal pressure hydrocephalus (iNPH) may face. The role of a biomarker is to confirm a diagnosis, serve for epidemiological studies, assess for prediction, monitoring the progression and response to treatment and studying brain–behavior relationships. Any marker will need to be validated against a definite diagnosis.

The first attempts to develop biomarkers specific for idiopathic normal pressure hydrocephalus (iNPH) to distinguish it from other neurodegenerative conditions were by Sørensen et al. in 1983 [3,4], Ahlberg et al. [5] and Albrechtsen et al. in 1985 [6]. Kudo et al. in 2000 were the first to measure the ventricular levels of tau protein, comparing it with orthopedic controls and hence investigating the role of tau protein as a potential marker of severity of the condition [7]. Four years later Lins et al. in 2004 assessed the levels of amyloid beta peptide (1–42) (Aβ (1–42)) and total tau protein (t-tau) in a group with the idiopathic form of NPH [8]. Theirs was the first group to realize the potential of using the two most commonly assessed cerebrospinal fluid (CSF) biomarkers for dementia patients for assessing the CSF biochemistry of an iNPH group. Two literature reviews in 2006 and 2009 [9,10] highlighted the potential of establishing biomarkers for this condition. Since then further studies have been published attempting to establish diagnostic or prognostic biomarkers in iNPH by exploring the possibility of other neurodegenerative processes coexisting in a cohort of the elderly population.

Rationale for their use

The case for emerging biomarkers in iNPH has arisen because of similar developments in other common causes of dementia and the increasing awareness of both the epidemiology of NPH [11,12] and its impact on the quality of life of elderly patients [13]. Geriatricians and

Adult Hydrocephalus, ed. Daniele Rigamonti. Published by Cambridge University Press.

neurologists are often faced with the difficult task of identifying those patients with a probable diagnosis of NPH to refer them to a neurosurgeon to consider surgical CSF diversion. Up to 90% of patients can improve within 6 months [14].

Over the years, different diagnostic tests have been developed to improve the shunt-response prediction and, subsequently, guidelines were developed for selecting the patients for shunt surgery [15]. However, none of these tests achieved 100% sensitivity or specificity and it was thought that a combination of tests, rather than a single one, was needed to increase the chances of selecting the right patients to offer a surgical CSF diversion procedure [16]. Changes in the neurochemical composition of CSF due to hydrocephalus have been widely documented and reviewed and therefore analysis of the biochemical milieu in the CSF is becoming an attractive, yet invasive method of developing markers of sufficient accuracy to either help establish a diagnosis (a diagnostic marker) or be able to predict the prognosis of surgical CSF diversion (a prognostic marker) [17].

Comorbidities may affect surgical outcomes adversely [18]. The probable coexistence of AD and NPH has been raised in the past by various authors. A recent large series of autopsies of 563 cases with dementia found an average 1.6% of autopsied cases with a clinical picture of NPH [19]. The combination of abnormally low CSF Aβ (1–42) level and abnormally high CSF tau level is a hallmark of AD pathology. Such markers may be measured reliably in CSF by commonly used and fairly affordable laboratory methods such as ELISA. Amyloid plaques and hyperphosphorylated tau in cortical brain biopsies are reflected by low CSF Aβ (1–42) and high CSF total tau and phosphorylated form of tau protein (p-tau) levels, respectively [20]. In addition, altered CSF dynamics impair amyloid beta clearance in experimental NPH models [21]. The implications of such research findings mean that we can use commonly assessed markers to help us with the differential diagnosis of different pathologies with similar phenotypes.

Diagnostic versus prognostic biomarkers

CSF biomarkers in the differential diagnosis with Alzheimer's dementia

The problem with identifying diagnostic biomarkers between NPH and AD is that NPH was used in those studies more as a comparative control group rather than as the primary studied group, apart from a few exceptions [22–24]. In addition, it is well recognized that idiopathic and secondary NPH represent entities with different pathophysiological backgrounds and response to surgery [25,26]; therefore any attempts to identify diagnostic biomarkers in NPH should focus on the idiopathic form. A successful biomarker able to distinguish between NPH and AD would be able to reflect the pathological changes characteristic of AD and in particular abnormal phosphorylation of the tau protein [27], the synaptic and axonal degeneration, and the aggregation of amyloid with resulting deposition in plaques [28]. So far only the results of one study by Kapaki et al. [22] have reached clinical significance. The authors identified a cut-off level of the p-tau greater than 47 (pg/ml) which is able to distinguish between AD and idiopathic NPH with a sensitivity of 88.7% and specificity of 88.6%. The authors used a commercial ELISA assay (Innotest, Innogenetics, Gent, Belgium) to determine the total tau and p-tau, and Aβ (1–42). The authors also found that total tau was increased in both conditions when compared with controls, whereas β-amyloid levels were decreased in both. The diagnosis of iNPH was based on history, examination, and relevant imaging but no external lumbar drainage or tap test. A lumbar puncture was performed but the authors do not mention the pressures obtained.

Increased tau levels when compared with a control group (orthopedic subjects) were also detected by Kudo et al. [7] in a mixed NPH group using the same commercial assay (Innotest, Belgium). However, their results contradict the studies of Agren-Wilsson [23], Zemlan [29], Lins [8] and Gloeckner [30], where the levels of tau were either lower than the control group or within the normal range. Agren-Wilsson et al. used an "in-house" ELISA published previously [31], using patients undergoing orthopedic surgery as controls. This sample (n = 62) of iNPH patients is of value in providing a more accurate reflection of the markers' value because of its size and its proper selection (lumbar infusion test and tap test performed in patients with relevant history and imaging). In the study by Zemlan et al. the levels of the cleaved form of the tau protein were barely detectable with their in-house ELISA and Western Blot assays. Lins et al. used a commercial assay (Innotest, Belgium) to measure amyloid as well as total tau immunoreactivities. They formed a combined evaluation of Aβ (1–42) and total tau protein-immunoreactivities (TTIR) plot described previously

Table 15.1 Mean values of total tau protein (pg/ml) in five studies using the same commercial ELISA kit compared with patients with AD and controls (numbers of subjects studied in brackets)

Reference	Author	Year	iNPH	AD	Controls
7	Kudo	2000	391 (20)		138 (13)
8	Lins	2004	266 (12)	728 (12)	224.4 (12)
22	Kapaki	2007	219[a] (18)	571[a] (67)	166[a] (72)
30	Gloeckner	2008	302 (13)	488 (23)	231 (19)
32	Miyajima	2012	152 (46)	536 (10)	216 (8)
			266 (109)	580.7 (112)	195.1 (124)

[a] Only median values presented in the paper.

Table 15.2 Mean values of Aβ (1–42) protein (pg/ml) in three studies using the same commercial ELISA kit compared with patients with AD and controls (numbers of subjects studied in brackets)

Reference	Author	Year	iNPH	AD	Controls
8	Lins	2004	402.7 (12)	454.4 (12)	648.5 (12)
22	Kapaki	2007	400 (18)	422 (67)	721 (72)
30	Gloeckner	2008	563 (13)	378 (23)	887 (19)
			455.23 (43)	418.13 (102)	752.16 (103)

[8], which discriminated all NPH from the AD samples. They concluded that the combined use of both markers rather than one separately is of diagnostic use. No separate sensitivity or specificity figures were provided though. TTIR was not higher when compared with controls. Gloeckner et al. in their study using the same commercial assay found lower tau levels than controls [30].

Miyajima et al. assessed the levels of lumbar CSF of total tau (t-tau), phosphorylated tau (p-tau), soluble amyloid precursor protein (sAPP) sAPPa, sAPPb, and Aβ (1–42) in 46 iNPH subjects and compared the levels with AD patients and healthy controls [32]. All proteins except Aβ (1–42) were statistically different between AD and iNPH patients. Receiver operating characteristic (ROC) analysis revealed that sAPPa is the most reliable marker to distinguish iNPH from AD and normal controls (NC), with an area under the curve (AUC) of 0.994, which suggests high accuracy. With a cut-off of 234.5 ng/ml, sensitivity and specificity were 95.5% and 100%, respectively, thus allowing differentiation of iNPH from AD and NC.

In patients with NPH, the average value of total tau levels of the five studies that used the same commercial assay (Innotest, Belgium) [7,8,22,30,32] was 266 pg/ml (see Table 15.1). The range of total tau in two studies was 75–1040 pg/ml. The average level of total tau from control subjects was 195.1 pg/ml and in AD subjects it was 580.7 pg/ml in the four studies that reported AD levels.

With regard to Aβ (1–42) levels, these were assayed in three studies using the same commercial ELISA [8,22,30] (Table 15.2). The average value for patients with NPH was 455.23 pg/ml, whereas that of the control subjects was 752.16 pg/ml and 418.13 pg/ml in AD subjects. If we examine the ratio of total tau/Aβ (1–42), this was 0.58 in iNPH, 0.25 in control subjects, and 1.38 in patients with AD.

Other studies that provided significant differences in levels of CSF markers were those of Mazurek [33] who found that levels of vasopressin were normal in NPH when compared with AD; however, this study lacked an accurate description of its NPH subjects. Cacabelos et al. also detected significantly higher levels of interleukin-1 in NPH when compared with AD [34]. Nooijen et al. [35] proposed that lactate could act as a diagnostic marker since levels in NPH were much higher than they were in AD. However in the study by Malm et al., although lactate in both NPH and AD was significantly lower than in controls, there was no difference between NPH and AD [36]. Futakawa et al. assessed the CSF levels of two isoforms of transferrin (Tf-1 and Tf-2). The Tf-2/Tf-1 ratios of iNPH patients were significantly higher than those of controls

($p = 0.0019$) and AD patients ($p = 0.0010$), suggesting this ratio as a useful marker to distinguish iNPH from AD, and possibly other dementias [37].

CSF biomarkers in the differential diagnosis with vascular dementia

The problems of clinically distinguishing NPH patients from those with subcortical ischemic vascular dementia (SIVD) are clear since the clinical phenotype of the cognitive profile, as well as the gait disturbance noted, is similar in both conditions. In this sense, it is more difficult to distinguish a patient who has NPH from one who has SIVD than from a patient who has features of AD, since careful clinical or neuropsychological evaluation will distinguish the latter group. So far similar CSF markers to the ones used to differentiate between iNPH and AD have been assayed. This is a reflection of the design of most studies, which included both patients with AD and SIVD as the primary studied cohorts and patients with NPH were used as a comparative control group. Besides, there are no condition-specific CSF biomarkers for patients with vascular dementia as there has been significant overlap with patients with AD in published results to date.

Only a few studies focused on studying the NPH and SIVD conditions separately, namely those of Tullberg et al. [38,39] and Agren-Wilsson et al. [23]. The former group found that a cut-off level of sulfatide equal to 400 nmol/l can distinguish between cases of SIVD with a sensitivity of 74% and specificity of 94%; the same lower sulfatide values in a mixed NPH group when compared with SIVD were reported in a later study [39] by the same group. However, the latter group [23] did not find any significant difference in levels; they explained this difference in their results by suggesting that this is due to their cohort being composed purely of idiopathic cases, whereas that of the former group contained both idiopathic and secondary cases.

With regard to tau no significant difference was found in the study by Tullberg et al. [38], whereas in the study by Agren-Wilsson et al. [23] tau was found to be significantly lower than in patients with SIVD. The latter group devised a multinomial logistic regression model to calculate the probability of diagnosing NPH by combining the concentrations of neurofilament light chain protein (NFL), p-tau, and Aβ (1–42); the model provided a high overall accuracy of 84.5% [23].

NFL is found mostly in large unmyelinated axons. In a meta-analysis NFL levels appear higher in patients with vascular dementia when compared with control subjects. Tullberg et al. found that NFL is increased in NPH patients when compared with patients with Binswanger's disease (BD, or subcortical leukoencephalopathy, a rare form of multi-infarct dementia) [39]. Higher NFL in NPH (854 ng/l) and SAE (subcortical arteriosclerotic encephalopathy of Binswanger's type) patients (1268 ng/l) when compared with controls (395 ng/l) were detected by Agren-Wilsson et al. [23]. There was not a statistical significant difference between NPH and SAE NFL levels in this latter study. Unfortunately, neither of those studies provided a cut-off value to calculate sensitivity and specificity of the marker.

Vasoactive intestinal peptide (VIP) has been consistently lower in NPH when compared with SIVD groups [38,40]. However, neither of those studies provides us with a cut-off value. The difference in VIP levels might be attributed to VIP's neuroprotective and anti-inflammatory role which has been highlighted recently [41]. Ferrero et al. found higher levels of the diazepam binding inhibitor receptor when compared with AD and SIVD groups [42]. 5-HIAA, NPY, and GABA were significantly lower in NPH when compared with SAE [38]. Lipocalin-type prostaglandin D synthase was also found to be lower in NPH patients than in patients with SIVD [43].

CSF biomarkers in the differential diagnosis with Parkinson's disease

Gait disorders are frequent among neurological patients. Up to 93% of patients with Parkinson's disease (PD) may exhibit gait disorder. The difficulty in the differential diagnosis of PD with patients with NPH lies in the features of the gait disorder. Therefore NPH and vascular dementia have been described as the two causes of "lower parkinsonism" [44]. Symptoms similar to those of extrapyramidal disturbance are frequent in patients with iNPH [45]. Up to 86% of patients with iNPH have demonstrated symptoms of akinesia, tremor, hypertonia, or hyperkinesia [46]. External visual or auditory cues improve walking in iNPH only slightly, but are more effective in PD [44].

Reduced stride length and reduced step height characterize the gait of iNPH together with a disturbance of balance leading to loss of the dynamic equilibrium required for normal gait. The normal variability of step width and foot angles appears decreased, leading to an insufficient compensation of body sway, which is of particular importance during obstacle avoidance [47].

The study by Beal et al. that assessed somatostatin-like immunoreactivity provided no help in discriminating between these two conditions [48]. Ferrero et al. also compared the levels of diazepam binding inhibitor receptor and found higher levels of the marker in NPH and depressed PD patients when compared with other groups [42]. Arai et al. in their first study investigating tau as a marker found increased levels in NPH when compared with PD and other control groups [49]. Although this marker may prove useful, its use must be evaluated against latest research that shows clear pathogenic links between mutations in α-synuclein, tau or leucine-rich repeat kinase 2 (LRRK2), and a familial form of PD. LRRK2 PD is phenotypically similar to the sporadic form of PD, and therefore any future research would have to distinguish between sporadic or familial types of PD [50].

Lins et al. investigated both tau and Aβ (1–42) as a means of discriminating between AD, SIVD, PD, and NPH [6]. NPH patients showed no significant TTIR (total tau immunoreactivities) changes compared with SIVD, PD, and controls. Aβ (1–42) 42-immunoreactivity (IR) in the NPH group was significantly lower compared with PD. However, using a TTIR by Aβ (1–42) 42 plot, all NPH, PD, and control samples were within the non-AD plot region, therefore not offering any help in the differential diagnosis between NPH and PD [8]. Rota et al. studied a group of cytokines comparing patients with probable PD, AD, and SIVD with patients with NPH. None of the cytokines was of aid as a diagnostic marker [51].

Prognostic biomarkers

There have been much fewer studies developing prognosis biomarkers when compared with those assessing diagnostic biomarkers. Even though CSF is an easily accessed biological fluid by lumbar puncture or ventricular cannulation, the follow-up and measurement of outcomes is more difficult to monitor and therefore development of prognostic biomarkers becomes more cumbersome. There can of course be no prognostic biomarkers for presymptomatic individuals stratifying the risk of developing the syndrome, but only prognostic of surgical outcome if the individual undergoes surgical treatment. Multidisciplinary collaboration among physicians dealing with the diagnosis, treatment, and further follow-up of patients with iNPH is more problematic. Often there is no set protocol among different teams on how to follow up these patients; in real life practice surgical teams tend to focus less on established outcome scales and more on monitoring of surgical complications. Besides, elderly patients with other chronic conditions may fail to attend follow-up clinics. The average age of patients having surgery is early to mid seventies, therefore achieving a 10-year follow-up is proving to be more difficult than with other conditions. Other chronic conditions that may develop in time (e.g. degenerative spinal and cardiovascular conditions) may add to the overall medical burden of an individual and therefore influence overall outcomes. We discuss below studies that have focused only on surgical outcomes.

Miyajima et al. in their study of lumbar CSF for 46 patients with iNPH attempted to predict outcomes by analyzing cognitive outcomes (using the mini-mental state examination [MMSE]) after 6 months of follow-up [32]. Total tau and p-tau levels proved to be lower in patients who showed improved cognitive function after surgery. Also in groups that had MMSE ≥25 both p-tau and sAPPa were significantly lower than in the worse performing group. The only marker with the highest sensitivity and specificity (≥80%) for predicting a better cognitive outcome, MMSE ≥25, was sAPPAa [32].

Patel et al. studied 39 patients and evaluated their outcomes at 4 months using a disease-specific outcomes scale, and a psychometric battery [52]. Higher p-tau/Aβ (1–42) ratios were associated with poorer improvement in both cognition and gait after shunting. The finding that patients with high p-tau/Aβ (1–42) ratios show less recovery of gait after shunting is accounted for at least partly by their higher baseline gait performance compared with patients lacking comorbid AD pathology. Patients with high p-tau/Aβ (1–42) ratios showed poorer post-shunt improvement mainly on tests of memory (immediate and delayed word list recall) and visuospatial function (clock copy) – cognitive domains that are typically impaired in patients with AD [52].

Leinonen et al. analyzed seven markers in total and in particular total tau, p-tau181, Aβ (1–42), NFL, TNF-α, TGF-β1, and VEGF in lumbar CSF of 35 patients with suspected NPH and correlated the findings with the outcomes of external lumbar drainage (ELD) rather than surgical CSF diversion. It is known that ELD is a useful ancillary test in predicting surgical outcomes because it simulates the physiological changes occurring with permanent surgical CSF diversion. To that effect, the authors found that none of the markers studied in lumbar CSF could predict which patients would respond to ELD [53]. It would be important for this team to study the surgical outcomes of the cohort that was selected for surgical CSF diversion and report on them in a future study.

In a study of 22 patients Tarnaris et al. found that a combination of Aβ (1–42) levels and total tau protein levels predicted favorable surgical outcomes at 6 months with acceptable accuracy to be of clinical use [54]. The authors used a disease-specific outcome scale to record the outcomes. Although neither Aβ (1–42) nor t-tau levels had sufficient sensitivity or specificity, their combined calculation predicted favorable outcomes in more than 80% of cases.

Scollato et al. analyzed the proteome of 17 patients with NPH selected by ICP monitoring. They found no differences in the proteome of nonresponders compared with improved patients [55]. The overexpression of alpha-2HS glycoprotein, alpha-1-antichymotrypsin, and alpha-1-beta glycoprotein and the underexpression of glial fibrillary acidic protein, apolipoproteins (AIV, J, and E), complement C3c, antithrombin, alpha-2-antiplasmin, and albumin appeared to be associated with a positive response to surgery [55].

Nakajima et al. assessed the levels of tau protein and leucine-rich α-2-glycoprotein (LGR) in the lumbar CSF of 52 patients and correlated the results with cognitive outcomes at 12 months. A combination of higher LGR and lower tau protein values predicted a positive response in the tap test in over 90% of patients and all shunt responders. Their cut-offs of LRG concentrations of 67 ng/ml or higher gave 81.6% sensitivity and 78.6% specificity [56]. Interestingly tau protein levels in the CSF did not differ significantly between the shunt responders (167.4 ± 105.4 pg/ml) and the nonresponder group (264.9 ± 209.5 pg/ml; $p > 0.05$).

Summary of current evidence

When neurologists with an interest in dementia assess patients they base their diagnosis of the condition mostly on clinical grounds, and any biomarkers will then serve an auxiliary role. Out of the most studied CSF proteins, Aβ (1–42), is decreased in the CSF of AD patients possibly because of the deposition of fibrillar Aβ (1–42) in senile plaques. Tau protein is increased in the CSF of AD patients as a reflection of the release of tau in CSF with neuronal loss. P-tau stems finally from tangle deposition. The pooled sensitivities and specificities for Aβ (1–42) in AD versus controls is 86% and 89% and for tau 81% and 91%, respectively [57]. There are no exclusive biomarkers for patients with vascular dementia and so the aforementioned have been studied. In the case of vascular dementia versus AD the combination rather than the use of a single biomarker appears useful. Having reviewed the current literature we have seen that none of the studied proteins can fulfill the role of a biomarker for iNPH according to the criteria set by the Consensus Report of the Working Group on Molecular and Biochemical Markers of Alzheimer's Disease (sensitivity and specificity greater than 80% and validated by two independent studies) [2].

Summary of currently available evidence

- No CSF biomarker has fulfilled the criteria required to aid in the diagnosis or differential diagnosis of the condition.
- Lower than AD total tau levels and comparable Aβ (1–42) levels to AD may aid in the differential diagnosis from patients with AD.
- sAPPa appears in one study as a single marker (cut-off of 234.5 ng/ml), with high sensitivity and specificity to differentiate between iNPH, AD, and normal controls.
- A combination of the light chain of neurofilament protein (NFL), p-tau, and Aβ (1–42) has provided high accuracy in distinguishing iNPH from SIVD in one study and again may act as a platform for future prospective studies.
- No CSF marker has shown currently any promise to distinguish between NPH and patients with PD.
- The evidence for prognostic biomarkers is at present weak since there are too few studies, with small numbers of patients. A combination of p-tau and Aβ (1–42) or t-tau and Aβ (1–42) appears promising and should be replicated in further studies by different groups.

Experimental problems

Any diagnostic biomarkers need to reflect the pathological changes characterizing the condition. In iNPH, because of the small number of autopsy cases, it is impossible to conclude whether anatomicopathological alterations are present in all cases, or differ depending on the severity or the chronicity of the condition. The pathological changes observed have resulted mainly from cortical biopsies and selected autopsy studies from research that predates modern diagnostic criteria and have not been replicated in a cohort of idiopathic NPH. However, it is thought that in NPH changes similar to those found in arteriosclerotic encephalopathy or Alzheimer's dementia are common. In a prospective study of 56 patients who underwent ventriculoperitoneal shunting for iNPH and cortical biopsy no specimen biopsy showed inflammation, neoplasm, neurons with Lewy bodies, Pick bodies, or glial cells with silver-positive inclusions [58]. Amyloid angiopathy and neuropil threads were detected in only a few specimens and sparse accumulations of neurofibrillary tangles were seen in six (10.7%). Neuritic plaques were found in 23 (41%) biopsies, whereas 12 (21.4%) patients showed only diffuse plaques. A diagnosis of definite Alzheimer's disease could be made in seven cases (12.5%), probable disease in nine (16%), and possible disease in seven (12.5%) [58].

There are firstly technical details that need to be considered such as the fast transfer of the CSF sample to the lab from theaters or the ward, proper spinning and storage to proper polypropylene tubes and freezing. The CSF volume taken can influence the concentration of biomarkers [59]. If storage is required for later investigation this can be done at 4–8°C (short-term) or at –20°C (long-term). If storage is required, 12 ml of CSF should be partitioned into three to four sterile tubes [60]. Also avoidance of thawing of the CSF, which may affect the accuracy of protein measurement, is paramount. If ventricular CSF is collected, the first few ml need to be discarded as they may "contaminate" the CSF sample. This is because the sample obtained may contain proteins from the cerebral tissue encountered during cannulation, thus not reflecting the ventricular CSF levels. When one measures ventricular or lumbar levels of a biomarker one needs to be aware that there are rostrocaudal variations in the markers and the lumbar levels do not always reflect the ventricular levels and vice versa. It is important to collect matched serum and/or plasma samples for evaluation of CSF biomarkers because the concentration of the marker in blood often influences that in CSF. In addition, serum/plasma pairs are essential to study the intrathecal origin of a biomarker and its central nervous system specificity.

Standardization of laboratory methods and adherence to published guidelines are also of importance. A recent meta-analysis showed considerable differences in absolute concentrations of Aβ (1–42) and tau between laboratories, even when the same test kit was used.

Quo vadis?

It has taken the medical community 40 years to provide internationally accepted and evidence-based guidelines for the diagnosis and treatment of the syndrome [61]. As seen at the beginning of the chapter, it took 20 years from the description of the syndrome for the first studies in CSF markers to be published and almost 40 years until the first study that looked into amyloid beta and tau as potential markers for the condition.

It has been emphasized on many occasions in the past that collaborative studies across multiple centers are needed to ensure a large enough number of participants. This is more feasible in studies that explore diagnostic markers using patients with AD or other forms of neurodegenerative disorders as the control group because these conditions are more common than iNPH. Such studies will require robust diagnostic criteria and inclusion criteria as well as validated outcome scales which at best should be condition specific. The follow-up should also be much longer than the most commonly used period of 12 months. Various studies have shown that the beneficial effects of shunt implantation can last more than 5 years, so it is important to be able to select those patients that will most likely benefit from a surgical procedure. One of these studies is the European multicenter study on iNPH [62], which it is hoped will give us further insight into potential biomarkers of the condition.

Ideally biomarkers should combine findings from multiple disciplines, including neuropsychological testing, blood tests, CSF biochemistry, and brain imaging. It is difficult to evaluate whether diagnostic or prognostic biomarkers would be of most value in the effective treatment of our patients. Currently CSF biomarkers are assessing the "load" of comorbid conditions in a single patient, thus highlighting what we currently know about the unfavorable surgical outcomes in patients who may harbor AD or vascular ischemic pathologies. Researchers should focus on markers that have showed promise so far such as t-tau, p-tau, and Aβ (1–42), reproducing results of previous studies in the hope that some of these proteins will fulfill the definition of a biomarker. No condition-specific biomarker has been so far developed because our insight into the pathology of the syndrome is still at an early stage. It is hoped that once biomarkers have been established, they will form part of any future diagnostic guidelines for the syndrome. Using the noninvasive biomarkers that are being developed and taking into account the heterogeneity of the syndrome, we may then move towards a stratified or personalized approach to treatment of our patients.

References

1. Atkinson AJ, Colburn WA, DeGruttola VG, et al. Biomarkers and surrogate endpoints: preferred definitions and conceptual framework. *Clin Pharmacol Ther* 2001;69(3):89–95.
2. Radebaugh T, Khachaturian ZS. Consensus report of the working group on: "Molecular and Biochemical Markers of Alzheimer's Disease." *Neurobiol Aging* 1998;19(2):109–16.
3. Sørensen PS, Hammer M, Vorstrup S, Gjerris F. CSF and plasma vasopressin concentrations in dementia. *BMJ* 1983;46(10):911–16.
4. Sørensen PS, Gjerris F, Ibsen S, Bock E. Low cerebrospinal fluid concentration of brain-specific protein D2 in patients with normal pressure hydrocephalus. *J Neurol Sci* 1983;62(1–3):59.
5. Ahlberg J, Blomstrand C, Ronquist G, Wikkelsø C. Dementia-and adenylate kinase activity in cerebrospinal fluid. *Acta Neurol Scand* 1985;72(5):525–7.
6. Albrechtsen M, Sørensen PS, Gjerris F, Bock E. High cerebrospinal fluid concentration of glial fibrillary acidic protein (GFAP) in patients with normal pressure hydrocephalus. *J Neurol Sci* 1985;70(3):269–74.
7. Kudo T, Mima T, Hashimoto R, et al. Tau protein is a potential biological marker for normal pressure hydrocephalus. *Psychiatry Clin Neurosci* 2000;54(2):199–202.
8. Lins H, Wichart I, Bancher C, et al. Immunoreactivities of amyloid beta peptide ((1–42)) and total tau protein in lumbar cerebrospinal fluid of patients with normal pressure hydrocephalus. *J Neural Transm* 2004;111(3):273–80.
9. Tarnaris A, Watkins LD, Kitchen ND. Biomarkers in chronic adult hydrocephalus. *Cerebrospinal Fluid Res* 2006;3(1):11.
10. Tarnaris A, Toma AK, Kitchen ND, Watkins LD. Ongoing search for diagnostic biomarkers in idiopathic normal pressure hydrocephalus. *Biomarkers* 2009;3(6):787–805.
11. Tisell M, Höglund M, Wikkelsø C. National and regional incidence of surgery for adult hydrocephalus in Sweden. *Acta Neurol Scand* 2005;112(2):72–5.
12. Trenkwalder C, Schwarz J, Gebhard J, et al. Starnberg trial on epidemiology of Parkinsonism and hypertension in the elderly. Prevalence of Parkinson's disease and related disorders assessed by a door-to-door survey of inhabitants older than 65 years. *Arch Neurol* 1995;52(10):1017–22.
13. Gelling L, Iddon J, McVicar A, Pickard JD. CSF circulation disorders: measuring progress in patients through quality of life and hope. *J Clin Nurs* 2004;13(5):589–600.
14. Poca MA, Solana E, Martinez-Ricarte FR, et al. Idiopathic normal pressure hydrocephalus: results of a prospective cohort of 236 shunted patients. *Acta Neurochir Suppl* 2012;114:247–53.
15. Relkin N, Marmarou A, Klinge P, Bergsneider M, Black PM. Diagnosing idiopathic normal-pressure hydrocephalus. *Neurosurgery* 2005;57(3 Suppl):S4–16; discussion ii–v.
16. Marmarou A, Bergsneider M, Klinge P, Relkin N, Black PM. The value of supplemental prognostic tests for the preoperative assessment of idiopathic normal-pressure hydrocephalus. *Neurosurgery* 2005;57(3 Suppl):S17–28; discussion ii–v.
17. Del Bigio MR. Hydrocephalus-induced changes in the composition of cerebrospinal fluid. *Neurosurgery* 1989;25(3):416–23.
18. Lemcke J, Meier U. Idiopathic normal pressure hydrocephalus (iNPH) and co-morbidity: an outcome analysis of 134 patients. *Intracranial Pressure and Brain Monitoring XIV*. 255–9.
19. Cabral D. Frequency of Alzheimer's disease pathology at autopsy in patients with clinical normal pressure hydrocephalus. Thesis, The University of Arizona College of Medicine; 2011.
20. Seppälä TT, Nerg O, Koivisto AM, et al. CSF biomarkers for Alzheimer disease correlate with cortical brain biopsy findings. *Neurology* 78(20):1568–75.
21. Silverberg GD, Miller MC, Machan JT, et al. Amyloid and Tau accumulate in the brains of aged hydrocephalic rats. *Brain Res* 2010;1317:286–96.
22. Kapaki EN, Paraskevas GP, Tzerakis NG, et al. Cerebrospinal fluid tau, phospho-tau181 and beta-amyloid1–42 in idiopathic normal pressure hydrocephalus: a discrimination from Alzheimer's disease. *Eur J Neurol* 2007;14(2):168–73.
23. Agren-Wilsson A, Lekman A, Sjoberg W, et al. CSF biomarkers in the evaluation of idiopathic normal pressure hydrocephalus. *Acta Neurol Scand* 2007;116(5):333–9.
24. Wikkelsø C, Blomstrand C. Cerebrospinal fluid proteins and cells in normal-pressure hydrocephalus. *J Neurol* 1982;228(3):171–80.
25. Vanneste JA. Three decades of normal pressure hydrocephalus: are we wiser now? *BMJ* 1994;57(9):1021–5.
26. Black PM, Ojemann RG, Tzouras A. CSF shunts for dementia, incontinence, and gait disturbance. *Clin Neurosurg* 1985;32:632.
27. Grundke-Iqbal I, Iqbal K, Tung YC, et al. Abnormal phosphorylation of the microtubule-associated protein

(tau) in Alzheimer cytoskeletal pathology. *Proc Natl Acad Sci USA* 1986;83(13):4913–17.

28. Braak H, Braak E. Neuropathological staging of Alzheimer-related changes. *Acta Neuropathol* 1991;82(4):239–59.
29. Zemlan FP, Rosenberg WS, Luebbe PA, et al. Quantification of axonal damage in traumatic brain injury: affinity purification and characterization of cerebrospinal fluid tau proteins. *J Neurochem* 1999;72(2):741.
30. Gloeckner SF, Meyne F, Wagner F, et al. Quantitative analysis of transthyretin, tau and amyloid-β in patients with dementia. *J Alzheimer's Dis* 2008; 14(1):17–25.
31. Blennow K, Wallin A, Agren H, et al. Tau protein in cerebrospinal fluid: a biochemical marker for axonal degeneration in Alzheimer disease? *Mol Chem Neuropathol* 1995;26(3):231.
32. Miyajima M, Nakajima M, Ogino I, et al. Soluble amyloid precursor protein α in the cerebrospinal fluid as a diagnostic and prognostic biomarker for idiopathic normal pressure hydrocephalus. *Eur J Neurol* 2013;20(2):236–42.
33. Mazurek MF. CSF vasopressin concentration is reduced in Alzheimer's disease. *Neurology* 1986;36(8):1133–7.
34. Cacabelos R, Barquero M, Garcia P, Alvarez XA, Varela de Seijas E. Cerebrospinal fluid interleukin-1 beta (IL-1 beta) in Alzheimer's disease and neurological disorders. *Methods Findings Exp Clin Pharmacol* 1991;13(7):455.
35. Nooijen PT, Schoonderwaldt HC, Wevers RA, Hommes OR, Lamers KJ. Neuron-specific enolase, S-100 protein, myelin basic protein and lactate in CSF in dementia. *Dement Geriatr Cogn Disord* 1997;8(3):169–73.
36. Malm J, Kristensen B, Ekstedt J, Adolfsson R, Wester P. CSF monoamine metabolites, cholinesterases and lactate in the adult hydrocephalus syndrome (normal pressure hydrocephalus) related to CSF hydrodynamic parameters. *J Neurol Neurosurg Psychiatry* 1991;54(3):252–9.
37. Futakawa S, Nara K, Miyajima M, et al. A unique N-glycan on human transferrin in CSF: a possible biomarker for iNPH. *Neurobiol Aging* 2012;33(8):1807–15.
38. Tullberg M, Mansson JE, Fredman P, et al. CSF sulfatide distinguishes between normal pressure hydrocephalus and subcortical arteriosclerotic encephalopathy. *J Neurol Neurosurg Psychiatry* 2000;69(1):74–81.
39. Tullberg M, Hultin L, Ekholm S, et al. White matter changes in normal pressure hydrocephalus and Binswanger disease: specificity, predictive value and correlations to axonal degeneration and demyelination. *Acta Neurol Scand* 2002;105(6):417–26.
40. Wikkelsø C, Ekman R, Westergren I, Johansson B. Neuropeptides in cerebrospinal fluid in normal-pressure hydrocephalus and dementia. *Eur Neurol* 1991;31(2):88–93.
41. Delgado M, Varela N, Gonzalez-Rey E. Vasoactive intestinal peptide protects against beta-amyloid-induced neurodegeneration by inhibiting microglia activation at multiple levels. *Glia* 2008;56(10):1091–103.
42. Ferrero P, Benna P, Costa P, et al. Diazepam binding inhibitor-like immunoreactivity (DBI-LI) in human CSF: correlations with neurological disorders. *J Neurol Sci* 1988;87(2–3):327–49.
43. Mase M, Yamada K, Shimazu N, et al. Lipocalin-type prostaglandin D synthase (beta-trace) in cerebrospinal fluid: a useful marker for the diagnosis of normal pressure hydrocephalus. *Neurosci Res* 2003;47(4):455–9.
44. Espay AJ, Narayan RK, Duker AP, Barrett ET, de Courten-Myers G. Lower-body parkinsonism: reconsidering the threshold for external lumbar drainage. *Nat Clin Pract Neurol* 2008;4(1):50–5.
45. Mandir AS, Hilfiker J, Thomas G, et al. Extrapyramidal signs in normal pressure hydrocephalus: an objective assessment. *Cerebrospinal Fluid Res* 2007;4(1):7.
46. Krauss JK, Regel JP, Droste DW, et al. Movement disorders in adult hydrocephalus. *Mov Disord* 1997;12(1):53–60.
47. Stolze H, Kuhtz-Buschbeck JP, Drucke H, et al. Comparative analysis of the gait disorder of normal pressure hydrocephalus and Parkinson's disease. *J Neurol Neurosurg Psychiatry* 2001;70(3):289–97.
48. Beal MF. CSF somatostatin-like immunoreactivity in dementia. *Neurology* 1986;36(2):294–7.
49. Arai H, Terajima M, Miura M, et al. Tau in cerebrospinal fluid: a potential diagnostic marker in Alzheimer's disease. *Ann Neurol* 1995;38(4):649–52.
50. Dawson TM, Dawson VL. Molecular pathways of neurodegeneration in Parkinson's disease. *Am Assoc Adv Sci* 2003:819–22.
51. Rota E, Bellone G, Rocca P, et al. Increased intrathecal TGF-α1, but not IL-12, IFN-α and IL-10 levels in Alzheimer's disease patients. *Neurol Sci* 2006;27(1):33–9.
52. Patel S, Lee EB, Xie SX, et al. Phosphorylated tau/amyloid beta 1–42 ratio in ventricular cerebrospinal fluid reflects outcome in idiopathic normal pressure hydrocephalus. *Fluids Barriers CNS* 2012;9(1):7.
53. Leinonen V, Menon LG, Carroll RS, et al. Cerebrospinal fluid biomarkers in idiopathic normal pressure hydrocephalus. *Int J Alzheimers Dis* 2011; doi:10.4061/2011/312526.

54. Tarnaris A, Toma AK, Chapman MD, et al. Use of cerebrospinal fluid amyloid-β and total tau protein to predict favorable surgical outcomes in patients with idiopathic normal pressure hydrocephalus. *J Neurosurg* 2011;115(1):145–50.

55. Scollato A, Terreni A, Caldini A, et al. CSF proteomic analysis in patients with normal pressure hydrocephalus selected for the shunt: CSF biomarkers of response to surgical treatment. *Neurol Sci* 2010;31(3):283–91.

56. Nakajima M, Miyajima M, Ogino I, et al. Leucine-rich α-2-glycoprotein is a marker for idiopathic normal pressure hydrocephalus. *Acta Neurochir (Wien)* 2011;153(6):1339–46.

57. Blennow K. Cerebrospinal fluid protein biomarkers for Alzheimer's disease. *NeuroRx* 2004;1(2):213–25.

58. Golomb J, Wisoff J, Miller DC, et al. Alzheimer's disease comorbidity in normal pressure hydrocephalus: prevalence and shunt response. *J Neurol Neurosurg Psychiatry* 2000;68(6):778–81.

59. Teunissen CE, Petzold A, Bennett JL, et al. A consensus protocol for the standardization of cerebrospinal fluid collection and biobanking. *Neurology* 2009;73(22):1914–22.

60. Deisenhammer F, Bartos A, Egg R, et al. Guidelines on routine cerebrospinal fluid analysis. Report from an EFNS task force. *Eur J Neurol* 2006;13(9):913–22.

61. Marmarou A, Bergsneider M, Relkin N, Klinge P, Black PM. Development of guidelines for idiopathic normal-pressure hydrocephalus: introduction. *Neurosurgery* 2005;57(3 Suppl):S1–3; discussion ii–v.

62. Klinge P, Hellström P, Tans J, Wikkelsø C. One-year outcome in the European multicentre study on iNPH. *Acta Neurol Scand* 2012;126(3):145–53.

Chapter 16

Hydrocephalus shunt procedures

Benjamin D. Elder, C. Rory Goodwin, Thomas A. Kosztowski, and Daniele Rigamonti

Introduction

Cerebrospinal fluid (CSF) shunting is one of the most common neurosurgical procedures performed, and has been used for many years with excellent results in the treatment of multiple forms of hydrocephalus in both pediatric and adult patients. However, despite many advances in shunt technology over the years, the rate of shunt failure requiring revision or replacement has remained unacceptably high. This chapter will describe many of the techniques and protocols that can be used to minimize the risk of shunt failure, with a specific focus on the surgical procedure at each anatomic location for proximal and distal catheter placement. Therefore, extended discussions of ventricular and lumbar proximal catheters, and peritoneal, atrial, pleural, and other distal catheters are included. For each shunt location, a description of our preferred surgical protocol is presented, followed by a review of the literature to discuss why we have selected our current protocols. Furthermore, the indications and complications for the different shunt locations will be addressed.

Valves

Over 100 different shunt valves are currently available from a multitude of manufacturers. Although different valve types and their characteristics will be discussed in detail elsewhere in this publication and have been reviewed in detail previously [1], they can essentially be divided into four different categories: differential pressure valves, flow-regulated valves, antisiphon valves, and adjustable valves. Differential pressure valves allow drainage once a pressure gradient across the valve is established, allowing for a linear correlation of flow rate with intracranial pressure (ICP), which can result in overdrainage in some situations such as coughing or straining that may transiently increase ICP. Flow-regulated valves allow for a constant flow rate with no dependence on ICP, although they generally have a safety mechanism that is activated at very high ICPs when their function converts to that of a differential pressure system. Additionally, flow control valves have increased flow rates with increased distance from the proximal catheter tip, so generally they need to be placed close to above the vertical location of the proximal catheter tip [2]. Horizontal-vertical valves (Integra Life-Sciences, Plainsboro, NJ), a modification of flow control valves, are used in conjunction with lumbar shunts, and include two valves for differential control of drainage in the upright or supine positions. Antisiphon valves add an antisiphon component to differential pressure valves to prevent the effects of siphoning when a patient is upright. These will be discussed in further detail below. Finally, adjustable shunt valves allow for percutaneous adjustment of the pressure setting, often with the use of a magnet. As such, some of them must be reprogrammed following an MRI and can be affected by some household magnets placed nearby, although some newer designs have locking mechanisms and don't require reprogramming following MRI.

In general, underdrainage of CSF leads to persistence or recurrence of the initial symptoms while overdrainage of CSF leads to complications such as subdural hematomas or hygromas, overdrainage headaches, slit ventricle syndrome, or restricted head growth in pediatric patients. As such, the optimal shunt setting is usually the highest setting that still allows for the patient's improvement. Therefore, at initial placement, we generally prefer using a midrange setting for normal pressure hydrocephalus (NPH) patients and a setting in the higher range for patients with pseudotumor cerebri (PTC). Along these lines, Bergsneider et al. [3] placed adjustable valves in 13 patients with idiopathic

NPH along with intraparenchymal ICP monitors to assess the effects of patient position on ICP and determine an optimal valve setting. They found that lower pressure settings caused a significant reduction in ICP when the patient was in the supine position, which potentially explains why there can be a high incidence of overdrainage complications in patients with NPH. Additionally, based on optimizing the shunt setting with ICP monitoring, the median setting at discharge of the Codman Hakim adjustable valve (Codman & Shurtleff Inc/Johnson & Johnson Co, Raynham, MA) was 140 mmH_2O (range, 30–200 mmH_2O).

Valve and manufacturer choice can be of personal preference and is beyond the scope of this chapter, but we prefer adjustable valve placement as the setting can be adjusted and optimized postoperatively percutaneously, without requiring additional surgery to replace a valve with an ineffective fixed opening pressure. However, it must be noted that adjustable valves do have a significantly higher cost. Additionally, a recent retrospective review comparing Hakim differential pressure valves (NMT Neurosciences GmbH, Frankfurt, Germany) and Codman Hakim adjustable valves found no significant difference in rates of valve replacement for over- or underdrainage, although interestingly, the fixed pressure valves had a significantly lower rate of nontraumatic subdural hematomas and hygromas [4].

Antisiphon devices (ASD)

As described above, antisiphon valves are used to prevent the siphoning of CSF into the distal compartment. The different available antisiphon valves and their advantages have been reviewed in detail previously [5], but a brief discussion of these devices will be presented here.

In normal physiology, blood and CSF within the craniospinal compartment remain at the same hydrostatic level. In shunting, CSF is diverted outside of the craniospinal compartment, into the peritoneum, atrium, or pleural space. When the patient is horizontal, these spaces remain at the same hydrostatic pressure as the craniospinal compartment, but the hydrostatic pressure will change as the patient is mobilized. Therefore, the greatest pressure gradient is formed when the patient is upright, potentially leading to siphoning of CSF as the distal compartment is at a lower hydrostatic pressure than the craniospinal space. This effect is especially pronounced when distal catheters are placed in the pleural cavity, where negative intrapleural pressures occur with each respiratory cycle.

The effects of siphoning can lead to the various complications of overdrainage which have been described above. Therefore, ASDs are primarily used in management of NPH patients in the adult population to prevent the formation of subdural hematomas and hygromas, and in the management of hydrocephalus in the pediatric population to prevent the slit ventricle syndrome and proximal catheter obstruction. For instance, Gruber and Roehrig [6] found a significant reduction in ventricular catheter obstruction in pediatric patients, with proximal obstruction rates of approximately 0.2% over approximately 10 years when an antisiphon device was used. In a different study, Khan et al. [7] found a decrease in shunt obstruction from 20% to 15% over the 5-month follow-up, though this was not a significant difference.

As was mentioned above for flow-control valves, the placement as well as orientation of antisiphon devices has an effect on the performance of the antisiphon device. In general, the antisiphon device blocks drainage once the distal suction pressure exceeds the ICP. In bench studies using Delta valves with siphon control devices, it was found that CSF flow increased with increasing distance between the valve and level of the foramen of Monro [8]. In our practice, we believe that a vertical orientation of the antisiphon device placed in a retro-auricular location under the galea, approximately at the level of the foramen of Monro, has produced the optimal function of the device. This positioning has also been supported in pediatric patients [6]. However, other groups have found that placement as low as 10 cm below the foramen of Monro is optimal [9].

General surgical principles and postoperative care

At our institution, preparation for shunt insertion is performed as follows: a limited shave is performed with a clipper, if necessary, over the area of the incision. The sites of the incisions and tunneling are then scrubbed with povidone-iodine for 5 minutes, followed by application of Duraprep and draping with double layers of drapes with plastic povidone-iodine impregnated sheets overlying the areas of the incisions and tunneling path, to decrease the risk of contaminating the field. Local anesthesia, generally 0.25% Marcaine with 1/200 000 epinephrine), is then injected over the course of the incisions. All patients receive a dose of prophylactic antibiotics, generally cefazolin or clindamycin (if penicillin allergy), and antibiotics are continued for 24 h postoperatively.

Additionally, all shunt procedures at our institution involve closure as follows: the valve is secured in its subcutaneous pocket using 4–0 Nurolon sutures. The wounds are then irrigated with antibiotic solution. For closure of the tissue, 0 Vicryl sutures are used for the fascia, 3–0 Vicryl sutures are used for the deep layers, and a 3–0 nylon running, non-locking suture is used for the skin.

For all routine shunt placements, patients are generally brought to the post anesthesia care unit (PACU) and admitted to the neurosurgical floor for overnight observation. A set of shunt survey X-rays is performed on all patients postoperatively as a baseline and to confirm that all connections remain intact. Additionally, a baseline head CT is obtained to verify ventricular catheter location, ascertain presence of hemorrhage, and serve as a baseline for further care. Depending on distal catheter placement site, additional imaging is obtained. For atrial and pleural distal catheter placement, a chest X-ray is obtained while the patient is in the PACU to check for pneumothorax. For peritoneal catheter placement, an abdominal X-ray is obtained approximately 12 h after the shunt survey is performed to verify movement of the distal catheter, thus confirming that the catheter is in fact in the peritoneum and not in a loculated space. Finally, an erythrocyte sedimentation rate (ESR) and C-reactive protein (CRP) are also sent for all patients postoperatively to serve as a baseline value for comparison if a later concern for shunt infection arises.

Proximal catheter placement

Ventricular catheter insertion

In general, there are three anatomical approaches that can be used for ventricular catheter placement. The frontal approach usually incorporates a burr hole overlying Kocher's point, which is approximately 1 cm anterior to the coronal suture in the mid-pupillary line. The catheter is then placed into the frontal horn of the lateral ventricle in order to avoid the choroid plexus that arises more posteriorly. This same area of the frontal horn can be accessed from a posterior approach in the parieto-occipital region, again with avoidance of the choroid plexus. A final approach is used to target the atrium of the ventricle from a parietal burr hole, as the atrium is often the most dilated portion of the ventricular system. For the past several years we have inserted the proximal catheter using image guidance, because of our preference to use a posterior approach.

Procedure

The general procedure is illustrated in Figure 16.1. The patient is positioned depending on the location of the incision. For a frontal insertion, a curvilinear incision is made approximately overlying Kocher's point. An additional retro-auricular or cervical incision is also often required as the frontal location requires a longer tunneling path. For a parieto-occipital placement, a single comma-shaped retro-auricular incision is made behind and above the pinna.

For both procedures, a 10 blade scalpel and the Bovie, in cutting and coagulator mode, are used to make the incision through the skin and galea, while preserving the pericranium. A subgaleal pocket is then made to house the valve and reservoir away from where the incision is located. A cerebellar self-retaining retractor is inserted. Next, using a perforator drill, a burr hole is made. The dura is then coagulated and cut using the Bovie knife at power of 18. The pia-arachnoid is then gently coagulated with the bipolar coagulator.

Following tunneling of the catheter from the distal site to the proximal incision, the valve is secured to the proximal and distal catheters with silk ties, and is positioned in the aforementioned subgaleal pocket. The ventricles are then again outlined using the CT-based wand and the best trajectory to enter the ventricles is again confirmed. Next, the wand, which is covered by a 9 French peel-away sheath, is advanced gently into the lateral ventricle, while confirming optimal trajectory in real time with the stereotactic system. For most patients with parieto-occipital trajectories, we cross midline with the wand to enhance communication between the lateral ventricles, maximize drainage, and minimize proximal catheter obstruction or differential ventricle collapse. Once the optimal location is found and CSF is obtained, the wand is removed, leaving the peel-away sheath in place. The appropriately sized ventricular catheter (generally 5 ± 2 cm for frontal approach and 9 ± 2 cm for parieto-occipital approach), which is already connected to the valve, is then advanced into the peel-away sheath. The peel-away sheath is then stripped away. Next, 4–0 Nurolon sutures are used to anchor the new valve to the pericranium. Pumping of the valve is then performed, and the exit of CSF from

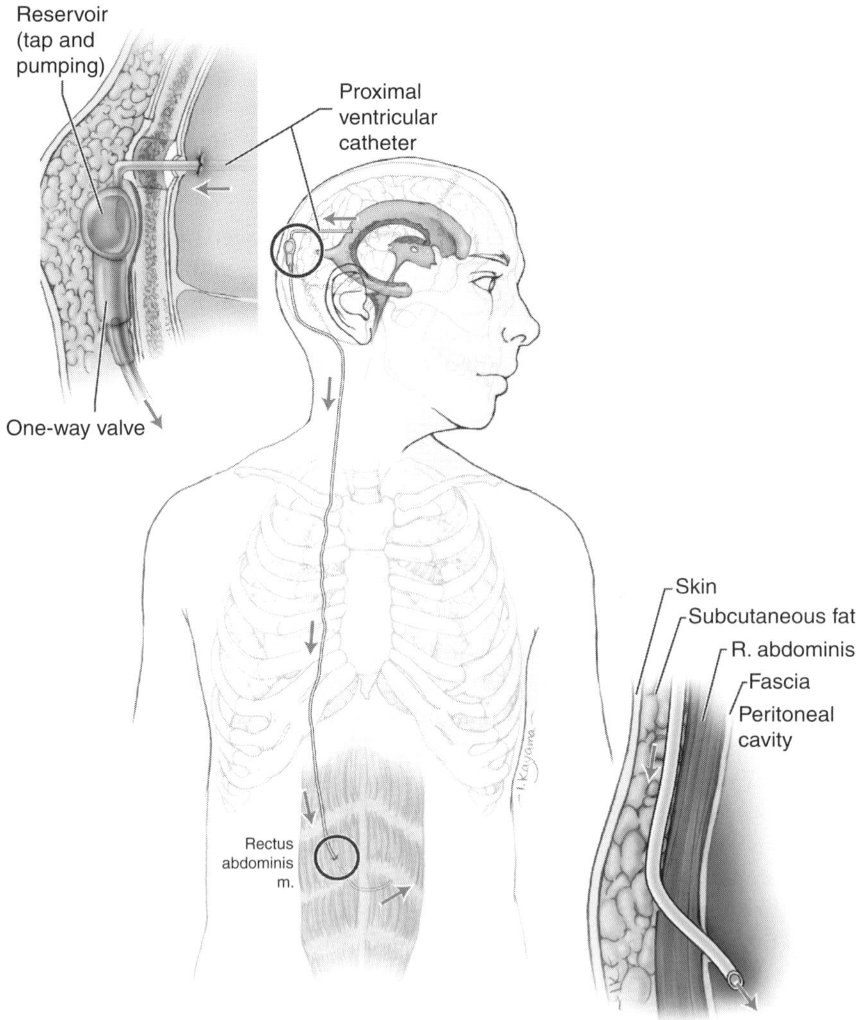

Figure 16.1 Ventriculoperitoneal shunt insertion. The distal catheter generally is inserted off midline, through the rectus abdominis muscle and fascia, although many other techniques can be used. A full-color version is included in the color plate section.

the distal end is confirmed prior to insertion of the distal catheter. The incisions are then closed as described previously.

Discussion and complications

It has been demonstrated that the location of the catheter tip has a significant correlation with the rates of shunt malfunction, as a catheter tip entirely in CSF space had a failure rate of around 20%, compared to around 33% for a catheter tip only partially surrounded by CSF [10]. Wan et al. [11] studied different factors that affected optimal ventricular catheter placement in a retrospective study of 141 patients of all ages who underwent freehand catheter placement, and found that, as expected, patients with ventriculomegaly had better catheter placement. Additionally, they found that patients who underwent a frontal burr hole approach to the frontal horn had better catheter placement than patients who underwent a parieto-occipital burr hole approach to the frontal horn. Lind et al. [12] demonstrated similar results in patients over age 16 using a freehand method, as frontal catheters were found to be in the frontal horn target zone at a significantly higher rate than parieto-occipital catheters, with rates of 64% and 42%, respectively. The same group also performed a morphometric study based on imaging of normal adults and those with acute hydrocephalus to determine the margin of error of the different ventricular catheter approaches [13]. They found that the parieto-occipital placement had a significantly smaller margin of error than the frontal or parietal approaches, with mean range of successful trajectories of 8° in the sagittal plane and 11° in the coronal plane for parieto-occipital placement, compared to 42° in the sagittal plane and 30° in the coronal plane for frontal placement, and 23° in the sagittal plane and 36° in the coronal plane for parietal placement. They also found that there was no significant difference in successful trajectories with slight variations in the burr hole location. However, even with the wide range of successful trajectories with frontal placement, there was only an 86% chance of successful catheter placement.

As such, the authors advocated the use of image guidance or stereotactic navigation for catheter placement, particularly for the parieto-occipital burr hole. We agree with this recommendation at our institution and perform the majority of our adult shunts using stereotactic navigation with the Vector Vision BrainLab software (Heimstetten, Germany). All patients receive preoperative CT scans with thin (2–3 mm) slices of the brain and skull with six radiopaque fiducial markers in place. MRI can be used alternatively, but is generally more difficult and time-consuming and at a greater cost than CT. The patient is positioned in the Mayfield clamp, and a reference star is then used to register the navigation system. As described above, the wand, surrounded by a peel-away catheter, is then passed into the ventricle. This protocol was described previously by our group in the treatment of PTC, in which patients typically have small ventricles [14]. MRI guidance was used to place frontal ventricular catheters, and all catheters were successfully placed in slit ventricles with a single pass, with no shunt malfunction due to proximal obstruction found over the 24-month follow-up period. A similar setup was used by Gil et al. [15] in a small series of children with slit ventricle syndrome or small ventricles, and had no complications during surgery; additionally, none of the patients required revision of the proximal catheter during the 8-month follow-up period. A different group utilized an alternative CT-based negative system, the Stealth Station (Medtronic Sofamor-Danek), which does not require the placement of fiducial markers preoperatively. In a series of 26 adult and pediatric patients with ventricles of varying sizes, the operative time was still short at an average of 46 min, and 20 of the 21 patients had excellent catheter positioning while 1 patient had acceptable catheter positioning [16].

Although there has been success with stereotactic guidance for ventricular catheter placement, other methods have been used to improve proximal catheter location. For instance, Villavicencio et al. [17] utilized direct visualization of catheter placement using an endoscope system in which a semi-rigid endoscope was used as the catheter stylet. In a retrospective review of pediatric patients who underwent shunt placement with or without the endoscope, they demonstrated that endoscopic placement did not affect overall shunt survival, but did significantly decrease the rate of proximal catheter failure, with no increase in the infection rate. Additionally, although the use of intraoperative guidance has been used previously for insertion of ventricular catheters in infants with an open fontanelle [18], Whitehead et al. [19] adapted the procedure for use in older children with closed fontanelles. They made 1.5–2 cm burr holes that were large enough for placement of the ultrasound transducer head and catheter tip simultaneously, allowing for catheter placement under ultrasound guidance. In their series of 10 children, all catheters were placed with a single pass, postoperative CT scans confirmed good catheter placement within the ventricle, and there was no evidence of intraventricular hemorrhage postoperatively.

As mentioned above, we advocate the use of a peel-away sheath to aid with placement of the proximal catheter. This serves two functions: it prevents obstruction of the ventricular catheter perforations with brain tissue during passage into the ventricle, and it allows for passage of the catheter through the exact trajectory that the wand is passed under image guidance. The use of a similar system, though with a stylet in place of the wand in the peel-away sheath, led to a reduction in proximal ventricular catheter obstruction in the first year postoperatively from 18% to 5%, though this result was not significant due to the small sample size.

The most common cause of proximal shunt malfunction is obstruction of the catheter tip with choroid plexus and ependymal tissue [20]. This can cause additional problems during proximal shunt revision as the catheter is often difficult to remove from the ventricle, and more forceful removal will often result in intraventricular hemorrhage. Although the use of a peel-away sheath as described above can diminish the risk of occlusion of the catheter perforations with brain tissue, an alternative solution was proposed recently in which a metal guidewire inside a plastic sheathed 21-gauge needle was passed percutaneously through a Rickham reservoir and then coagulated with a monopolar in

5 s bursts to coagulate any debris or choroid plexus obstructing the catheter tip. This technique relieved the ventricular catheter blockage in their entire series of seven patients [21]. A downside to this approach is that it requires a Rickham reservoir as the reservoir access point is directly in line with the proximal catheter. We have adapted a similar approach that aids with proximal catheter removal during shunt revision or removal [22]. In our approach, intraoperatively, the proximal catheter is disconnected from the reservoir, and a stylet is passed down the proximal tubing. The stylet is then coagulated with a monopolar as described above, and the proximal catheter can then generally be removed with minimal force.

If the proximal catheter removal or placement does result in intraventricular hemorrhage, there are several approaches in management. If there is severe intraventricular hemorrhage, often placement of a ventriculostomy catheter is required. Simultaneously, if there is an adjustable shunt valve, the valve can be dialed up to the highest setting in an attempt to encourage drainage of the intraventricular blood through the ventriculostomy in an attempt to salvage the shunt. Before the ventriculostomy is removed, the shunt should be accessed to check for proximal flow, or alternatively, a radionuclide shunt patency test can be performed to verify the patency of the shunt. If a shunt revision is required, as the blood clears, the CSF can be sampled serially for protein level. We generally refrain from revising the shunt until the protein level drops below a level of 100, as levels above 100 tend to lead to shunt obstruction.

Distal catheter insertion

Peritoneal catheter insertion

The historical first-line approach for distal catheter placement has been the peritoneal cavity due to the familiarity with the anatomy, lower risk of complications, and ease of revision if needed.

Procedure

We make a paramedian incision in the upper quadrant, just lateral to the midline. The skin and subcutaneous layers are incised, and a self-retaining retractor is inserted. Next, the fascia is incised parallel to the direction of the rectus muscle fibers. The fibers of the rectus muscle are then separated bluntly, followed by incising the inner fascia of the muscle and the parietal peritoneum. When this is done, small mosquito clamps are used to hold the edges of the incision. After inserting an Olivecrona dissector in the peritoneum to verify the proper location, a purse-string suture is applied to the incision. The distal peritoneal catheter can then be tunneled to the proximal incision site. Once the valve is in place and catheters are attached and secured, the distal catheter is advanced into the peritoneal incision, and the wound is closed as described previously (Figure 16.1).

Discussion and complications

Although we typically utilize an open approach to peritoneal shunt placement due to comfort with the procedure, other groups have utilized laparoscopic insertion of the peritoneal catheter, either alone or in conjunction with general surgeons. For instance, Stoddard and Kavic [23] described an approach in which a small incision was made for passage of a Veress needle, and a separate small incision was used to place a trocar to pass an endoscope. The distal catheter was then passed into the peritoneal cavity with a Hickman introducer kit. This offered the advantage of a less invasive incision, as well as visual confirmation of distal shunt placement and drainage of CSF from the distal catheter. Furthermore, due to the smaller fascial incision, there is theoretically a lower risk of distal catheter withdrawal and hernia formation, though this has not been studied in detail yet. Other variations of this technique using a single trocar and access hole have been described as well [24,25].

Although the most common complications result from distal catheter infection, obstruction, or fracture, and management of these is described elsewhere in this chapter, a multitude of other more obscure complications have been documented in isolated case reports. Some of these complications include volvulus [26], bowel obstruction [27], inguinal hernia or hydrocele [28], pleural effusion/hydrothorax [29], or migration and erosion into other organs such as the bladder [30] and heart [31].

Atrial catheter insertion

Placement of the distal catheter in the right atrium is often a second choice following complications with peritoneal placement or when peritoneal placement is contraindicated. For instance, it is often pursued in patients who have undergone multiple prior abdominal surgeries or peritoneal shunt placements with significant adhesions, have severe ascites, prior peritonitis, frequent distal catheter obstruction or malfunction, or when body habitus precludes peritoneal shunt placement. Although the internal jugular vein has traditionally been accessed with a venous cut-down procedure, many groups, including our own, have moved to a percutaneous ultrasound-guided approach. The average percutaneous procedure was 22 min faster than the cut-down procedure [32].

Procedure

Our approach has been described in detail previously [32], and is illustrated in Figure 16.2. The patient is placed in slight Trendelenburg position to minimize the risk of air embolism. The optimal location of the incision is determined using ultrasound to visualize the carotid artery medially and the internal jugular vein laterally prior to preparation of the skin and draping. A 1 cm incision is then made over the vein using a 10 blade scalpel and the Bovie in coagulator mode through the skin and underlying soft tissues. Under ultrasound guidance, an introducer needle attached to a syringe is then passed, medial to the sternocleidomastoid muscle edge and pointing slightly laterally, into the vein while gently aspirating venous blood. The syringe is then removed and the straightened "J" tip of guidewire is then inserted into the needle and advanced until some electrocardiographic changes are noted, at which point it is pulled back slightly. The needle is then removed and the guidewire is anchored. At this point, the distal catheter is tunneled to the proximal incision and connected to the proximal valve system prior to proceeding, with confirmation of distal CSF flow obtained.

Next, the vessel dilator and sheath introducer are passed together over the guidewire using a rotational motion. The length of the distal catheter is calculated as described previously [33], using a preoperative chest X-ray. The guidewire and vessel dilator are then removed from the peel-away introducer, and the atrial catheter is then passed through the peel-away introducer into the superior vena cava. At this point, the peel-away introducer is stripped away and gentle pressure is applied over the neck incision to stop the venous oozing. The incision is then closed as described previously.

Discussion and complications

The main complications occur from the development of a fibrous capsule and eventually occlusion of the distal catheter or vessel thrombosis if the catheter length is too short [34], or risk of intra-atrial clot formation and subsequent shunt occlusion, pulmonary embolism, or congestive heart failure if the catheter is too long. As such, we have adopted our approach as outlined above. Using this approach with preoperative chest X-ray measurement, 14 patients in the series had catheter placement within 0.4 cm of the cavoatrial junction, and no patients required distal revision for a malpositioned catheter tip [34]. Other groups have used intraoperative transesophageal echocardiography to confirm distal catheter location with similarly positive results [35], although the patients are subjected to a more invasive echocardiogram with inherent risks of its own. Typically, duplex ultrasound of the internal jugular vein is obtained preoperatively to ensure patency for passage of the distal catheter; however, if difficult placement is encountered intraoperatively due to anatomical variations, thrombosis, or large venous valves, we have previously used intraoperative venography to navigate around the obstruction [36]. There is an additional risk of pneumothorax or carotid artery cannulation, though this risk is mitigated with a postoperative chest X-ray and the use of ultrasound guidance during venipuncture.

Pleural catheter insertion

Placement of the distal shunt in the pleural space has been considered a third-line treatment in most situations when peritoneal or atrial placement is contraindicated, due to the concern for pneumothorax and pleural effusion from drainage of CSF. Pleural shunting generally has a siphoning effect due to the negative intrapleural pressure, although this is mitigated with the use of some of the newer antisiphon devices.

Procedure

Our approach is demonstrated in Figure 16.3. A curvilinear incision is made laterally to the breast, centered on the anterior axillary line and following along the course of the underlying rib (often the seventh). The skin and subcutaneous layers are incised. The most anterolateral attachment of the fascia (of the serratus anterior muscle) is then incised, and the attachments of the external intercostal muscle, intermedius intercostal muscle and internal intercostal muscle are separated from the upper margin of the rib using the Bovie knife. The parietal pleura is then visualized and the lung can be observed moving underneath it with each respiratory cycle. A tunneler is then used to pass the distal catheter from the proximal incision to the chest incision. The

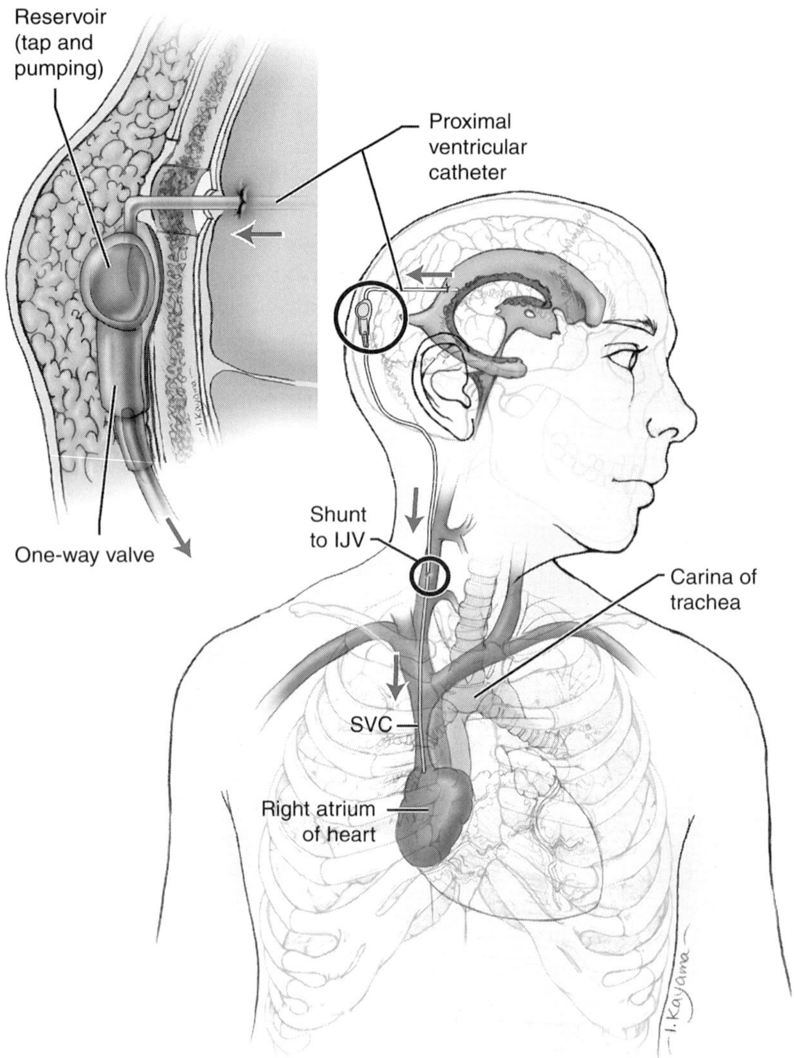

Figure 16.2 Ventriculoatrial shunt insertion. The distal catheter is introduced through the internal jugular vein (IJV), with a goal termination at the cavoatrial junction. SVC, superior vena cava. A full-color version is included in the color plate section.

distal end of the new catheter is inserted into the pleural cavity, with closure as described above.

Discussion and complications

Tension hydrothorax is the most severe complication following placement of a pleural distal catheter [37]. Following a shunt malfunction or decreased drainage of CSF from the pleural space, fluid accumulation can occur generally subacutely, leading to tachycardia, hypotension, desaturation, and eventually cardiopulmonary collapse if not recognized. Treatment is with emergent chest tube placement to decompress the fluid, and often shunt externalization and distal revision once the patient is stabilized. As such, a patient with a pleural distal catheter with any concern for malfunction should have an urgent chest X-ray.

Other distal catheter locations

In cases of shunting where distal catheter failure has occurred at the above locations, other locations

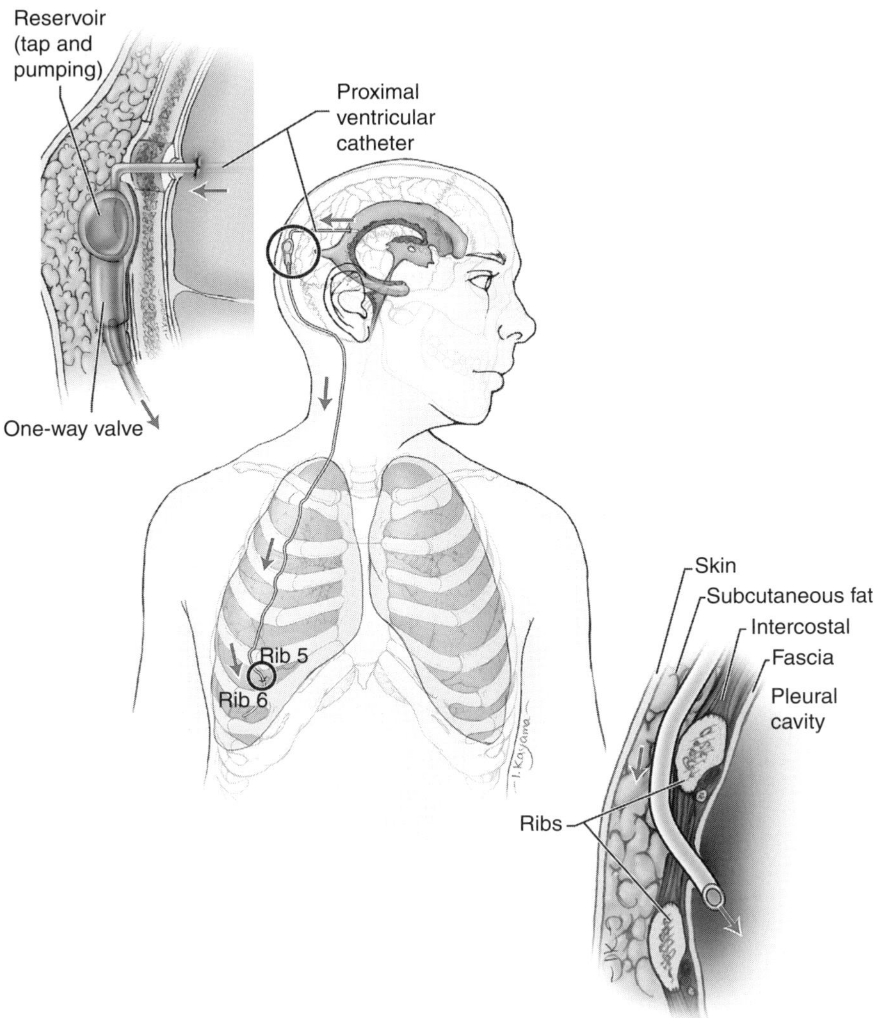

Figure 16.3 Ventriculopleural shunt insertion. The distal catheter is introduced above the sixth rib in order to avoid the intercostal vessels and nerve. A full-color version is included in the color plate section.

have been utilized, including gallbladder placement, as reviewed in detail previously [38], and ureteral placement, although these locations have had mixed results and are often considered end-stage locations. These methods are exceedingly rarely used at our institution.

Lumbar catheter insertion

Lumbar shunts have been used in the treatment of communicating hydrocephalus, pseudomeningocele, and CSF leaks, but are predominantly used in the treatment of PTC, and are contraindicated in the treatment of obstructive hydrocephalus.

Procedure

Our approach is illustrated in Figure 16.4. The patient is positioned to minimize the risk of injury during surgery on a bean bag in a lateral position, as is done to perform a spinal tap. The first incision is made in the midline in the lumbar region, and the fascia is exposed. A special Touhy needle is then advanced between two adjacent spinous processes into the subarachnoid space, until good return of CSF is obtained. After removal of the stylet, the proximal catheter is advanced in the subarachnoid space for at least 5 cm and the Touhy needle is withdrawn. Next, the catheter is tunneled to a separate incision in the flank, where a special pocket is created in the subcutaneous tissue to accept the valve.

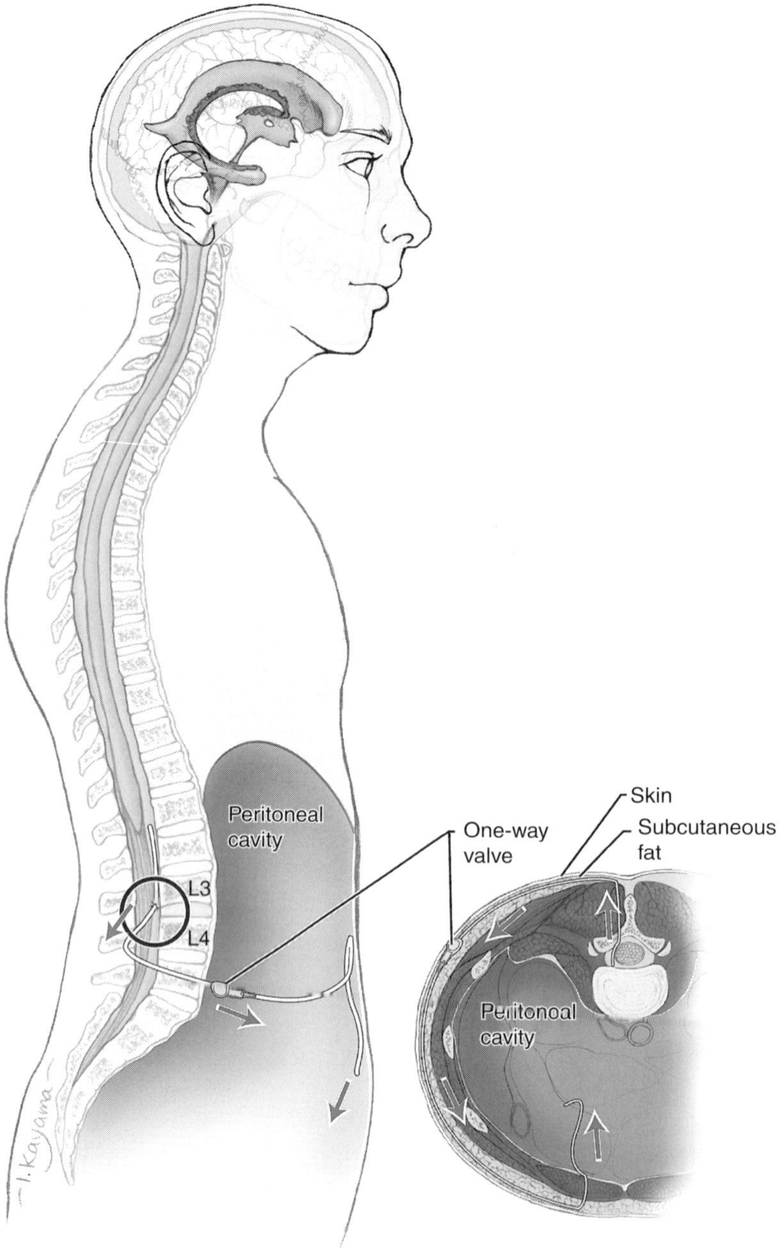

Figure 16.4 Lumboperitoneal shunt insertion. The proximal catheter is often introduced at the L3–4 level, although adjacent levels are also used commonly. A full-color version is included in the color plate section.

A third incision is made in the abdomen for the distal shunt. The proximal and distal catheters are then connected to the valve, and a silk tie is used to secure the connections. The catheter can then be tunneled to its intended destination, with wound closure as described above.

Discussion and complications

Lumbar shunting holds some advantages over ventricular catheterization, including a decreased risk of parenchymal injury as no catheter is passed through the brain. Additionally, since drainage occurs through the lumbar cistern for communicating hydrocephalus, drainage occurs symmetrically throughout the entire ventricular system without the risk of unilateral ventricular collapse leading to shunt malfunction that can be seen with ventricular catheters. Furthermore, there is some evidence that lumbar shunts are associated with a lower rate of infection than ventricular shunts [39]. Finally, lumbar shunts are often easier to place than ventricular shunts, particularly in PTC patients who typically have small slit ventricles. Additionally, a lower rate of subdural hematomas and hygromas has been noted with lumbar catheter placement compared to some of the series examining ventricular catheter placement [40,41]. Finally, lumbar shunts are believed to have a lower risk of siphoning as the distal catheter is typically at a similar height as the proximal catheter.

However, lumbar catheter placement is not without complications. Catheter obstruction is the predominant complication that has been noted with lumbar shunt placement, and was the cause of 65% of the revisions in one series [40]. Additionally, lumbar shunting may lead to overdrainage causing intracranial hypotension. Overdrainage was responsible for 15% of the revisions in a series [40], although this could be alleviated somewhat with the use of adjustable valves. This overdrainage has even led to an increased risk of Chiari malformations in the pediatric population [42,43], resulting in a 4% rate of suboccipital decompression for symptomatic Chiari. However, this complication does not seem to be as significant in the adult population [40,41]. Furthermore, lumbar radiculopathy and back pain has been noted in patients with lumbar shunts, and was responsible for 4.5% of the revisions in a series [40]. Also, although lumbar catheterization is generally less invasive than ventricular catheterization, patients with lumbar stenosis often require a partial laminectomy in order to pass the catheter in the subarachnoid space. There is an additional risk of spinal cord injury or extra-axial hematoma formation, though these complications are rarely seen with proper technique. Another major drawback of lumbar shunting is that the shunts are often inserted without a reservoir, or the reservoir is difficult to access given the patient's body habitus; thus, it is much more difficult to assess shunt function with a shunt tap or radionuclide shunt patency study, and opening pressure often must be assessed with a lumbar puncture. This is especially problematic in PTC patients who frequently present with worsening headaches and concern for shunt malfunction. Finally, in a series of 76 patients who underwent lumbar shunt placement, a complication of lumbar shunt placement with a horizontal-vertical valve included malposition of the valve, as it requires the components to be in a horizontal and vertical orientation for proper functioning [41]. This complication was addressed by suturing the valve in place, although this method is not always foolproof especially in PTC patients who tend to have a larger body habitus.

There is not a consensus on which type of shunt to use for communicating hydrocephalus, although many groups advocate the use of lumbar shunting for PTC, particularly given their typically difficult-to-access slit ventricular system. Although we previously demonstrated that ventricular catheterization could be reliably performed under image guidance for PTC patients [14], we have progressed to generally using lumbar shunts in this patient population due to the greater ease of this procedure and minimization of siphoning effects. Tarnaris et al. [44] compared the outcomes of ventricular versus lumbar catheterization in PTC patients, and found similar outcomes in visual symptoms and headache improvement between the two locations, with no significant difference in the length of time of catheter patency. However, Abubaker et al. [45] found a higher revision rate of lumbar shunts compared to ventricular shunts. Similarly, McGirt et al. [46] showed that lumbar shunts had a 2.5-fold increase in shunt revision and 3-fold increase in shunt obstruction compared to ventricular shunts. Based on the conflicting data, it is difficult to make a final recommendation regarding the ideal shunt type for PTC, though if ventricular catheterization is selected, it should always be performed under image guidance.

Shunt infections

Shunt procedures have a high rate of infection, with a recent review of the literature documenting an average infection rate of 5.4% [47], although an older study documented an infection rate of almost 10% [48]. In general, shunt infections are found within the first 4 months postoperatively [49,50], although other studies have defined shunt infection as those occurring within the first 6 months postoperatively [51]. Shunt infections are suspected when there is evidence of meningismus or ventriculitis, erythema or inflammation along the catheter tract, or new discharge from or dehiscence of the wound. Additional abdominal findings including pain or distension, cysts or collections of CSF can be indicative of shunt infection.

As reviewed previously [52], shunt infection likely arises from bacterial colonization of the hardware intraoperatively, potentially from contact with the skin or skin edges. As the shunt is a foreign body, some of the normal immune response is blunted and eventually a biofilm develops on the shunt hardware, reducing or eliminating response to antibiotic therapy without hardware removal. The majority of shunt infections are caused by *Staphylococcus* species, although species such as *Enterococcus*, *Pseudomonas*, *Haemophilus influenzae*, *Escherichia coli*, and several other species, can cause infection, as described in a prior review [47].

To decrease the infection rate, Choux et al. [51] developed a shunt insertion protocol in which procedures were completed in under 40 min, presterilization packages were opened just prior to implantation and shunt materials were immersed in a gentamicin bath, a minimal area needed to complete the procedure was exposed under adhesive sterile drapes, and the abdominal dissection was completed first to decrease the amount of time that the cranial incision was open to air. Although these factors were not assessed individually, the authors were able to decrease their infection rate from 7.75% to 0.17% using this protocol. Faillace [53] developed a similar protocol for shunt insertion and decreased the shunt infection rate from 9.1% to 2.9%. Some modifications of that protocol included the same scrub team was kept throughout the case, traffic in and out of the operating room was limited during the procedure, and all staff received in-service education on the protocol. Additionally, preoperative vancomycin and gentamicin were given and continued 48 h postoperatively, a wide shave and 5 min scrub with povidone-iodine scrub solution was performed followed by povidone-iodine painting, two layers of iodine-impregnated adhesive sheets and a double layer of drapes were applied to avoid contact with the skin as much as possible, and wide draping was used as a barrier between the surgical field and the anesthesia area. Furthermore, Faillace [53] utilized a no-touch technique in which all personnel double-gloved, contact with the skin edges was avoided, the shunt materials were handled minimally and only with forceps, a separate table and instruments were used for handling the shunt after skin incision, and the equipment was opened immediately before use and placed in a bacitracin solution. At our institution, we utilize and advocate a very similar protocol, with modifications of using Duraprep rather than povidone-iodine painting, and preoperative cefazolin or clindamycin, given within 1 h of incision, and continued for only 24 h postoperatively.

In terms of perioperative antibiotics, we advocate the use of perioperative antibiotics for 24 h only, as described above. Along these lines, for ventriculostomy placement, there was no difference in infection rates between patients receiving 24 h of antibiotics starting immediately prior to placement compared to patients receiving antibiotics for the entire time the drain was in place. Additionally, Ratilal et al. [52] performed a meta-analysis of the literature and found no support for continuing prophylactic antibiotics for more than 24 h postoperatively.

An additional important method for shunt infection control has been the development of antibiotic-impregnated shunts (AIS), in which the proximal and distal shunt catheters are impregnated with antibiotics. The AIS in use at our institution is the Bactiseal (Codman, Johnson & Johnson, Boston, MA), which is impregnated with 0.54% rifampicin and 0.15% clindamycin. The predominant function of the AIS is prevention of bacterial adherence and colonization of the shunt hardware.

In a retrospective analysis of pediatric patients at our institution, Sciubba et al. [54] compared the infection rates of Bactiseal AIS catheters versus non-AIS catheters, and found that AIS catheter use significantly decreased the infection rate, from 12% to 1.4%, over the 6-month period of follow-up. In a similar retrospective analysis of adult patients at our institution, Farber et al. [55] also demonstrated a significant decrease in infection rate with Bactiseal AIS catheter use, decreasing the infection rate from 4.0% to 1.2%. However, a different series of 258 adult and pediatric patients found no significant difference in infection rate between AIS and non-AIS catheters, although their baseline infection rate with AIS catheters was somewhat higher than has been encountered at our institution [56]. One concern with the use of AIS has been the selection of resistant organisms, but similar rates of oxacillin-resistant *S. aureus* infections were noted when using the AIS compared to regular catheters [57].

Once shunt infection is encountered, intravenous antibiotics are usually insufficient to eradicate the organism, and revision or replacement of the shunt hardware is required. A common practice in the treatment of shunt infection is shunt externalization, near the clavicle or cranially, with external drainage and initiation of intravenous antibiotics. CSF is then sampled serially until negative cultures are obtained, at which point the entire shunt system is removed and replaced. Patients are often continued on a prolonged course of intravenous antibiotics postoperatively as well. This treatment often results in a prolonged hospital stay and a significant expense. For instance, Attenello et al. [58] found that in pediatric patients with an admission for shunt infection, the mean hospital stay was 12 days, an average of 3 shunt surgeries, 4 CT scans, and 6 X-rays were performed, and an average antibiotic course of 3 weeks was prescribed, all at a mean hospital cost of almost $50 000 per patient. Similarly, a study of shunt infection in adult patients found a mean hospital cost per shunt infection of $40 000 [59]. Although the AIS catheters have a significantly higher initial cost, the direct cost savings from a lower infection rate have been estimated to range from $25 000 per 100 patients [60] to $50 000 per 100 patients [59]. Based on all of these results, we strongly recommend the use of AIS catheters in shunt surgery.

Conclusion

Although there has been significant success in optimizing shunt placement in order to decrease the rates of shunt failure, clearly there is still work to be done in this arena as there is still a non-negligible rate of shunt failure. As such, along with encouraging the development of new and more advanced shunt technology, we must strive to continue to revise and optimize our surgical procedures and management of hydrocephalus.

References

1. Garton HJ. Cerebrospinal fluid diversion procedures. *J Neuroophthalmol* 2004;24(2):146–55.
2. Francel PC, Honeycutt J, Tompkins P. The effect of alignment on the pressure/flow characteristics of flow control shunt valves. *Childs Nerv Syst* 2001;17(8):467–70; discussion 471.
3. Bergsneider M, Yang I, Hu X, et al. Relationship between valve opening pressure, body position, and intracranial pressure in normal pressure hydrocephalus: paradigm for selection of programmable valve pressure setting. *Neurosurgery* 2004;55(4):851–8; discussion 858–9.
4. Ringel F, Schramm J, Meyer B. Comparison of programmable shunt valves vs standard valves for communicating hydrocephalus of adults: a retrospective analysis of 407 patients. *Surg Neurol* 2005;63(1):36–41; discussion 41.
5. Kurtom KH, Magram G. Siphon regulatory devices: their role in the treatment of hydrocephalus. *Neurosurg Focus* 2007;22(4):E5.
6. Gruber RW, Roehrig B. Prevention of ventricular catheter obstruction and slit ventricle syndrome by the prophylactic use of the Integra antisiphon device in shunt therapy for pediatric hypertensive hydrocephalus: a 25-year follow-up study. *J Neurosurg Pediatr* 2010;5(1):4–16.
7. Khan RA, Narasimhan KL, Tewari MK, Saxena AK. Role of shunts with antisiphon device in treatment of pediatric hydrocephalus. *Clin Neurol Neurosurg* 2010;112(8):687–90.
8. Hassan M, Higashi S, Yamashita J. Risks in using siphon-reducing devices in adult patients with normal-pressure hydrocephalus: bench test investigations with Delta valves. *J Neurosurg* 1996;84(4):634–41.
9. Tokoro K, Chiba Y. Optimum position of the antisiphon device. *Neurosurgery* 1990;27(2):332–4.
10. Tuli S, O'Hayon B, Drake J, Clarke M, Kestle J. Change in ventricular size and effect of ventricular catheter placement in pediatric patients with shunted hydrocephalus. *Neurosurgery* 1999;45(6):1329–33; discussion 1333–5.
11. Wan KR, Toy JA, Wolfe R, Danks A. Factors affecting the accuracy of ventricular catheter placement. *J Clin Neurosci* 2011;18(4):485–8.
12. Lind CR, Tsai AM, Lind CJ, Law AJ. Ventricular catheter placement accuracy in non-stereotactic shunt surgery for hydrocephalus. *J Clin Neurosci* 2009;16(7):918–20.
13. Lind CR, Tsai AM, Law AJ, Lau H, Muthiah K. Ventricular catheter trajectories from traditional shunt approaches: a morphometric study in adults with hydrocephalus. *J Neurosurg* 2008;108(5):930–3.
14. Woodworth GF, McGirt MJ, Elfert P, Sciubba DM, Rigamonti D. Frameless stereotactic ventricular shunt placement for idiopathic intracranial hypertension. *Stereotact Funct Neurosurg* 2005;83(1):12–16.
15. Gil Z, Siomin V, Beni-Adani L, Sira B, Constantini S. Ventricular catheter placement in children with hydrocephalus and small ventricles: the use of a frameless neuronavigation system. *Childs Nerv Syst* 2002;18(1–2):26–9.
16. Reig AS, Stevenson CB, Tulipan NB. CT-based, fiducial-free frameless stereotaxy for difficult ventriculoperitoneal shunt insertion: experience in 26 consecutive patients. *Stereotact Funct Neurosurg* 2010;88(2):75–80.
17. Villavicencio AT, Leveque JC, McGirt MJ, et al. Comparison of revision rates following endoscopically versus nonendoscopically placed ventricular shunt catheters. *Surg Neurol* 2003;59(5):375–9; discussion 379–80.

18. Babcock DS, Barr LL, Crone KR. Intraoperative uses of ultrasound in the pediatric neurosurgical patient. *Pediatr Neurosurg* 1992;18(2):84–91.

19. Whitehead WE, Jea A, Vachhrajani S, Kulkarni AV, Drake JM. Accurate placement of cerebrospinal fluid shunt ventricular catheters with real-time ultrasound guidance in older children without patent fontanelles. *J Neurosurg* 2007;107(5 Suppl):406–10.

20. Collins P, Hockley AD, Woollam DH. Surface ultrastructure of tissues occluding ventricular catheters. *J Neurosurg* 1978;48(4):609–13.

21. Gnanalingham KK, Lafuente J, Brew S, et al. Percutaneous coagulation of choroid plexus to unblock the ventricular catheter using the Seldinger technique: preliminary report. *Surg Neurol* 2005;64(5):440–3.

22. Steinbok P, Cochrane DD. Removal of adherent ventricular catheter. *Pediatr Neurosurg* 1992;18(3):167–8.

23. Stoddard T, Kavic SM. Laparoscopic ventriculoperitoneal shunts: benefits to resident training and patient safety. *JSLS* 2011;15(1):38–40.

24. Goitein D, Papasavas P, Gagne D, et al. Single trocar laparoscopically assisted placement of central nervous system-peritoneal shunts. *J Laparoendosc Adv Surg Tech A* 2006;16(1):1–4.

25. Tepetes K, Tzovaras G, Paterakis K, et al. One trocar laparoscopic placement of peritoneal shunt for hydrocephalus: a simplified technique. *Clin Neurol Neurosurg* 2006;108(6):580–2.

26. Sakoda TH, Maxwell JA, Brackett CE, Jr. Intestinal volvulus secondary to a ventriculoperitoneal shunt. Case report. *J Neurosurg* 1971;35(1):95–6.

27. Agha FP, Amendola MA, Shirazi KK, Amendola BE, Chandler WF. Unusual abdominal complications of ventriculo-peritoneal shunts. *Radiology* 1983;146(2):323–6.

28. Agarwal T, Pandey S, Niranjan A, et al. Unusual complication of ventriculoperitoneal shunt surgery. *J Pediatr Neurosci* 2009;4(2):122–3.

29. Kupeli E, Yilmaz C, Akcay S. Pleural effusion following ventriculopleural shunt: case reports and review of the literature. *Ann Thorac Med* 2010;5(3):166–70.

30. Pohlman GD, Wilcox DT, Hankinson TC. Erosive bladder perforation as a complication of ventriculoperitoneal shunt with extrusion from the urethral meatus: case report and literature review. *Pediatr Neurosurg* 2011;47(3):223–6.

31. Nguyen HS, Turner M, Butty SD, Cohen-Gadol AA. Migration of a distal shunt catheter into the heart and pulmonary artery: report of a case and review of the literature. *Childs Nerv Syst* 2010;26(8):1113–16.

32. Sheth SA, McGirt M, Woodworth G, Wang P, Rigamonti D. Ultrasound guidance for distal insertion of ventriculo-atrial shunt catheters: technical note. *Neurol Res* 2009;31(3):280–2.

33. Metellus P, Hsu W, Kharkar S, et al. Accuracy of percutaneous placement of a ventriculoatrial shunt under ultrasonography guidance: a retrospective study at a single institution. *J Neurosurg* 2009;110(5):867–70.

34. Pudenz RH. Experimental and clinical observations on the shunting of cerebrospinal fluid into the circulatory system. *Clin Neurosurg* 1957;5:98–114; discussion 114–15.

35. Machinis TG, Fountas KN, Hudson J, Robinson JS, Troup EC. Accurate placement of the distal end of a ventriculoatrial shunt with the aid of real-time transesophageal echocardiography. Technical note. *J Neurosurg* 2006;105(1):153–6.

36. Momin EN, Recinos PF, Coon AL, Rigamonti D. Use of intraoperative venography to guide the distal portion of a ventriculoatrial shunt past an obstruction in the central veins: technical case report. *Neurosurgery* 2010;66(6 Suppl Operative):370–1; discussion 371.

37. Wu TS, Kuroda R. Tension hydrothorax in a pediatric patient with a ventriculopleural shunt. *J Emerg Med* 2011;40(6):637–9.

38. Girotti ME, Singh RR, Rodgers BM. The ventriculo-gallbladder shunt in the treatment of refractory hydrocephalus: a review of the current literature. *Am Surg* 2009;75(8):734–7.

39. Aoki N. Lumboperitoneal shunt: clinical applications, complications, and comparison with ventriculoperitoneal shunt. *Neurosurgery* 1990;26(6):998–1003; discussion 1004.

40. Eggenberger ER, Miller NR, Vitale S. Lumboperitoneal shunt for the treatment of pseudotumor cerebri. *Neurology* 1996;46(6):1524–30.

41. Wang VY, Barbaro NM, Lawton MT, et al. Complications of lumboperitoneal shunts. *Neurosurgery* 2007;60(6):1045–8; discussion 1049.

42. Chumas PD, Kulkarni AV, Drake JM, et al. Lumboperitoneal shunting: a retrospective study in the pediatric population. *Neurosurgery* 1993;32(3):376–83; discussion 383.

43. Chumas PD, Armstrong DC, Drake JM, et al. Tonsillar herniation: the rule rather than the exception after lumboperitoneal shunting in the pediatric population. *J Neurosurg* 1993;78(4):568–73.

44. Tarnaris A, Toma AK, Watkins LD, Kitchen ND. Is there a difference in outcomes of patients with idiopathic intracranial hypertension with the choice of cerebrospinal fluid diversion site: a single centre experience. *Clin Neurol Neurosurg* 2011;113(6):477–9.

45. Abubaker K, Ali Z, Raza K, Bolger C, Rawluk D, O'Brien D. Idiopathic intracranial hypertension: lumboperitoneal shunts versus ventriculoperitoneal shunts – case series and literature review. *Br J Neurosurg* 2011;25(1):94–9.

46. McGirt MJ, Woodworth G, Thomas G, et al. Cerebrospinal fluid shunt placement for pseudotumor cerebri-associated intractable headache: predictors of treatment response and an analysis of long-term outcomes. *J Neurosurg* 2004;101(4):627–32.

47. Parker SL, Anderson WN, Lilienfeld S, Megerian JT, McGirt MJ. Cerebrospinal shunt infection in patients receiving antibiotic-impregnated versus standard shunts. *J Neurosurg Pediatr* 2011;8(3):259–65.

48. Gardner P, Leipzig T, Phillips P. Infections of central nervous system shunts. *Med Clin North Am* 1985;69(2):297–314.

49. George R, Leibrock L, Epstein M. Long-term analysis of cerebrospinal fluid shunt infections. A 25-year experience. *J Neurosurg* 1979;51(6):804–11.

50. Ronan A, Hogg GG, Klug GL. Cerebrospinal fluid shunt infections in children. *Pediatr Infect Dis J* 1995;14(9):782–6.

51. Choux M, Genitori L, Lang D, Lena G. Shunt implantation: reducing the incidence of shunt infection. *J Neurosurg* 1992;77(6):875–80.

52. Ratilal B, Costa J, Sampaio C. Antibiotic prophylaxis for surgical introduction of intracranial ventricular shunts: a systematic review. *J Neurosurg Pediatr* 2008;1(1):48–56.

53. Faillace WJ. A no-touch technique protocol to diminish cerebrospinal fluid shunt infection. *Surg Neurol* 1995;43(4):344–50.

54. Sciubba DM, Stuart RM, McGirt MJ, et al. Effect of antibiotic-impregnated shunt catheters in decreasing the incidence of shunt infection in the treatment of hydrocephalus. *J Neurosurg* 2005;103(2 Suppl):131–6.

55. Farber SH, Parker SL, Adogwa O, McGirt MJ, Rigamonti D. Effect of antibiotic-impregnated shunts on infection rate in adult hydrocephalus: a single institution's experience. *Neurosurgery.* 2011;69(3):625–9; discussion 629.

56. Ritz R, Roser F, Morgalla M, et al. Do antibiotic-impregnated shunts in hydrocephalus therapy reduce the risk of infection? An observational study in 258 patients. *BMC Infect Dis* 2007;7:38.

57. Parker SL, Attenello FJ, Sciubba DM, et al. Comparison of shunt infection incidence in high-risk subgroups receiving antibiotic-impregnated versus standard shunts. *Childs Nerv Syst* 2009;25(1):77–83; discussion 85.

58. Attenello FJ, Garces-Ambrossi GL, Zaidi HA, Sciubba DM, Jallo GI. Hospital costs associated with shunt infections in patients receiving antibiotic-impregnated shunt catheters versus standard shunt catheters. *Neurosurgery* 2010;66(2):284–9; discussion 289.

59. Farber SH, Parker SL, Adogwa O, Rigamonti D, McGirt MJ. Cost analysis of antibiotic-impregnated catheters in the treatment of hydrocephalus in adult patients. *World Neurosurg* 2010;74(4–5):528–31.

60. Eymann R, Chehab S, Strowitzki M, Steudel WI, Kiefer M. Clinical and economic consequences of antibiotic-impregnated cerebrospinal fluid shunt catheters. *J Neurosurg Pediatr* 2008;1(6):444–50.

Chapter 17

Hydrocephalus shunts

Principles, hardware, shunt testing

Zofia Czosnyka, Krzysztof Cieslicki, Hugh K. Richards, John D. Pickard, and Marek Czosnyka

Although the cause of hydrocephalus is much more complex than an abnormality of the CSF circulation, shunt surgery is still considered the treatment of choice in most types of communicating hydrocephalus. The role of a shunt is simple: to drain excess CSF from the fluid spaces of the cranial-spinal compartment into an extracranial compartment. Hydrocephalus is caused by different etiological factors, but the common final pathway creates a vicious circle of altered CSF circulation, cerebral blood flow, and metabolism that affects brain homeostasis. In communicating hydrocephalus, draining of CSF appears to be the simplest way of interrupting this circle by improving the CSF circulation. Similarly, in noncommunicating hydrocephalus, third ventriculostomy improves the CSF circulation by bypassing the block to the anatomical circulatory pathway. If other ways of treatment exist, they remain to be demonstrated.

It is believed that an ideal shunt should contribute to restoration of the normal circulation of CSF and regional cerebral blood flow in areas adjacent to ventricular surface [1], prevent excessive build-up of intracranial pressure, and encourage restitution of the cerebral mantle, comprising both gray and white matter. As shunting is a purely mechanistic treatment, which moreover dramatically changes the biomechanics of a patient's pressure–volume compensation, the CSF dynamics should be carefully examined before the shunt is implanted [2]. A shunt should correct the disturbances of CSF circulation by reducing the resistance to CSF outflow to about 5–10 mmHg/ml/min – the typical hydrodynamic resistance in normal brain [3]. Therefore, if a patient presenting with hydrocephalus-like symptoms has normal intracranial pressure, and a normal resistance to CSF outflow (6–10 mmHg/ml/min), a shunt theoretically cannot help because the resistance cannot be reduced further without the risk of overdrainage.

The ability to obtain variables that describe CSF dynamics before shunting allows clinicians to more categorically address some key questions in the clinical decision-making process:

- Scope for improvement with CSF shunting: shunts work by providing an alternative (normal resistance) pathway for CSF outflow.
- To determine which shunt system is the best to use for a patient and in the case of an adjustable valve, to choose initial shunt setting.
- In case of shunt failure, later on, a pre-shunting infusion test provides a baseline for post-shunt comparison.

For all the above points, knowledge of the hydrodynamic properties of hydrocephalus shunts is paramount.

Shunt failure occurs at a rate of approximately 20–30% in the first year, and 3–5% per annum subsequently [4]. Clinical symptoms of shunt malfunction can be diverse for different subjects. Deterioration can be gradual and subtle or sudden and dramatic; moreover, for patients with comorbidities it can be nonspecific. In such cases it can be difficult to justify revision without quantitative evidence and comparative analysis. Similarly, in patients presenting with persistent symptoms post-shunting, testing of CSF dynamics is a useful method of excluding revision, if relative normalization of CSF dynamics has been demonstrated [5]. Assessment of shunt functioning in vivo is impossible without detailed knowledge of the shunt's hydrodynamic properties.

The mathematical model of CSF pressure–volume compensation, introduced by A. Marmarou [6] and modified in later studies [7,8], provides a theoretical basis for the differential diagnosis of hydrocephalus. Shunt testing in vivo in hydrocephalus using physiological measurements requires the

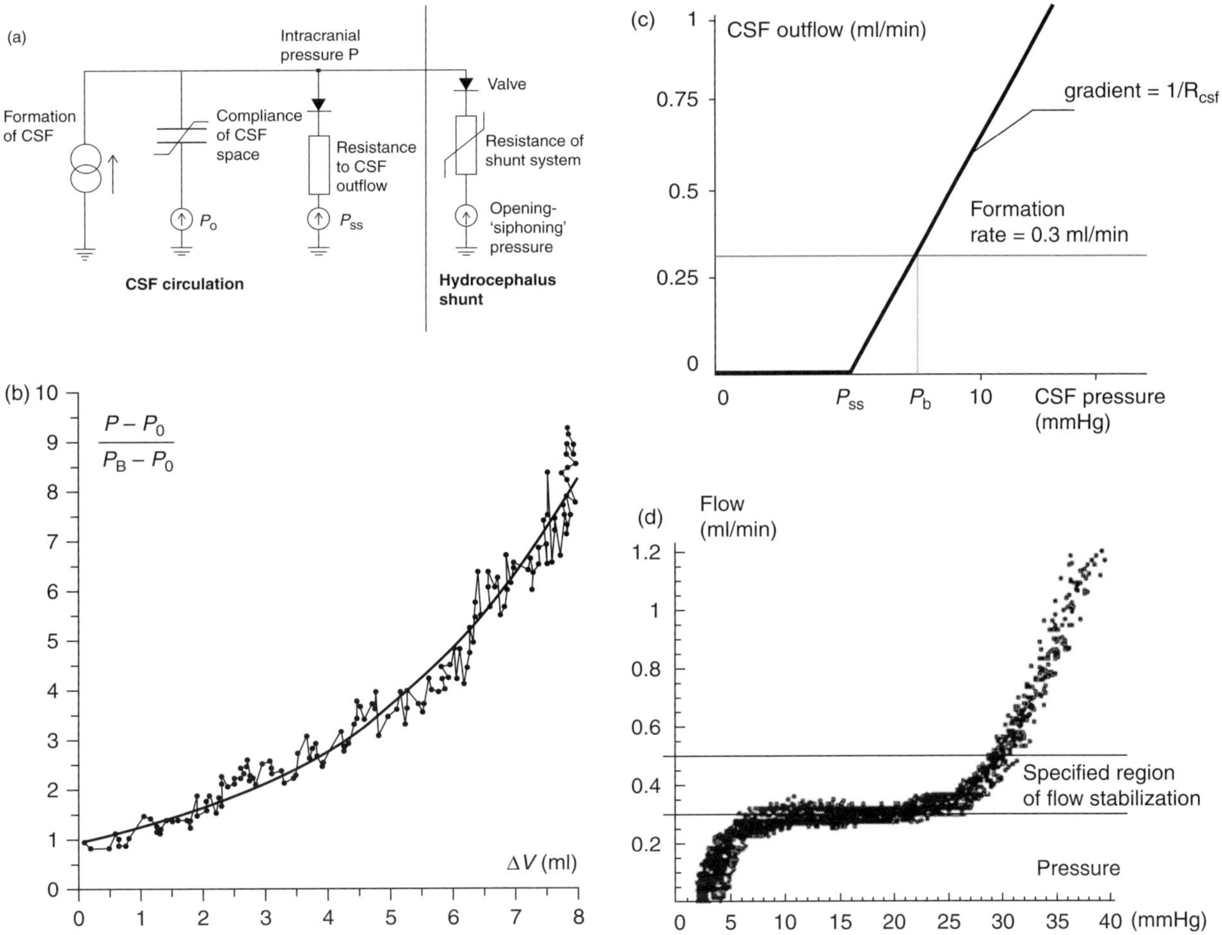

Figure 17.1 (a) Electrical model of CSF circulation and implanted shunt. All parameters are strongly nonlinear. The pressure–volume curve (b) has a linear-exponential character. Resistance to CSF outflow (c) is infinitely high when ICP is below sagittal sinus pressure level and constant (6–10 mmHg/[ml/min]) when it is greater than sagittal sinus pressure. On top of this nonlinearity, the assumption that sagittal pressure is constant may not be valid in some clinical situations. Finally, nonlinearity of shunt performance may be substantial (d) as in the case of the Orbis-Sigma valve. The combination of these three nonlinear elements (pressure–volume curve, resistance to CSF outflow, and shunt flow–pressure curve) may make analysis of stability of ICP in shunted patients quite complex.

model to be extended by a branch representing a shunt (Figure 17.1 – part of the circuit, to the right from vertical line). It is important to notice that the reference pressure here is not the same as in the branch representing the patient's physiological CSF reabsorption (i.e. sagittal sinus pressure). The hydrocephalus shunt bypasses the impaired physiological pathways of CSF circulation and creates a new nonphysiological connection between the CSF pools and the site of drainage (abdomen, right atrium, pleural space, etc.). Therefore, the reference pressure (outlet pressure) is that of the implantation site. Moreover, it could be grossly modified by the patient's body position: decreased (in vertical position) by still controversial "siphoning pressure" or almost atmospheric in horizontal position. Theoretically it represents the pressure exerted by a water column in a tubing connecting ventricles to receiving extracranial compartment and reflects the distance separating them. Therefore, siphoning is greater in ventriculoabdominal than ventriculoatrial shunts [9].

The resistance of most *passive* shunts is nonlinear. A diode with positive polarization voltage represents the valve: this can be of fixed or magnetically adjustable value. Hydrodynamic parameters of the shunt, i.e. its pressure–flow performance, hydrodynamic resistance to flow when the shunt is open, and opening/closing pressure, will be discussed in detail in this chapter. Knowledge of these parameters is important when choosing which valve to implant, and in adjustable valves choosing an appropriate setting; it is also important for confirming shunt function in vivo when adverse clinical symptoms occur after shunting.

Hardware

From the first documented cases of shunting in 1896 by Mikulicz, the attempts to develop a reliable internal CSF shunt turned into an avalanche in the second half of the twentieth century [10]. The recent technological improvements have been substantial: from the first rubber ventriculojugular valves invented by Nulsen and Spitz in 1952 to contemporary high-tech adjustable devices. New materials prevent bacterial adhesion and colonization, novel constructions help to avoid overdrainage. A wide variety of shunt products (over 80 generic types, having numerous subtypes and performance levels) are on the market, with little systematic knowledge available to help the practicing surgeon compare their comparative cost-effectiveness. Similarly, there is very little known about whether a specific type of shunt is better suited to correct an individual pattern of disturbed CSF circulation.

Classical differential-pressure valves: most contemporary valves are differential-pressure passive constructions. This means that the drainage of CSF is regulated by pressure difference between the inlet and the outlet of the valve. Consequently these valves control the pressure in the CSF compartment from where the fluid is drained. The opening pressure of the valve is the determining parameter. And this opening pressure can be fixed or (in the new generation devices) adjustable magnetically after implantation. There are only a few constructions that are designed to regulate the flow through the shunt in a range of differential pressures across the valve. Classification, construction principles, trade names, and hydrodynamic resistances of the most popular valves are listed in Table 17.1.

In a horizontal body position, the mathematical equation describing the drainage through the shunt is relatively simple to solve, providing the pressure–flow performance curve of the shunt is known. In the vertical position, everything is disturbed by the gravitation-induced pressure gradient in the long tubing (average 80 cm long), connecting the inflow and outflow sides of the shunt. This may accelerate CSF drainage and consequently an additional decrease in CSF pressure in the vertical position (on average by 10 mmHg), potentially causing symptoms related to postural overdrainage: headaches, subdural collections, or even hematoma. Another complication related to overdrainage is the "slit ventricle syndrome" [11] affecting mostly young patients. This condition, characterized by completely collapsed ventricles and elevated (30–40 mmHg) intraparenchymal ICP and responsible for severe symptoms of intracranial hypertension, is difficult to correct and in some cases even life-threatening.

Devices intended to attenuate the influence of postural changes on the drainage (antisiphon devices) can be incorporated in the valve body or can be added in line with the valve.

Lumboperitoneal shunts may produce similar posture-related problems. The difference is that the hydrostatic pressure does not produce pulling but rather pushing force in the vertical body position. Therefore, designated lumboperitoneal shunts have usually greater hydrodynamic resistance. If low hydrodynamic resistance valves are used in this arrangement, adverse effects such as tonsilar herniation are observed frequently [12].

The hydrodynamic performance of shunts is complex and determined predominantly by the design of the valve. Most modern constructions use either a ball-on-spring or silicone membrane to close the main CSF drainage aperture. For a summary of different constructions, see Figure 17.2a. Miter, distal/proximal slit, and cruciform valves are more common in the older generation of shunts. Some specific designs such as flow-regulating or referential pressure valves (so-called "Beverly Shunt," now discontinued), posture-compensating gravitational valves, etc., cannot readily be classified along traditional lines.

In the late 1980s the concept of *adjustable valves* was developed in the laboratories of major shunt manufacturers. Constructions used by then, and continued only with modest modifications until today, were ball-on-spring (Figure 17.2b). Adjustability is achieved by changing the pre-load of the spring. Moving a special rotor with an externally applied strong magnetic field changes the pre-load, producing matching different opening pressures of the valve. The range of adjustments usually varies within limits from 1 to 15 mmHg, in a variable number of steps from 3 to 20 (Table 17.2). In most constructions the hydrodynamic resistance of the valve remains constant when the operating pressure is changed. Once the valve is opened, it represents fixed low resistance to the flow.

Table 17.1 The Most common types of shunts and their hydrodynamic resistances (without distal drain)

Shunt name	Manufacturer	Functionality	Construction	Hydrodynamic resistance (mmHg/[ml/min])
Delta Valve	Medtronic PS Medical	cd + sp	Silicone membrane	1.9–2.2
Low Profile Valve	Heyer-Schulte	cd + sp	Silicone membrane	2.2–4.8
Pudenz-Flushing Valve with antisiphon device	Integra	cd + sp	Silicone membrane	1.6–1.7
In-Line Valve	Heyer-Schulte	cd	Miter	3.4–10.2
Contour Flex	Radionic Medical Products	cd	Silicone membrane	2.3–2.8
Holter Valve*	Codman	cd	Distal slit	3.9–5.2
Hakim Precision Valve	Codman	cd	Ball-on-spring	1.4–2.2
Accu-Flo	Codman	cd	Silicone membrane	3.1–4.6
Omni-Shunt	Integra	cd	Ball-on-spring	1.05
Uni-Shunt*	Codman	cd	Distal slit	2.4–11.4
CSF Flow Control Valve	Medtronic PS Medical	cd	Silicone membrane	2.7–4.6
Hakim Valve	Integra	cd	Ball-on-spring	4.3–4.6
CSF Lumboperitoneal Shunt	Medtronic PS Medical	cd	Distal slit	25
SinuShunt (no longer in production)*	CSF Dynamics	cd	Miter	9.6
Orbis-Sigma Valve	Integra	Flow-regulating	Moving diaphragm	Very high
Diamond Valve	Phoenix	Flow-regulating	Diamond aperture	Very high
Dual Switch	Aesculap-Miethke	Gravitational	Diaphragm and spring	2.2
PaediGav	Aesculap-Miethke	Gravitational	Ball on spring	3.3
Sophy Programmable	Sophysa	Adjustable	Ball on spring	2.8
Hakim Programmable	Codman	Adjustable	Ball on spring	1.4
Strata	Medtronic PS Medical	Adjustable + sp	Ball on spring	1.7
Strata NSC	Medtronic PS Medical	Adjustable	Ball on spring	2.1
Polaris Programmable	Sophysa	Adjustable	Ball on spring	1.6–11.2
ProSA + MiniNAV (Programmable ShuntAssistant)	Aesculap-Miethke	Adjustable + gravitational	Ball on spring	3.2–7.1
ProGav	Aesculap-Miethke	Adjustable + gravitational	Ball on spring	0.53
Certas*	Codman	Adjustable + sp	Ball on spring	1.4–3.7

cd, classic differential fixed pressure shunt; sp, membrane or other (SiphonGuard) siphon preventing mechanism included; * discontinued.

Adjustability theoretically facilitates fine-tuning of the valve's performance in vivo and better control of hydrocephalus, avoiding the need for revision. There are drawbacks: with the exception of a few of the newest constructions, adjustable devices can be accidentally affected by the external magnetic field.

Siphon-preventing devices can be divided into membrane, gravitational, and flow-regulating constructions

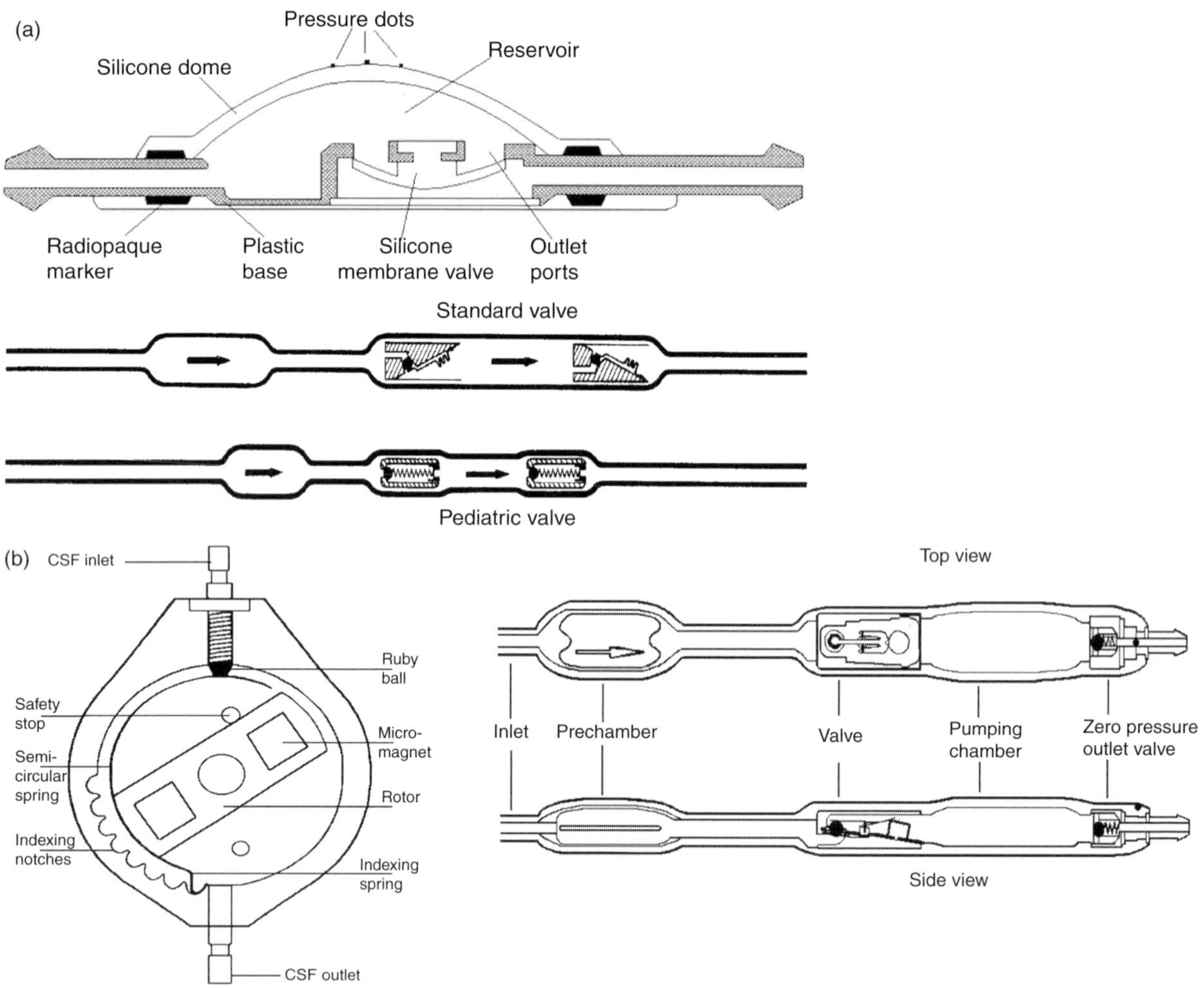

Figure 17.2 The most popular constructions of shunts and components. (a) Membrane valve (upper) and ball-on-spring design (bottom). (b) Adjustable valve: Sophy (left) and Codman Hakim adjustable (right). All adjustable shunts have ball-on-spring valves. (c) Siphon-control devices: membrane (upper) and gravitational (bottom).

(Figure 17.2c). Membrane constructions theoretically cut the flow through the shunt system when pulling (distal tube) pressure exceeds pushing pressure (ventricular) with a ratio 20:1 or so. They need a reference atmospheric pressure acting on the membrane, theoretically transmitted through the skin. However, in fat patients or in cases where scarring hardens skin above the membrane, these types of devices may become unreliable. Furthermore, increased membrane pressure may stop the flow through the shunt altogether. Gravitational devices (such as Shunt Assistant) increase opening pressure in upright body position by adding extra weight acting on the ball controlling flow in the device in-line with a shunt system.

Flow-regulating devices (such as SiphonGuard or Orbis-Sigma Valve) increase hydrodynamic resistance of the device when flow increases. This theoretically is able to limit overdrainage related both to body posture and to nocturnal vasocycling [13].

Laboratory shunt testing

Over the years, a number of independent laboratories, usually supported by academic institutions, have set the standard for shunt testing in vivo. Testing of shunts in Europe originated in the laboratory of Dr. A. Ashoff in Heidelberg over two decades ago [14]. The UK Shunt Evaluation Laboratory (Cambridge, UK) was established almost 20 years ago thanks to a grant from the Department of Health. Over this period, 26 shunts have been evaluated according to the ISO 7197 standard. Under the initial grant (1993–1998) all shunts in use in the UK were systematically evaluated with "blue

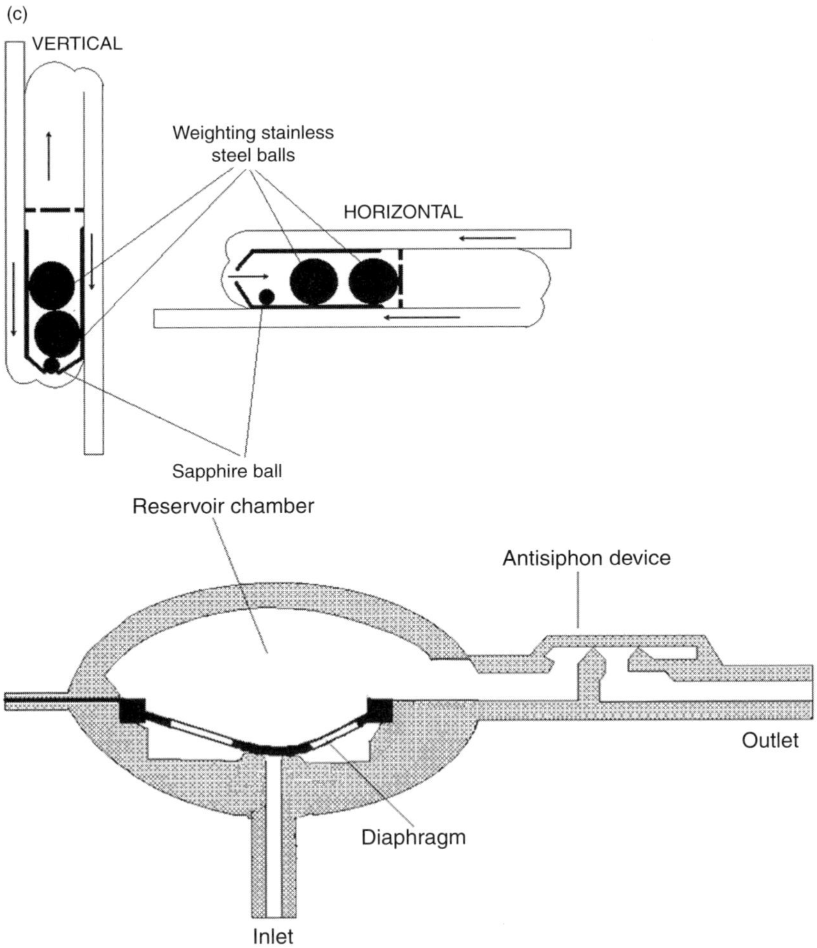

Figure 17.2 *(cont.)*

reports" printed by the Medical Devices Agency. New devices were tested as they appeared on the market (or as prototypes), and these results have been published in academic journals.

The Shunt testing rig is depicted in Figure 17.3a. Measurement is controlled by a standard IBM compatible personal computer that reads and zeroes the balance periodically (every 15 s) to calculate the drainage rate. In this way the weight of the outflowing fluid is measured incrementally, which cancels the influence of fluid vaporization from the outlet . The computer analyzes the pressure waveform from the pressure transducer and controls the rate of the infusion pump. The effect of changes in atmospheric pressure is compensated for by using the reference barometer.

The shunt and pressure transducer are placed on the same level. The water column in the fluid container (H), the degree of the shunt submersion, and the level of the outlet tubing (O) may be changed according to the test protocol.

The shunt is tested under two different regimes:

Flow–pressure test: Controlled fluid flow results in a differential pressure across the shunt (Figure 17.3b). Flow is the independent variable and the resulting differential pressure is the dependent variable. The computer controls flow by changing the rate of the infusion pump.

Pressure–flow test: Controlled differential pressure across the shunt causes fluid to flow (Figure 17.3c). Pressure is the independent variable and flow is the dependent variable. Pressure is controlled by means of a water column (height H) in the fluid container (with stopcock A open horizontally). This pressure decreases during the test as fluid flows out of the container.

Table 17.2 Comparison of most popular adjustable valves

	Sophy	Codman Hakim adjustable	Strata	Polaris	ProGAV
Number of steps	3 (8-SU8)	20	5	5	20
Range of pressures in mmHg	4.7–12.6	2.2–14.8	1.5–10.4	2.2–14.8	0–14.8
Resistance (without distal drain) in mmHg/(ml/min)	2.8	1.4	1.7	1.6–11.2 (dependent on performance level)	0.53
Siphon-control device integrated	No	Optional	Optional	No	Yes
Magnetic field sensitivity threshold	17 mT	40 mT	30 mT	3T	3T
Adjustment needs X-ray verification	No	Yes	No	No	No

The pressure–flow and flow–pressure relationships are plotted during every test (Figure 17.3d). The following parameters are calculated:

Closing pressure: differential pressure below which flow through the shunt ceases. The closing pressure is measured as the intercept of the regression line with the x-axis, drawn between pressure (independent variable) and flow (dependent variable) for flow from 0.2 to 0.05 ml/min.

Hydrodynamic resistance: the change in pressure divided by the change in flow decreasing from about 1.2 to 0.3 ml/min. The resistance is measured as a linear regression gradient between pressure and flow. It is the resistance of the permanently opened shunt and is expressed in mmHg/(ml/min). In adjustable valves the resistance is commonly confused with closing pressure.

Differential pressure for physiological flow (0.3 ml/min) – so-called "operating pressure."

Testing protocol

The testing protocol agrees with, but also extends beyond, requirements of the International Organization for Standardization Hydrocephalus Valves Testing Standard (ISO/DIS 7197). The protocol has been kept essentially fixed for all the previous tested shunts, therefore comparison between different types of devices is possible using retrospective datasets. Three shunts of the same type are tested simultaneously, filled with deionized and de-aerated water. The shunts are mounted in three identical cross-calibrated rigs and the testing protocol starts. The initial tests are used to observe whether the shunt starts to work properly immediately after first filling with water. When the calculated parameters are stable for two consecutive tests, the testing procedure recommences. Before each test the shunt is inspected for air bubbles, and if necessary, gently flushed. Each pressure transducer and the reference barometer are zeroed and recalibrated with the reference water column.

Usually tests start with assessment of the valve at constant, medium setting (for set or adjustable valves). The shape of the pressure–flow curve, its stability over time, basic hydrodynamic parameters (closing and opening pressure, hydrodynamic resistance of the valve) are tested over a long (18 days) period. Then the influence of change in bath temperature, changing residual resistance to CSF outflow, external pressure, magnitude of pulse waveform in inlet pressure, influence of outlet negative pressure, and distal drain of various lengths are tested. Then the variability of hydrodynamic parameters with different performance levels is assessed. The valves are exposed to a magnetic field in 3T MRI – safety, stability of adjustment, and volume of artifact on gradient echo and spin echo (T1) scans are assessed. For adjustable valves, basic hydrodynamic parameters are tested before and after MRI scan. Finally, reflux, durability of junctions, and drift of pressure–flow performance over the whole testing period are assessed.

Hydrodynamic properties of contemporary shunts

Eighteen nonprogrammable and eight programmable valves reveal the common hydrodynamic properties of contemporary shunts.

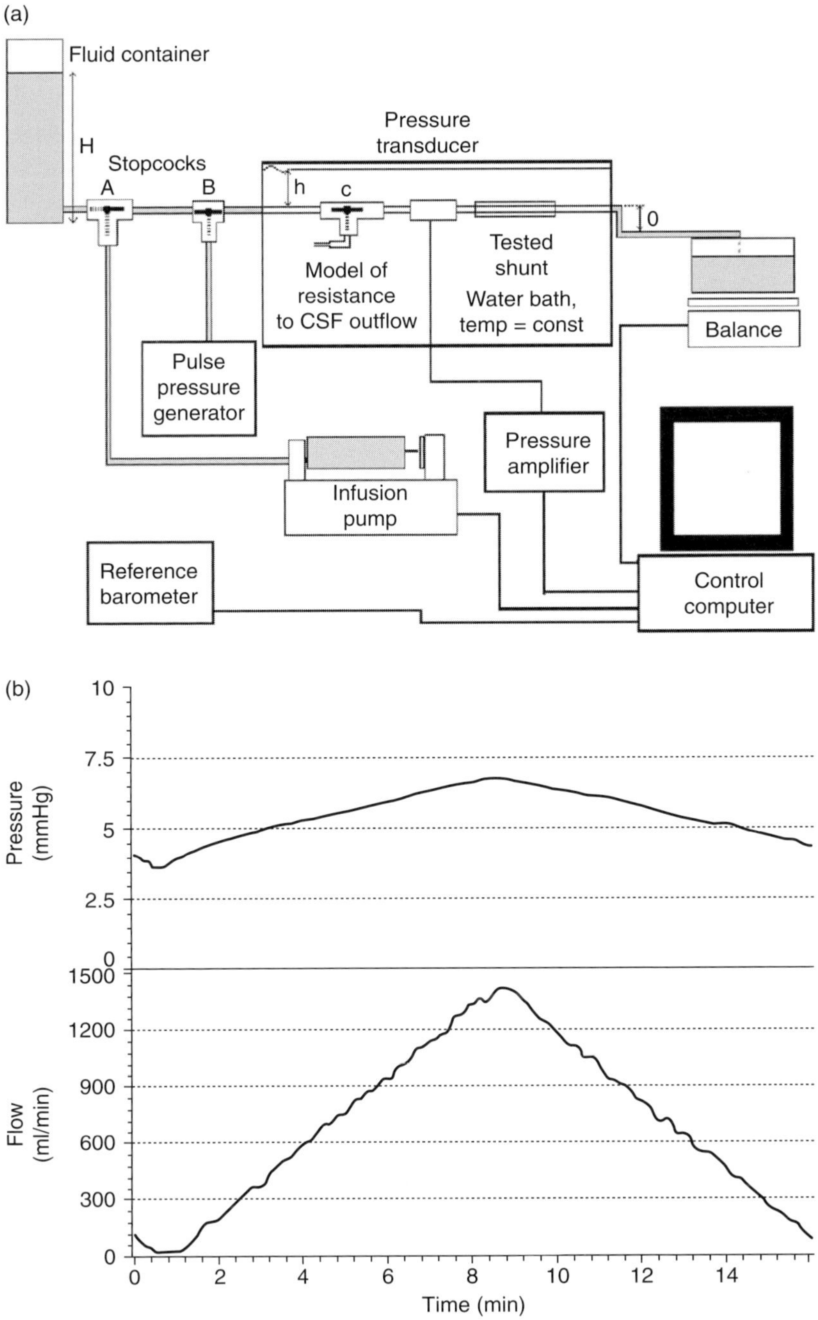

Figure 17.3 Principles and results of shunt testing in vitro: (a) Shunt testing rig. Computer controls measurement process. Shunt may be perfused with controlled rate (from infusion pump) or with decreasing pressure (from cylinder). (b) Flow–pressure (flow profile increasing and decreasing in a triangular manner) and (c) pressure–flow (pressure decreases as water head from cylinder decreases) tests. (d) Pressure–flow performance curves for fixed pressure shunts at three different performance levels (low, medium, high).

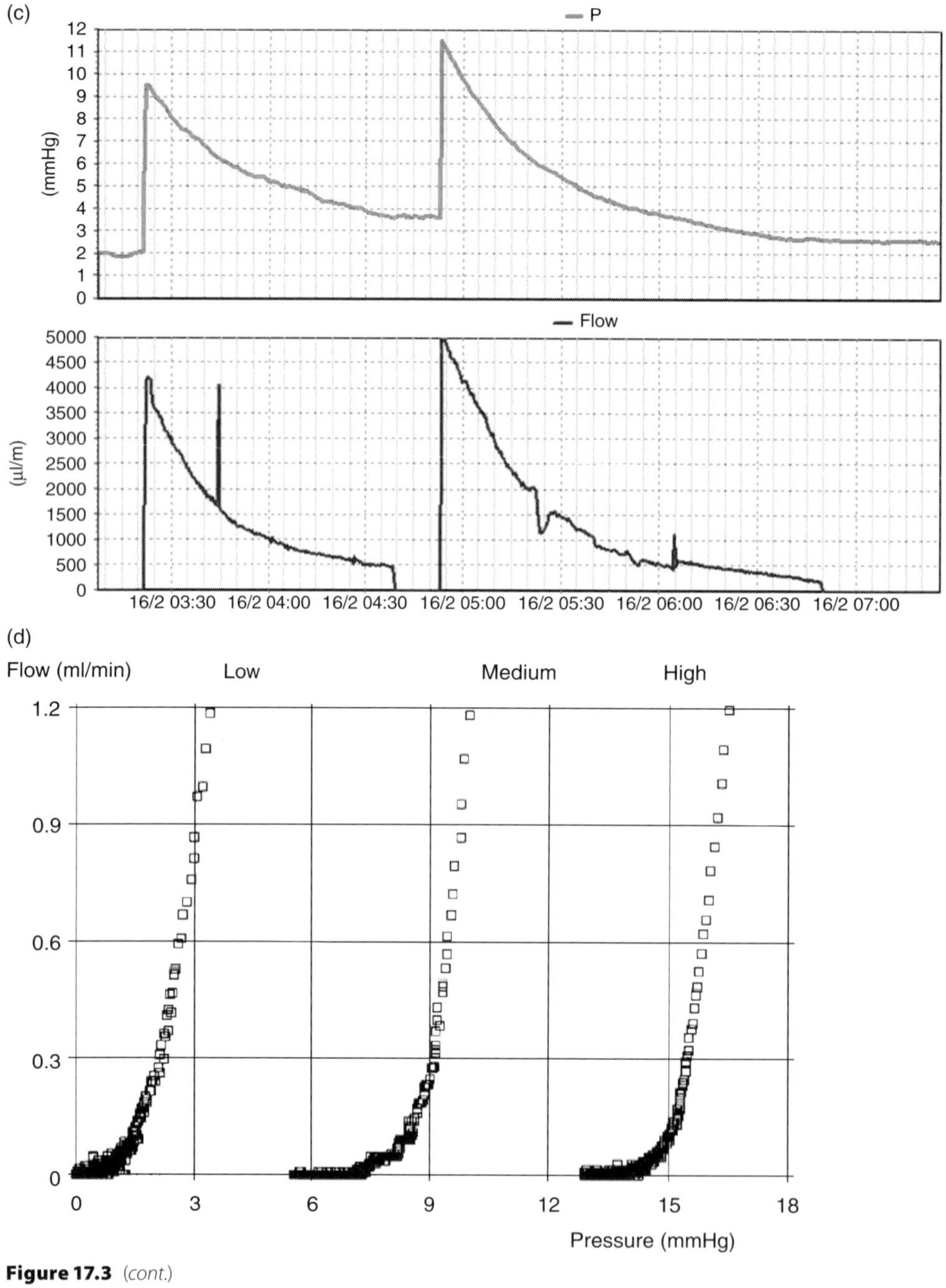

Figure 17.3 *(cont.)*

For different construction mechanisms, pressure–flow performance curves may have different shapes from completely linear (above opening pressure) to absolutely nonlinear (e.g. flow-regulating valves like Orbis-Sigma or Diamond). In some valves wide hysteresis of the performance curve can be seen, suggesting that measured differential pressure is dependent on flow through the shunt; silicone valves show particularly significant hysteresis whereas ball-on-spring valves are less susceptible. Ball-on-spring valves show usually better convergence of pressure–flow performance characteristics than membrane valves. Some constructions such as distal-slit valves may change their performance dramatically if distal arrangements change (wet or dry end, touching tissue at the outlet, or outlet being suspended in fluid).

Hydrodynamic resistance is calculated for pressures greater than valve opening pressure and is a well-defined parameter for valves with relatively linear pressure–flow performance curve; it cannot be evaluated for the Orbis-Sigma or Diamond valves (for these valves, stabilizing flow, hydrodynamic resistance is very high; theoretically infinite). In the literature, hydrodynamic resistance is commonly confused with operating pressure. The majority of the contemporary classic-differential shunts show low resistance to flow (as low as 1.05 mmHg/ml/min, which is substantially lower than physiological resistance to CSF drainage, measured at 6–10 mmHg/[ml/min] in normal subjects [15]). Low resistance is likely to result in overdrainage of CSF. Exceptions are the Medtronic Lumbo-Peritoneal Shunt, Codman Uni-Shunt, Sinu Shunt, and to some extent Holter Valve, of which the latter two have been discontinued. The resistance of the Uni-Shunt, however, may be strongly affected by conditions for flow at the distal end (e.g. in a peritoneal cavity).

Any repetitive variations of proximal pressure have a tendency to decrease the nominal operating pressure of shunts with unidirectional valves. This may lead to overdrainage in situations with regular vasogenic ICP waves or high respiratory fluctuations, particularly often seen in lumbopleural implantation. For this reason, lumbopleural shunts should be chosen from those with greater hydrodynamic resistance.

Long distal catheters increase resistance of the majority of classic-differential valves towards normal physiological values. It is important to remember that the resistance of a catheter is an inverse of the fourth power of its inner diameter and it is directly proportional to its length (Poisseuille's law). Therefore, a 1 m long catheter with a 1 mm inner diameter has a resistance of around 5 mmHg/(ml/min), while a similar length catheter of 1.2 mm inner diameter has a resistance of around 2.5 mmHg/(ml/min). A useful formula to calculate expected hydrodynamic resistance of the distal drain (it is always better to measure it – the resistance may be dependent on the materials used and the finish of the inner surface) is:

$$R = 5\frac{L}{D^4}$$

where D is an inner diameter expressed in millimeters and L is length expressed as a fraction of one meter (the above formula is valid for density and viscosity of CSF close to parameters of water).

By comparison, the resistance of the ventricular catheter is not greater than 1 mmHg/(ml/min). The number of patent holes in ventricular catheters does not usually change the resistance of the tubing as the resistance is mainly affected by the tube itself.

All valves with membrane siphon-preventing devices are sensitive to external pressure. External pressure exerted by tense skin or scar on the skin increases operating pressure of the valve. Increased external pressure (cap, headband) may close CSF drainage completely. External compression of the membrane is used in shunt testing in vivo to reveal patency of ventricular drain. All constructions without membrane siphon-preventing devices are not sensitive to external pressure up to 50 mmHg.

Negative outlet pressure decreases operating pressure by the same value in all valves without a siphon-preventing mechanism. When the resistance of the shunt system is low (4–6 mmHg/[ml/min]), negative outlet pressure of −15 mmHg may accelerate the drainage rate to a nonphysiological value of 2–4 ml/min. Overdrainage may also occur when a low resistance valve is subjected to repetitive cycling of proximal pressure (exceptions are Orbis-Sigma, Diamond Valve, and valves fitted with Codman SiphonGuard). Another rarely mentioned cause of overdrainage is "pumping" of proximal reservoir of the shunt [16], which is commonly performed in emergency departments when shunt dysfunction is suspected.

All adjustable valves can be reset in vivo by applying an external magnetic field. Most settings cover a range of operating pressures from 0 to 20 cmH_2O (0–15 mmHg). The number of steps varies from 5 to 20 (Table 17.2). In almost all valves, the levels are equally spaced, except for the Codman Certas Valve (Figure 17.4). In all valves except the Codman Hakim Programmable Valve, verification of the setting may be conveniently performed without the need for radiography using an external compass placed over the valve. Both measurement and adjustability may be affected if the valve rotates under the skin.

Magnetic fields can undesirably influence adjustable valve settings. The Sophy, Strata, Codman Hakim Programmable Valves can be readjusted by relatively weak fields (around 40 mT). Newer valves (Polaris, ProGAV, ProSA, and Certas) have mechanisms intended to prevent accidental readjustments, even in MRI scanners (up to 3T). All new valves tested were

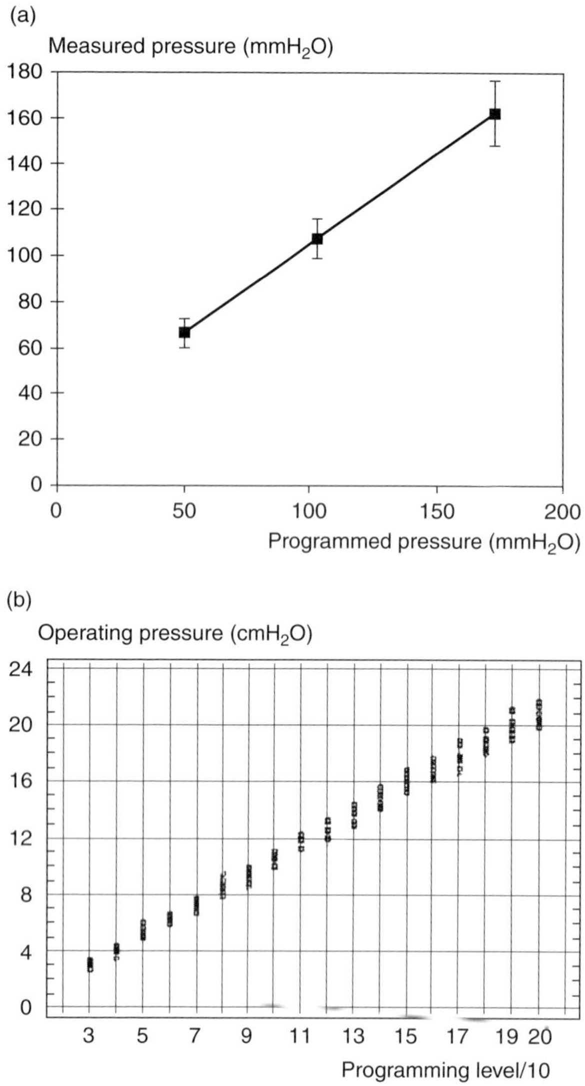

Figure 17.4 Shunt operating pressures assessed for different types of adjustable valves. (a) First adjustable valve Sophy (SU3), three levels adjusted magnetically. (b) Next generation Hakim-adjustable valve with 18 possible settings. This construction was much more precise, but a disadvantage was that the setting had to be confirmed with X-ray. Both constructions could be reset by a relatively weak magnetic field (20–40 milliteslas).

safe in MRI up to 3T (translational and torque forces are safe, heating is minimal), but cause significant distortion of the MR image. MR imaging of the brain is therefore unhelpful in these patients; however, it does facilitate MR imaging of other areas [17].

Small particles (10 μm, mimicking red blood cells) in the reagent tend to increase shunts' resistance or block them permanently. Large particles (25 μm) can block shunts, but sometimes tend to open them permanently (by suspending balls above surface of cone or membrane above the outlet orifice). However, it is not clear whether microspheres mimic the presence of particles in CSF.

Variations in temperature (30–40°C) have no meaningful effect on shunt functioning. Reflux was impossible in all tested valves up to 100 mmHg of reversal pressure difference. In abdominal placement of distal catheter, endoscopic laparoscopic procedure, when the abdomen is insufflated at high pressure (but definitely less than 100 mmHg), is safe. All junctions were free from leaks and breaks when tested according to ISO standard.

Shunt testing in vivo

Patients who never clinically improve, or improve and then worsen after CSF shunting, constitute a difficult group to manage, particularly with regard to establishing whether their clinical condition is due to shunt malfunction (under- or overdrainage) or any other overlapping diseases. It is believed that in adult patients across centers, 50–80% of shunted patients with a primary diagnosis of NPH improve after surgery (average probably around two-thirds). Whether shunt revision is necessary, and whether the repeated surgery can be recommended solely on the basis of clinical symptoms and brain imaging, is a notoriously difficult question to answer.

Various strategies exist, but in many circumstances clinical assessment, neuropsychological testing, and imaging are adequate to diagnose CSF shunt malfunction. However, in some clinical scenarios, particularly when the symptoms of shunt malfunction are insidious or subtle – such as in normal pressure hydrocephalus or partially compensated hydrocephalus overlapping with other diseases – other tools and techniques have been advocated with varying degrees of clinical usefulness. These include long-term monitoring of CSF pressure [18], shuntography [19], thermography [20], tympanometry [21], and transcranial Doppler ultrasonography [22]. If no additional tests are performed, patients usually end up with an excessive number of revisions, which hampers smooth management of the disease.

Variable or constant rate infusion studies of normal saline to evaluate a patient's CSF circulatory reserve have been previously described as useful in clinical practice. Using the model of CSF circulation in a shunted patient (Figure 17.1) and knowing the hydrodynamic parameters of an implanted shunt, it is possible to use the infusion test to assess the functioning of the shunt in vivo. Laboratory studies have supported the methodology and the choice of most relevant parameters and how to interpret their value [23–25]. This has been also confirmed by intraoperative findings [5].

It is important to remember that a shunt's opening (operating) pressure cannot be treated as an absolute determinant of intracranial pressure. The pressure on the site of drainage (peritoneum, atrium) has an impact. The effective pressure established on the proximal site of the shunt is affected by what is happening on the distal end, i.e. effective operating pressure should be increased by the pressure on the drainage side.

Proximal pressure = shunt operating pressure
+ distal outflow pressure
– "siphoning" in vertical body position.

In an obese patient or pregnant woman, the distal pressure can play a substantial role.

The methods of assessing CSF dynamics in shunted patients can be based on different techniques. The simplest and least invasive way is an infusion study through a previously implanted subcutaneous CSF reservoir. Lumbar puncture in communicating hydrocephalus or measurement of the pressure inside the chamber of the shunt is also possible. Pressure measurement and infusion into the shunt chamber is only possible with shunts having a CSF sampling reservoir proximal to the valve: therefore, the method is not applicable for the testing of some burr hole valves. Classic differential shunts should limit CSF pressure rise recorded during a constant rate infusion test [22,23] and hence abnormal pressure increase during the infusion is a crucial indicator of shunt underdrainage. The values of other parameters measured during the study are also meaningful, particularly the resistance to CSF outflow [24]. Also a comparison of results of the infusion study with those before the shunt insertion can be useful, especially with borderline results.

With pressure measurement via the shunt chamber the credibility of proper measurement of ICP should be confirmed. The presence of a CSF pressure pulse wave in the recorded signal and a pressure increase in response to coughing should confirm pressure transmission between the needle inserted in the shunt pre-chamber (25-gauge, not wider!) and the CSF space, consequently confirming the patency of the ventricular catheter.

For those valves with a low hydrodynamic resistance and a well-defined opening pressure, a sharp plateau of the pressure trend during infusion plateau phase should be seen at about 1–5 mmHg above the level of the shunt's critical pressure [25] (Figure 17.5a, b). The magnitude of this plateau should not exceed a value as defined by the equation:

$$\text{Critical pressure} = \text{shunt operating pressure} + (R_{shunt} \times \text{Infusion rate}) + 5\ \text{mmHg}$$

where R_{shunt} is the hydrodynamic resistance of the opened shunt.

Shunt operating pressure is the value of ICP that should be fixed when the opened shunt is draining CSF with the rate equal to that of its production. It is slightly higher than shunt opening pressure. Finally, constant of 5 mmHg is a "safety margin" also representing the value of non-zero abdominal pressure, which should be increased to 10–15 mmHg in obese people or pregnant women. Both shunt operating pressures and R_{shunt} can be measured in the laboratory (see above); these parameters provide guidelines for shunt testing in vivo [24,25].

When a shunted patient presents with low-pressure headache, small or slit ventricles, subdural collections, or chronic subdural hematomas, CSF overdrainage can be suspected. Reasons for overdrainage are diverse: the most common is postural overdrainage, but excessive dynamics of ICP (increased vasogenic waves, strong respiratory component) could result in excessive drainage even in the horizontal body position. In both situations different solutions would be recommended.

Overdrainage related to body posture may be assessed during the tilting test. Specific trends in pressure recording can be considered as signifying overdrainage. When the baseline pressure measured in the horizontal body position is low (usually negative) overdrainage is possible. A change to upright body position usually produces a further, excessive decrease in pressure. If the pressure decreases to a value lower than −10 mmHg (95% confidence limit for ICP in upright position in non-shunted patients is approximately −8 mmHg) overdrainage is likely (Figure 17.5c).

As the majority of contemporary valves usually have a low hydrodynamic resistance, this may cause overdrainage resulting from the periodic oscillations of cerebrovascular volume. The expanding vascular bed would act like the membrane of a water pump with a distal low-resistance valve. Early morning headache

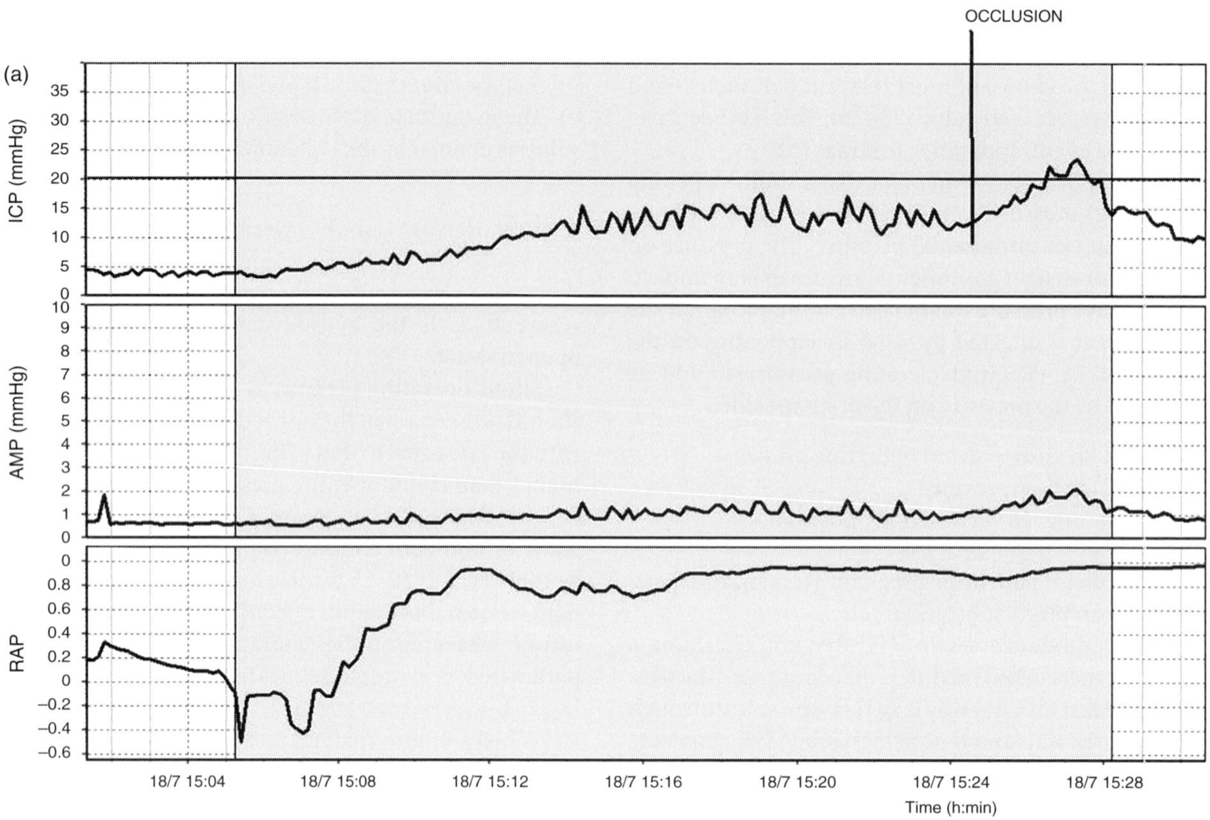

Figure 17.5 Examples of infusion studies performed in shunted patients through shunt pre-chamber with working (upper panel) and blocked (lower) shunt. (a) Patient with a Strata Valve set at 1.5. Pulse amplitude was low but clearly recordable, suggesting patency of ventricular drain. Opening pressure was low, and during infusion pressure increased to the value below the "critical threshold" for this valve (thick vertical line). During infusion, transcutaneous occlusion (external compression of siphon-control device) was performed (such a compression stops the drainage through the valve). Pressure started to rise immediately, confirming that shunt system was patent. Compensatory reserve was good at the baseline (RAP around 0). (b) Patient with Hakim-Programmable Valve set at 100 mmH_2O. Pressure increased well above "critical threshold" (horizontal line). Compensatory reserve was depleted at baseline (RAP >0.6). Pulse waveform was present in recording. There was distal obstruction of the shunt system confirmed during the revision of the shunt. (c) Tests for the posture-related overdrainage. Top: no overdrainage (patient with ASD put in-line with the shunt); pressure decreased in sitting position to −5 mmHg, Bottom: the overdrainage manifested by a decrease in ICP in sitting position below −10 mmHg. After the return to the horizontal position ICP was significantly lower than at baseline. (d) In patients with slit ventricles the pulse wave of ICP is rarely visible in recording. During infusion into a shunt pre-chamber all fluid is drained distally. Hence the recorded pressure is equivalent to the shunt operating pressure plus the pressure gradient along the distal tube plus the abdominal pressure. Respiratory waves may be visible, commonly transmitted from the abdominal space. In patients with a membrane siphon-preventing device, occlusion can be performed during pressure increases quickly to very high values (in this case above 70 mmHg), collapsed ventricles open within a relatively short time, pressure stabilizes at a lower level with a pulse wave clearly visible (arterial pulse from Finapress device is presented in the upper panel for comparison). The "stabilization pressure" is elevated as intraparenchymal ICP is usually high in slit ventricle syndrome. Ventricles may stay open over longer period of time, but more frequently they collapse again after the end of infusion (sharp decrease in recorded pressure after release of occlusion).

should not always be assumed to be high pressure: they may instead be a consequence of low pressure caused by nocturnal overdrainage [25].

In shunted patients with slit ventricles, baseline pressure recorded from the shunt pre-chamber would not comprise a pulse waveform, and should not be regarded as the patient's intracranial pressure. The walls of the ventricle would be collapsed around the catheter and thus no pressure transmission would take place. However, the pulse wave often appears after infusion is started, as the pressure builds up and opens up the ventricles (Figure 17.5d).

Shunt registry

The last but not least piece of "shunto-logy" is the possibility of tracing individual shunt function using a concept of "shunt registry" and converting it to a

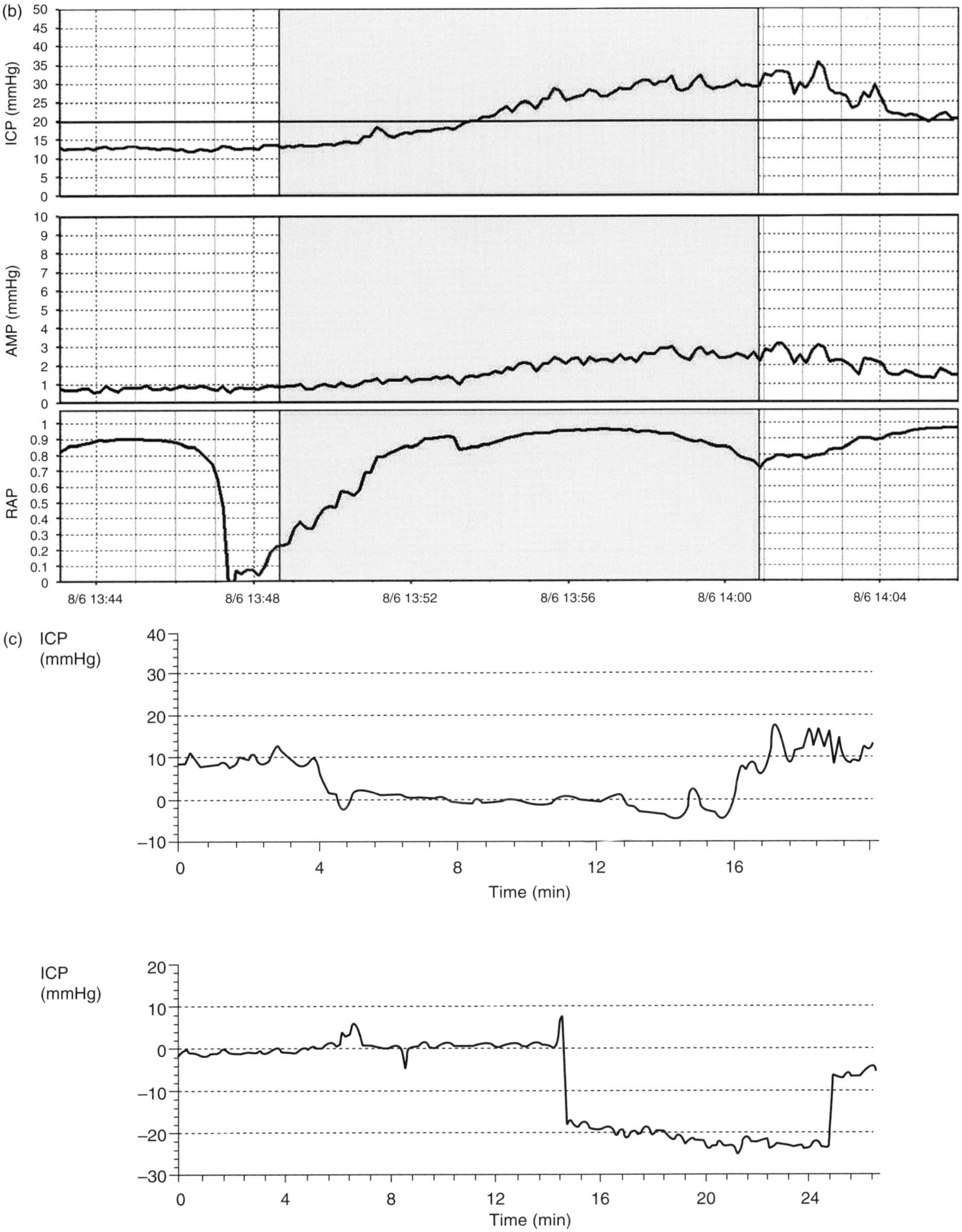

Figure 17.5 *(cont.)*

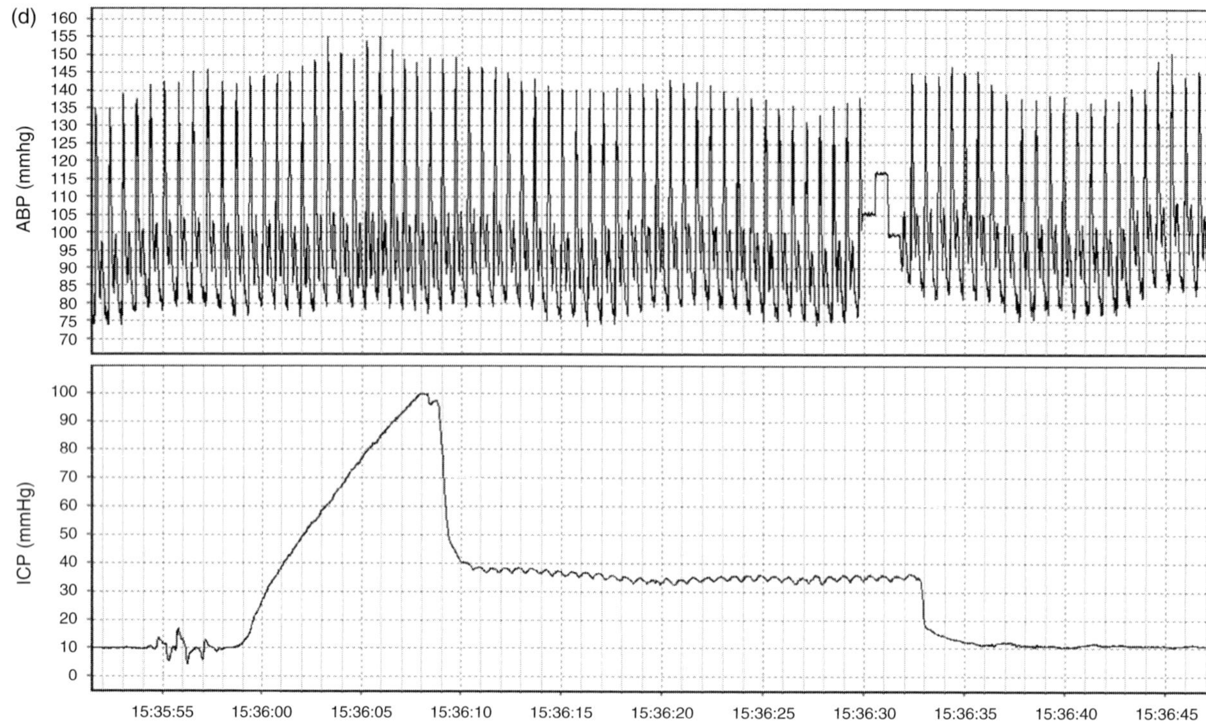

Figure 17.5 *(cont.)*

statistically justifiable picture through the mass entry of data from different centers.

Unlike pharmacological agents, medical devices do not require clinical trials before introduction to the market. It is therefore important that their performance in patients is carefully monitored. Apart from shunt evaluation in the laboratory, an effective way of achieving this is through national registries. The UK Shunt Registry has been active since May 1994, and now holds data on over 65 000 shunt and shunt-related procedures. The valves and shunts currently used in the UK appear to work to the manufacturers' specifications and hardware failures are rare. Recent years have seen the increased popularity of adjustable valves and the introduction of antibiotic-impregnated catheters. The performances of both these products are continuously being evaluated by the UK Shunt Registry [26] and, in combination with the information from the Shunt Evaluation Laboratory, should provide robust data on the efficacy of various shunt systems in specific pathophysiological circumstances.

The future of shunt technology

Shunting, particularly for normal pressure hydrocephalus in the elderly, is an empiric way of managing the disease process. Although the majority of patients improve, the improvement is sometimes questionable and might be short-lasting. It remains, however, an open question whether any other approach besides shunting may improve this situation.

The complications still accompanying shunting (infections, misplacement of ventricular drain, disconnections, overdrainage, and distal obstruction) remain a significant problem. Flow-regulating devices like the passive Orbis-Sigma valve were an interesting solution [4] in shunt technology. Unfortunately, the assumption that everyone has the same CSF production rate of 0.35 ml/min, without the possibility of adjusting this level in vivo as in differential-pressure adjustable valves, has proven detrimental. In the age of adjustable devices, few people would consider the fixed-flow valve as an ideal remedy.

Adjustable pressure, fixed flow; what about adjustable hydrodynamic resistance? This is still an unexplored idea and we only hope that someone will use it in construction of a new family of valves.

Probably, active valves, pumping CSF from ventricles or lumbar space (sometimes the end of the lumbar space is named "the fifth ventricle" – an interesting concept! Professor V. Varsos, personal communication), regardless of pressure gradients and body position, will be the valve of the future. It is interesting that active valves (i.e. active pumps) have never been tried seriously in clinical practice; however, the concepts were outlined in some detail in the scientific press [27]. Power supply seems to be a major obstacle here, as construction of bio-compatible micro-pumps based on MEMS technology seems to be possible nowadays [28].

Acknowledgments

We wish to express our gratitude to all colleagues who contributed to our shunt evaluation program, Dr. Helen Whitehouse, Dr. Steven Price, and our students: Rosie Taylor, Adam Bromby, David Alin, and A. Chari. We also want to thank Tim Rodwell from the Medical Device Agency and Dr. A. Aschoff from the Department of Neurosurgery at the University of Heidelberg for their helpful guidance.

References

1. Momjian S, Owler BK, Czosnyka Z, et al. Pattern of white matter regional cerebral blood flow and autoregulation in normal pressure hydrocephalus. *Brain* 2004;127(Pt 5):965–72.
2. Marmarou A, Shulman K, Rosende RM. A non-linear analysis of the CSF system and intracranial pressure dynamics. *J Neurosurg* 1978;48:332–44.
3. Ekstedt J. CSF hydrodynamic studies in man. Normal hydrodynamic variables related to CSF pressure and flow. *J Neurol Neurosurg Psychiatry* 1978;41:345–53.
4. Sainte-Rose C, Hooven MD, Hirsch JF. A new approach to the treatment of hydrocephalus. *J Neurosurg* 1987;66:213–26.
5. Petrella G, Czosnyka M, Smielewski P, et al. In vivo assessment of hydrocephalus shunt. *Acta Neurol Scand* 2009;120(5):317–23.
6. Marmarou A. A theoretical model and experimental evaluation of the cerebrospinal fluid system. Thesis, Drexel University, Philadelphia, PA; 1973.
7. Avezaat CJJ, Eijndhoven JHM. Cerebrospinal fluid pulse pressure and craniospinal dynamics. A theoretical, clinical and experimental study. Thesis, Jongbloed, The Hague; 1984.
8. Sliwka S. A clinical system for the evaluation of selected dynamic properties of the intracranial system. PhD thesis, Polish Academy of Sciences, Warsaw; 1980 (in Polish).
9. Czosnyka Z, Czosnyka M, Richards HK, Pickard JD. Posture-related overdrainage: comparison of the performance of 10 hydrocephalus shunts in vitro. *Neurosurgery* 1998;42(2):327–33.
10. Gjerris F, Snorrason E. The history of hydrocephalus. *J Hist Neurosci* 1992;1(4):285–312.
11. Sood S, Kumar CR, Jamous M, et al. Pathophysiological changes in cerebrovascular distensibility in patients undergoing chronic shunt therapy. *J Neurosurg* 2004;100(5 Suppl Pediatrics):447–53.
12. Chumas PD, Armstrong DC, Drake JM et al. Tonsillar herniation: the rule rather than exception after lumboperitoneal shunting in the paediatric population. *J Neurosurg* 1993;78:568–73.
13. Czosnyka ZH, Cieslicki K, Czosnyka M, Pickard JD. Hydrocephalus shunts and waves of intracranial pressure. *Med Biol Eng Comput* 2005;43(1):71–7.
14. Aschoff A, Kremer P, Benesch C, et al. Overdrainage and shunt technology. *Childs Nerv Syst* 1995;11:193–202.
15. Bromby A, Czosnyka Z, Allin D, et al. Laboratory study on "intracranial hypotension" created by pumping the chamber of a hydrocephalus shunt. *Cerebrospinal Fluid Res* 2007;4:2.
16. Lavinio A, Harding S, Van Der Boogaard F, et al. Magnetic field interactions in adjustable hydrocephalus shunts. *Neurosurg Pediatr* 2008;2(3):222–8.
17. Schuhmann MU, Sood S, McAllister JP, et al. Value of overnight monitoring of intracranial pressure in hydrocephalic children. *Pediatr Neurosurg* 2008;44(4):269–79.
18. May CH, Aurisch R, Kornrumpf D, Vogel S. Evaluation of shunt function in hydrocephalic patients with the radionuclide 99mTc-pertechnetate. *Childs Nerv Syst* 1999;15(5):239–44;
19. Caldarelli M, Di Rocco C, Cellini N, De Santis M. A technique for evaluation of CSF shunt patency using telethermography. *Neuropediatrics* 1981;12:303–7.
20. Samuel M, Burge DM, Marchbanks RJ. Tympanic membrane displacement testing in regular assessment of intracranial pressure in eight children with shunted hydrocephalus. *J Neurosurg* 1998;88:983–95.
21. Quinn MW, Pople IK. Middle cerebral artery pulsatility in children with blocked cerebrospinal fluid shunts. *J Neurol Neurosurg Psychiatry* 1992;55:325–7.
22. Taylor R, Czosnyka Z, Czosnyka M, Pickard JD. A laboratory model of testing shunt performance after implantation. *Br J Neurosurg* 2002;16:30–5.
23. Czosnyka ZH, Czosnyka M, Pickard JD. Shunt testing in-vivo: a method based on the data from the UK shunt evaluation laboratory. *Acta Neurochir Suppl* 2002;81:27–30.
24. Malm J, Kristensen B, Fagerlund M, Koskinen LO, Ekstedt J. Cerebrospinal fluid shunt dynamics

in patients with idiopathic adult hydrocephalus syndrome. *J Neurol Neurosurg Psychiatry* 1995;58(6):715–23.

25. Czosnyka Z, Czosnyka M, Richards HK, Pickard JD. Laboratory testing of hydrocephalus shunts – conclusion of the UK Shunt evaluation programme. *Acta Neurochir (Wien)* 2002;144(6):525–38.
26. Richards HK, Seeley HM, Pickard JD. Efficacy of antibiotic-impregnated shunt catheters in reducing shunt infection: data from the United Kingdom Shunt Registry. *J Neurosurg Pediatr* 2009;4(4):389–93.
27. Chung S, Kim JK, Wang KC, Han DC, Chang JK. Development of MEMS-based cerebrospinal fluid shunt system. *Biomed Microdevices* 2003;5(4):311–21.
28. Ezkerra A, Fernández LJ, Mayora K, Ruano-López JM. SU8 diaphragm micropump with monolithically integrated cantilever check valves. *Lab Chip* 2011;11(19):3320–5.

Chapter 18

Management of shunts in normal pressure hydrocephalus
Follow-up and late complications

Ahmed Mohyeldin, Ammar Shaikhouni, and John McGregor

Introduction

Normal pressure hydrocephalus (NPH) was classically defined by Solomon Hakim in his seminal thesis in 1964 and then later more formally with Raymond Adams in 1965 with the clinical triad of psychomotor retardation, gait apraxia and imbalance, and urinary incontinence [1,2]. When an identifiable risk factor such as inflammation, hemorrhage, infection, or traumatic brain injury has been implicated in the diagnosis of NPH it is often referred to as secondary NPH as opposed to idiopathic NPH (iNPH), the term used when no clear etiology is identified. A working diagnosis for NPH is made when then this constellation of symptoms is associated with clinical signs and radiographic evidence of ventricular system enlargement in the context of normal cerebrospinal fluid (CSF) opening pressures [3].

CSF diversion using the most common methods of ventriculoperitoneal or ventriculoatrial shunting has emerged as a useful tool in the management of this condition, carrying the potential for dramatic improvement in quality of life and reversal of the debilitating symptoms that so often characterize this disease process [3–5]. Several systematic reviews have reported improvement of symptoms in 30–50% of patients with idiopathic NPH and 50–70% of those with secondary NPH, underscoring the rising practice of CSF diversion in this disorder [5–7]. With increasing improvements in diagnostic testing and shunting equipment, the success rates for shunting procedures seem to have increased over time [8]. In addition, the incidence and prevalence of normal pressure hydrocephalus appear to be increasing as well. The incidence of shunt-responsive NPH has been reported in the past to be around 2.2 per million persons per year. With improvements in preoperative evaluations, heightened awareness, and an aging population, it is thought to be increasing [9]. Brean et al., in 2008, suggested that in Vestfold County, Norway, NPH had a prevalence of 21.9, and an incidence of 5.5 per 100 000 individuals based on the numbers of patient referrals with the appropriate diagnostic and clinical criteria. In addition, they noted that the highest prevalence of patients identified in their study was found in the 70- to 79-year-old age group (181.7/100 000), and second highest in the over 80 age group (93.3/100 000) [10,11]. While recognizing that this is a fairly homogeneous local population, it should be noted that those age groups are currently, and are projected to continue to be, among the fastest growing segments of the US population, based on the 2010 Census Data [12].

Due to the elderly demographic in whom this syndrome has been most often described, particularly between the sixth and eighth decades of life, establishing an accurate diagnosis distinguishing the syndrome from other potential comorbid medical conditions in the differential remains challenging. Ancillary tests such as high volume CSF spinal taps, external continuous lumbar drainage trials, and CSF outflow resistance studies have provided some tools with positive predictive values as to who will benefit from CSF shunting [13]. Unfortunately these tests have also been demonstrated to have low negative predictive values, and thus likely to fail to identify some patients who actually may benefit from shunting [14,15]. Meanwhile, neurosurgeons who offer a CSF diversion procedure to potential NPH patients are doubly challenged to evaluate the risk-to-benefit ratio of the procedure from the standpoint of the consequences of shunt-related complications associated with the procedure itself [9]. There is controversy surrounding the potential for complications

Adult Hydrocephalus, ed. Daniele Rigamonti. Published by Cambridge University Press.

from shunting. That, coupled with the variable results following CSF diversions which have been noted historically, has led some to believe that the overall morbidity rate for shunting NPH patients may even outweigh the benefits [9]. In addition, many studies have limited the analysis of risk and benefit to the early period following surgery, within the first months following the procedure. There are, however, important contributions that attempt to include the long-term results and possible complications following shunting. This chapter hopes to compile, compare, and place into context the incidence and the relevance of shunt-related complications, with special emphasis on infections. The chapter will review the types of late complications, their likelihood, and some clinical examples. We review here the late infection rates and identify key pathogens and associated risk factors that predispose to shunt infections. And lastly we review current strategies aimed at reducing the likelihood of shunt complications and shunt infection rates and discuss interventions at patient follow-up that can assist in maximizing benefit from shunt procedures, and help in maintaining symptomatic relief in patients following shunt surgery for NPH.

Types of shunt complications

CSF shunting and particularly ventriculoperitoneal shunting is a common procedure used to treat a variety of CSF flow dynamic pathologies including obstructive, communicating, and normal pressure hydrocephalus from a variety of etiologies. As with any treatment modality, and especially with any surgical procedure, there are inherent potential risks to treatment, which in the case of shunt surgery include infection, possible shunt-induced complications, and failure of the therapy to provide relief. In general there are several types of specific long-term complications associated with shunting procedures in addition to those more likely seen in the NPH population in particular. These include underdrainage of CSF, overdrainage of CSF, mechanical failures of the hardware such as alterations in valve resistance over time, malposition of the tubing, and frank breakage, CSF leak, subdural hemorrhage or hygroma, seizure, and infection.

Underdrainage and overdrainage

The symptoms of underdrainage tend to be those of return of the NPH triad. With either underdrainage or mechanical failure, the identification of these patients occurs when their symptoms return after a period of initial improvement following shunting. Patients who demonstrate initial improvement in gait, urinary continence, and cognition, who then deteriorate with return of their initial symptoms complex either partially or completely, are to be suspected of mechanical failure or underdrainage. Underdrainage conditions arise when shunt systems develop increased resistance across the valve over time, disconnection or kinking of the system components, or migration of the tubing out of an appropriate position for proper drainage and/or reabsorption. With the development of variable resistance valves that allow adjustment over time, patients are able to have their diversion rates changed based on symptoms of over- and underdrainage. It is not clear that any of these opportunities have decreased the need for subsequent revisions in this patient population over time as the revision rates remain fairly consistent across the studies over the years, but they may be associated with an improvement in general in the success rate in maintaining patients' symptomatic improvement [5,8].

The symptoms of overdrainage are also well described. Patients may complain of positional headaches or dizziness, imbalance, visual difficulties, or auditory changes. This clinical situation may need to be managed by changing the resistance in the shunt system, either by revision or adjustment. Adjustment of a programmable valve to a higher resistance, or revision of the valve system to a higher pressure, antisiphon device, or a valve with a decreased fixed flow rate may be warranted. Overdrainage does put patients at an increased risk for subdural hematoma or hygroma formation. Patients with these conditions present with new onset of headaches, unilateral or bilateral, mental status changes, motor or sensory impairments, or seizures. Imaging studies, either MRI or CT, can document the occurrence of extra-axial fluid collections. Management of the acute subdural hygroma/hematoma can be quite challenging. Acute intervention may be required and may run the gamut from simple adjustment of the shunt resistance, revision or occlusion of the shunt system, to burr hole evacuation, craniotomy and evacuation, and rarely complete craniectomy followed later by cranioplasty. Staged procedures may be necessary to complete the recovery of the more complicated clinical situations. Close follow-up is likely required with serial CT scans and/or MRI scans to assess for recovery and to gauge the advisability and timing of returning the patient back to a shunt in working order.

Imaging

Evaluation of the CSF diversion system may be accomplished by a combination of imaging and laboratory analyses. X-rays of the tubing system assess for position and continuity. A radiolucent gap along the path of the shunt is an indication of a possible disconnect. CT scans of the brain assess for shunt position and associated extra-axial fluid collection intracranially such as subdural hematoma or hygroma. CT scan of the abdomen will evaluate for tubing location, the possibility of intra-abdominal pseudocyst formation within the peritoneum, a clue to shunt infection, and extraperitoneal pseudomeningocele and/or coiling of the tubing suggestive of malposition of the catheter (as in Figure 18.1). CSF analysis via either a shunt reservoir aspiration or via a lumbar puncture may be needed to address the possibility of infection. MRI of the brain can document the proper location of the catheter within the ventricular system, can evaluate for extra-axial fluid, persistent periventricular white matter edema associated with underdrainage, and exuberant dural enhancement which may be indicative of an overdrainage condition (as in Figures 18.2 and 18.3) [16].

Shunt complication rates

Many studies have tried to address the overall complication rates for shunting procedures. Reddy et al. recently performed a retrospective review of 1015 ventriculoperitoneal shunts performed at their institution from 1961 to 2010 [17]; 70% were adults, 12% were NPH. In their study population, they identified 2239 total shunt procedures, of which 1224 were revision surgeries. It was noted, however, that in their adult patients only 39% of the surgeries were for revision, substantially less than for the general shunt population [17]. Others have demonstrated that 70–80% of patients with shunts, adult and children, and multiple diagnoses, will require at least one revision at some point in time [17–19]. Infections compromise a significant subset of shunt complications. They are associated with an increased risk of seizures, reduced intellectual performance, increased long-term mortality rate, and neurological disability and account for longer hospitalizations [20,21]. Studies that have looked at the overall complication rates of ventriculoperitoneal shunt have identified that despite the near universal use of preoperative and postoperative antibiotics, around 1–25% become infected [22,23]. A more specific number has been identified in two larger prospective trials with defined variables for infection in pediatric populations,

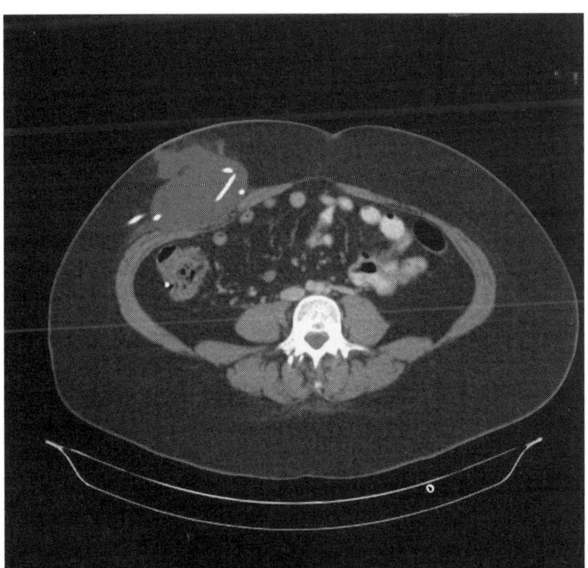

Figure 18.1 Abdominal CT scan in a patient with a ventriculoperitoneal shunt. Note migration of the abdominal catheter into the extraperitoneal space and a surrounding CSF collection.

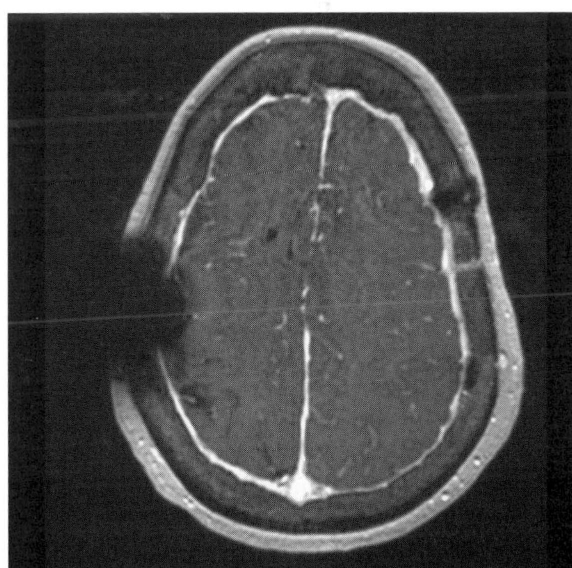

Figure 18.2 Contrast MRI shows exuberant dural enhancement suggestive of intracranial hypotension in a patient with NPH, a ventriculoperitoneal shunt, and a programmable valve (note the right parietal magnetic artifact). This finding is reversible. See Figure 18.3.

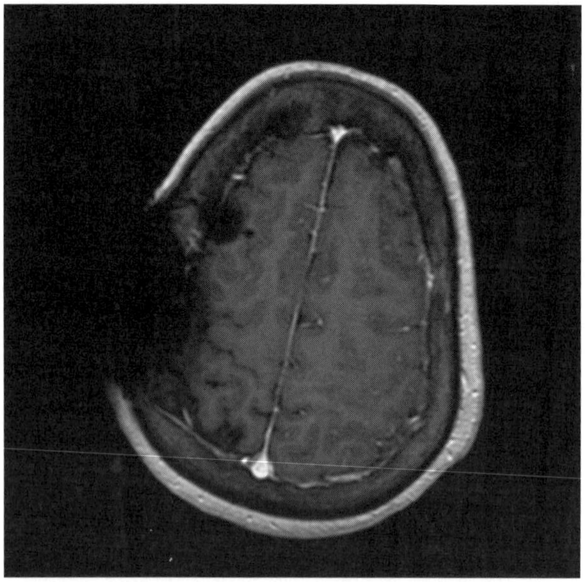

Figure 18.3 Contrast MRI in same patient as in Figure 18.2. This is the follow-up study 3 months after adjustment of the programmable valve. Normal dural enhancement suggestive of intracranial normotension is noted.

which reported rates ranging from 8% to 10% [24,25]. The recent review by Reddy et al. in 2012 also looked at long-term infection rates in their mixed adult and pediatric group of 1015 patients whose hydrocephalus was managed with a ventriculoperitoneal shunt. They demonstrated a per patient overall infection rate of 10.5%; however, only 2.4% were in patients with NPH [17].

Ventriculoperitoneal shunt complications and infections in NPH patients

CSF shunting for NPH patients has become increasingly common, and may be underutilized as a treatment modality [11]. Cognitive decline associated with NPH is a known cause of preventable dementia, and the at-risk population is increasing in number. Ancillary tests such as external continuous lumbar drainage trials, high volume CSF taps, and CSF outflow resistance studies have increased the preoperative positive predictive values as to who will benefit from CSF shunting [13]. As more is understood about the pathophysiology of this disorder, the decision as to which preoperative indicators might help predict those who will benefit from shunting will aid surgeons in assisting patients in their decisions about the benefits versus risks of placement of a shunt. The risks associated with surgery in this patient population have been studied over time. Table 18.1 presents the data from multiple recent series that attempted to give an estimate of the rate of complication associated with CSF diversion procedures in the population of patients with NPH.

Vanneste et al. reviewed their experience with shunting procedures from 1980 to 1989, and reviewed the literature from 1966 to 1980 [9]. They described up to a 27% overall complication rate within the first 2 months, but the long-term postsurgical morbidity and mortality from shunting in their NPH populations was 3% in patients with secondary NPH and 9% in patients they felt had true idiopathic NPH. These results included complications associated with all patients' comorbidities, and were not specifically limited to neurologic sequelae [9]. Boon et al. in 1997 [26] and 1998 [27] in the Dutch Normal-Pressure Hydrocephalus Study performed a prospective study enrolling 101 patients with NPH who underwent placement of a ventriculoperitoneal shunt and then underwent follow-up evaluations for one year. They noted that their population had extensive comorbidities, 48 past and current neurological and 190 non-neurological conditions. They observed 5 deaths in the first month from comorbidities, and 10 died over the next 11 months from comorbidities that included cerebral and cardiac ischemia and pneumonia. These data indicate the significance of comorbidities in the patient population at risk [26]. They also noted an increased risk of subdural effusions in patients receiving a low pressure shunt system (71%) compared to medium pressure systems (34%) [27].

Hebb and Cusimano performed their meta-analysis in 2001, which analyzed the literature to include all clinical trials of shunting in patients with NPH from 1966 through 2000 [28]. They identified 35 independent studies and a total patient population of 883. Their results are also included in the data presented in Table 18.1. The overall incidence of complications of any sort, acute or late, was 38% (of which 22% were shunt revisions), and they noted a 6% rate of long-term neurologic morbidity or mortality [28]. Since then, additional studies have added insight to help clarify long-term complication rates from CSF diversion procedures in patients with normal pressure hydrocephalus. Savolainen et al., in 2002, published their series of 51 patients, all less than 75 years of age, who were treated for NPH between 1993 and 1995, and then

Table 18.1 Complications from shunting in patients with NPH[a]

	Patients (n)	Follow-up (months)	Reoperation (%)	SDH	Hygroma	Infection	SDH surgery	Stroke	Distal failure	Proximal failure	Valve failure	Over-drainage	Lack of benefit	Seizure	Malfunction
Bloch and McDermott, 2012 [31]	33	19	27%	0	0	6%	0		1%	12%	6%	6%	0%		
Klinge et al., 2012 [8]	115	12	15%	6%	9%	1%	1%		4%	4%	4%	2%	17%		
Pujari et al., 2008 [5]	55	70	53%			10%							13%		46%
McGirt et al. 2005 [29]	132	18	33%	2%		6.7%	2%		21%	9%		15%	15%		33%
Marmarou et al., 2005 [30]	151	12		2%	2%	2%							9.5%		
Savolainen et al., 2002 [4]	51	60											50%		
Hebb and Cusimano, 2001 [28]	883	var.	17%	19%		5%		6%					41%	4%	18%
Boon et al., 1997 [26]	96	12	19%	53%		3%	8%	2%	10%	9%			41%	1%	19%
Vanneste et al., 1992 [9]	152	37		15%		4%		9%					63%	3%	21%

[a] Cells left blank if authors did not report the indicated data. See text for additional analysis.

followed for 5 years [4]. Their study used specific established criteria for proceeding with CSF diversion. Half of their patients underwent placement of a ventriculoperitoneal shunt and half did not. At 5-year follow-up eight patients with a shunt and nine patients without a shunt had died of complications associated with their comorbidities, none of which were shunt related according to the authors [4]. McGirt et al., in 2005, reviewed their single institution population of 132 patients with normal pressure hydrocephalus treated between 1993 and 2003, who underwent shunting procedures. They describe a 33% revision rate, a 2% late complication rate, and 1% mortality [29]. Marmarou et al. also in 2005 reviewed their series of 151 patients who were evaluated for idiopathic NPH between 1993 and 2003 of which 102 were treated with shunt surgery and then followed for 12 months [30]. They noted that 24 patients had complications overall, of which 10 (9.8%) were major complications including infection, subdural hematoma, and a venous sinus thrombosis. All but the patient with the sinus thrombosis had partial or complete recovery [30]. Pujari et al., in a 2008 retrospective analysis, reviewed the revision rates for their series of 55 patients who had 3 or more years of follow-up after an initial shunt procedure for the treatment of NPH [5]. They reported a revision rate of 53%, in this group, half of these after the first year of follow-up, the majority of revisions being for shunt malfunction. However, they noted that revisions, sometimes multiple over the study period in some patients, were still associated with a 74% incidence of symptomatic improvement. They concluded that with attention to follow-up, and monitoring for possible shunt obstructions or dysfunctions, there is a better chance of sustaining symptomatic improvement in this patient population [5]. Klinge et al. published in 2012 their results from the European multicenter study on idiopathic normal pressure hydrocephalus [8]. The series consisted of 115 patients who had undergone ventriculoperitoneal shunt placement for idiopathic NPH and who had completed their 1-year follow-up. The authors noted an overall complication rate requiring further surgery of 15% and 1% infection rate. They noted a complication rate not requiring surgery of 13%. They also noted that with the use of an adjustable shunt valve system they were able to make a total of 76 adjustments over the year in 36 patients (31%). Such attention to adjustments may help to minimize the complication rate due to over- or underdrainage [8]. For comparison, Bloch and McDermott performed a retrospective analysis of patients with idiopathic normal pressure hydrocephalus treated only with a lumboperitoneal shunt [31]. The review consisted of 33 patients in this report. They were followed annually for an average of 19 months (1–94). Nine patients (27%) required at least one revision. Two patients developed shunt infections. No patients developed subdural hematomas. The authors suggest that a shunt in the lumboperitoneal configuration is not more likely to need further surgery than a shunt in the ventricular configuration [31].

Shunt infections

Infection-related complications of CSF diversion for hydrocephalus, while not as common as shunt malfunction, are potentially serious developments in this population. In patients with shunts placed for any cause, those that develop infections suffer almost twice the risk of death and are three times more likely to undergo multiple shunt revision surgeries as patients who don't develop infections [32,33]. In Hebb and Cusimano's review, overall infection rate was 5% with a range of 0–18% [28]. Recent reports from large long-term outcome studies on patients who underwent CSF diversion for normal pressure hydrocephalus show similar infection rates [34]. Zemack and Romner described their experience implanting adjustable shunts in 218 NPH patients with an infection rate of 6.4% [34]. McGirt et al. included 132 patients who underwent shunt implantations for normal pressure hydrocephalus with an overall infection of 6.7% [29]. Pujari et al. reported a shunt infection rate of 10% in their series of 55 NPH patients [5].

Also as noted above, results from Reddy et al. in their large single institution study showed that first time shunt infection rates in adults are lower than those in children. Interestingly the same study showed shunts implanted to treat normal pressure hydrocephalus were associated with a lower infection rate (2.4%) in comparison to shunts implanted to treat other hydrocephalus etiologies (10.5%) [17]. Aside from age, other described risk factors for the development of shunt infections include placement of a shunt after previous shunt infections and the neurosurgeon's experience [35,36].

Common pathogens and common sources of shunt infections and their sequelae

The mechanisms that explain shunt infections are not completely understood. The most common source of infection is colonization of the shunt catheter at time of implantation [35,37]. This can be due to improper handling of the catheter by surgeon or operating room staff or improper sterilization and preparation of the skin prior to implantation of the shunt. Other causes of shunt infection include retrograde infection of the system from the distal catheter. This can occur at time of insertion of the catheter by inadvertent bowel injury or later on due to spontaneous infection or perforation of viscera. This becomes important in the NPH patient population due to the risk for diverticulosis and diverticulitis in this age group [38]. A third important source of shunt infection is local irritation, infection, and skin erosion around the shunt material. This can be due to erosion of the valve itself through the skin, which is more common in older patients with reduced skin thickness. However, most commonly this occurs through skin infection over the shunt tract either due to infection of a pressure ulcer or the development of spontaneous cellulitis. These are more common in the older patient in general, the less mobile, the gait impaired, and the patient at risk for soiling, which often describes the NPH patient. Furthermore, NPH patients commonly suffer from other comorbidities placing them at high risk to receive surgical procedures in the areas traversed by shunt hardware, such as stimulators, pacemakers, central venous catheters, tracheotomies, hernia repairs, laparoscopic procedures, or feeding tubes, which subject their shunt to potential contact with contamination or infected fluids leading to secondary infections [35].

Based on the above mechanisms it is not surprising that the most common pathogens related to shunt infection are from skin flora or abdominal species. These likely infect the shunt through direct seeding and colonization during shunt manipulation and placement or retrograde contamination or infection of the intra-abdominal distal catheter. One study in particular has identified common pathogens that were isolated from a large series of adult patients with infected implanted shunts [39]. Similar results were described in other studies [32,35,40,41]. Many of the implicated bacteria are biofilm formers. These bacteria irreversibly attach to the catheter material, forming a colonization of the catheter [42]. Within this ecosystem, the bacteria that are colonized in the catheter material become resistant to treatment and over time migrate proximally or distally along the catheter tract or shed bacterial emboli. The development of antibiotic-impregnated shunts (AIS) shows promise as an effective way to prevent the development of these biofilms. Studies have shown that these catheters are associated with decreased infection rates [41].

Once infection develops, the symptoms are nonspecific except for the rare classic cases that represent medical emergencies. The most common presenting symptom is fever, present in 14–90% of cases [35,39]. Other symptoms include general malaise, headache, neck stiffness, photophobia, and possibly meningismus associated with meningitis or ventriculitis. Symptoms of shunt failure, which for the NPH patient could mean return of the preoperative symptoms, and cellulitis overlying any portion of the shunt components, could also be indicative of shunt infection. Abdominal pain, distension, nausea, vomiting, and intraperitoneal pseudocyst formation or pleuritic discomfort and shortness of breath may also be associated with infection of the distal peritoneal or pleural portion of the shunt system, depending on the location of the distal catheter. Rarely symptoms of sepsis including multisystem organ insufficiency may be noted. Due to the nonspecific nature of the symptoms and signs of shunt infection, the physician has to remain vigilant. Unfortunately diagnosis of shunt infections is difficult even with laboratory analysis. CSF studies are not as sensitive or as specific for shunt infections as one would hope, particularly in the situation of a distal tubing infection [35]. Microbiological analyses of infected material including shunt hardware, adjacent fluid collections, and CSF obtained either from a spinal tap or by way of a reservoir tap or both are thought to be the most reliable tests to aid in the identification of a shunt infection. Still, Gram stains and CSF cultures can remain negative, even in cases of shunt infection or become falsely positive due to contamination [35,39].

Treatment strategies aimed at reducing shunt infection rates

Several strategies have emerged over the years aimed at curbing shunt-related infection rates. The use of preoperative and postoperative antibiotics, advances in surgical technique, surgeon experience in shunt placement, and developments in shunt technology have reduced shunt-related infection but unfortunately have not eliminated them [41,43].

The development of antibiotic-impregnated shunt (AIS) catheters became possible when early in vitro and in vivo studies demonstrated that antibiotics incorporated into silicone catheters withstood sterilization procedures and provided local antimicrobial activity [44–46]. The clinical introduction of AIS catheters was based on sound empiric rationale, and the shunt catheters were initially evaluated in the pediatric population where benefit was noted [43,47]. Subsequently there have been numerous clinical studies that have demonstrated varying degrees of efficacy and safety in the literature. Many of these studies have either been too small or underpowered and predominantly retrospective in nature. Parker et al., in 2011, performed a systematic literature review and meta-analysis of all 11 studies to that date that directly compared the infection rates between AIS and non-AIS catheter cohorts [41]. The studies were performed in pediatric populations, adult populations, and a mixture of the two. In the 11 studies, 5613 shunt procedures were identified. There was an overall infection rate of 5.4%, but there was a significant reduction in shunt-related infections using AIS catheters versus non-AIS catheters (3.3% vs. 7.2%) and furthermore the use of AIS catheters was not associated with an increased incidence of antibiotic-resistant organisms. Additionally, a subset analysis of adult and pediatric populations revealed a similar reduction in infections in both subsets when the AIS catheters were used: adults (0.9% vs. 5.8%) and pediatric (5.0% vs. 11.2%) [41].

The use of AIS catheters has predominately been studied in pediatric patients, where it has demonstrated a significant reduction in the absolute and relative risk of shunt infections. Several investigators have been able to suggest similar efficacy in adults [48,49]. Farber et al. in 2011 reviewed their institutional experience from 2004 to 2009 having uniformly converted to AIS catheters in 2006 [49]. They analyzed infection rates within the first year after shunt placement in adult cohorts taken from each period. The mean age of the study population was 60 ± 18 years. Five hundred patients were compared in this study (250 AIS vs. 250 non-AIS catheter placements). Hydrocephalus had various etiologies in their cohorts, but 76% of the patients underwent surgery for NPH and they were reasonably distributed between cohorts (73% in the AIS vs. 78% in the non-AIS cohorts). The overall infection rate was 2.6%, and the incidence was decreased in AIS patients (1.2%) compared to non-AIS patients (4.0%) (p = 0.0492). The most common organism in this group was *Staphylococcus epidermidis* [49]. Parker et al., in their meta-analysis of AIS versus non-AIS

Table 18.2 Organism prevalence in shunt infections in the era of antibiotic-impregnated shunt (AIS) catheters (see text for further analysis)

	Farber et al. [49]		Parker et al. [41]	
	n = 13		n = 301	
	AIS	Non-AIS	AIS	Non-AIS
Staphylococcus aureus		2	26	64
Staphylococcus epidermidis	2	6	11	29
Streptococci			2	2
Enterococcus spp.		1	5	6
Pseudomonas spp.	1		3	3
Haemophilus influenzae			2	
Escherichia coli			1	3
Corynebacterium spp.		1		2
Klebsiella spp.		1	1	
Propionibacterium spp.				1
Others			4	3

cohort studies from 2002 to 2010 reviewed 5613 shunt procedures, with infections noted in 301 cases (5.4%) [41]. The most common pathogen in both AIS and non-AIS catheter groups was *Staphylococcus aureus* (29.5% in the AIS and 30% in the non-AIS groups). Other pathogens identified were *S. epidermidis* (13.3%), *Enterococcus* spp. (3.7%), and *Pseudomonas* spp. (2.0%) [41] (Table 18.2).

Although prospective, randomized trials are needed to confirm the direct association of reduced infection rates and AIS catheters, the available data are compelling. Some have speculated that reluctance to adopt AIS catheters has been due to the initial indirect cost associated with their use, as they may be $400 more than conventional catheter systems [50]. However, Attenello et al. performed a cost analysis of their treatment of patients with shunt infections at their institution [50]. In their review of 608 shunt surgeries, they demonstrated a 2.4-fold decreased likelihood of shunt infection in patients who had an AIS catheter implanted compared to the patients without. Given that their average hospitalization cost to treat a patient with a shunt infection was $48 454 they were able to realize a direct cost saving of $402 133 per 100 shunts placed by using AIS catheters, including the added cost of the catheter itself. The scope of the problem of shunt infections was indicated by Patwardhan and Nanda, who analyzed the Nationwide Inpatient Sample Database for the year 2000, a period before the widespread availability of AIS catheters, and who were able to estimate the cost of treating patients with implanted ventricular shunts [51]. They noted 5574 admissions for patients needing ventricular shunt procedures, of which 7.2% were for underlying infection. Given the database represents a sample size of 20% of the US admissions, the data project the annual admissions for shunt infections alone at over 2000 patients. They found an average cost per patient for treating all admitted patients with shunt complications, infection or otherwise, at $35 816, which is similar to the Attenello figure of $48 454, and would translate into an annual direct cost of over $70 million in the period prior to the institution of AIS catheters [50,51]. These figures presented are represented as estimates, but they are probably gross underestimates of the total cost of shunt infections as they only address fixed hospital costs. They do not take into account any economic costs attributable to shunt infections such as lost time, lost educational opportunity, lost wages, and costs associated with extended care, all of which are fixtures of the increased acuity associated with patients hospitalized with shunt infections.

Conclusion

The use of CSF diversion in NPH has come a long way from its humble initial applications. As we review the literature we can get the sense that the long-term complication rates from placement of ventriculoperitoneal shunts in patients with NPH are improving. The ability to maintain patients in symptomatic relief with shunts is improving. The risk of infection from shunt placement is falling. These successes are a result of a combination of better awareness of the condition we are trying to treat, improved equipment available for the treatment, in particular programmable valves and antibacterial impregnated catheters, increased opportunities to intervene in follow-up to help maintain patients' symptom-free status, and vigilance by the healthcare providers to continue with ongoing follow-up so as to make needed adjustments and recommend surgical revision when indicated. Still, moving forward into the future, the risk-to-benefit ratio for shunting in patients with NPH can be substantially improved by realizing the opportunity to address both risk and benefit. Better understanding of the most appropriate and predictive preoperative evaluations will allow the offering of surgery particularly to those patients most likely to improve their symptoms with shunting. The population at risk with this disease is at present likely underserved, and at the same time growing in number. Public awareness about NPH has dramatically increased and many patients and their families now inquire about the disorder with the hope of possible intervention. On the other side of the analysis, the decision to shunt patients with NPH adds a known set of risks to the therapy for this patient population, one which often comes with significant comorbidities. Improvement in the risk profile will occur in the future from continued evolution of the process of patient management: accurate perioperative assessments, improved attention to safety and quality at the time of surgical placements, advances in hardware, and vigilant long-term follow-up evaluations, intervening when necessary to maintain the patient with optimal CSF diversion and by extension optimal symptomatic relief.

References

1. Adams RD, Fisher CM, Hakim S, et al. Symptomatic occult hydrocephalus with "normal" cerebrospinal-

fluid pressure. A treatable syndrome. *N Engl J Med* 1965;273:117–26.

2. Wallenstein MB, McKhann GM, 2nd. Salomon Hakim and the discovery of normal-pressure hydrocephalus. *Neurosurgery* 2010;67(1):155–9.
3. Gallia GL, Rigamonti D, Williams MA. The diagnosis and treatment of idiopathic normal pressure hydrocephalus. *Nat Clin Pract Neurol* 2006;2(7):375–81.
4. Savolainen S, Hurskainen H, Paljarvi L, et al. Five-year outcome of normal pressure hydrocephalus with or without a shunt: predictive value of the clinical signs, neuropsychological evaluation and infusion test. *Acta Neurochir (Wien)* 2002;144(6):515–23.
5. Pujari S, Kharkar S, Metellus P, et al. Normal pressure hydrocephalus: long-term outcome after shunt surgery. *J Neurol Neurosurg Psychiatry* 2008;79(11):1282–6.
6. Black PM, Ojemann RG, Tzouras A. CSF shunts for dementia, incontinence, and gait. *Clin Neurosurg* 1985;32:632–51.
7. Vanneste JA. Three decades of normal pressure hydrocephalus: are we wiser now? *J Neurol Neurosurg Psychiatry* 1994;57(9):1021–5.
8. Klinge P, Hellström P, Tans J, et al. One-year outcome in the European multicentre study on iNPH. *Acta Neurol Scand* 2012;126(3):145–53.
9. Vanneste J, Augustijn P, Dirven C, et al. Shunting normal-pressure hydrocephalus: do the benefits outweigh the risks? A multicenter study and literature review. *Neurology* 1992;42(1):54–9.
10. Brean A, Eide PK. Prevalence of probable idiopathic normal pressure hydrocephalus in a Norwegian population. *Acta Neurol Scand* 2008;118(1):48–53.
11. Brean A, Fredø HL, Sollid S, et al. Five-year incidence of surgery for idiopathic normal pressure hydrocephalus in Norway. *Acta Neurol Scand* 2009;120(5):314–16.
12. Howden LM, Meyer JA. Age and Sex Composition: 2010. *2010 Census Briefs*. US Department of Commerce Economics and Statistics Administration. US Census Bureau. Washington, DC 20233 May 2011. www.census.gov/prod/cen2010/briefs/c2010br-03.pdf. (Accessed January 25, 2013.)
13. Marmarou A, Bergsneider M, Klinge P, et al. The value of supplemental prognostic tests for the preoperative assessment of idiopathic normal-pressure hydrocephalus. *Neurosurgery* 2005;57(3 Suppl):S17–28.
14. Panagiotopoulos V, Konstantinou D, Kalogeropoulos A, et al. The predictive value of external continuous lumbar drainage, with cerebrospinal fluid outflow controlled by medium pressure valve, in normal pressure hydrocephalus. *Acta Neurochir (Wien)* 2005;147(9):953–8.
15. Walchenbach R, Geiger E, Thomeer RT, et al. The value of temporary external lumbar CSF drainage in predicting the outcome of shunting on normal pressure hydrocephalus. *J Neurol Neurosurg Psychiatry* 2002;72(4):503–6.
16. Fishman RA, Dillon WP. Dural enhancement and cerebral displacement secondary to intracranial hypotension. *Neurology* 1993;43(3 Pt 1):609–11.
17. Reddy GK, Bollam P, Caldito G. Ventriculoperitoneal shunt surgery and the risk of shunt infection in patients with hydrocephalus: long-term single institution experience. *World Neurosurg* 2012;78(1–2):155–63.
18. Vinchon M, Fichten A, Delestret, I, et al. Shunt revision for asymptomatic failure: surgical and clinical result. *Neurosurgery* 2003;52(2):347–56.
19. Blount JP, Campbell JA, Haines, SJ. Complications in ventricular cerebrospinal fluid shunting. *Neurosurg Clin N Am* 1993:4(4):633–56.
20. Jeelani NU, Kulkarni AV, Desilva P, et al. Postoperative cerebrospinal fluid wound leakage as a predictor of shunt infection: a prospective analysis of 205 cases. Clinical article. *J Neurosurg Pediatr* 2009;4(2):166–9.
21. McGirt MJ, Zaas A, Fuchs HE, et al. Risk factors for pediatric ventriculoperitoneal shunt infection and predictors of infectious pathogens. *Clin Infect Dis* 2003;36(7):858–62.
22. Steinbok P, Milner R, Agrawal D, et al. A multicenter multinational registry for assessing ventriculoperitoneal shunt infections for hydrocephalus. *Neurosurgery* 2010;67(5):1303–10.
23. Bayston R, Lambert E. Duration of protective activity of cerebrospinal fluid shunt catheters impregnated with antimicrobial agents to prevent bacterial catheter-related infection. *J Neurosurg* 1997;87(2):247–51.
24. Drake JM, Kestle JR, Milner R, et al. Randomized trial of cerebrospinal fluid shunt valve design in pediatric hydrocephalus. *Neurosurgery* 1998;43(2):294–303.
25. Kestle JR, Drake JM, Cochrane DD, et al. Lack of benefit of endoscopic ventriculoperitoneal shunt insertion: a multicenter randomized trial. *J Neurosurg* 2003;98(2):284–90.
26. Boon AJ, Tans JT, Delwel EJ, et al. Dutch normal-pressure hydrocephalus study: prediction of outcome after shunting by resistance to outflow of cerebrospinal fluid. *J Neurosurg* 1997;87(5):687–93.
27. Boon AJ, Tans JT, Delwel EJ, et al. Dutch normal-pressure hydrocephalus study: randomized comparison of low- and medium- pressure shunts. *J Neurosurg* 1998;88:490–5.
28. Hebb AO, Cusimano MD. Idiopathic normal pressure hydrocephalus: a systematic review of diagnosis and outcome. *Neurosurgery* 2001;49(5):1166–84.

29. McGirt MJ, Woodworth G, Coon AL, et al. Diagnosis, treatment, and analysis of long-term outcomes in idiopathic normal-pressure hydrocephalus. *Neurosurgery* 2005;57(4):699–705.

30. Marmarou A, Young HF, Aygok GA, et al. Diagnosis and management of idiopathic normal-pressure hydrocephalus: a prospective study in 151 patients. *J Neurosurg* 2005;102(6):987–97.

31. Bloch O, McDermott MW. Lumboperitoneal shunts for the treatment of normal pressure hydrocephalus. *J Clin Neurosci* 2012;19(8):1107–11.

32. Schoenbaum SC, Gardner P, Shillito J. Infections of cerebrospinal fluid shunts: epidemiology, clinical manifestations, and therapy. *J Infect Dis* 1975;131(5):543–52.

33. Wong JM, Ziewacz JE, Ho AL, et al. Patterns in neurosurgical adverse events: cerebrospinal fluid shunt surgery. *Neurosurg Focus* 2012;33(5):E13:1–7.

34. Zemack G, Romner B. Adjustable valves in normal-pressure hydrocephalus: a retrospective study of 218 patients. *Neurosurgery* 2008;62(Suppl 2):677–87.

35. Gutiérrez-González R, Boto GR, Pérez-Zamarrón A. Cerebrospinal fluid diversion devices and infection. A comprehensive review. *Eur J Clin Microbiol Infect Dis* 2012;31(6):889–97.

36. Borgbjerg BM, Gjerris F, Albeck MJ, et al. Risk of infection after cerebrospinal fluid shunt: an analysis of 884 first-time shunts. *Acta Neurochir (Wien)* 1995;136(1–2):1–7.

37. Bayston R, Lari J. A study of the sources of infection in colonised shunts. *Dev Med Child Neurol* 1974;16(6 Suppl 32):16–22.

38. Conn HO. Normal pressure hydrocephalus: new complications and concepts. *Pract Neurol* 2007;7(4):252–8.

39. Conen A, Walti LN, Merlo A, et al. Characteristics and treatment outcome of cerebrospinal fluid shunt-associated infections in adults: a retrospective analysis over an 11-year period. *Clin Infect Dis* 2008;47(1):73–82.

40. Tuan TJ, Thorell EA, Hamblett NM, et al. Treatment and microbiology of repeated cerebrospinal fluid shunt infections in children. *Pediatr Infect Dis J* 2011;30(9):731–5.

41. Parker SL, Anderson WN, Lilienfeld S, et al. Cerebrospinal shunt infection in patients receiving antibiotic-impregnated versus standard shunts. *J Neurosurg Pediatr* 2011;8(3):259–65.

42. Braxton EE, Ehrlich GD, Hall-Stoodley L, et al. Role of biofilms in neurosurgical device-related infections. *Neurosurg Rev* 2005;28(4):249–55.

43. Sciubba DM, Stuart RM, McGirt MJ, et al. Effect of antibiotic-impregnated shunt catheters in decreasing the incidence of shunt infection in the treatment of hydrocephalus. *J Neurosurg* 2005;103(2 Suppl):131–6.

44. Bayston R, Grove N, Siegel J, et al. Prevention of hydrocephalus shunt catheter colonisation in vitro by impregnation with antimicrobials. *J Neurol Neurosurg Psychiatry* 1989;52(5):605–9.

45. Hampl J, Schierholz J, Jansen B, et al. In vitro and in vivo efficacy of a rifampin-loaded silicone catheter for the prevention of CSF shunt infections. *Acta Neurochir (Wien)* 1995;133(3–4):147–52.

46. Bayston R, Lambert E. Duration of protective activity of cerebrospinal fluid shunt catheters impregnated with antimicrobial agents to prevent bacterial catheter-related infection. *J Neurosurg* 1997;87(2):247–51.

47. Aryan HE, Meltzer HS, Park MS, et al. Initial experience with antibiotic-impregnated silicone catheters for shunting of cerebrospinal fluid in children. *Childs Nerv Syst* 2005;21(1):56–61.

48. Albanese A, De Bonis P, Sabatino G, et al. Antibiotic-impregnated ventriculo-peritoneal shunts in patients at high risk of infection. *Acta Neurochir (Wien)* 2009;151(10):1259–63.

49. Farber SH, Parker SL, Adogwa O, et al. Effect of antibiotic-impregnated shunts on infection rate in adult hydrocephalus: a single institution's experience. *Neurosurgery* 2011;69(3):625–9.

50. Attenello FJ, Garces-Ambrossi GL, Zaidi HA, et al. Hospital costs associated with shunt infections in patients receiving antibiotic-impregnated shunt catheters versus standard shunt catheters. *Neurosurgery* 2010;66(2):284–9.

51. Patwardhan RV, Nanda A. Implanted ventricular shunts in the United States: the billion-dollar-a-year cost of hydrocephalus treatment. *Neurosurgery* 2005;56(1):139–44.

Chapter 19

Endoscopic third ventriculostomy

Indications, technique, outcome, and complications

Steffen Fleck, Jörg Baldauf, and Henry W. S. Schroeder

Indications and outcome

Although the first endoscopic third ventriculostomy (ETV) was performed by Mixter back in 1923 [1], ETV has only become established over the past 20 years as the preferred therapeutic option for obstructive hydrocephalus. This is largely the result of improved endoscopic optics, cold light fountains, and miniaturized CCD cameras [2–10].

Overall ETV success rates range from 33% to 95% and are excellent in both (1) obstructive hydrocephalus caused by aqueductal stenosis (>75%) and (2) third ventricle outflow obstructions caused by benign space-occupying lesions (95%) [2,4–15]. O'Brien and coworkers also noted that primary ETV was highly successful in treating hydrocephalus related to spina bifida (88%), aqueductal stenosis (69%), and arachnoid cysts (100%). In a secondary ETV group (after shunt malfunction), the highest success rates were described for arachnoid cysts (100%) followed by aqueductal stenosis (68%) and spina bifida (55%) [16]. The procedure is also successful in treating tetraventricular hydrocephalus [13].

ETV has also been used in communicating hydrocephalus with conflicting results. Though it may be an effective treatment in certain patients [17], ETV success rates appear substantially lower in communicating than occlusive hydrocephalus.

Studies that have assessed nonobstructive hydrocephalic patients with a history of hemorrhage and/or infection have reported ETV success rates ranging from 0 to 100% [8,9,17–20]. In general, however, poor primary ETV outcomes were observed in patients with intraventricular hemorrhage (IVH)-induced hydrocephalus and hemorrhage and infection-induced hydrocephalus [16,20].

The discussion concerning factors that influence ETV success rate is ongoing. Factors that might affect ETV outcome include the type of hydrocephalus, age of the patient at the time of intervention, previous shunt placement, previous brain radiation, intraventricular tumor, and accompanying cerebrospinal fluid (CSF) infections. Dlouhy et al. demonstrated the predictive value of preoperative ventricular bowing for ETV success, but 33% of patients without bowing were also successfully treated with ETV [21]. The bowing may be absent due to a decreased ventricular compliance, e.g. in slit ventricle syndrome.

Moreover, relevant anatomical structures for the ETV approach and their maintained integrity following ETV, such as massa intermedia, mammillary bodies, basilar artery, clivus, and the extent of Liliequist's membrane, also play an important role in outcome estimation [11].

ETV in adult patients

ETV is an effective treatment option for adult patients with noncommunicating hydrocephalus. Dusick et al. demonstrated an overall long-term shunt independence in 79% of 108 patients with idiopathic aqueductal stenosis, mass lesions causing noncommunicating hydrocephalus, and other miscellaneous obstructive etiologies [2]. These findings corroborate success rates reported in other studies with adult patient subsets – ranging from 66% to 88% [6,22–25]. A recent summary by Sacko et al. reported an overall success rate of 77% in adults with a higher failure risk in hemorrhage-related and idiopathic chronic hydrocephalus than in other types of hydrocephalus [26] (Table 19.1).

ETV in children and the role of age and etiology dependence

The roles that (1) age at the time of treatment and (2) etiology of the hydrocephalus play in ETV outcome in

Table 19.1 Reported indications for ETV

	Related to/associated with
Obstructive hydrocephalus	Aqueductal stenosis
	Dandy–Walker malformation
	Syringomyelia/Chiari malformation
	Myelomeningocele
	Encephalocele
	Arachnoid cyst
	Tectomesencephalic tumor
	Posterior fossa tumor
	Cerebellar infarction (space-occupying)
	Multiloculated
	Craniosynostosis (syndromic)
	Shunt malfunction
	Slit ventricle syndrome
	Intraventricular hemorrhage
	After shunt failure (post-hemorrhagic/infectious)
Communicating hydrocephalus	Post-hemorrhagic
	Postinfectious (meningitis; ventriculitis)
	Idiopathic normal pressure hydrocephalus (iNPH)

children are currently being discussed [8–10,12,27–29]. The following pathophysiological explanations have been offered in light of higher ETV failure rates in children.

The immaturity of arachnoid granulations leads to decreased CSF absorption in newborns, and the open fontanelle with splayed sutures prevents an increase of intracranial pressure of more than 5 mmHg, which would be necessary for a sufficient absorption through the sagittal sinus [30–34]. Cinalli et al. showed that long-term ETV outcomes were the same across children younger and older than 6 months of age, and postulated that this procedure is not contraindicated in this patient group. Furthermore, repeated ETV is a useful management technique for a delayed failure in cases of stoma obstruction [12]. In a recent retrospective study, Costa Val et al. noted that the effectiveness of ETV is more likely due to hydrocephalus etiology rather than age. They found that ETV treatment of aqueductal stenosis had a 90% success rate in comparison with 50% for Chiari-II-related hydrocephalus [35].

On the other hand, many studies have assessed ETV failure rates in very young infants compared with children older than 6–12 months [5,8,10,29,36–41]. Patients under 6 months of age had a 5-fold increase in risk of ETV failure compared with older patients [26]. Beems and Grotenhuis favored the role of etiology for estimating ETV success in children younger than 2 years of age. Though they found an overall success rate of 53% in 66 children younger than 2 years, success varied across etiologies, ranging from 20% to 88% [10]. Siomin et al. found that ETV was not beneficial in premature newborns and patients with IVH-induced hydrocephalus. However, in this multicenter study, the authors reported that secondary ETV following shunt malfunction had a high rate of success in patients harboring a triventricular hydrocephalus [20].

Kombogiorgas and Sgouros reported an overall ETV success rate of 42% in a series of 33 hydrocephalic children with a mean age of 76 months. They concluded that ETV may not be suitable for patients with a complicated shunt history due to previous CSF or shunt infection. CSF leakage following ETV in patients without previous shunt implantation or in children under 2 years of age was strongly associated with ETV failure [42].

The ETV success score (ETVSS) attempts to predict ETV success and failure in the treatment of childhood hydrocephalus by taking age, cause of hydrocephalus, and history of previous shunt placement into account [43].

Warf concluded after a series of 300 consecutive hydrocephalic children (81.3% younger than 1 year of age), usually caused by CSF infection, that ETV can be performed with acceptable results in a developing country in spite of the difficulties regarding shunt dependence [44].

ETV in previously shunted patients

Results pertaining to ETV efficacy in previously shunted patients are conflicting. On the one hand, Hopf et al. reported a success rate of 84% in previously shunted patients, a finding that several studies have corroborated [6,45].

Teo and Jones showed a statistically significant success rate of ETV for previously shunted patients with myelomeningocele (84%) in comparison with patients without previous shunt implantation (29%) [46].

On the other hand, the failure rates of ETV across previously shunted and non-shunted patients were 20.8% and 20.5% in a series of 63 adult patients. The authors pointed out that the history of three or more shunt revisions was a statistically significant risk factor for ETV failure [15]. Kombogiorgas and Sgouros concluded that ETV may not be suitable in young pediatric patients with a complicated shunt history due to previous CSF or shunt infection [42].

However, studies by O'Brien et al., Cinalli et al., and Mallucci et al. have reported success following secondary ETV in obstructive hydrocephalus after IVH who present with ventriculoperitoneal (VP) shunt malfunction [16,47,48]. Furthermore, O'Brien et al. reported a high ETV success rate in patients with infection-induced obstructive hydrocephalus [16].

ETV in communicating hydrocephalus

ETV has been reported to be an effective treatment for communicating hydrocephalus in certain patients [17]. The precise underlying mechanisms of communicating hydrocephalus remain unknown. Ransohoff et al. suggested a nomenclature with "intraventricular obstructive hydrocephalus" including obstruction of aqueduct and outlet foramina of the fourth ventricle, and "extraventricular obstructive hydrocephalus" [30]. Recently, Rekate investigated the basal cisterns as a source of CSF flow blockage and suggested that all hydrocephalus is to some extent obstructive. Thus, the modified bulk flow theory might explain ETV's effectiveness in certain types of communicating hydrocephalus [17,49].

The low primary ETV success rate and encouraging secondary ETV results following shunt failure in patients with hemorrhage and/or infection were described as follows. Initially, a communicating hydrocephalus due to the debris in the subarachnoid space and arachnoid granulations occurs and shunting allows for the re-expansion and normalization of the subarachnoid spaces. Aqueductal stenosis may then be acquired during the following course. This seems to explain ETV's usefulness at a later period and the high failure rate in the initial phase. Thus, the endoscopic approach might be an alternative to be discussed in patients after shunt malfunction and infection [16].

ETV in idiopathic normal pressure hydrocephalus

The first reported patient series using ETV to treat idiopathic normal pressure hydrocephalus (iNPH) was performed by Mitchell and Mathew, and Meier and coworkers [50–52].

Mitchell and Mathew reported improvement in three out of four cases after performing ETV, and suggested that the relief of periventricular tissue stress improved local blood flow.

Meier et al. compared 15 patients who underwent ETV with 60 patients who were shunted and observed that though immediate results were similar, the ETV patients had better long-term outcomes. They additionally suggested that ETV might be particularly beneficial in those patients with increased resistance following the ventricular infusion test but normal lumbar infusion test results. This indicates that obviously patients with both communicating and noncommunicating hydrocephalus have been included in this study. Gangemi et al. found an overall rate of neurological improvement of 72% following ETV in a series of 25 patients with clinical preoperative history of NPH of up to one year [53]. The authors concluded that ETV and shunt implantation offer similar results in patients with iNPH who present with a short duration of symptoms, prevalence of gait disturbance, and slight mental impairment. Furthermore, they suggested that these results indirectly confirm that CSF absorption is at least sufficient in these selected patients. Typical complications of shunting, like subdural hematoma and effusion, are significantly diminished after ETV due to only slight decrease in intracranial pressure (ICP) after ETV.

The following pathophysiological explanations (hydrodynamic concept) may play a role when choosing ETV as a therapeutic option in iNPH.

Communicating hydrocephalus is caused by decreased intracranial compliance which increases systolic pressure and fluid transmission into the brain parenchyma rather than CSF absorption. The increased systolic pressure in the brain distends the brain towards the skull and compresses the periventricular region against the ventricles. These factors lead to a predominant enlargement of the ventricles and narrowing of the subarachnoid space [54]. The parenchyma is chronically damaged due to continuous systolic pulsations and periventricular edema, leading to a decrease of cerebral blood flow. Thus, communicating hydrocephalus is a disorder of intracranial pulsations caused by decreased compliance [55,56]. ETV results in a reduction of the increased systolic pressure by venting ventricular CSF through a stoma, leading to an improvement of the cerebral blood flow and perfusion pressure and abolition of transependymal resorption, whereas the patent aqueduct is too narrow to sufficiently vent the CSF [53,54,57].

Longatti et al. suggested possible factors that could explain good outcomes in 3 of 14 patients with NPH, namely, a partial fourth ventricle outlet obstruction, and a functionally compressed aqueduct [58]. Therefore, a full exploration of the fourth ventricle with flexible endoscopes is suggested to exclude unexpected blockages of the outlet not assessed in MR studies. In addition, the authors postulated the mechanism that intermittent aqueductal squeezing may occur because it is easier for the brainstem to slip upwards through the tentorial notch than the cerebellum thereby leading to a functionally constricted aqueduct. Particular attention should be paid to any slight deformation of the third ventricle floor suggestive of a functional aqueductal stenosis [58].

Hailong and coworkers have shown an overall proportion of 65.6% of excellent/good (≥50% clinical improvement) clinical outcomes after ETV in 32 patients (including 17 patients with iNPH). The authors found a high correlation of Kiefer scores and patient age with favorable outcomes, and determined that the preoperative mental state plays an important role in the prediction of outcome after ETV [17]. Gangemi et al. [59] retrospectively reviewed 110 patients with idiopathic normal pressure hydrocephalus who underwent ETV in four Italian neurosurgical centers. Clinical improvement occurred in 69.1% of patients after 2 years. The authors found no correlation between success rate and patient age, or type of ventricular enlargement (normal or enlarged fourth ventricle). Conversely, the rate of neurological improvement was higher in patients with shorter clinical history, better preoperative neurological score, and clinical onset with gait disturbances. Moreover, sudden intraoperative reappearance of normal cerebral pulsations and significant downward and upward movements of the third ventricular floor after ETV were also correlated with good outcome [59]. A systematic review has been planned to evaluate the possible evidence of ETV in iNPH [60].

In summary, the published series show inconsistent clinical results after ETV for iNPH. In our experience, ETV for iNPH is not successful in the long term. A short-lasting effect is seen similar to the effect after lumbar puncture. It is our impression that the good results of most studies are due to the fact that not only true iNPH was included but also forms of obstructed hydrocephalus with a patent aqueduct which resembled iNPH, for example the extraventricular intracisternal obstructive hydrocephalus described by Kehler and Gliemroth [61]. The hypothesis of (distal and proximal) intracisternal obstructive hydrocephalus may be helpful in patient selection for ETV in cases of so-called "communicating hydrocephalus." The authors suggested an indication for ETV in cases of *proximal* intracisternal obstruction with documented downward bulging of the third ventricle floor in MR images [61]. Based on our results, we do not recommend ETV for the treatment of iNPH.

Intraoperative factors influencing the success of ETV

Intraoperative factors, such as hemorrhage, size of stoma, thickness of the third ventricular floor [62], and flow through the stoma, may play a role in ETV success rates. Some studies have found a correlation between success rate and presence of prepontine adhesions, thickened floor of the third ventricle, and small size of stoma in children. Kombogiorgas and Sgouros, however, did not find such a correlation. They evaluated a stoma diameter of over 30% of the distance between posterior clinoid and basilar artery as a possible association with success of ETV in children without previous shunting but pointed out the possible increased risk of basilar artery injury during the creation of a very large stoma [34]. Floating tissue has to be carefully coagulated or resected to avoid a stoma obstruction [7].

Factors leading to the obstruction of the ETV stoma are important for the ETV failure rate: gliotic tissue or arachnoid membranes have been described [7,11,15,63]. Liliequist's membrane has to be opened as it acts as a barrier of supra- and infratentorial cisterns and may cause a failure of ETV [63,64]. Intraoperative ventriculography may help to evaluate the patency of the stoma and of the intracisternal CSF pathways [65].

Definition of success after ETV and diagnosis of ETV failure

Shunt independence has often been cited as a criterion for the success of an ETV [2,7,14,66]. However, symptomatic improvement has been considered the main criterion. Therefore, the diagnosis of ETV failure is primarily based on clinical and not radiological aspects. It is difficult to define success, for instance, in patients with only minimal clinical improvement after the endoscopic procedure. In many cases, patients present with vague symptoms of possible recurrent hydrocephalus such as headache without specific clinical signs indicating a raised intracranial pressure [14].

The volumes of the third and lateral ventricles are usually reduced after ETV, but up to 20% of patients (especially those with longstanding ventriculomegaly) show little or no changes in ventricular size despite good outcomes [67,68]. The reduction of ventricular volume is much less evident than in imaging following shunt placement. Especially in very young children, ETV rarely results in a major reduction of the ventricles [16].

MRI studies may clearly show the stoma and the flow through the stoma. However, they do not predict the clinical success, as patients may have a combination of obstructive and communicating hydrocephalus. This means that despite a patent stoma with a good flow void the procedure may fail [4]. Furthermore, patients with subtle symptoms and chronic ventriculomegaly may not experience dramatic clinical improvements, or improvements may be delayed [2].

Possible causes of an ETV failure are (re-)obstruction of the stoma due to hemorrhage, debris or scar tissue, not opened membranes within the perimesencephalic cisternal space, decreased absorption due to infection, hemorrhage, or longstanding VP shunt history.

The time of ETV failure is unpredictable and may occur days to years after the operation, leading even to an abrupt and life-threatening deterioration [2,12,14,69].

Management of ETV failure

If the primary ETV fails to improve the patient's symptoms, the patency of the stoma has to be checked. If MR imaging shows that the stoma is obstructed, a redo ETV should be performed if during the first surgery no negative predictors such as severe arachnoid scarring of the prepontine cistern were observed. The chance of a successful outcome after a re-ETV in our series was 80% [70]. If the stoma is patent and MR imaging shows a flow void signal, the hydrocephalus is obviously not only obstructive but has a CSF resorption component. Then, shunting is usually necessary to treat the hydrocephalus successfully. Our experience corresponds with reports in the literature. In a series of 20 patients, a re-ETV was shown to be safe with a success rate of 65% [71]. Additionally, Koch et al. concluded that ETV has to be considered as a sufficient treatment option after an initial successful ETV in cases of later stoma occlusion [72].

Advantages/disadvantages of ETV compared to VP shunt placement

The main advantage of ETV is that no foreign material has to be inserted. This decreases the risks of infection and malfunction – namely, obstruction or disconnection. Studies confirm that the risk of infection following a neuroendoscopic operation is lower than with shunting (approximately 0–2% vs. 5–10%) [16,73,74]. ETV's main disadvantage is that it is not effective in most types of communicating hydrocephalus. Unfortunately, no tests are currently available to accurately predict the success of an ETV. Shunt placement is an effective therapy for obstructive and communicating hydrocephalus in all age groups, but carries the risk of infection and/or malfunction of 25–40% in the first year after shunt placement and the risk remains at 4–5% each year thereafter [16,74–76]. Long-term data show a revision rate of 81% in 12 years [77]. Triventricular hydrocephalus treatment with ETV has been shown to have a success rate of 72% over 6 years [12]. Other types of hydrocephalus treated with ETV are reported to have less successful outcomes [19,47]. Slit ventricles and diminished reabsorption due to peritoneal adhesions may present difficulties for shunted patients but do not pose any problems for ETV patients.

Preoperative planning and anatomic eligibility for ETV

ETV success and complication avoidance during/following the operative procedure depends on precise preoperative planning, and is usually based on MR imaging. Certain aspects have to be considered when planning an ETV (see Table 19.2).

First, the ventricular size must allow handling of the endoscope without an increased risk to the surrounding structures. Furthermore, the width of the foramen of Monro must be estimated to allow the passage of the endoscope. Because it is the bottleneck of the approach to the third ventricle, the foramen will

Table 19.2 MR findings to be considered preoperatively

Width of ventricles (right/left)
Width of foramen of Monro (right/left)
Bulging of the third ventricle floor, lamina terminalis, pineal recess, infundibular recess
Dilation of prestenotic aqueduct
Narrowness of basilar artery to clivus/side predominance of branches
Massa intermedia
Perimesencephalic membranes

essentially influence the choice of endoscope used in the procedure. An endoscope with a diameter larger than the foramen of Monro may cause damage to surrounding anatomical structures like the fornix, veins, and choroid plexus. Smaller endoscopes are recommended particularly for newborns and young children. If narrow, it is useful to view the foramina of Monro on coronal and sagittal MR images to determine the optimal approach [16].

Furthermore, the perimesencephalic cisternal anatomy should be carefully evaluated. Patients in whom the brainstem and distal basilar artery were judged to be too close to the clivus (in general 2 mm space) have not been considered to be eligible for an ETV [2]. On the other hand, however, the prepontine space will be widened due to the normalization of the supratentorial pressure after drainage of the CSF. We agree with O'Brien et al. who suggested that there is rarely a contraindication to perform an ETV [16].

Navigation systems help to plan the trajectory in patients without significantly enlarged ventricles. Moreover, navigation is helpful if anatomic landmarks on the floor of the third ventricle are distorted – a situation that could lead to decreased or absent orientation. Chen and Nakaji have suggested after trajectory views of 53 patients that the optimal entry point for ETV is 30.1 ± 7 mm perpendicular to the midline and 8.9 ± 14.1 mm behind the coronal suture. Furthermore, they stated that the entry point is highly variable and image guidance should be used in all patients whenever available [78].

Kehler has introduced a grading system to classify eligible patients for ETV on a 5-point scale: (1) presence of imaging evidence of obstruction, (2) degree of bulging of the third ventricular floor, and (3) the presence of progression in preoperative symptoms within the 12 months preceding the ETV. This standardized grading system predicts the outcome of ETV and helps in decision-making for ETV versus VP shunting [79]. Another grading system, the ETV success score (ETVSS), includes age, cause of hydrocephalus, and history of previous shunt placement to model ETV success and failure in the treatment of childhood hydrocephalus [43]. However, to date, no test can precisely predict the success in an individual patient.

An externalization of the shunt 48 to 72 hours before the operation under strict ICP monitoring can help to enlarge the ventricles in patients with shunt-related slit ventricles [80].

MRI: flow dynamics measurement

CSF flow can qualitatively be described as the flow-void signal on T2-weighted images. CSF flow is best appreciated in narrow areas within the ventricular system such as aqueduct or after third ventriculostomy within the stoma site. To evaluate the dynamics of the CSF flow, the technique of cardiac-gated cine phase-contrast MR imaging has been increasingly used over the past 15 years. This extremely sensitive imaging technique allows the visualization and quantification of CSF flow noninvasively, even in slow flow and, therefore, allows considerable information on the physiology of the normal CSF circulation. Furthermore, information about flow disturbances is possible in certain pathological circumstances: communicating and obstructive hydrocephalus, Chiari malformation, cystic lesions, and cervical stenosis. Cine MR imaging has been recommended for evaluating third ventriculostomy patency [81–83]. For this measurement, technical considerations include: a high field MR unit (1.5T or greater) with a circular polarized head-array coil and a gradient system capable of acquiring standard axial (5 mm slice thickness) T1-weighted images. CSF flow can be visualized with flow sensitive T2-weighted images, e.g. T2-weighted turbo inversion-recovery spin-echo sequence (TE 4300 ms, TE 60 ms, and 2 mm slice thickness). For phase-contrast MR imaging, a two-dimensional fast low-angle shot (FLASH) T1-sequence can be used. Velocity encoding should be set at 6–10 cm/s. The imaging plane should be placed in the middle of the ventriculostomy or the aqueduct and slice thickness should be 4 mm. For flow quantification, the axial plane with through-plane velocity encoding in the craniocaudal direction, and for qualitative assessment, the sagittal plane with in-plane velocity encoding in the craniocaudal direction can be used [84].

Surgical technique of ETV, avoidance of complications

We use the LOTTA® (Karl Storz GmbH & Co. KG, Tuttlingen, Germany) rod-lens ventriculoscopic system which includes a larger (Standard LOTTA) and a smaller (Little LOTTA) ventriculoscope (Figures 19.1 and 19.2) [85]. For ETV, we usually use the smaller scope (diameter 3.6 mm). We prefer rigid rod-lens scopes with HD cameras because of the excellent image quality and ease of guidance. Flexible scopes are rarely used. The endoscope can either be guided "freehand" or fixed using a holding device (e.g. Point Setter pneumatic arm, Mitaka Co., Tokyo, Japan), which is, in our opinion, preferable.

We always administer antibiotic prophylaxis (cefuroxime) as a single shot intravenous medication around 30 minutes before skin incision. The head of the supine positioned patient should be anteflexed 30° to avoid CSF loss. The burr hole is placed in front of the coronal suture and about 2.5 cm paramedian [86]. Usually, we place the entry point on the right side. If the right foramen of Monro or the right ventricle is significantly smaller than on the left side, we make the approach on the left side. Depending on the need for further procedures (e.g. tumor biopsy, inspection of the aqueduct, septostomy), the burr hole must be placed more anteriorly, posteriorly, or laterally. It is essential to plan the trajectory before the skin incision. In most cases of hydrocephalus, the ventricles are clearly dilated and allow an uneventful puncture of the frontal horn.

We only use navigation in patients in whom we expect anatomical variations which make orientation difficult, such as ventriculitis, or to approach narrow ventricles.

After having placed the burr hole, the dura is coagulated and incised. The cortex is coagulated and the ventricle punctured bluntly using a Cushing needle to confirm the trajectory. A small amount of CSF is taken for laboratory examination. The endoscopic sheath is introduced with the aid of the trocar into the frontal horn. Usually, the frontal horn is reached at a depth of 4–5 cm. Then, the trocar is removed and the endoscope introduced. Excessively deep introduction of the endoscope or endoscopic sheath into the lateral ventricle may cause thalamic contusion or midbrain injury. Tiny hemorrhages always disappear within minutes with continuous irrigation.

The choroid plexus, the veins, and the foramen of Monro are then identified and the endoscope is carefully advanced through the foramen into the third ventricle. The fornix structures should not be touched. Therefore, the endoscope is moved on the top of the plexus and the plexus is gently pressed down if the interventricular foramen is narrow. It is also essential to see and control the edges of the endoscopic sheath (endoscope pulled back into the trocar) during movements within the ventricle, especially when passing the foramen of Monro. Limitations of a very narrow foramen are obvious. Once the trajectory to the floor of the third ventricle is not optimal, maneuvering the device within the foramen is difficult and may cause an injury to the fornix.

The mammillary body and the infundibular recess are identified. The typical point for fenestration of the third ventricular floor is the midpoint of a triangle formed by the mammillary bodies and the infundibular recess, just posterior to the infundibular blush. Usually, this point is halfway between mammillary bodies and infundibular recess, just behind the clivus. However, the anatomic landmarks may be distorted. Sometimes, the floor of the third ventricle is thick and non-translucent, e.g. in the event of acute hydrocephalus or after chronic inflammation. If the basilar artery is not seen through the floor, the position of the basilar artery and the distance to the mammillary

(a) (b)

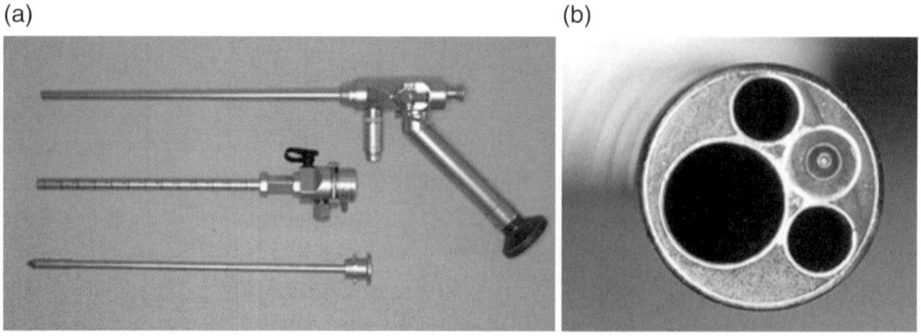

Figure 19.1 (a) LOTTA ventriculoscope, sheath and trocar. (b) Tip of the endoscope including lens, working and irrigation channels.

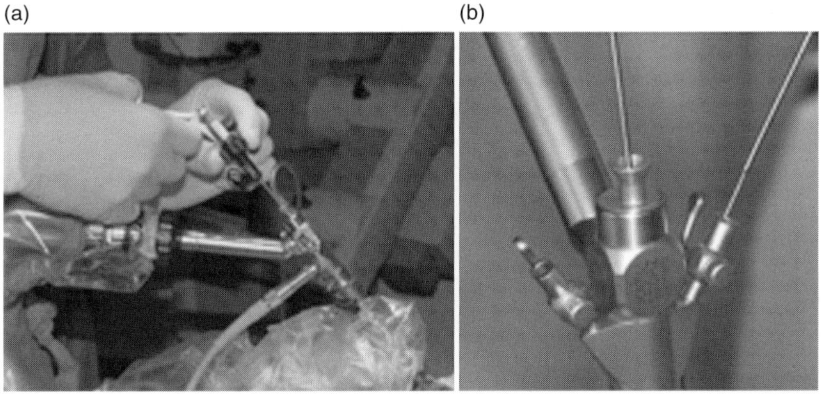

Figure 19.2 (a) Endoscope fixed with the pneumatic holding arm allowing a bimanual manipulation of the instruments. (b) Bimanual dissection with two instruments inserted through the main working channel (middle) and one side channel that alternatively can be used for irrigation.

bodies and clivus is obtained from MR imaging. We prefer to perforate the floor bluntly using a closed "Decq" forceps. During this step, the basilar artery and perforators are at the greatest risk for injury and, therefore, we do not advise fenestrating nearer to the mammillary bodies than the triangle midpoint described above. The perforation is then enlarged by inflating the balloon of a 3-French-Fogarty catheter. The catheter should be inflated with saline instead of air to prevent the "pop-up" phenomenon and assure a slow and constant enlargement of the balloon. Usually, pulsation of the floor can be observed after the fenestration has been achieved. The premesencephalic and prepontine cisternal space has to be inspected to confirm that the subarachnoid space has been reached and a patent premesencephalic and prepontine subarachnoid space is present. The basilar artery should be seen (Figure 19.3a–e). If there are arachnoid membranes which might interfere with CSF flow, such as Liliequist's membrane, these membranes have to be opened too. Sometimes, several membranes have to be cut with scissors. To enhance the safety of this procedure, the endoscopic sheath of the Little LOTTA scope is inserted through the ventriculostomy into the prepontine cistern. Then, under good visual control, the membranes are cut with the sharp-pointed scissors. If intraoperative hemorrhage occurs, it will be important to maintain the position of the endoscope and to irrigate (lactated Ringer's solution at 37°C) to improve the visualization. Especially in difficult procedures where long irrigation and substitution of the CSF is needed, this fact is noticeable, because the alternative use of saline solution may lead to prolonged awakening after surgery, hyperventilation, and transient confusion of the patient as observed by the authors. Rarely, the use of the bipolar rod or forceps is necessary. Usually, minor hemorrhages stop after a few minutes of irrigation. Mild bleeds of the rim of the fenestrated membrane may be controlled simply by leaving the dilated Fogarty balloon within the stoma for a minute for compression. While irrigating, the surgeon has to make sure that the outflow canal for the irrigation fluid is not closed to avoid a critical increase of ICP. Additionally, air bubbles causing a diminished view have to be avoided during the irrigation.

After a sufficient ETV has been achieved, the endoscope is withdrawn from the third ventricle into the lateral ventricle and the foramen is inspected. While the endoscope is removed from the brain, the cortical puncture channel is visualized for potential active bleeding. In most cases, the dura is not closed. We simply place a piece of Gelfoam® in the burr hole. The galea is sutured and the skin is closed with an atraumatic running suture. In premature newborns and newborns, we try to achieve a water-tight dural closure because of the higher risk of CSF fistula. We suture the dura, if possible the periosteum too, and place a piece of Tachosil® (Nycomed, Konstanz, Germany) over the suture line. We particularly mention not to use autologous bone dust to close the bony defect. For cosmetic reasons, a titanium burr hole plate can be used to cover the burr hole.

Usually, we do not place a reservoir after having performed an ETV. However, Aquilina and coworkers recommend the routine placement of a ventricular reservoir after ETV due to the fact of unpredictable timing of a possible failure and its unexpected, abrupt, and life-threatening course [73]. It allows emergency therapeutic CSF aspiration which assists in the diagnosis of ETV failure, and intrathecal drug administration without an increased operative risk. For cosmetic reasons, a circular depression in the outer table of the

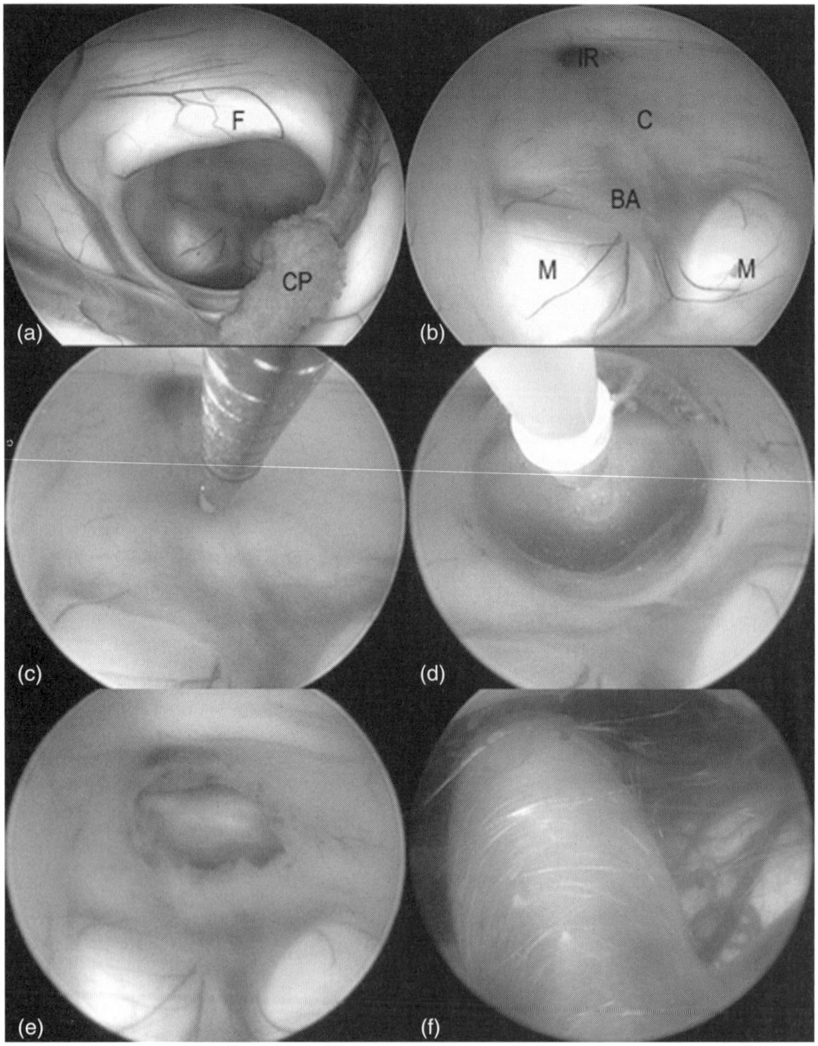

Figure 19.3 Endoscopic third ventriculostomy. (a) View through the foramen of Monro (CP, choroid plexus; F, fornix). (b) Floor of the third ventricle (BA, basilar artery; M, mammillary bodies; C, clivus; IR, infundibular recess). (c) Blunt perforation of the floor of the third ventricle with the Decq forceps. (d) Dilation of the stoma by inflating the balloon of the Fogarty catheter. (e) Sufficient open stoma after ETV. (f) Inspection of the prepontine cistern showing the basilar artery. A full-color version is included in the color plate section.

cranium can be made to countersink the burr hole reservoir [73].

Reported complications

The rate of complications varies between 0% and 31.2% with an overall complication rate of 8.5% according to a literature review by Bouras and Sgouros [87]. The technique as described in detail within this chapter covers different intraoperative steps that have to be completed very carefully to avoid damage to the intra- and paraventricular structures.

Herniation syndromes following increased ICP due to a closed endoscope outflow channel have been observed and result in a transient decrease of consciousness and permanent confusion. Although unusual, it has also been reported that in a patient with very narrow foramina of Monro who underwent ETV because of hydrocephalus related to aqueductal stenosis, bilateral occlusion of the foramina of Monro had occurred 30 months after ETV [88].

Inflating the balloon within the ambient cistern and then pulling the balloon through the tuber cinereum may risk incorporating a branch of the posterior circulation [89]. Major subarachnoid hemorrhages due to basilar artery injuries and its branches may be underreported, but happen and frequently lead to death [90]. Apart from vascular injuries, transient and permanent damage to the oculomotor nerve has been reported [91].

Furthermore, hormonal disturbances following ETV are closely related to hypothalamic injuries. It is possible that an eccentric stoma creation is responsible for the traumatization of the hypothalamus [87]. Transient diabetes insipidus has been frequently observed [23,24,91]. Also, abnormalities of prolactin levels, postoperative hyperkalemia, and inappropriate secretion of antidiuretic hormone after ETV have been reported [92–94].

During the postoperative period, CSF leaks may occur due to inappropriate skin closure or increased intracranial pressure in 1.61% [87]. Occasionally, it is an early sign of a failure of ETV. Infectious complications such as meningitis or ventriculitis are seen rarely but have to be treated with antibiotics [87,91].

Although subarachnoid hemorrhage after ETV has already been mentioned as a deadly complication, due to injury of the basilar artery or its branches, other intracranial hemorrhages such as intraventricular, subdural, or epidural hematomas can also be found. Subdural hematomas may develop because of a decrease of the intracranial pressure after ETV related to the CSF drainage during the procedure itself or as a result of tiny cortical bleeds into the subdural space due to the corticotomy [89,95,96].

Sudden late deterioration is a rare but probably underestimated complication in patients after ETV. The largest series was reported by Drake et al. and included 16 children with a mean age of 7.6 years [97]. The time to ETV failure ranged from 5 weeks to 7.8 years. Thirteen patients died due to a closed stoma as verified at the autopsy. We concur with other colleagues that the mechanism of a closure of a stoma is likely influenced by multiple factors such as a poor fenestration of the floor of the third ventricle, prepontine remnants of arachnoid membranes, or CSF absorptive problems by arachnoid granulations especially seen in cases of infection or hemorrhage [89]. Bone dust used for filling the burr hole may migrate via the cortical channel through the ventricles and occlude the aqueduct or stoma resulting in an acute increase in ICP [98].

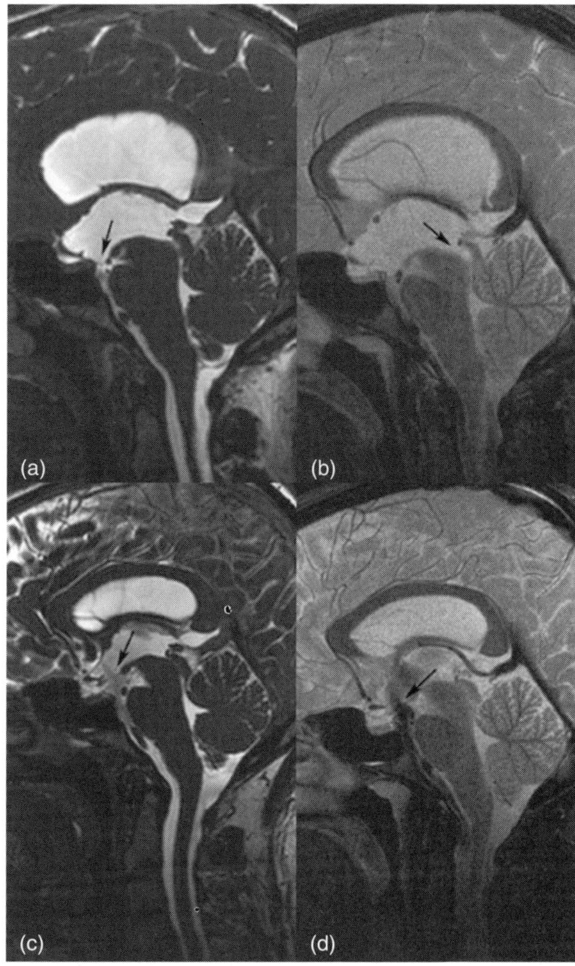

Figure 19.4 MR images show a typical patient with hydrocephalus due to aqueductal stenosis. (a, CISS sequence) and (b, IRTSE) demonstrate the preoperative state with enlargement of the lateral and third ventricle with a typical bulging of the floor of the third ventricle (arrow, image a) and the widened prestenotic aqueduct without a flow within the lumen (arrow, image b). Postoperative images after successful ETV reveal a decrease of the size of the ventricles and the elevated floor of the third ventricle with the fenestration site (arrow, image c). The typical flow void can be seen within the stoma between the third ventricle and the prepontine cistern (arrow, image d).

Postoperative care and follow-up

Most failures occur early, but long-term follow-up is vital as mentioned above. In our institution, all patients receive MR imaging with flow studies 1 day postoperatively to assess the patency of the stoma (Figure 19.4). Measurement of ICP during the immediate postoperative course can be performed but is not standard in our ETV protocol [99,100].

Usually, we recommend a clinical examination 10 to 14 days after discharge. The next follow-up examination including MR imaging with flow studies is performed 3 months after surgery and then annually with an uneventful course.

Summary

ETV has been established as the therapy of choice for obstructive hydrocephalus and is considered to be straightforward and safe. At this point, there is insufficient evidence to suggest that ETV is also effective in communicating hydrocephalus. Because our experience with about 300 ETVs showed that ETV frequently failed as a treatment for communicating hydrocephalus, we do not recommend ETV in these cases. The preferred initial treatment of premature hemorrhagic hydrocephalus is still VP shunt placement. The same is true for iNPH.

ETV patients should have follow-up checks similar to shunt patients. They and/or caregivers should be advised that rapid deterioration with the need for emergency admission can occur at any time.

References

1. Mixter W. Ventriculoscopy and puncture of the floor of the third ventricle. *Boston Med Surg J* 1923;188:277–8.
2. Dusick JR, McArthur DL, Bergsneider M. Success and complication rates of endoscopic third ventriculostomy for adult hydrocephalus: a series of 108 patients. *Surg Neurol* 2008;69(1):5–15.
3. Murshid WR. Endoscopic third ventriculostomy: towards more indications for the treatment of non-communicating hydrocephalus. *Minim Invasive Neurosurg* 2000;43(2):75–82.
4. Tisell M, Almström O, Stephensen H, Tullberg M, Wikkelsö C. How effective is endoscopic third ventriculostomy in treating adult hydrocephalus caused by primary aqueductal stenosis? *Neurosurgery* 2000;46(1):104–10; discussion 10–11.
5. Koch D, Wagner W. Endoscopic third ventriculostomy in infants of less than 1 year of age: which factors influence the outcome? *Childs Nerv Syst* 2004;20(6):405–11.
6. Hopf NJ, Grunert P, Fries G, Resch KD, Perneczky A. Endoscopic third ventriculostomy: outcome analysis of 100 consecutive procedures. *Neurosurgery* 1999;44(4):795–804; discussion 804–6.
7. Feng H, Huang G, Liao X, et al. Endoscopic third ventriculostomy in the management of obstructive hydrocephalus: an outcome analysis. *J Neurosurg* 2004;100(4):626–33.
8. Buxton N, Macarthur D, Mallucci C, Punt J, Vloeberghs M. Neuroendoscopic third ventriculostomy in patients less than 1 year old. *Pediatr Neurosurg* 1998;29(2):73–6.
9. Brockmeyer D, Abtin K, Carey L, Walker ML. Endoscopic third ventriculostomy: an outcome analysis. *Pediatr Neurosurg* 1998;28(5):236–40.
10. Beems T, Grotenhuis JA. Is the success rate of endoscopic third ventriculostomy age-dependent? An analysis of the results of endoscopic third ventriculostomy in young children. *Childs Nerv Syst* 2002;18(11):605–8.
11. Iantosca MR, Hader WJ, Drake JM. Results of endoscopic third ventriculostomy. *Neurosurg Clin N Am* 2004;15(1):67–75.
12. Cinalli G, Sainte-Rose C, Chumas P, et al. Failure of third ventriculostomy in the treatment of aqueductal stenosis in children. *J Neurosurg* 1999;90(3):448–54.
13. Gangemi M, Donati P, Maiuri F, et al. Endoscopic third ventriculostomy for hydrocephalus. *Minim Invasive Neurosurg* 1999;42(3):128–32.
14. Fukuhara T, Vorster SJ, Luciano MG. Risk factors for failure of endoscopic third ventriculostomy for obstructive hydrocephalus. *Neurosurgery* 2000;46(5):1100–9; discussion 1009–11.
15. Buxton N, Ho KJ, Macarthur D, et al. Neuroendoscopic third ventriculostomy for hydrocephalus in adults: report of a single unit's experience with 63 cases. *Surg Neurol* 2001;55(2):74–8.
16. O'Brien DF, Javadpour M, Collins DR, Spennato P, Mallucci CL. Endoscopic third ventriculostomy: an outcome analysis of primary cases and procedures performed after ventriculoperitoneal shunt malfunction. *J Neurosurg* 2005;103(5 Suppl):393–400.
17. Hailong F, Guangfu H, Haibin T, et al. Endoscopic third ventriculostomy in the management of communicating hydrocephalus: a preliminary study. *J Neurosurg* 2008;109(5):923–30.
18. Goumnerova LC, Frim DM. Treatment of hydrocephalus with third ventriculocisternostomy: outcome and CSF flow patterns. *Pediatr Neurosurg* 1997;27(3):149–52.
19. Jones RF, Stening WA, Brydon M. Endoscopic third ventriculostomy. *Neurosurgery* 1990;26(1):86–91; discussion 91–2.
20. Siomin V, Cinalli G, Grotenhuis A, et al. Endoscopic third ventriculostomy in patients with cerebrospinal fluid infection and/or hemorrhage. *J Neurosurg* 2002;97(3):519–24.
21. Dlouhy BJ, Capuano AW, Madhavan K, Torner JC, Greenlee JD. Preoperative third ventricular bowing as a

predictor of endoscopic third ventriculostomy success. *J Neurosurg Pediatr* 2012;9(2):182–90.

22. Bognar L, Markia B, Novak L. Retrospective analysis of 400 neuroendoscopic interventions: the Hungarian experience. *Neurosurg Focus* 2005;19(6):E10.
23. Grunert P, Charalampaki P, Hopf N, Filippi R. The role of third ventriculostomy in the management of obstructive hydrocephalus. *Minim Invasive Neurosurg* 2003;46(1):16–21.
24. Kadrian D, van Gelder J, Florida D, et al. Long-term reliability of endoscopic third ventriculostomy. *Neurosurgery* 2005;56(6):1271–8; discussion 1278.
25. Santamarta D, Diaz Alvarez A, Goncalves JM, Hernandez J. Outcome of endoscopic third ventriculostomy. Results from an unselected series with noncommunicating hydrocephalus. *Acta Neurochir* 2005;147(4):377–82; discussion 382.
26. Sacko O, Boetto S, Lauwers-Cances V, Dupuy M, Roux FE. Endoscopic third ventriculostomy: outcome analysis in 368 procedures. *J Neurosurg Pediatr* 2010;5(1):68–74.
27. Scarrow AM, Levy EI, Pascucci L, Albright AL. Outcome analysis of endoscopic III ventriculostomy. *Childs Nerv Syst* 2000;16(7):442–4; discussion 445.
28. Kim SK, Wang KC, Cho BK. Surgical outcome of pediatric hydrocephalus treated by endoscopic III ventriculostomy: prognostic factors and interpretation of postoperative neuroimaging. *Childs Nerv Syst* 2000;16(3):161–8; discussion 169.
29. Javadpour M, Mallucci C, Brodbelt A, Golash A, May P. The impact of endoscopic third ventriculostomy on the management of newly diagnosed hydrocephalus in infants. *Pediatr Neurosurg* 2001;35(3):131–5.
30. Ransohoff J, Shulman K, Fishman RA. Hydrocephalus: a review of etiology and treatment. *J Pediatr* 1960;56:399–411.
31. Olivero WC, Rekate HL, Chizeck HJ, Ko W, McCormick JM. Relationship between intracranial and sagittal sinus pressure in normal and hydrocephalic dogs. *Pediatr Neurosci* 1988;14(4):196–201.
32. Cutler RW, Page L, Galicich J, Watters GV. Formation and absorption of cerebrospinal fluid in man. *Brain* 1968;91(4):707–20.
33. Jones RF, Kwok BC, Stening WA, Vonau M. Third ventriculostomy for hydrocephalus associated with spinal dysraphism: indications and contraindications. *Eur J Pediatr Surg* 1996;6(Suppl 1):5–6.
34. Kombogiorgas D, Sgouros S. Assessment of the influence of operative factors in the success of endoscopic third ventriculostomy in children. *Childs Nerv Syst* 2006;22(10):1256–62.
35. Costa Val JA, Scaldaferri PM, Furtado LM, de Souza Baptista G. Third ventriculostomy in infants younger than 1 year old. *Childs Nerv Syst* 2012;28(8):1233–5.
36. Balthasar AJ, Kort H, Cornips EM, et al. Analysis of the success and failure of endoscopic third ventriculostomy in infants less than 1 year of age. *Childs Nerv Syst* 2007;23(2):151–5.
37. Etus V, Ceylan S. Success of endoscopic third ventriculostomy in children less than 2 years of age. *Neurosurgical Rev* 2005;28(4):284–8.
38. Fritsch MJ, Kienke S, Ankermann T, Padoin M, Mehdorn HM. Endoscopic third ventriculostomy in infants. *J Neurosurg* 2005;103(1 Suppl):50–3.
39. Gorayeb RP, Cavalheiro S, Zymberg ST. Endoscopic third ventriculostomy in children younger than 1 year of age. *J Neurosurg* 2004;100(5 Suppl Pediatrics):427–9.
40. O'Brien DF, Seghedoni A, Collins DR, Hayhurst C, Mallucci CL. Is there an indication for ETV in young infants in aetiologies other than isolated aqueduct stenosis? *Childs Nerv Syst* 2006;22(12):1565–72.
41. Yadav YR, Jaiswal S, Adam N, Basoor A, Jain G. Endoscopic third ventriculostomy in infants. *Neurology India* 2006;54(2):161–3.
42. Kombogiorgas D, Sgouros S. Removal of subdural-peritoneal shunts in infants. *Childs Nerv Syst* 2005;21(6):458–60.
43. Kulkarni AV, Drake JM, Kestle JR, et al. Predicting who will benefit from endoscopic third ventriculostomy compared with shunt insertion in childhood hydrocephalus using the ETV Success Score. *J Neurosurg Pediatr* 2010;6(4):310–15.
44. Warf BC. Hydrocephalus in Uganda: the predominance of infectious origin and primary management with endoscopic third ventriculostomy. *J Neurosurg* 2005;102(1 Suppl):1–15.
45. St George E, Natarajan K, Sgouros S. Changes in ventricular volume in hydrocephalic children following successful endoscopic third ventriculostomy. *Childs Nerv Syst* 2004;20(11–12):834–8.
46. Teo C, Jones R. Management of hydrocephalus by endoscopic third ventriculostomy in patients with myelomeningocele. *Pediatr Neurosurg* 1996;25(2):57–63; discussion 63.
47. Cinalli G, Salazar C, Mallucci C, et al. The role of endoscopic third ventriculostomy in the management of shunt malfunction. *Neurosurgery* 1998;43(6):1323–7; discussion 1327–9.
48. Mallucci C, Buxton N, Vloeberghs M, Punt J. Neuroendoscopic third ventriculostomy: the first line of treatment for blocked ventriculoperitoneal shunts? *Eur J Pediatr Surg* 1997;7(Suppl 1):65.

49. Rekate HL. Comments on the article by D. Greitz "Paradigm shift in hydrocephalus research in legacy of Dandy's pioneering work: rationale for third ventriculostomy in communicating hydrocephalus". *Childs Nerv Syst* 2007;23(11):1227–8; author reply 1229–31.

50. Meier U, Zeilinger FS, Schonherr B. Endoscopic ventriculostomy versus shunt operation in normal pressure hydrocephalus: diagnostics and indication. *Acta Neurochir Suppl* 2000;76:563–6.

51. Mitchell P, Mathew B. Third ventriculostomy in normal pressure hydrocephalus. *Br J Neurosurg* 1999;13(4):382–5.

52. Meier U. [Shunt operation versus endoscopic ventriculostomy in normal pressure hydrocephalus: diagnostics and outcome]. *Zentralbl Neurochir* 2003;64(1):19–23.

53. Gangemi M, Maiuri F, Buonamassa S, Colella G, de Divitiis E. Endoscopic third ventriculostomy in idiopathic normal pressure hydrocephalus. *Neurosurgery* 2004;55(1):129–34; discussion 134.

54. Greitz D. Paradigm shift in hydrocephalus research in legacy of Dandy's pioneering work: rationale for third ventriculostomy in communicating hydrocephalus. *Childs Nerv Syst* 2007;23(5):487–9.

55. Egnor M, Zheng L, Rosiello A, Gutman F, Davis R. A model of pulsations in communicating hydrocephalus. *Pediatr Neurosurg* 2002;36(6):281–303.

56. Greitz D, Hannerz J, Rahn T, Bolander H, Ericsson A. MR imaging of cerebrospinal fluid dynamics in health and disease. On the vascular pathogenesis of communicating hydrocephalus and benign intracranial hypertension. *Acta Radiol* 1994;35(3):204–11.

57. Hakim CA, Hakim R, Hakim S. Normal-pressure hydrocephalus. *Neurosurg Clin N Am* 2001;12(4):761–73, ix.

58. Longatti PL, Fiorindi A, Martinuzzi A. Failure of endoscopic third ventriculostomy in the treatment of idiopathic normal pressure hydrocephalus. *Minim Invasive Neurosurg* 2004;47(6):342–5.

59. Gangemi M, Maiuri F, Naddeo M, et al. Endoscopic third ventriculostomy in idiopathic normal pressure hydrocephalus: an Italian multicenter study. *Neurosurgery* 2008;63(1):62–7; discussion 67–9.

60. Tudor MTK, Car J. Endoscopic third ventriculostomy (ETV) for idiopathic normal pressure hydrocephalus (iNPH) (Protocol). *The Cochrane Library* 2012(8).

61. Kehler U, Gliemroth J. Extraventricular intracisternal obstructive hydrocephalus – a hypothesis to explain successful 3rd ventriculostomy in communicating hydrocephalus. *Pediatr Neurosurg* 2003;38(2):98–101.

62. Faggin R, Calderone M, Denaro L, Meneghini L, d'Avella D. Long-term operative failure of endoscopic third ventriculostomy in pediatric patients: the role of cine phase-contrast MR imaging. *Neurosurg Focus* 2011;30(4):E1.

63. Buxton N, Vloeberghs M, Punt J. Liliequist's membrane in minimally invasive endoscopic neurosurgery. *Clin Anat* 1998;11(3):187–90.

64. Brasil AV, Schneider FL. Anatomy of Liliequist's membrane. *Neurosurgery* 1993;32(6):956–60; discussion 960–1.

65. Hellwig D, Grotenhuis JA, Tirakotai W, et al. Endoscopic third ventriculostomy for obstructive hydrocephalus. *Neurosurg Rev* 2005;28(1):1–34; discussion 35–8.

66. Beems T, Grotenhuis JA. Long-term complications and definition of failure of neuroendoscopic procedures. *Childs Nerv Syst* 2004;20(11–12):868–77.

67. Schwartz TH, Ho B, Prestigiacomo CJ, et al. Ventricular volume following third ventriculostomy. *J Neurosurg* 1999;91(1):20–5.

68. Dalrymple SJ, Kelly PJ. Computer-assisted stereotactic third ventriculostomy in the management of noncommunicating hydrocephalus. *Stereotact Funct Neurosurg* 1992;59(1–4):105–10.

69. Javadpour M, May P, Mallucci C. Sudden death secondary to delayed closure of endoscopic third ventriculostomy. *Br J Neurosurg* 2003;17(3):266–9.

70. Baldauf J, Oertel J, Gaab MR, Schroeder HWS. Probability of shunt independence after endoscopic third ventriculostomy. May 2009. www.egms.de/static/en/meetings/dgnc2009/09dgnc105.shtml (accessed July 26, 2013).

71. Siomin V, Weiner H, Wisoff J, et al. Repeat endoscopic third ventriculostomy: is it worth trying? *Childs Nerv Syst* 2001;17(9):551–5.

72. Koch D, Grunert P, Filippi R, Hopf N. Re-ventriculostomy for treatment of obstructive hydrocephalus in cases of stoma dysfunction. *Minim Invasive Neurosurg* 2002;45(3):158–63.

73. Aquilina K, Edwards RJ, Pople IK. Routine placement of a ventricular reservoir at endoscopic third ventriculostomy. *Neurosurgery* 2003;53(1):91–6; discussion 96–7.

74. Drake JM, Kestle JR, Milner R, et al. Randomized trial of cerebrospinal fluid shunt valve design in pediatric hydrocephalus. *Neurosurgery* 1998;43(2):294–303; discussion 303–5.

75. Bierbrauer KS, Storrs BB, McLone DG, Tomita T, Dauser R. A prospective, randomized study of shunt function and infections as a function of shunt placement. *Pediatr Neurosurg* 1990;16(6):287–91.

76. Piatt JH, Jr., Carlson CV. A search for determinants of cerebrospinal fluid shunt survival: retrospective analysis of a 14-year institutional experience. *Pediatr Neurosurg* 1993;19(5):233–41; discussion 242.

77. Sainte-Rose C, Piatt JH, Renier D, et al. Mechanical complications in shunts. *Pediatr Neurosurg* 1991;17(1):2–9.

78. Chen F, Nakaji P. Optimal entry point and trajectory for endoscopic third ventriculostomy: evaluation of 53 patients with volumetric imaging guidance. *J Neurosurg* 2012;116(5):1153–7.

79. Kehler U, Regelsberger J, Gliemroth J, Westphal M. Outcome prediction of third ventriculostomy: a proposed hydrocephalus grading system. *Minim Invasive Neurosurg* 2006;49(4):238–43.

80. Boschert JM, Krauss JK. Endoscopic third ventriculostomy in the treatment of shunt-related over-drainage: preliminary experience with a new approach how to render ventricles navigable. *Clin Neurol Neurosurg* 2006;108(2):143–9.

81. Schroeder C, Fleck S, Gaab MR, Schweim KH, Schroeder HW. Why does endoscopic aqueductoplasty fail so frequently? Analysis of cerebrospinal fluid flow after endoscopic third ventriculostomy and aqueductoplasty using cine phase-contrast magnetic resonance imaging. *J Neurosurg* 2012;117(1):141–9.

82. Joseph VB, Raghuram L, Korah IP, Chacko AG. MR ventriculography for the study of CSF flow. *AJNR Am J Neuroradiol* 2003;24(3):373–81.

83. Kulkarni AV, Drake JM, Armstrong DC, Dirks PB. Imaging correlates of successful endoscopic third ventriculostomy. *J Neurosurg* 2000;92(6):915–19.

84. Nitz WR, Bradley WG, Jr., Watanabe AS, et al. Flow dynamics of cerebrospinal fluid: assessment with phase-contrast velocity MR imaging performed with retrospective cardiac gating. *Radiology* 1992;183(2):395–405.

85. Schroeder HW. A new multipurpose ventriculoscope. *Neurosurgery* 2008;62(2):489–91; discussion 491–2.

86. Kanner A, Hopf NJ, Grunert P. The "optimal" burr hole position for endoscopic third ventriculostomy: results from 31 stereotactically guided procedures. *Minim Invasive Neurosurg* 2000;43(4):187–9.

87. Bouras T, Sgouros S. Complications of endoscopic third ventriculostomy. *J Neurosurg Pediatr* 2011;7(6):643–9.

88. El Refaee E, Baldauf J, Schroeder HW. Bilateral occlusion of the foramina of Monro after third ventriculostomy. *J Neurosurg* 2012;116(6):1333–6.

89. Chowdhry SA, Cohen AR. Intraventricular neuroendoscopy: complication avoidance and management. *World Neurosurg* 2013;79(2 Suppl):S15. e1–10.

90. Schroeder HW, Warzok RW, Assaf JA, Gaab MR. Fatal subarachnoid hemorrhage after endoscopic third ventriculostomy. Case report. *Neurosurg Focus* 1999;6(4):e4.

91. Schroeder HW, Niendorf WR, Gaab MR. Complications of endoscopic third ventriculostomy. *J Neurosurg* 2002;96(6):1032–40.

92. Fritsch MJ, Bauer M, Partsch CJ, Sippell WG, Mehdorn HM. Endocrine evaluation after endoscopic third ventriculostomy (ETV) in children. *Childs Nerv Syst* 2007;23(6):627–31.

93. Anandh B, Madhusudan Reddy KR, Mohanty A, Umamaheswara Rao GS, Chandramouli BA. Intraoperative bradycardia and postoperative hyperkalemia in patients undergoing endoscopic third ventriculostomy. *Minim Invasive Neurosurg* 2002;45(3):154–7.

94. Vaicys C, Fried A. Transient hyponatriemia complicated by seizures after endoscopic third ventriculostomy. *Minim Invasive Neurosurg* 2000;43(4):190–1.

95. Kamel MH, Murphy M, Aquilina K, Marks C. Subdural haemorrhage following endoscopic third ventriculostomy. A rare complication. *Acta Neurochir* 2006;148(5):591–3.

96. Sgaramella E, Castelli G, Sotgiu S. Chronic subdural collection after endoscopic third ventriculostomy. *Acta Neurochir* 2004;146(5):529–30.

97. Drake J, Chumas P, Kestle J, et al. Late rapid deterioration after endoscopic third ventriculostomy: additional cases and review of the literature. *J Neurosurg* 2006;105(2 Suppl):118–26.

98. Kafadar A, Abuzayed B, Kucukyuruk B, Cetin E, Gazioglu N. Intracranial migration of bone dust after intraventricular neuroendoscopy complicating acute hydrocephalus and removal of bone dust: case report. *Neurosurgery* 2010;67(2):E503–4.

99. Cinalli G, Spennato P, Ruggiero C, et al. Intracranial pressure monitoring and lumbar puncture after endoscopic third ventriculostomy in children. *Neurosurgery* 2006;58(1):126–36; discussion 126–36.

100. Santamarta D, Martin-Vallejo J. Evolution of intracranial pressure during the immediate postoperative period after endoscopic third ventriculostomy. *Acta Neurochir Suppl* 2005;95:213–17.

Chapter 20

Outcome of idiopathic normal pressure hydrocephalus

Gunes A. Aygok

Introduction

Hakim et al. [1] introduced a unique triad of clinical symptoms defining normal pressure hydrocephalus (NPH), which included gait disturbance, dementia, and incontinence in association with enlarged ventricles and normal cerebrospinal fluid (CSF) pressure in his thesis "Some observations on CSF pressure: hydrocephalic syndrome in adults with 'normal' CSF pressure" and later in an article published by Hakim and Adams [2]. He reported that diversion of fluid using a shunt relieved the symptoms, and this has remained the primary treatment modality. Following shunting, many authors have reported that with appropriate diagnosis, the range of improvement varies from 24% to 90% [3–6].

However, studies had extreme ranges of follow-up periods from a few months to many years post-shunting in which long-term outcomes of shunted patients are few, partly due to the inherent loss of follow-up. The comorbidity which is a major confounder in outcome assessment in the elderly idiopathic normal pressure hydrocephalus (iNPH) patient population is seldom reported. There is a lack of standardized outcome scales, which makes such reporting difficult. The outcome results are graded based on clinical judgment by the physician as well as patient and caregiver opinions and are relatively subjective in nature and not quantified. Most importantly, there are no Class I data which address the best diagnostic strategy, surgical versus conservative management of iNPH, identifying one valve or configuration as superior to another, and reporting of shunt-related complications and malfunctions.

In a prospective study of 42 iNPH patients, Malm et al. [4] reported an overall improvement of 64% at 3 months compared with 26% at 3 years. At 3 months, 74% of his patients were independent, at 3 years the independent group was only 28%. Aygok et al. [5] reported from a prospective series of 50 iNPH patients that at 3-year follow-up, even though there was a slight decline, patients still retained a 75% improvement in gait. Moreover, 80% retained their improvement in memory and incontinence at 3 years post-shunt. These diverse findings are not only challenging but also are confusing for physicians, patients, and families when making diagnostic and treatment decisions. The following list represents the key steps which will hopefully serve as a guide to achieving a favorable outcome in iNPH patients:

- proper selection criteria for diagnosis of iNPH;
- deficiencies in identifying the degree of clinical impairment and therefore clinical improvement;
- standardized management protocols related to outcome;
- impact of complications after surgery;
- impact of comorbidities.

Proper selection criteria for diagnosis of iNPH

Since the 1960s, great efforts have been made to improve diagnosis and management of NPH and achieve better selection of patients with idiopathic NPH (iNPH) and NPH of known cause (secondary NPH). Despite these efforts, there was a lack of Class I evidence for proper diagnosis and management, so the experts in the field assembled evidence-based guideline groups and published the first editions of international and Japanese guidelines for diagnosis and management of iNPH in 2005 and 2004, respectively, followed by the second edition of the Japanese guidelines in 2011 [7–13].

Adult Hydrocephalus, ed. Daniele Rigamonti. Published by Cambridge University Press.

Based on these guideline recommendations, it is now essential to differentiate idiopathic NPH (iNPH) from other pathologies and to provide a multidimensional/multidisciplinary diagnostic approach which includes taking a detailed clinical history, assessing the triad of symptoms (gait/balance, cognition, urinary incontinence), and obtaining brain imaging [7,13,14]. Additionally, complementary diagnostic tests such as CSF infusion testing, CSF tap test or external lumbar drainage (ELD) when utilized in conjunction with clinical and radiological criteria, were found to identify iNPH patients more accurately and therefore better outcomes were achieved more efficiently [9,15].

In a prospective study of 43 iNPH patients, Walchenbach et al. [16] reported a positive predictive value of 87% with ELD for shunt outcome. Patients admitted to the Medical College of Virginia (MCV) who were diagnosed with iNPH according to a fixed protocol using diagnostic criteria based on gait disturbance, dementia, and incontinence in combination with ventriculomegaly without antecedent cause underwent a 3-day ELD procedure, and selection for surgery was made based on the improvement after ELD. The results indicated that ELD was the best prognostic indicator of a positive shunt outcome, with an accuracy of prediction greater than 90% [17]. The Study of Idiopathic Normal Pressure Hydrocephalus on Neurological Improvement: SINPHONI was conducted as a multicenter prospective study to evaluate the utility of MRI-based diagnosis for determining the 1-year outcome [18]. One hundred patients aged between 60 and 85 years with one or more iNPH symptoms (gait, cognitive, and urinary problems) and MRI evidence of disproportionately enlarged subarachnoid space hydrocephalus (DESH), i.e. tight high convexity and medial subarachnoid spaces and enlarged sylvian fissure associated with ventriculomegaly, received ventriculoperitoneal (VP) shunts with the Codman Hakim Programmable Valve. A favorable outcome was achieved in 69% of patients on the modified Rankin Scale whereas this rate was increased to 77% using the iNPH grading scale. The authors concluded that the MRI features of disproportionately enlarged subarachnoid space hydrocephalus (DESH) were useful for the diagnosis of iNPH. Advanced imaging modalities, measurement of regional cerebral blood flow (rCBF), acetazolamide challenge rCBF, and magnetic resonance spectroscopy (MRS) were also found to assist the selection of shunt responders [19].

It is clear that the increased chance of improvement after shunting was due to the proper selection of patients using dedicated clinical and radiological criteria and supplemental tests such as external lumbar drainage, which still remains the gold standard for predicting iNPH patients. Considering the fact that without surgery, most iNPH patients had measurable deterioration as early as 3 months following initial assessment, it is important to utilize standardized and validated criteria for proper diagnosis and conduct multicenter, randomized, placebo or cross-over designed clinical studies to obtain Class I evidence.

Deficiencies in identifying the degree of clinical impairment and therefore clinical improvement

Currently, there are neither standardized impairment nor standardized outcome scales that can be used for iNPH, such as the Glasgow Coma and Glasgow Outcome Scales that are used for head injury management [20]. Despite this fact, there are an increasing number of centers of excellence for iNPH management where clinicians have the opportunity to follow patients from baseline diagnosis to the plateau of improvement after surgery. These unique settings providing care for large numbers of iNPH patients enable clinicians to use and develop impairment and outcome scales for the management of iNPH even though validation and standardization of these tools is still limited (Table 20.1).

In an attempt to resolve the deficiencies in identifying the degree of clinical impairment in iNPH patients, the Kubo iNPH scale, Kiefer clinical grading, and iNPH scale (Tables 20.2–20.6) were introduced which measure impairment in the three major domains of iNPH symptoms: gait/balance, cognitive, and urinary continence [21– 23]. Furthermore, scales were developed to measure the impairment of individual iNPH symptoms only. For example, gait impairment can be measured using the iNPH MCV gait grade (Table 20.7), timed up and go test, and Tinetti tool, which all capture the key characteristics of iNPH gait pattern [17,24,25]. Cognitive impairment can be assessed with a commonly used outpatient test, the mini-mental state examination (MMSE), in addition to various neuropsychological tests of executive function (Stroop test), memory (Rey Auditory Verbal Learning Test [RAVLT]), and psychomotor function (Grooved

Table 20.1 Summary of publications for assessment of outcome of iNPH treatment

Author	Title of publication	Diagnostic criteria	Mean age (# of patients, n)	Follow-up	Outcome assessment	Deaths	Conclusion
Aygok et al. [5], 2005, USA	Three-year outcome of shunted idiopathic NPH patients	Clinical and radiological assessment followed by CSF bolus infusion test and 3-day external lumbar drainage (ELD)	70.4 (n = 50)	3 months and 3 years after shunting	Marmarou Outcome Scale	4	From 3 months to 3 years post-shunting, a slight decline in gait performance (from 91% to 75%), a retention of memory improvement (80% and 80%), and an improvement in incontinence occurred over time (70% to 82.5%) in iNPH patients
Black [3], 1980, USA	Idiopathic normal-pressure hydrocephalus. Results of shunting in 62 patients	Clinical and radiological assessment followed by isotope cisternography	67.8 (n = 62)	3 years after shunting	Stein and Langfitt Scale, Black Outcome Scale	5	With the author's classification, an improvement rate of 50% was noted in contrast to 33% for the same group of iNPH patients when measured by the Stein and Langfitt Scale. An "obstructive" cisternographic radioisotope pattern was not significantly different from a "normal" pattern in predicting a response to shunting
Cage et al. [43], 2011, USA	Self-reported functional outcome after surgical intervention in patients with idiopathic normal pressure hydrocephalus	Patient demographics, familial factors, comorbidities, quality of life, and treatment complications related to the treatment of hydrocephalus	Age range: 46–90 years (n = 252)	30 years after diagnosis	Patient's assessment of their functioning and debilitation	Not reported	In surgically treated iNPH patients, the rate of improvement in gait (81.1%), urinary incontinence (55.9%), and dementia (64.4%) and a return to independence through improved functional and social outcomes were achieved

Chen et al. [19], 2008, Japan	Normal pressure hydrocephalus: cerebral hemodynamic, metabolism measurement, discharge score, and long-term outcome	Clinical and radiological assessment	Not reported (n = 28)	3 months, 1, 2, and 3 years after shunting	Karnofsky Performance Scale	1	Karnofsky Performance Scale was found to be a reliable tool for the short- and long-term follow-up. Additionally, the authors suggested that for the patient with suspected NPH, measurement of regional cerebral blood flow (rCBF), acetazolamide challenge rCBF, and MRS may be helpful in selecting shunt responders
Hashimoto et al. [18], 2010, Japan	Diagnosis of idiopathic normal pressure hydrocephalus is supported by MRI-based scheme: a prospective cohort study	iNPH Grading Scale (iNPHGS), and radiological findings	74.5 (n = 100)	3, 6, and 12 months after shunting	Modified Rankin Scale (mRS), iNPHGS, timed 3 meter "up and go" test (TUG), and the mini-mental state examination (MMSE) at one year after surgery	2	The MRI features of disproportionately enlarged subarachnoid space hydrocephalus (DESH), i.e. tight high-convexity and medial subarachnoid spaces and enlarged sylvian fissure associated with ventriculomegaly, were useful for the diagnosis of iNPH
Kiefer et al., 2010 [6], Germany	Does idiopathic normal pressure hydrocephalus always mean a poor prognosis?	Kiefer Index (KI), and a comorbidity index (CMI)	Not reported (n = 125)	5.1 years		Not reported	The authors concluded that iNPH patients with favorable preconditions may have a similar or better prognosis than patients with any other kind of hydrocephalus. The worse overall clinical results of iNPH result from late recognition and in most instances worse preconditions

Table 20.1 *(cont.)*

Author	Title of publication	Diagnostic criteria	Mean age (# of patients, n)	Follow-up	Outcome assessment	Deaths	Conclusion
Klinge et al. [35], 2012, Europe	One year outcome in the European multi-centre study on iNPH	iNPH scale and radiological findings	71 (n = 142)	1, 3, and 12 months after shunting	Modified Rankin Scale (mRS) and iNPH scale	3	69% of patients were improved according to the mRS whereas 84% of the same patients were improved according to the iNPH scale at one year after surgery
Lemcke et al. [48], 2012, Germany	Idiopathic normal pressure hydrocephalus (iNPH) and co-morbidity: an outcome analysis of 134 patients	Comorbidity index (CMI)	Not reported (n = 134)	2 years after shunting	Kiefer Index (KI) and NPH recovery rate were compared using the preoperative CMI	Not reported	Data in this report affirm that comorbidity is a statistically significant predictor of the clinical outcome for patients with iNPH undergoing shunt therapy. According to these data, a successful outcome in patients with a CMI of 6 or more is not to be expected
Lundin et al. [44], 2012, Sweden	How active are patients with idiopathic normal pressure hydrocephalus and does activity improve after shunt surgery? A controlled actigraphic study	Clinical and radiological assessment	73 (n = 33)	12 months after shunting	Time needed for a 10 m walk in seconds (w10mt) and number of steps (w10ms); timed up and go test in seconds (TUGt) and steps (TUGs), MMSE	Not reported	The iNPH patients improved in the gait tests 3 months after surgery, but the actigraphy parameters indicated that these patients did not use their improved capacity in their daily life

Malm et al. [4], 2000, Sweden	Three-year survival and functional outcome of patients with idiopathic adult hydrocephalus syndrome	Clinical and radiological assessment	71.8 (n = 42)	3 years after shunting	Improvement in gait and cognitive function, Barthel ADL Index	12	The authors reported an overall improvement in 64% of patients at 3 months compared with 26% at 3 years. At 3 months, 74% of iNPH patients were independent, but at 3 years the independent group was only 28%
Mirzayan et al. [46], 2010, Germany	Extended long-term (>5 years) outcome of cerebrospinal fluid shunting in idiopathic normal pressure hydrocephalus	Clinical and radiological assessment followed by CSF removal	70.2 (n = 51)	18.8 months and 80.9 months after shunting	Krauss Improvement Index	29	Shunt surgery for treatment of iNPH may yield sustained improvement even after 7 years or longer. Outcome depends mainly on the selection of patients. The major cause of death was vascular comorbidity
Poca et al. [15], 2012, Spain	Idiopathic normal pressure hydrocephalus: results of a prospective cohort of 236 shunted patients	Clinical, radiological, neuropsychological, and functional assessment	75 (n = 236)	6 months after shunting		Not reported	The authors concluded that a high percentage of patients with iNPH can improve after shunting, with early and late complication rates of less than 12%
Pujari et al. [36], 2008, USA	Normal pressure hydrocephalus: long-term outcome after shunt surgery	Clinical and radiological assessment followed by 2 days of continuous CSF pressure (P_{csf}) monitoring and 3-day external lumbar drainage (ELD) procedures	Not reported (n = 55)	1, 3, 6, and 12 months after shunting	Mini-mental state examination (MMSE) and Tinetti gait scores	Not reported	Clinical improvement of patients with NPH can be sustained for 5–7 years, even if shunt revision surgery is needed multiple times. Monitoring, identification, and treatment of shunt obstruction is a key management principle

Table 20.1 *(cont.)*

Author	Title of publication	Diagnostic criteria	Mean age (# of patients, n)	Follow-up	Outcome assessment	Deaths	Conclusion
Tisell et al. [31], 2011, Sweden	Shunt surgery in patients with hydrocephalus and white matter changes	Clinical and radiological assessment followed by CSF resistance and CSF tap test	Not reported (n = 14)	3 and 6 months after shunting	Identical Forms, Bingley Visual Memory Test, Reaction Time Test, and the time in seconds needed to walk 10 m	3	Patients with enlarged ventricles, extensive vascular white matter changes, and symptoms compatible with NPH showed improved motor and psychometric functions after shunt surgery despite an R_{out} <12 mmHg/ml/min and no response after a CSF tap test
Toma et al. [14], 2011, UK	Natural history of idiopathic normal-pressure hydrocephaus	Literature review	Not reported (n = 102)	3 months to 7.2 years	Literature review	Not reported	Although quality of studies was poor and numbers were small, this review showed that without surgery, most INPH patients had measurable deterioration as early as 3 months following initial assessment

Table 20.2 Conversion of results on gait tests of the iNPH scale

Ordinal rating of gait		Walk 10 m free pace (steps)		Walk 10 m free pace (time)	
Gait quality	**Score**	**No. of steps**	**Score**	**Time (s)**	**Score**
Normal	100	<15.50	100	<8.75	100
Slight disturbance of tandem walk and turning	86	15.50–16.50	90	8.75–9.25	90
Wide-based gait with sway, without foot corrections	71	16.75–17.25	80	9.50–9.75	80
Tendency to fall, with foot corrections	57	17.50–18.00	70	10.00–10.25	70
Walking with cane	43	18.25–19.25	60	10.50–10.75	60
Bi-manual support needed	29	19.50–20.25	50	11.00–11.50	50
Aided	14	20.50–21.25	40	11.75–13.00	40
Wheelchair bound	0	21.50–23.75	30	13.25–16.00	30
		24.00–27.25	20	16.25–19.25	20
		27.50–40.00	10	19.50–27.00	10
		>40 or fail	0	>27 or fail	0

The domain score is the mean value of the available converted scores.

Table 20.3 Conversion of results on neuropsychological tests of the iNPH scale

Grooved Pegboard (time needed for the fastest trial)		RAVLT (the sum of recalled words on the five learning trials)		Stroop, color naming (time needed for completion)		Stroop, interference (time needed for completion)	
Time (s)	**Score**	**No. of words**	**Score**	**Time (s)**	**Score**	**Time (s)**	**Score**
<79	100	>44	100	<68	100	<132	100
79–87	90	38–44	90	68–77	90	132–160	90
88–96	80	32–37	80	78–81	80	161–188	80
97–105	70	30–31	70	82–87	70	189–210	70
106–114	60	28–29	60	88–96	60	211–239	60
115–128	50	26–27	50	97–106	50	240–298	50
129–144	40	22–25	40	107–121	40	299–385	40
145–173	30	19–21	30	122–134	30	386–600	30
174–245	20	15–18	20	135–171	20	> 600	20
246–600	10	11–14	10	172–300	10	fail	10
>600 or fail	0	<11 or fail	0	>300 or fail	0		

The domain score is the mean value of the available converted scores.

Table 20.4 Conversion of results on balance rating of the iNPH scale

Balance rating	Score
Able to stand independently for more than 30 s on either lower extremity alone	100
Able to stand independently for <30 s on either lower extremity alone	83
Able to stand independently with the feet together (at the heels) for more than 30 s	67
Able to stand independently with the feet together for <30 s	50
Able to stand independently with the feet apart (one foot length) for more than 30 s	33
Able to stand independently with the feet apart for <30 s	17
Unable to stand without assistance	0

Table 20.5 Conversion of results on continence rating of the iNPH scale

Continence rating	Score
Normal	100
Urgency without incontinence	80
Infrequent incontinence without napkin	60
Frequent incontinence with napkin	40
Bladder incontinence	20
Bladder and bowel incontinence	0

Pegboard [Lafayette Instrument Co., Lafayette, IN]). A depression scale such as the Beck Depression Inventory (BDI) can also be incorporated in the cognitive assessment [26–30]. For incontinence, validated questionnaires about urinary incontinence, overactive bladder, and quality of life related to urinary tract symptoms can be administered and, when necessary, urodynamics tests should be offered to obtain objective measures of urinary problems.

When used both pre- and postoperatively, these measures serve as a reliable tool in identifying the degree of clinical impairment and therefore the clinical improvement post-shunting. The difference between the preoperative and post-shunting follow-up scores on these scales has been able to provide an accurate means of outcome assessment. In addition, the increased certainty in diagnosing iNPH by using these dedicated scales has resolved the misinterpretation of

Table 20.6 Total score of the iNPH scale

$$\frac{2 \times \text{Gait} + \text{Neuropsychology} + \text{Balance} + \text{Continence}}{5 \text{ (or number of available domain scores)}}$$

The total score, the domain scores, and the scores on within-domain assessments/tasks all have a min–max range from 0 to 100 where 100 represent normal performance among healthy individuals in an iNPH typical age range of 70–74 years

atypical findings on imaging and challenged the common belief that very old age (above 80 years) has a negative impact on outcome. In a recent randomized study on hydrocephalus patients who had abundant white matter changes, which was generally thought to be a negative predictor for prognosis, the results indicated that these patients significantly improved after surgery if they were properly diagnosed [31]. Similarly, patients aged over 80 achieve a high degree of clinical improvement, despite the increased rate of comorbidities and complications that are mostly due to aging.

Standardized management protocols related to outcome

Since the publication of the international and Japanese guidelines, the establishment of common diagnostic criteria and measurement of characteristic features of iNPH have improved the management of iNPH patients [7,12]. Standardized protocols in the areas of shunt management, clinical outcome grading, time to follow-up after surgery, and clinical judgment are now under development which will enable comparability and reproducibility.

Shunt management

The pathophysiology of NPH secondary to other causes has been investigated in conjunction with the primary etiology. However, the pathophysiology of iNPH is still unclear, including the hypotheses of dysfunctional CSF absorption through arachnoid granulations or anomalies in the venous sinuses or iNPH being a "two hit" disease starting in infancy as "benign external hydrocephalus" followed by deep white matter ischemia (DWMI) in late adulthood [32]. Therefore, the purpose of surgical diversion of CSF via shunt in iNPH is to alleviate symptoms that have an unknown mechanism

Table 20.7 iNPH MCV gait grade

Characteristics of gait pattern	Clinical impairment		Clinical improvement
	Pre	Post	[1] N/A, [2] No Deficit, [3] Improvement, [4] No Improvement, [5] Worse
	Yes/No	Yes/No	
Magnetic			
Shuffling			
Wide base			
Postural instability			
Need assistance			
	E/D/I*	**E/D/I**	
Standing up			
Tandem gait			
Turning			
	Number	**Number**	
# of Steps to turn 180° – mean (SD)			
# of Steps/s for 30 feet walk – mean (SD)			
iNPH MCV gait grade			

iNPH MCV gait grade:
Grade 1 Normal
Grade 2 Impossible tandem gait only
Grade 3 Wide-base gait or short-step gait and impossible tandem
Grade 4 Both wide-base gait and short-step gait and impossible tandem
Grade 5 Help is necessary for walking
Grade 6 Walking is impossible
*Easy/Difficult/Impossible

with high expectations of improvement after shunt surgery. In this regard, the exploration of the in vivo hydrodynamics of CSF shunts before making decisions between different shunt configurations and valve types and antisiphon devices plays a vital role.

Fixed differential pressure valves emerged as the first generation of treatment, to be followed by the introduction of flow-regulated and adjustable (programmable) valves. Adjustable valves have advantages for the management of improvement in triad symptoms and for resolving the problems of underdrainage and overdrainage noninvasively and thus better outcomes can be achieved without surgical intervention [10,33,34]. In the European iNPH study in which adjustable valves were implanted in all patients, one-third of the patients had shunt adjustments due to either over- or underdrainage [35]. In addition, standardized follow-up with control of shunt function and opening pressure in case of no or only partial improvement is important in order to achieve the benefit from shunting, as already pointed out by the same group and by various authors. Klinge et al. [35] reported from the same European iNPH study that 11% of their unimproved patients had "silent" shunt dysfunctions and were converted to improvers after noninvasive readjustments. A similar approach is also recommended in the Japanese guidelines [13] that for possible shunt dysfunction, two settings of reductions each for 30 mmH_2O should be performed before considering a shunt revision. Furthermore, setting the postoperative shunt pressure to a higher setting and then gradually lowering the pressure after surgery will help elderly brains to cope better with the continuous CSF drainage through the shunt. An antisiphon device also serves as a siphon guard where excessive CSF flow may occur due to a positional siphoning effect.

In regard to shunt function, the standard approach is to obtain a cerebral image while exploring the in vivo CSF shunt dynamics. The imaging should be performed the day after surgery or just before discharge to serve as a baseline, and should be followed by further imaging 6 months to 1 year after surgery to show the effect of shunting. The type of imaging depends on the problem that needs to be identified. If an image is required for routine follow-up or if a shunt malfunction is suspected, a non-contrast head CT can be performed. However, if comorbidities such as dementia, atrophy, or organic etiologies need to be ruled out, then MRI is a better imaging modality. In addition, the utilization of routine shunt series should be considered when there is a suspected lack of physical integrity of the shunt or when there is a possibility of the distal end migration or abscess formation preceding overt shunt malfunction. Nevertheless, a CSF infusion test or a CSF tap test through the shunt chamber, even though they are relatively invasive in nature, provide the most accurate information in identifying the shunt malfunction [10–13,36].

In conclusion, it is now well understood that the shunt devices have a tremendous impact on the outcome of iNPH patients, therefore the valve type, configuration, opening and maintenance pressures, and auxiliary devices have to be properly selected with standard protocols. Any type of shunt malfunction has to be explored immediately by determining the best diagnostic approach available in that particular clinical setting. Only then, will the outcome in iNPH patients be accurately assessed and the rate of improvement after surgery be objectively determined.

Standardized outcome assessment

The commonly used outcome scales for iNPH, the modified Rankin Scale (mRS) and Barthel ADL Index (BI), measure the overall improvement or change in activities of daily living of people who mostly have suffered a stroke, which therefore makes it difficult to draw a clear picture for iNPH outcome [37–39]. In 1974, Stein and Langfitt [40] introduced an assessment of outcome in NPH patients based on activities of daily living – the Stein and Langfitt Scale. However, in the early studies, there was no consensus on which of these scales was most suitable for outcome assessment, therefore many authors decided to develop their own outcome measurement tool.

Boon et al. [41] used the Rankin Scale as a disability score and then developed a "Dutch NPH Scale." Using Stein and Langfitt's scale, Black et al. [42] reported an improvement in 33% of 62 iNPH patients. Simultaneously, they also assessed the improvement, which was graded based on the preoperative and postoperative changes in gait, dementia, and incontinence. They then created their own outcome scale using the above criteria and with their classification, the improvement rate was 50% in contrast to the 33% noted in the same group of patients using Stein and Langfitt's scale. In the Medical College of Virginia, since 1992, preoperative and postoperative gait videos have been captured and analyzed to identify the impairment as well as the improvement of gait features in iNPH using the iNPH MCV gait grade presented in Table 20.7 [5,17]. For cognitive assessment, the mini-mental state examination (MMSE) and various neuropsychological tests were administered before and after surgery. For incontinence, the assessment was previously based on the patient's and family's own judgment. Since 2007, validated questionnaires about urinary incontinence, overactive bladder, and quality of life related to urinary tract symptoms have been administered before and after shunt treatment. If necessary, urodynamic tests were offered to obtain objective measures of urinary problems as well. A final conclusion about outcome was made based on the pre- and postoperative comparison of the triad symptoms using the above-mentioned assessments followed by classification of the overall improvement as "Excellent," "Good," "Partial," or "None" using the Marmarou outcome scale [5].

More recently, a group of investigators developed a continuous, calibrated, and norm-based scale for grading the severity of symptoms and assessment of treatment outcome in iNPH [23]. This iNPH scale (Tables 20.2–20.6) was designed for the assessment of the four domains of gait, neuropsychology, balance, and continence, using ordinal ratings and continuous measures. The investigators reported that guidelines and papers discussing the prominent clinical features of iNPH, in conjunction with their clinical experience with iNPH patients, had served as the backbone for their development. In addition, data from normative studies were used to determine the limits for normal scores. Simultaneously, a prospective European multicentre study was conducted using this new iNPH scale as a diagnostic tool along with the radiological findings, and the primary outcome was measured as the difference between the preoperative and 12-month scores on the iNPH scale [35]. The presence of the four major domains (gait, neuropsychological, balance, and continence problems) in 142 patients with iNPH in the European multicenter study confirmed that this new iNPH scale provides proper diagnosis which distinguishes well between patients with different levels of symptom severity, and also between iNPH patients and healthy individuals. In regard to outcome, 84% of patients were improved one year after shunt treatment according to the new iNPH scale. In contrast, the change after surgery as measured by MRI showed an improvement in only 69% of these patients.

These findings are in agreement with the guideline recommendations that if ordinal and insensitive scales developed for other pathophysiological conditions are utilized to assess the outcome in iNPH patients, it will be impossible to accurately capture the improvement in the entire iNPH patient population. Therefore, preoperative and postoperative grading of the patient symptoms via gait analysis, neuropsychological testing, and internationally validated questionnaires for incontinence in conjunction with urodynamic studies are recommended for accurate diagnosis and outcome assessment. Other domains such as balance, dizziness, and headache scales can be incorporated if needed.

The time period for short-term and long-term outcome

The time for follow-up in iNPH patients had extreme ranges from months to years post-shunting, with short term referring to 3–6 months after surgery and long term to one year and more and even as long as 10–15 years post-surgery. For many years, investigators reported mixed results without identifying the specific time spans for follow-up. This resulted in various rates of improvement and therefore made it difficult to justify the long-term maintenance of favorable outcome after shunt surgery. Aygok et al. [5] reported that 3 months after shunt placement in 50 iNPH patients, 41% of patients had excellent/good recovery in gait whereas 50% had partial gait improvement. In general, overall gait improvement equaled 91%. For memory impairment, 40% of patients had excellent/good recovery and another 40% had partial recovery. For incontinence, 44% had improved dramatically and another 26% had partial improvement. At the end of 3 years, 92% of patients had survived. At three years, the improvement in gait was preserved for 75% of patients. Better results were seen in memory improvement at 3 years compared with 3 months; 80% of patients with memory impairment had sustained their recovery after 3 years and 20% had even reached a better improvement category. More than 80% of improvement was observed in incontinence in excellent/good/partial improvement categories.

The conclusion is that, if there is standardization of diagnosis and treatment and if all patients are being followed post-surgery within the same time intervals, then it is possible to see the positive effect of shunting in iNPH patients. Therefore, since the publication of the international and Japanese guidelines, there has been a consensus about obtaining regular follow-up assessments and reporting the time periods in which the outcome is assessed post-surgery [7,12]. Considering the fact that some iNPH patients have temporary improvements which are not long-lasting, 3–6 months post-surgery has to be considered as the short term and any time point after 6 months post-surgery has to be considered as the long-term follow-up.

Clinical judgment

The outcome results are graded based on clinical judgment performed by the physician since the investigators agree that this task mostly falls to the neurosurgeon, neurologist, geriatrician or sometimes the primary care physician. The patient and caregiver opinion is also being valued; however, it is important to remember that this could be relatively subjective in nature [43,44].

The standards regarding the frequency and nature of follow-up visits have now been established in the centers of excellence for iNPH management. Based on these suggestions, the neurosurgeon who performs the shunt operation should be seen within 2 weeks of surgery for suture removal and also for detecting any early complications. Then based on the type of implanted valve and the degree of improvement in iNPH symptoms, patients are scheduled for follow-up visits two to four times for the first year followed by bi-annual or annual visits afterwards. These assessments can be performed by a neurosurgeon, a neurologist, or a geriatrician and the consulting team should share the information with all the corresponding physicians who are involved in the patient's care.

Impact of complications after surgery

Complications after shunting which impact the quality of clinical outcome include:

(a) major (subdural hematoma [SDH]/hygroma, shunt infection, and shunt failure); and
(b) minor (orthostatic headache, double vision, and hearing loss).

There is a strong correlation between outcome of shunted iNPH patients and complications after surgery. Even though shunting will eventually help to improve the symptoms of iNPH patients, complications if not treated will not only delay but also complicate the clinical improvement. Additionally, the different treatment options for various complications have major impacts on outcome post-shunting. The type of complication reversed noninvasively by resetting the shunt pressures mostly causes minor delays in clinical improvement. However, the surgical treatment of an SDH with a mass effect or a shunt removal for a serious shunt infection, recovery from which may take weeks to months, can cause major delays in achieving a favorable outcome. In a series of 50 iNPH patients treated with adjustable shunts, major (SDH, hygroma) and minor complications (headache, hearing loss, double vision) due to surgery totaled 6% and 14%, respectively [5]. All these patients improved without surgical intervention by adjusting the opening pressures. Hashimoto et al. (SINPHONI) [18] found there was a 3% incidence of serious events and 20% incidence of less serious events.

In conclusion, preventing complications during and after surgery before it occurs is crucial. To decrease the risk of over/underdrainage problems, valve and auxiliary device settings and configurations have to be properly selected based on the patient's height, weight, and physical condition. For the risk of infection, the precautions have to be taken in the operating room and if infection is suspected then early detection is necessary. If adjustable valves are the choice of treatment, the goal is to have standardized protocols for managing the shunt opening pressures. One way is to set the pressure setting at a higher level during the shunt operation then to start reducing the opening pressure gradually. The same approach can be applied when treating the overdrainage complications: SDH, hygroma, headache, hearing loss, and double vision. Once these complications are resolved, then the shunt opening pressures can be gradually decreased. Nevertheless, if there is a serious risk such as mass effect and severe deterioration in clinical symptoms because of a complication, then patients have to be taken to the operating room for surgical intervention.

Impact of comorbidities

Comorbidity is a major confounder in outcome assessment in the iNPH patient population [45–47]. There is no doubt that health conditions like coexisting Parkinson's disease, or spine, hip or knee problems in iNPH can affect the patient's gait, and prostate problems may worsen the incontinence. Memory impairment can also be a part of vascular disease or Alzheimer's disease.

Meier et al. [48] proposed a critical question in diagnosis and treatment of iNPH patients about whether preoperative factors can most reliably predict outcomes following shunt insertion. The results of the prospective follow-up examination (Kiefer Score, NPH Recovery Rate) of 82 out of 100 shunted iNPH patients were compared with the preoperative comorbidity index (CMI). Of the patients with a CMI score of 0–1, 67% experienced an excellent outcome, whereas a score of 4–5 was related to only 14% excellent. Remarkably, the excellent outcome of the patients between 6 and 8 on the CMI was 0%. The authors concluded that comorbidity is a statistically significant predictor of the clinical outcome for patients with iNPH undergoing shunt therapy. In a series reported by Aygok et al. [5], 24% (12/50) of the patients had comorbidities not related to surgery, including stroke, cardiac problems, vertigo, and psychiatric problems. Of these, stroke affected the independence in activities of daily living, whereas dementia and depression affected cognitive function, therefore improvement due to shunting became compromised. Since these comorbid conditions in the iNPH patient population have an influence on the clinical outcome after shunting, it is important to diagnose and treat these conditions.

Conclusion

With proper identification of iNPH patients and precise determination of the most suitable valve type and configuration, the improvement in outcome seen immediately after shunting is reasonably sustained over a period of years and provides a favorable risk/benefit profile of shunting in this elderly population. In addition, using standardized and validated iNPH scales that measure the clinical impairment before surgery and the clinical improvement after surgery will improve the outcome assessment during both short-term and long-term follow-up.

References

1. Hakim S. Some observations on CSF pressure: Hydrocephalic syndrome in adults with "normal" CSF pressure. PhD thesis no. 957. Javeriana University School of Medicine, Bogota; 1964.
2. Hakim S, Adams RD. The special clinical problem of symptomatic hydrocephalus with normal cerebrospinal fluid pressure observations on cerebrospinal fluid hydrodynamics. *J Neurol Sci* 1965;2:307–27.
3. Black PM. Idiopathic normal-pressure hydrocephalus. Results of shunting in 62 patients. *J Neurosurg* 1980;52(3):371–7.
4. Malm J, Kristensen B, Stegmayr B, Fagerlund M, Koskinen LO. Three-year survival and functional outcome of patients with idiopathic adult hydrocephalus syndrome. *Neurology* 2000;55(4):576–8.
5. Aygok GA, Marmarou A, Young HF. Three year outcome of shunted idiopathic NPH patients. *Acta Neurochir Suppl* 2005;95:241–5.
6. Kiefer M, Meier U, Eymann R. Does idiopathic normal pressure hydrocephalus always mean a poor prognosis? *Acta Neurochir Suppl* 2010;106:101–6.
7. Marmarou A, Bergsneider M, Relkin N, Klinge P, Black PM. Development of guidelines for idiopathic normal-pressure hydrocephalus: introduction. *Neurosurgery* 2005;57(Suppl):S1–3.
8. Relkin N, Marmarou A, Klinge P, Bergsneider M, Black PM. Diagnosing idiopathic normal-pressure hydrocephalus. *Neurosurgery* 2005;57(3 Suppl):S4–16.
9. Marmarou A, Bergsneider M, Klinge P, Relkin N, Black PM. The value of supplemental prognostic tests for the preoperative assessment of idiopathic normal-pressure hydrocephalus. *Neurosurgery* 2005;57(3 Suppl):S17–28.
10. Bergsneider M, Black PM, Klinge P, Marmarou A, Relkin N. Surgical management of idiopathic normal-pressure hydrocephalus. *Neurosurgery* 2005;57(Suppl):S29–39.
11. Klinge P, Marmarou A, Bergsneider M, Relkin N, Black PM. Outcome of shunting in idiopathic normal pressure hydrocephalus and the value of outcome assessment in shunted patients. *Neurosurgery* 2005;57(3 Suppl):S40–52.
12. Ishikawa M, Hashimoto M, Kuwana N, et al. Guidelines for management of idiopathic normal pressure hydrocephalus: Guidelines from the Guidelines Committee of Idiopathic Normal Pressure Hydrocephalus, the Japanese Society of Normal Pressure Hydrocephalus. *Neurol Med Chir (Tokyo)* 2008;48(Suppl):S1–S23.
13. Mori E, Ishikawa M, Kato T, et al. Guidelines for management of idiopathic normal pressure hydrocephalus: Second Edition. *Neurol Med Chir (Tokyo)* 2012;52:775–809.
14. Toma AK, Stapleton S, Papadopoulos MC, Kitchen ND, Watkins LD. Natural history of idiopathic normal-pressure hydrocephalus. *Neurosurg Rev* 2011;34(4):433–9.
15. Poca MA, Solana E, Martínez-Ricarte FR, et al. Idiopathic normal pressure hydrocephalus: results of a prospective cohort of 236 shunted patients. *Acta Neurochir Suppl* 2012;114:247–53.
16. Walchenbach R, Geiger E, Thomeer RTWM, Vanneste JAL. The value of temporary external lumbar CSF drainage in predicting the outcome of shunting on normal pressure hydrocephalus. *J Neurol Neurosurg Psychiatry* 2002;72:503–6.
17. Marmarou A, Young HF, Aygok GA, et al. Diagnosis and management of idiopathic normal-pressure hydrocephalus: a prospective study in 151 patients. *J Neurosurg* 2005;102:987–97.
18. Hashimoto M, Ishikawa M, Mori E, Kuwana N. The study of INPH on neurological improvement (SINPHONI). Diagnosis of idiopathic normal pressure hydrocephalus is supported by MRI-based scheme: a prospective cohort study. *Cerebrospinal Fluid Res* 2010;7:18.
19. Chen YF, Wang YH, Hsiao JK, et al. Normal pressure hydrocephalus: cerebral hemodynamic, metabolism measurement, discharge score, and long-term outcome. *Surg Neurol* 2008;70(S1):69–77.
20. American Association of Neurological Surgeons, Joint Section of Neurotrauma and Critical Care, Brain Trauma Foundation. Guidelines for the management of severe head injury. *J Neurotrauma* 1996;13(11):641–734.
21. Kubo Y, Kazui H, Yoshida T, et al. Validation of grading scale for evaluating symptoms of idiopathic normal-pressure hydrocephalus. *Dement Geriatr Cogn Disord* 2008;25:37–45.
22. Kiefer M, Eymann R, Komenda Y, Steudel W. A grading system for chronic hydrocephalus. *Zentralbl Neurochir* 2003;64:109–15.
23. Hellström P, Klinge P, Tans J, Wikkelsø C. A new scale for assessment of severity and outcome in iNPH. *Acta Neurol Scand* 2012;126:229–37.
24. Podsiadlo D, Richardson S. The timed "Up & Go": a test of basic functional mobility for frail elderly persons. *J Am Geriatr Soc* 1991;39:142–8.

25. Abbruzzese LD. The Tinetti performance-oriented mobility assessment tool. *Am J Nursing* 1998;98:16J–16L.
26. Folstein MF, Folstein SE, McHugh PR. "Mini-mental State". A practical method for grading the cognitive state of patients for the clinician. *J Psychiatr Res* 1975;12:189–98.
27. Stroop JD. Studies of interference in serial verbal reactions. *J Exp Psychol* 1935;18 (6):643–62.
28. Schmidt M. *Rey Auditory Verbal Learning Test: A Handbook (RAVLT)*. Los Angeles, CA: Western Psychological Services; 1996.
29. Beck AT, Steer RA, Ball R, Ranieri W. Comparison of Beck depression inventories -IA and -II in psychiatric outpatients. *J Pers Assess* 1996;67(3):588–97.
30. Thomas G, McGirt MJ, Woodworth G, et al. Baseline neuropsychological profile and cognitive response to cerebrospinal fluid shunting for idiopathic normal pressure hydrocephalus. *Dement Geriatr Cogn Disord* 2005;20(2–3):163–8.
31. Tisell M, Tullberg M, Hellström P, et al. Shunt surgery in patients with hydrocephalus and white matter changes. *J Neurosurg* 2011;114(5):1432–8.
32. Bradley WG, Bahl G, MD, Alksne JF. Idiopathic normal pressure hydrocephalus may be a "two hit" disease: benign external hydrocephalus in infancy followed by deep white matter ischemia in late adulthood. *J MRI* 2006;24:747–55.
33. Pollack IF, Albright AL, Adelson PD. A randomized, controlled study of a programmable shunt valve versus a conventional valve for patients with hydrocephalus. Hakim-Medos Investigator Group. *Neurosurgery* 1999;45:1399–408.
34. Ringel F, Schramm J, Meyer B. Comparison of programmable shunt valves vs. standard valves for communicating hydrocephalus of adults: a retrospective analysis of 407 patients. *Surg Neurol* 2005;63:36–41.
35. Klinge P, Hellström P, Tans J, Wikkelsø C. One-year outcome in the European multi-centre study on iNPH. *Acta Neurol Scand* 2012;126(3):145–53.
36. Pujari S, Kharkar S, Metellus P, et al. Normal pressure hydrocephalus: long-term outcome after shunt surgery. *J Neurol Neurosurg Psychiatry* 2008;79(11):1282–6.
37. Rankin J. Cerebral vascular accidents in patients over the age of 60. II. Prognosis. *Scott Med J* 1957;2(5):200–15.
38. van Swieten J, Koudstaal P, Visser M, et al. Interobserver agreement for the assessment of handicap in stroke patients. *Stroke* 1988;19(5):604–7.
39. Mahoney FI, Barthel DW. Functional evaluation: the Barthel Index. *MD State Med J* 1965;14:61–5.
40. Stein SC, Langfitt TW. Normal-pressure hydrocephalus. Predicting the results of cerebrospinal fluid shunting. *J Neurosurg* 1974;41(4):463–70.
41. Boon AJ, Tans JT, Delwel EJ, et al. Dutch normal pressure hydrocephalus study: prediction of outcome after shunting by resistance to outflow of cerebrospinal fluid. *J Neurosurg* 1997;87:687–93.
42. Black PM, Ojemann RG, Tzouras A. CSF shunts for dementia, incontinence, and gait disturbance. *Clin Neurosurg* 1985;32:632–51.
43. Cage TA, Auguste KI, Wrensch M, Wu YW, Gupta N. Self-reported functional outcome after surgical intervention in patients with idiopathic normal pressure hydrocephalus. *J Clin Neurosci* 2011;18(5):649–54.
44. Lundin F, Ulander M, Svanborg E, Wikkelsø C, Leijon G. How active are patients with idiopathic normal pressure hydrocephalus and does activity improve after shunt surgery? A controlled actigraphic study. *Clin Neurol Neurosurg* 2013;115(2):192–6.
45. Raftopoulos C, Massager N, Baleriaux D, et al. Prospective analysis by computed tomography and long-term outcome of 23 adult patients with chronic idiopathic hydrocephalus. *Neurosurgery* 1996;38(1):51–9.
46. Mirzayan MJ, Luetjens G, Borremans JJ, Regel JP, Krauss JK. Extended long-term (>5 years) outcome of cerebrospinal fluid shunting in idiopathic normal pressure hydrocephalus. *Neurosurgery* 2010;67(2):295–301.
47. Lemcke J, Meier U. Idiopathic normal pressure hydrocephalus (iNPH) and co-morbidity: an outcome analysis of 134 patients. *Acta Neurochir Suppl* 2012;114:255–9.
48. Meier U, Lemcke J. Co-morbidity as a predictor of outcome in patients with idiopathic normal-pressure hydrocephalus. *Acta Neurochir Suppl* 2010;106:127–30.

Chapter 21

Normal pressure hydrocephalus syndrome secondary to hemorrhage, infection, and malignancy

C. Rory Goodwin, Benjamin D. Elder, Thomas A. Kosztowski, and Daniele Rigamonti

Normal pressure hydrocephalus (NPH) is characterized by the presence of ventriculomegaly associated with the triad of gait, memory, and urinary problems in the absence of a detectable cause. There is a group of individuals with longstanding compensated hydrocephalus that might develop a clinical picture similar to idiopathic NPH (iNPH) at an age younger than the typical age of presentation of iNPH. The syndromes of hydrocephalus in young and middle-aged adults, SHYMA, or longstanding overt ventriculomegaly, also known as LOVA, specifically refer to this phenomenon. This characteristic clinical presentation of iNPH, however, also accompanies the insidious onset of hydrocephalus secondary to other processes, such as infection, malignancy, and hemorrhage. In this chapter, we discuss the clinical features, evaluation, and management of secondary and/or compensated hydrocephalus.

The syndrome of compensated hydrocephalus

Compensated hydrocephalus is usually associated with macrocephaly and copper cranium. Other common radiologic features include: herniation of the third ventricle into the sella turcica, empty sella, less prominent temporal horns and atrophy of the corpus callosum. These patients commonly have mild symptoms that can manifest in frequent mild to moderate headaches, clumsiness, or difficulty concentrating. Literature would suggest that these other forms of chronic or compensated hydrocephalus are subsets of normal pressure hydrocephalus; however, there are enough distinctive features to suggest that some of these syndromes represent an entirely separate clinical entity based on the same pathophysiologic mechanism (Figure 21.1).

Late-onset idiopathic aqueductal stenosis (LIAS)

LIAS can result in hydrocephalus and typically presents in young adults as headaches. While ventriculography was the standard diagnostic tool used when LIAS was first described, advances in imaging techniques and specifically the advent of magnetic resonance imaging (MRI) allowing clearer visualization of the cerebral aqueduct has resulted in easier diagnosis of LIAS [1,2]. Typically, there is no pathognomonic sign for LIAS, but it is generally associated with a "small fourth ventricle" and cine MR imaging has been shown to be sensitive for blockage of cerebrospinal fluid (CSF) flow at the cerebral aqueduct [3,4]. One study reported that cine imaging was useful in cases of mild hydrocephalus, but reported that seven out of nine patients with significant dilation of the ventricles demonstrated CSF flow at the cerebral aqueduct. The pathophysiologic mechanism in LIAS patients is attributed to partial obstruction with minimal flow through the aqueduct, because a complete obstruction would present with symptomatology that is more rapid and severe. In terms of treatment, CSF drainage via a shunt was the primary modality used when LIAS was first described; however, advances in neuroendoscopy and specifically third ventriculostomy have slowly changed the treatment method of choice [5–7].

The syndrome of longstanding overt ventriculomegaly (LOVA) and the syndrome of hydrocephalus in young and middle-aged adults (SHYMA)

The syndrome of longstanding overt ventriculomegaly describes the association of congenital aqueductal

Adult Hydrocephalus, ed. Daniele Rigamonti. Published by Cambridge University Press.

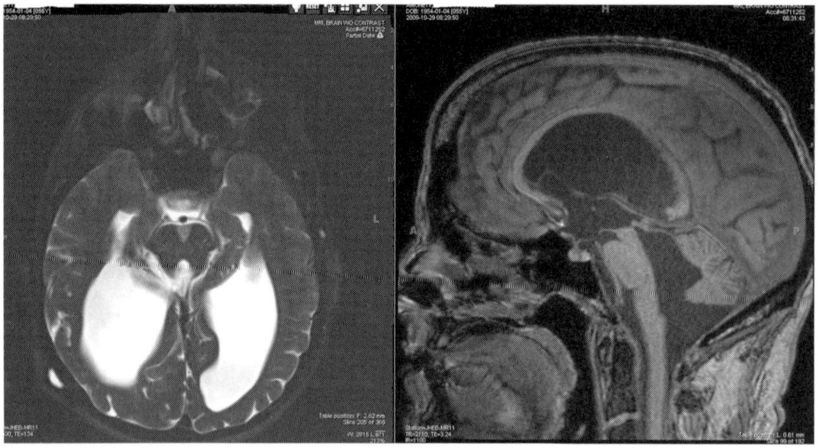

Figure 21.1 This 54-year-old patient experienced chronic headaches for many years. He always had trouble walking (he never biked and could not roller skate either; he was always uncoordinated when playing baseball). He had a large head: his head circumference is 62 cm (greater than the 97th percentile). According to his wife, he had been falling and forgetting things at work insidiously over a few years. Note the macrocephaly, herniation of the third ventricle into the sella turcica and its outward bulging walls, the less prominent temporal horns, and the atrophy of the corpus callosum.

stenosis with headaches and macrocephaly. SHYMA is a clinical syndrome affecting young and middle-aged adults and is associated with either decompensated hydrocephalus, acquired hydrocephalus, or idiopathic hydrocephalus [8]. Age appears to be the main determinant of the clinical syndrome. While the primary symptoms are similar to those of NPH, the main predicament of these patients is the impact on their everyday functional activities in spite of the subtlety of their symptoms. These patients most often have difficulty in performing job-related tasks, with some clumsiness, difficulty with uneven surfaces, and difficulty with stairs in the context of notably absent gait ataxia. In terms of urinary symptoms, patients with SHYMA in Cowan et al.'s study [8] often complained of urinary urgency or frequency but stated that urinary incontinence was rare. The most consistent symptom in this cohort was headache, which was present in 70% of patients. In terms of functional activities, almost 84% of patients in this series reported job performance impairment before a diagnosis was made, with many of these patients facing disciplinary action or job loss. The duration of their symptoms was on average almost 6 years. The majority of patients with SHYMA benefited from surgical intervention, either third ventriculostomy or CSF shunting, with 93% of patients showing at least partial improvement and 56% of patients demonstrating complete recovery. While 29 underwent primary shunting, and 11 underwent third ventriculostomy, interestingly, 6 of the 11 third ventriculostomy patients ultimately required a shunt [8] (Figure 21.2).

Hydrocephalus secondary to other processes

Hydrocephalus can occur under any situation in which the ventricular system is obstructed, CSF production is increased or CSF absorption is impaired. As such, hydrocephalus can be a secondary process that results from a primary lesion. Most commonly obstruction from either aneurysmal subarachnoid hemorrhage, brain malignancy (whether a primary brain tumor or metastases), spinal malignancy, or an infectious etiology can precipitate or directly lead to hydrocephalus.

Hydrocephalus and malignancies

Hydrocephalus secondary to malignancy is a common phenomenon that occurs in adults and children, alike. Patients can present initially with signs and symptoms of hydrocephalus, which prompts radiological imaging that leads to the diagnosis of the underlying tumor. It is estimated that greater than 50% of pediatric patients with brain tumors also have associated hydrocephalus [9]. In this subset of patients almost 95% of pediatric brain tumor patients had obstructive hydrocephalus, with the remainder being communicating hydrocephalus. Greater than 90% of these patients presented with hydrocephalus at diagnosis [9]. Blockage of CSF can occur at several levels depending on tumor location. Cerebral hemisphere tumors, thalamic tumors, tumors of the sellar region, and tumors in the region of the third ventricle can cause blockage on one or both sides of the foramen of Monro, whereas thalamic neoplasms, pineal region tumors and midbrain tumors

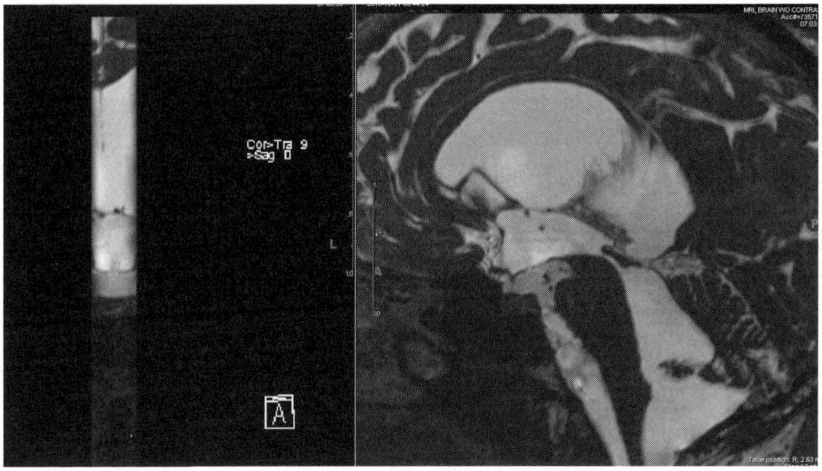

Figure 21.2 T2-weighted images in the coronal and sagittal planes. Note the patent endoscopic third ventriculostomy (ETV) and the normal shape of the third ventricle after the ETV.

can block the foramen of Monro or the cerebral aqueduct (Figure 21.3). At the level of the posterior fossa, blockage of the fourth ventricle can lead to obstructive hydrocephalus.

In contrast, communicating hydrocephalus is thought to occur in the context of increased CSF production, such as in the case of choroid plexus tumors (Figure 21.4) [9], or impaired CSF absorption, secondary to leptomeningeal disease or tumor bleeding. Carcinomatous meningitis is associated with various tumor types, including lung and breast cancer metastases. Liaw et al. reported that hydrocephalus was present in 62% of such patients [10]. In another series of three patients with meningeal carcinomatosis, symptoms of hydrocephalus were the presenting complaints with gait disturbance in all three, headaches in two of the patients, and altered mentation in one patient. Resolution of the symptoms of hydrocephalus occurred in all three patients with the insertion of a ventriculoperitoneal shunt. Although tumor responsiveness to radiation and/or chemotherapy as well as the burden of systemic disease ultimately influence survival in this patient population, placement of a ventriculoperitoneal shunt in patients who exhibit signs of hydrocephalus is beneficial, because it allows maintenance of a more meaningful quality of life. Lumboperitoneal shunts can be used in selective cases where CSF overproduction is a prominent feature.

Obstructive hydrocephalus secondary to a neoplasm is most commonly treated with surgical resection with or without external ventricular drainage, which is commonly temporary. Baroncini et al. described 284 adult and pediatric cases of tumors of the lateral ventricle in which two-thirds of the cases had some associated CSF disorder [11]. This group noted that neuropsychological deficits were the most frequent sequelae (22.8%) secondary to hydrocephalus [11]. Ventriculoperitoneal shunt implantation is the most common shunting procedure performed in patients with pediatric brain tumors, although endoscopic third ventriculostomy is often utilized in patients with tumors originating from the pineal region, thalamus, tectum, or pons.

Hydrocephalus can be a complication following radiation treatment secondary to radiation-induced edema. Following radiation, stiffening of the ventricles and effacement of the ventricular system can lead to increased intracranial pressure. More commonly this occurs in the setting of metastases to the posterior fossa with blockage of the fourth ventricle causing impaired CSF circulation. Hydrocephalus following radiation treatment can occur at any tumor location where the ventricular system has the potential to be obstructed secondary to mass effect from the underlying lesion or surrounding edema.

The association between spinal cord tumors and hydrocephalus was first described by Nonne in 1900 [12,13]. Kyrieleis described the first thoracolumbar tumor presenting with symptoms of hydrocephalus, headache, and papilledema, in 1931, and reported that removal of the tumor alleviated the symptoms [14,15]. With the development and implementation of CT and MR imaging the number of cases reported in the literature has grown to over 300. Mirone et al. contend that 1% of patients with intraspinal tumors will have some degree of hydrocephalus at initial presentation [15].

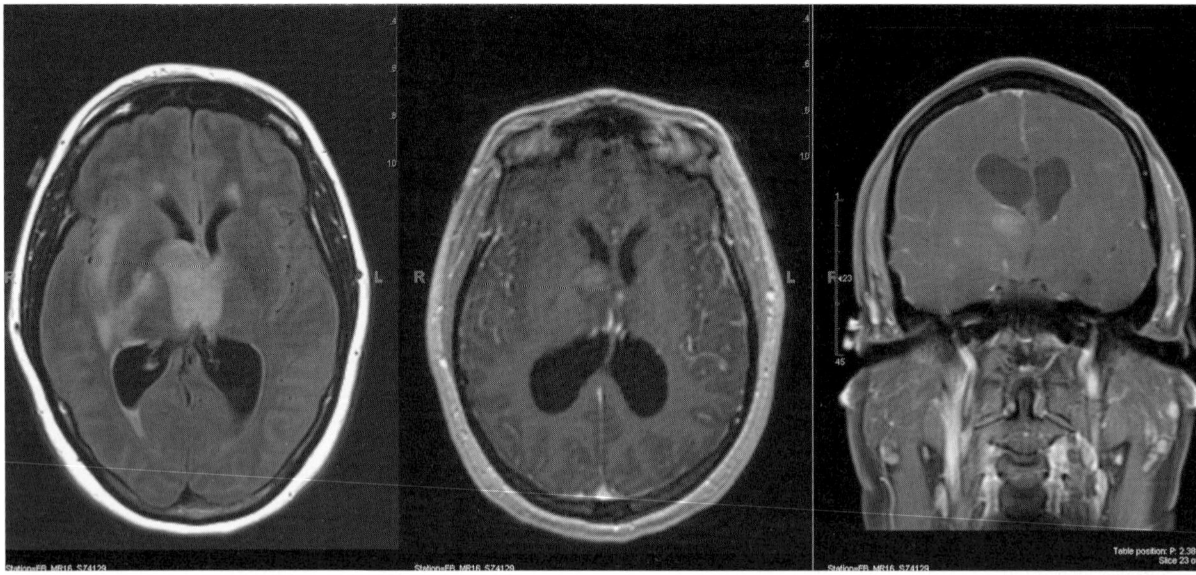

Figure 21.3 This 48-year-old woman presented with an episode of loss of consciousness and work-up in the emergency department demonstrated hydrocephalus secondary to a large mass involving the thalamus. The patient was well until 10 days prior when she began experiencing frequent, severe headaches, of which she had no prior history. MRI TE and T1-weighted images with contrast enhancement show a centrally necrotic, peripherally enhancing nodule within the ventricle, heterogeneous, prominently T2 hyperintense, component of the mass within the right anteromedial and midmedial thalamus, vasogenic edema and infiltrating tumor within the right striatocapsular region, leftward convex bowing of the third ventricle which is slit like, and dilation of the lateral ventricles. Pathological examination of the surgical specimen revealed an infiltrating astrocytoma.

Rifkinson-Mann et al. described a series of 171 patients with intramedullary spinal cord tumors, in which 15% of the patients had symptomatic hydrocephalus. In this series, the authors also conclude that the patients with malignant intramedullary astrocytoma with associated hydrocephalus have a shorter survival time than patients with high grade lesions without hydrocephalus [16]. Astrocytomas and ependymomas are more frequently associated with hydrocephalus than other spinal tumor types and intramedullary tumors were associated with hydrocephalus almost 75% of the time[15]. Maroulis et al. analyzed the 269 patients with spinal cord tumors and hydrocephalus in the literature and concluded that in 47% of the cases, the two disease processes were diagnosed at the same time [17]. In this series, a history of either back pain, transient sphincter disturbance, or peripheral neurological signs raised suspicion of an underlying spinal lesion.

The pathophysiologic mechanism leading to hydrocephalus in patients harboring malignant intraspinal lesions is postulated to be secondary to the meningeal infiltration which increases resistance to CSF flow and absorption in the subarachnoid space. Several hypotheses have been suggested for the mechanism leading to hydrocephalus in patients with benign lesions: they range from alterations in the CSF pressure and flow from spinal obstruction, decreased CSF resorption around the spinal nerve sheaths, increased CSF viscosity secondary to increased protein content, increased deposition of fibrin, or outflow obstruction at the cervicomedullary junction [12]. While Rifkinson-Mann et al. concluded that rostral tumor cyst extension to the cervicomedullary junction was the predominant cause of the resultant hydrocephalus [16], Cinalli et al. contend that this most likely only represents a subset of tumor cases [12].

Surgical resection of the spinal lesion should be the first treatment when hydrocephalus and the intraspinal tumor are diagnosed at the same time, because removal of the lesion may resolve the hydrocephalus. Prior to surgical resection, a pan neuraxis MRI with contrast should be utilized to identify the extent of intracranial and spinal leptomeningeal seeding and other potential causes of hydrocephalus. In cases where leptomeningeal seeding is diffuse, hydrocephalus is likely to persist after tumor resection, making a shunting procedure necessary. This may be true in spite of the fact that certain authors contend that surgical trauma and/or the existence of a shunt could enhance tumor spread most likely due to changes in dissemination of neoplastic

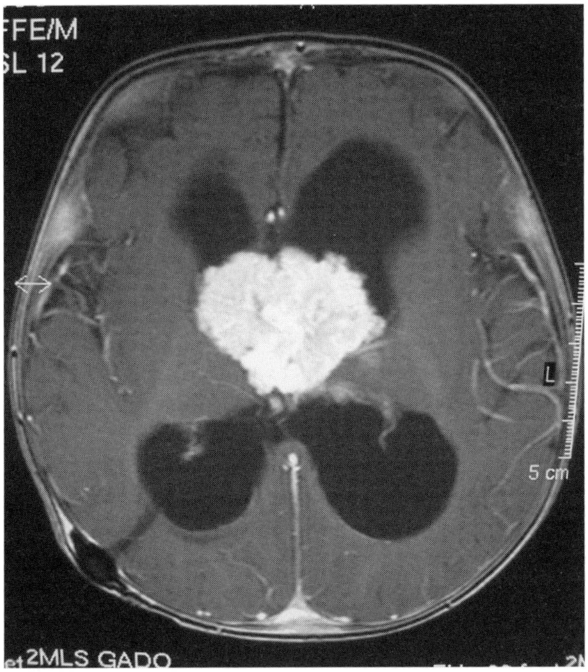

Figure 21.4 A young patient presenting with signs of increased intracranial pressure underwent MRI that showed an intensely enhancing mass originating in the third ventricle causing obstructive hydrocephalus. Pathological examination of the surgical specimen revealed a choroid plexus papilloma.

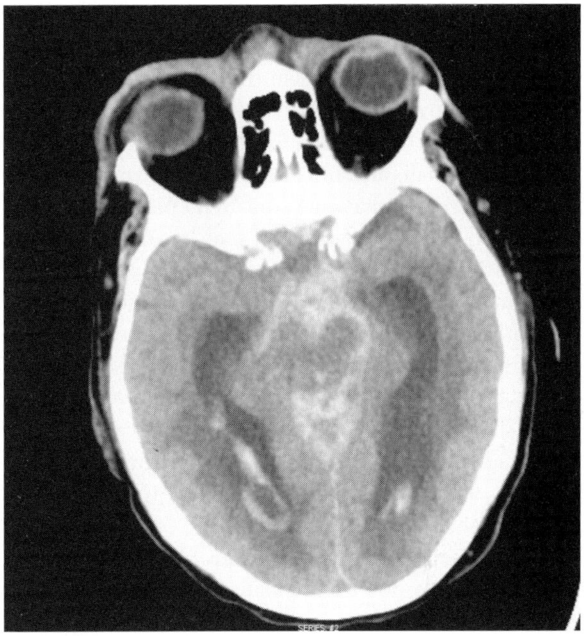

Figure 21.5 This 71-year-old woman was emergently admitted to the hospital after she suddenly lost consciousness. CT showed extensive intraventricular and subarachnoid hemorrhage causing moderate to severe hydrocephalus.

cells in the subarachnoid pathways and increase leptomeningeal seeding [15].

Hydrocephalus following subarachnoid hemorrhage (SAH)

Subarachnoid hemorrhage following aneurysmal rupture is a common disease process, first described by Bagley in 1928, that results in significant morbidity and mortality. Post-SAH hydrocephalus can be classified as either acute, occurring within 72 hours, subacute occurring over a few weeks, or chronic, occurring more than one month after the initial injury, resulting in permanent hydrocephalus often treated via CSF diversion. The development of hydrocephalus acutely can result in significant neurological disability, coma, and even death. Risk factors that predispose individuals to hydrocephalus include poor Hunt–Hess grade, intraventricular hemorrhage, history of hypertension, and aneurysms in the posterior circulation that can lead to obstruction of the fourth ventricle (Figure 21.5) [18–20].

Acute hydrocephalus following SAH is a common complication that is estimated to affect 20–30% of SAH patients [19,21,22]. The pathophysiological mechanism for the development of acute hydrocephalus is most often due to associated intraventricular hemorrhage which results in obstruction of CSF flow through the ventricular system and subarachnoid. In certain instances the increased subarachnoid blood and/or clot results in mass effect on the brain and ventricular system. The most common symptoms include headache, nausea, vomiting, impaired eye movements (particularly upward gaze), or impaired or decreased level of consciousness. The most significant symptom requiring intervention is decreased level of consciousness. Development of acute hydrocephalus is correlated with poor prognosis following subarachnoid hemorrhage [23]. In the acute setting, placement of an external ventricular drainage catheter is indicated. One study reported that approximately 29.6% of patients had acute hydrocephalus that resolved spontaneously within 48 hours of development, and 37.0% (10/27) of patients required intervention with external ventricular drainage due to either increased hydrocephalus or clinical deterioration [24].

Once the hydrocephalus moves past 72 hours, it enters the subacute or chronic phase. Under these circumstances patients generally undergo some type of shunting procedure. During surgery for aneurysmal subarachnoid hemorrhage, the lamina terminalis is typically opened to increase the operative exposure, but it also allows for increased drainage [25,26]. It has been suggested by Sindou et al. that fenestration of the lamina terminalis and Liliequist's membrane improves overall prognosis in aneurysmal SAH patients [25,26]. Tomasello et al. demonstrated that lamina terminalis fenestration during aneurysm clipping in patients with subarachnoid hemorrhage resulted in a rate of 4.2% of postoperative hydrocephalus compared to the average of 20% [27]. The mechanism for decreased rates of hydrocephalus in these patients is thought to be related to the direct drainage of CSF from the lateral and third ventricles into the subarachnoid space, bypassing the cisterns of the base where scarring prompted by the blood might have occurred [28].

In patients requiring ventriculostomy for treatment of hydrocephalus, the criteria for weaning off an external ventricular drainage (EVD) system to ultimate removal versus placement of a shunt must also be considered. Klopfenstein et al. conducted a randomized controlled prospective study comparing gradual, multi-step EVD weaning versus rapid weaning [29]. This group demonstrated that a 96-hour trial, in which the external ventricular system was raised sequentially over every 24-hour period until the drain could be closed, provided no advantage in terms of preventing the need for permanent CSF diversion in comparison to a rapid wean, exemplified by immediate clamping of the EVD. The rate of shunting in both groups was ~60% [29].

Hydrocephalus following infection (post-infective)

Post-infective hydrocephalus is more commonly found in developing countries and has been reported to occur in 30–40% of hydrocephalus cases [30]. Post-infective hydrocephalus is commonly caused by either tuberculous or pyogenic meningitis [30].

In neonates, the most common organisms responsible for meningitis are *E. coli* and group B streptococci. The meningitis is usually acquired through maternal infection in neonates who have undergone a complicated labor or delivery with premature or prolonged rupture of membranes. More commonly the neonate suffers from generalized sepsis and the underlying meningitis is not recognized until later [31]. In preterm infants to children 3 months of age, group B streptococci, *Staphylococcus* species and *Haemophilus influenzae* are predominantly implicated, whereas in adolescents and young adults *Neisseria meningitidis* is the commonest organism responsible (Figure 21.6) [30].

In pyogenic cases, the pathophysiologic mechanism for the resultant hydrocephalus is the increased

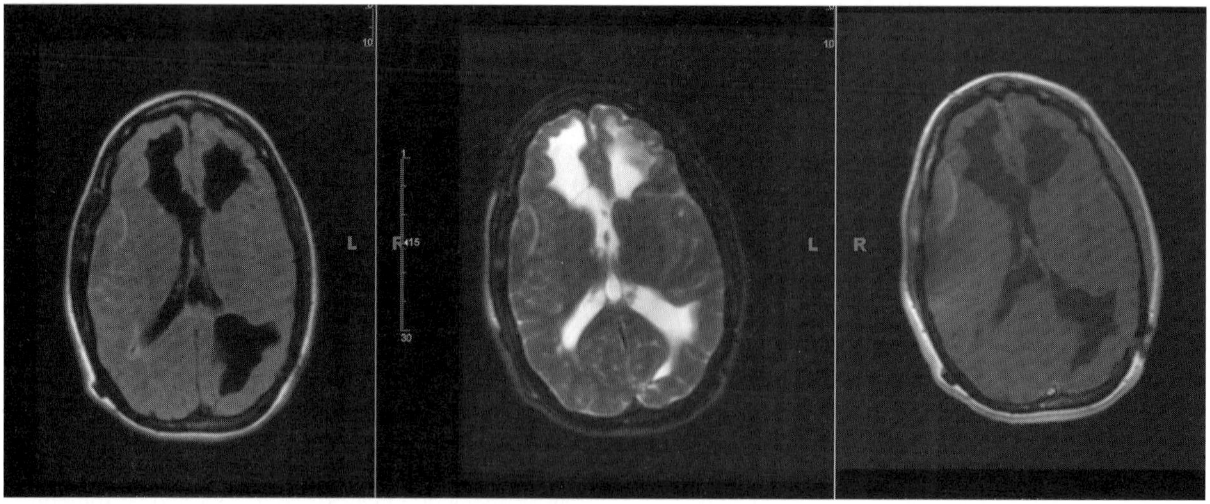

Figure 21.6 This 27-year-old mentally retarded woman was born premature at 36 weeks. At 6 days after birth she developed *Citrobacter* meningitis and brain abscesses. She then developed hydrocephalus at 6 weeks and underwent shunt at about 2 months of age. She had a shunt revision in 1984 aged 6, another one in 1986 aged 8, one in 1996, and one in 1998. Since that surgery she had experienced intense dizziness. She had several shunt revisions between 2005 and 2006. MRI showed multiple porencephalic cysts in the bilateral frontal region, and left parietal region with ex-vacuo dilatation of the associated ventricles, and minimal gliotic change in the surrounding white matter without abnormal enhancement.

cellularity and fibrotic adhesions that form on the arachnoid secondary to the inflammatory response of the offending organism. When meningitis occurs, the vessels become congested resulting in exudative material in the basal cisterns and ventricular system. As the fluid becomes more congested and turbid, the choroid and arachnoid tissue become covered in pus, which leads to leukocyte and plasma cell migration into the CSF circulation. In turn, the increased cellularity coupled with the fibrosis, adhesions, and septations that develop in the ventricles, cisterns, and arachnoid granulations impede CSF circulation and reabsorption causing hydrocephalus [30].

Toxoplasmosis is caused by the intracellular protozoan *Toxoplasma gondii* and most commonly occurs, in developed and developing countries alike, as a secondary infection in immunocompromised hosts, particularly those with HIV/AIDS. Congenital toxoplasmosis typically occurs in the infants of HIV/AIDS infected mothers [32]. *T. gondii* was described in 1908 in rodents and the first human case was later discovered in the retina of an infant who had hydrocephalus, seizures, and a unilateral ocular anomaly. On neuroimaging, single or multiple ring-enhancing mass lesions localized at the corticomedullary junction, in the white matter, or the basal ganglia are commonly seen, although cerebellar lesions have also been reported. Parenchymal involvement often causes extensive brain tissue necrosis and surrounding inflammation, which can potentially occlude the ventricular system, through mass effect on the cerebral aqueduct, foramen of Monro or fourth ventricle, or it can cause a ventriculitis. Similar to other disease processes, treatment should be directed at the underlying causative agent. In emergent situations where acute hydrocephalus is diagnosed, an external ventricular drainage device should be utilized to temporize the patient until anti-toxoplasma therapy can be initiated. For toxoplasma infection the most important method for treating and/or preventing the secondary effects of this disease is treating the immunocompromised state, particularly with HAART therapy in HIV/AIDS patients.

Ingestion of eggs from the tapeworm *Taenia solium* can lead to infection of the brain and covering meninges (neurocysticercosis). Once the oncospheres hatch in the intestine and penetrate the intestinal wall, the organism has an affinity for the central nervous system. Although epilepsy is the most common manifestation of neurocysticercosis, once the organism invades the ventricular system, acute hydrocephalus can occur. It is estimated that anywhere from 15% to 54% of cases present with the intraventricular form [33]. Neurocysticercosis most commonly affects the fourth ventricle (53%), followed by the third (27%) and then the lateral ventricle (11%) and cerebral aqueduct (9%). Once a cyst migrates to the fourth ventricle it can cause an obstructive hydrocephalus that can lead to rapid clinical deterioration. In one series, over 30% of patients presented with clinical deterioration and/or sudden death secondary to acute hydrocephalus. Scarring of the leptomeninges or arachnoiditis can lead to communicating hydrocephalus.

Intraventricular neurocysticercosis is diagnosed by the clinical presentation and imaging findings. Computed tomography (CT) is often used to initially diagnose the lesion, although its sensitivity is much lower given that the cyst contents and the CSF share the same density. As such, the cyst and the scolex may not be visible on CT. Cysts in the third ventricle often have the same appearance as a colloid cyst [34]. On MRI intraventricular cysts are identified 80% of the time with a spherical lesion seen on T1-weighted imaging with a hyperintense cyst wall and the scolex appearing as a mural nodule (Figure 21.7), whereas on T2-weighted imaging the cyst contents are isointense with a hyperintense scolex. Treatment for parasitic lesions is based on the clinical presentation and location of the cyst in the

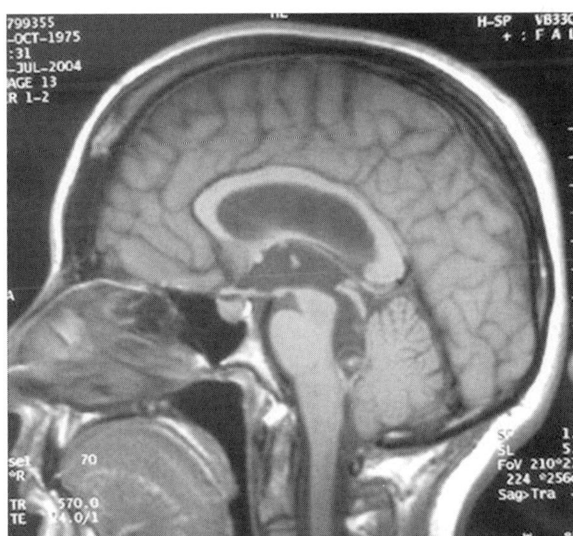

Figure 21.7 This 29-year-old woman from Bolivia developed headache, nausea and vomiting, and gait ataxia after a trip to her country. Sagittal T1-weighted image with gadolinium enhancement showed neurocysticercosis causing obstructive hydrocephalus.

ventricular system. Emergent ventriculostomy should be the first treatment in cases of acute hydrocephalus as this procedure has the potential to be life-saving. Other interventions include ventriculoperitoneal shunt placement for obstructive hydrocephalus, and endoscopic or open surgical removal of the cyst. Although the cysts may be removed, ventriculoperitoneal shunting may be required afterwards [34]. In cases where shunting is required, the rate of revision can be as high as 30–67%, especially in cases complicated by ventriculitis [35,36]. Endoscopic treatment of ventricular neurocysticercosis has the advantage of allowing easy navigation through the ventricular system with minimal postoperative complications [37]. Several approaches and techniques have been described using endoscopic intervention for this disease process. Intraoperative rupture of the cyst may lead to ventriculitis necessitating continuous irrigation through the endoscope intraoperatively to help clear the contents and a potential shunting procedure postoperatively. Clinical outcomes from endoscopic treatment of neurocysticercosis are better than outcomes after open surgical procedures [33].

Conclusion

Compensated hydrocephalus or the syndromes of LIAS or SHYMA are clinical entities that are most likely underdiagnosed secondary to the subtlety of the findings. Advancements in neuroimaging have allowed for the correct diagnosis and potential treatment of these patients. These syndromes represent chronic disorders with symptoms that are typically easily missed, because they are understated, but have been shown to improve following shunt implantation. In contrast, hydrocephalus that develops secondary to either malignancy, post-hemorrhage, or in conjunction with an infectious etiology can have acute symptoms that can be life-threatening. When the ventricular system is obstructed, CSF production is increased or CSF absorption is impaired. In the setting of acute clinical deterioration, the first line of treatment is usually an external ventricular drainage device. Shunt implantation can also be indicated depending on the extent of residual effects from the primary process.

References

1. Bennett RT, Allen PB, Miller JD. Non-tumoral stenosis of the aqueduct in adults. *Surg Neurol* 1975;4(6):523–7.
2. Vertosick F, Jr., Sekhar L. Adult aqueductal stenosis presenting as double incontinence: a case report with magnetic resonance imaging. *Surg Neurol* 1989;31(5):387–9.
3. Quencer RM. Intracranial CSF flow in pediatric hydrocephalus: evaluation with cine-MR imaging. *AJNR Am J Neuroradiol* 1992;13(2):601–8.
4. Quencer RM, Post MJ, Hinks RS. Cine MR in the evaluation of normal and abnormal CSF flow: intracranial and intraspinal studies. *Neuroradiology* 1990;32(5):371–91.
5. Drake JM. Ventriculostomy for treatment of hydrocephalus. *Neurosurg Clin N Am* 1993;4(4):657–66.
6. Fukuhara T, Vorster SJ, Luciano MG. Risk factors for failure of endoscopic third ventriculostomy for obstructive hydrocephalus. *Neurosurgery* 2000;46(5):1100–9; discussion 1109–11.
7. Kelly PJ. Stereotactic third ventriculostomy in patients with nontumoral adolescent/adult onset aqueductal stenosis and symptomatic hydrocephalus. *J Neurosurg* 1991;75(6):865–73.
8. Cowan JA, McGirt MJ, Woodworth G, Rigamonti D, Williams MA. The syndrome of hydrocephalus in young and middle-aged adults (SHYMA). *Neurol Res* 2005;27(5):540–7.
9. Wong TT, Liang ML, Chen HH, Chang FC. Hydrocephalus with brain tumors in children. *Childs Nerv Syst* 2011;27(10):1723–34.
10. Liaw CC, Ng KT, Huang JS, et al. Meningeal carcinomatosis from solid tumors: clinical analysis of 42 cases. *Journal of the Formosan Medical Association = Taiwan yi zhi* 1992;91(3):299–303.
11. Baroncini M, Peltier J, Le Gars D, Lejeune JP. [Tumors of the lateral ventricle. Review of 284 cases]. *Neuro-Chirurgie* 2011;57(4–6):170–9.
12. Cinalli G, Sainte-Rose C, Lellouch-Tubiana A, et al. Hydrocephalus associated with intramedullary low-grade glioma. Illustrative cases and review of the literature. *J Neurosurg* 1995;83(3):480–5.
13. Nonne. Ueber einen Fall von intramedullärem ascendirendem Sarcom sowie drei Fälle von Zerstörung des Halsmarks. Weitere Beiträge zur Lehre von Verhalten der Sehnenreflexe bei hoher Querläsion des Rückenmarks. *Arch Psychiat Nervenkrank* 1900;83:393–430.
14. Kyrieleis. *Die Augenveranderungen bei den entzundlichen Erkrankungen des Zentralnervensystem.* Berlin: Springer 1931.
15. Mirone G, Cinalli G, Spennato P, Ruggiero C, Aliberti F. Hydrocephalus and spinal cord tumors: a review. *Childs Nerv Syst* 2011;27(10):1741–9.

16. Rifkinson-Mann S, Wisoff JH, Epstein F. The association of hydrocephalus with intramedullary spinal cord tumors: a series of 25 patients. *Neurosurgery* 1990;27(5):749–54; discussion 754.

17. Maroulis H MW, Leone E, Cinalli G. *Hydrocephalus and Spinal Tumors*. Milan: Springer; 2004.

18. Dorai Z, Hynan LS, Kopitnik TA, Samson D. Factors related to hydrocephalus after aneurysmal subarachnoid hemorrhage. *Neurosurgery* 2003;52(4):763–9; discussion 769–71.

19. Hellingman CA, van den Bergh WM, Beijer IS, et al. Risk of rebleeding after treatment of acute hydrocephalus in patients with aneurysmal subarachnoid hemorrhage. *Stroke* 2007;38(1):96–9.

20. Lin CL, Kwan AL, Howng SL. Acute hydrocephalus and chronic hydrocephalus with the need of postoperative shunting after aneurysmal subarachnoid hemorrhage. *The Kaohsiung Journal of Medical Sciences* 1999;15(3):137–45.

21. Germanwala AV, Huang J, Tamargo RJ. Hydrocephalus after aneurysmal subarachnoid hemorrhage. *Neurosurg Clin N Am* 21(2):263–70.

22. van Asch CJ, van der Schaaf IC, Rinkel GJ. Acute hydrocephalus and cerebral perfusion after aneurysmal subarachnoid hemorrhage. *AJNR Am J Neuroradiol* 2010;31(1):67–70.

23. Bakker AM, Dorhout Mees SM, Algra A, Rinkel GJ. Extent of acute hydrocephalus after aneurysmal subarachnoid hemorrhage as a risk factor for delayed cerebral infarction. *Stroke* 2007;38(9):2496–9.

24. Lu J, Ji N, Yang Z, Zhao X. Prognosis and treatment of acute hydrocephalus following aneurysmal subarachnoid haemorrhage. *J Clin Neurosci* 2012;19(5):669–72.

25. Komotar RJ, Olivi A, Rigamonti D, Tamargo RJ. Microsurgical fenestration of the lamina terminalis reduces the incidence of shunt-dependent hydrocephalus after aneurysmal subarachnoid hemorrhage. *Neurosurgery* 2002;51(6):1403–12; discussion 1412–13.

26. Sindou M. Favourable influence of opening the lamina terminalis and Lilliequist's membrane on the outcome of ruptured intracranial aneurysms. A study of 197 consecutive cases. *Acta Neurochir* 1994;127(1–2):15–16.

27. Tomasello F, d'Avella D, de Divitiis O. Does lamina terminalis fenestration reduce the incidence of chronic hydrocephalus after subarachnoid hemorrhage? *Neurosurgery* 1999; 45(4):827–31; discussion 831–2.

28. Mura J, Rojas-Zalazar D, Ruiz A, Vintimilla LC, Marengo JJ. Improved outcome in high-grade aneurysmal subarachnoid hemorrhage by enhancement of endogenous clearance of cisternal blood clots: a prospective study that demonstrates the role of lamina terminalis fenestration combined with modern microsurgical cisternal blood evacuation. *Minim Invasive Neurosurg* 2007;50(6):355–62.

29. Klopfenstein JD, Kim LJ, Feiz-Erfan I, et al. Comparison of rapid and gradual weaning from external ventricular drainage in patients with aneurysmal subarachnoid hemorrhage: a prospective randomized trial. *J Neurosurg* 2004;100(2):225–9.

30. Chatterjee S, Chatterjee U. Overview of post-infective hydrocephalus. *Childs Nerv Syst* 2011;27(10):1693–8.

31. Stoll BJ, Schuchat A. Maternal carriage of group B streptococci in developing countries. *Pediatr Infect Dis J* 1998;17(6):499–503.

32. Ibebuike K, Mantanga L, Emereole O, et al. Cerebellar toxoplasmosis in HIV/AIDS infant: case report and review of the literature. *Neurol Sci* 2012;33(6):1423–8.

33. Sinha S, Sharma BS. Intraventricular neurocysticercosis: a review of current status and management issues. *Br J Neurosurg* 2012;26(3):305–9.

34. Couldwell WT, Chandrasoma P, Apuzzo ML, Zee CS. Third ventricular cysticercal cyst mimicking a colloid cyst: case report. *Neurosurgery* 1995;37(6):1200–3.

35. Cuetter AC, Andrews RJ. Intraventricular neurocysticercosis: 18 consecutive patients and review of the literature. *Neurosurg Focus* 2002;12(6):e5.

36. Kelley R, Duong DH, Locke GE. Characteristics of ventricular shunt malfunctions among patients with neurocysticercosis. *Neurosurgery* 2002;50(4):757–61; discussion 761–2.

37. Anandh B, Mohanty A, Sampath S, Praharaj SS, Kolluri S. Endoscopic approach to intraventricular cysticercal lesions. *Minim Invasive Neurosurg* 2001;44(4):194–6.

Chapter 22

Low-pressure syndromes and cerebrospinal fluid leaks

Diagnosis and management

Debraj Mukherjee and Wouter I. Schievink

Epidemiology

Cerebrospinal fluid (CSF) leaks are increasingly considered an important cause of low-pressure headaches, particularly among younger patients [1]. While rigorous epidemiological evidence is lacking, several series have documented the relative incidence of CSF leak from varying etiologies. Approximately 80% of CSF fistulae with rhinorrhea have been reported to be caused by nonsurgical trauma and 16% by surgical trauma, with the remaining 4% having nontraumatic etiology [2]. Of course, for patients with spontaneous intracranial hypotension, the underlying CSF leak should be looked for in the spine and not at the level of the skull base [3]. Spontaneous intracranial hypotension has been estimated to range between 1 per 50 000 to 5 per 100 000 persons in community-based and emergency department based settings, respectively [4,5]. Spontaneous intracranial hypotension affects women twice as frequently as men and typically presents in the fourth or fifth decade of life, though the specific pathophysiological reason for this demographic trend is currently unknown [6–16].

Pathogenesis

The specific etiology underlying spontaneous CSF leaks remains largely unknown, but underlying structural weakness of the spinal meninges is suspected, though a history of trauma may be elicited in up to a third of patients [14,17–19]. This dural weakness, ranging from simple dural tears to meningeal diverticula, allows CSF to leak into the epidural [20,21]. Ventral spinal CSF leaks are often seen at the level of the disk space and may be associated with degenerative disk disease.

Varying connective tissue disorders may play a role in the development of spontaneous spinal CSF leaks, with two-thirds of patients having some physical exam features consistent with such disorders, inclusive of joint hypermobility or subtle skeletal manifestations of Marfan syndrome [22]. These patients with some skeletal manifestations consistent with Marfan syndrome have been found to have a defect in microfibrils, an important component of the extracellular matrix associated with fibrillin, rather than a mutation in fibrillin-1 itself that is characteristic of Marfan syndrome [23]. Less frequently, spontaneous intracranial hypotension has occurred in well-described connective tissue disorders including Ehlers–Danlos syndrome type II, autosomal dominant polycystic kidney disease, neurofibromatosis, Lehman syndrome, and true Marfan syndrome [24–28].

Some authors have suggested that spontaneous intracranial hypotension results from decreased CSF secretion or generalized CSF hyperabsorption, though no significant data support such alternate mechanisms. It seems that the final common pathway is likely not CSF hypovolemia but rather altered distribution of craniospinal elasticity due to spinal loss of CSF [29].

Clinical presentation

Positional headaches

Spontaneous intracranial hypotension typically manifests as an orthostatic headache, often worst within 15 minutes of assuming an upright position, though the lag period may be as long as several hours after assuming an upright position. Improvement of the headache upon lying supine is less variable and generally occurs within 15 to 30 minutes of lying flat. These headaches may be throbbing or not, are generally bilateral, and are most commonly in the occipital or suboccipital

Adult Hydrocephalus, ed. Daniele Rigamonti. Published by Cambridge University Press.

region. The severity of the headache varies widely, with mild cases likely often remaining undiagnosed while others may be incapacitated while upright [30]. These positional headaches are thought to be a direct result of downward displacement of the brain due to loss of CSF buoyancy, with resultant traction on pain-sensitive structures inclusive of the dura, or from compensatory dilation of pain-sensitive intracranial venous structures.

Other patterns of headache have also been found in those with low pressure headaches. Rarely, non-positional headaches may precede the typical orthostatic headache. Additionally, some patients do not have posture-related headaches, but rather develop headaches upon exertion or at the end of the day. Intermittent headaches, thought to be caused by intermittent spinal CSF leaks, may even occur as infrequently as over the course of weeks or months. Some patients deny headaches at all, though these patients often present with other symptoms consistent with spontaneous intracranial hypotension.

Miscellaneous symptoms

In addition to headaches, other symptoms have been reported in spontaneous intracranial hypotension including neck pain or stiffness, nausea, and emesis. In total, these symptoms have been reported to be present in up to 50% of patients [15]. Additional symptoms include changes in hearing, with some patients describing echoing, a feeling of being underwater, tinnitus, or a disturbed sense of balance. Such symptoms may be the result of abnormal CSF pressure relative to that of the perilymph or alternatively from stretching of the eighth nerve complex [31]. Downward displacement of the brain in patients with spontaneous CSF leak has been associated with myriad miscellaneous symptoms including visual blurring, diplopia, and facial numbness/pain/weakness [32–35]. Severe displacement of the brain has even been implicated in a decreased level of consciousness due to diencephalic herniation [36,37], dementia [38,39], and parkinsonism [40].

Diagnosis

Cranial computed tomography

Brain computed tomography (CT) does not provide as many cardinal features as magnetic resonance (MRI), though CT scans may show features suggestive of CSF leak, including bilateral subdural hygromas/hematomas, effacement of the subarachnoid cisterns, and ventricular collapse. Thus, CT scans may be a helpful initial diagnostic tool, for instance in the outpatient or emergency department setting, prior to more definitive imaging.

Cranial magnetic resonance imaging

While some findings of CSF leak in MRI can be variable, there are generally five characteristic imaging features most often associated with spontaneous intracranial hypotension: subdural fluid collections, enhancement of the meninges, engorgement of venous structures, pituitary hyperemia, and sagging of the brain (mnemonic, SEEPS) [1] (Figure 22.1).

Subdural fluid collections are common in spontaneous intracranial hypotension, are thought to be caused by tearing of subdural bridging veins, and occur in approximately 50% of such patients [41]. Most of these collections are bilateral hygromas located over convexities and do not cause any significant mass effect or midline shift. True subdural hematomas are less common, affecting approximately one-quarter of all patients [41]. Most subdural hematomas in this setting can be managed by primarily treating the underlying spinal CSF leak, either with treatment via interventional radiology or with open spinal surgery; only a minority of patients required craniotomy for direct surgical evacuation of blood [41]. Improvement in this MRI finding can be expected within days to weeks of successful treatment for small subdural collections, while larger subdural hematomas may require up to 3 months to fully resolve. Clinical improvement generally precedes radiographic improvement in most spontaneous intracranial hypotension patients.

Diffuse enhancement of both the supra- and infratentorial meninges is the best-known imaging finding in spontaneous intracranial hypotension, with the dilation of thin-walled blood vessels of the subdural zone thought to be the mechanism for contrast enhancement. However, up to 20% of patients do not develop enhancement on MRI [42].

Engorgement of venous structures is also a common finding in spontaneous intracranial hypotension, with findings most evident in the large cerebral veins and/or dural sinus. Such findings may be relatively subtle and may require the comparison of post- versus pre-gadolinium images to help identify them.

Pituitary hyperemia has additionally been described as an often cardinal feature of spontaneous

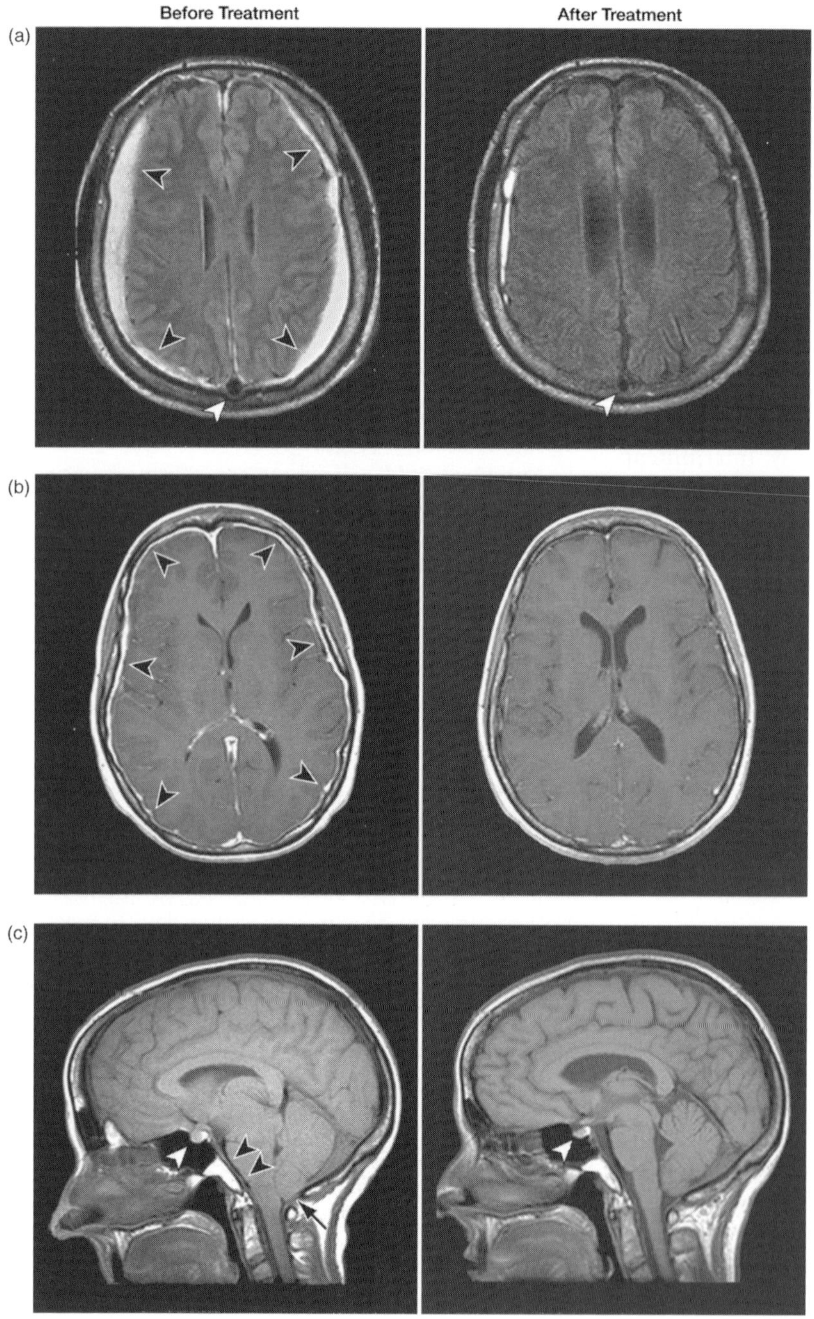

Figure 22.1 Pretreatment and posttreatment magnetic resonance imaging. (a) Axial FLAIR imaging shows resolution of bilateral subdural hematomas (black arrowheads) and engorgement of the superior sagittal sinus (white arrow). (b) Axial post-gadolinium contrast, T1-weighted imaging shows resolution of meningeal enhancement (black arrowheads). (c) Sagittal T1-weighted imaging without contrast shows resolution of brain sag inclusive of less flattening of the pons/effacement of the prepontine cistern (black arrowheads), less displacement of the cerebellar tonsils within the posterior fossa (black arrow), and less hyperemia of the pituitary gland (white arrows). Used with permission from Schievink WI. Spontaneous spinal cerebrospinal fluid leaks and intracranial hypotension. *JAMA* 2006;295:2286–96.

intracranial hypotension. The relative hyperemia in such cases may at times mimic a pituitary adenoma or hyperplasia, and requires some clinical correlation of radiographic findings.

Sagging of the brain is thought to be due to loss of CSF buoyancy and may be accompanied by ventricular collapse. This brain sag is associated with several key features including effacement of perichiasmatic cisterns, bowing of the optic chiasm, flatting of the pituitary stalk, effacement of the prepontine cisterns, flattening of the pons, and descent of the cerebellar tonsils within the posterior fossa. This latter feature may be mistaken for a Chiari malformation. As noted above, subdural fluid collection may be seen, though the degree of brain sagging is generally out of proportion to any mass effect caused by these subdural collections.

Myelography

The study of choice to define CSF leaks of the spine has been myelography, either with iodinated contrast followed by thin-cut CT or with gadolinium followed by MRI of the entire spine [43]. A majority of such CSF leaks are found at the cervicothoracic junction or within the thoracic spine. Frequently, multiple CSF leaks are demonstrated, although it should be noted that multiple spinal meningeal diverticula are frequently mistaken for multiple spinal CSF leaks. In some cases, delayed imaging may be required to visualize slow or intermittent leaks, but the yield of such endeavors is strikingly low. Conversely, ultra-early CT imaging may be required to identify high-volume leaks. The most effective method of demonstrating high flow ventral CSF leaks is digital subtraction myelography [44].

The risk of cerebral herniation during myelogram has never been documented as such risk would appear to be markedly low, as the dural hole made by lumbar puncture is small and CSF pressure is already low. Likewise, worsening symptoms from a dural puncture are quite rare in patients with spontaneous intracranial hypotension and such an occurrence should instill some doubt regarding the diagnosis.

Radionuclide cisternography

Radionuclide cisternography has been used in the evaluation of spontaneous intracranial hypotension but has demonstrated only limited usefulness as the site of CSF leak remains unknown in up to one-third of patients [45]. Typical findings include slow ascent along the spinal axis and a relative lack of activity over the convexities. This modality of imaging does maintain some usefulness when the diagnosis of intracranial hypotension remains in doubt following normal myelography.

Spinal MRI

Although spinal MRI has not been as effective at localizing CSF leaks as CT myelography, more recent work has demonstrated some specific spinal manifestations of spontaneous intracranial imaging in spinal MR imaging. Such findings include dilated epidural and intradural veins, dural enhancement, and meningeal diverticula [46,47]. MR myelography is particularly well-suited to demonstrating spinal meningeal diverticula and dural ectasia. Also, plain MRI is an excellent method of demonstrating the extent of ventral spinal CSF leaks (Figure 22.2).

Lumbar puncture

Although lumbar puncture can introduce a small dural opening as mentioned above, additional diagnostic information can be ascertained from such intervention. Generally, opening pressures are less than 60 mmH_2O, whereas normal values range from 65 to 195 mmH_2O. Occasionally, pressures have been unremarkable or even negative. Other spontaneous intracranial hypotension patients can consistently have normal CSF opening pressures despite multiple lumbar punctures. Microscopic examination often demonstrates a lymphocytic pleocytosis of up to 200 cells/mm^3, an elevated protein content of up to 1000 mg/dl, or xanthochromia, all thought to be caused by a combination of increased permeability of meningeal blood vessels and decreased CSF flow in the lumbar subarachnoid space.

Diagnostic criteria

Several iterations of diagnostic criteria for spontaneous intracranial hypotension have been developed over the past decade, with some variations in inclusion and exclusion criteria used including varying clinical symptoms and radiographic evidence. Perhaps the most widely cited set of diagnostic criteria are those established by the Headache Classification Subcommittee of the International Headache Society [48]. This set of criteria included a positional headache with at least one additional clinical symptom, at least one radiographic or diagnostic criterion, no history of dural puncture or other cause of CSF fistula, and a headache that resolves within 72 hours of epidural blood patch, as outlined in Table 22.1.

A more recently proposed classification scheme allows for a three-step approach to the diagnosis. For instance, patients may either have a demonstrated spinal CSF leak (for instance, via CT or MR myelography) or may fulfill one of two separate sets of criteria. The first of these two sets of criteria include having MR brain imaging findings consistent with CSF leak in addition to having either a low opening pressure (less than or equal to 60 mmH_2O), the presence of spinal meningeal diverticula, or improvement in symptoms

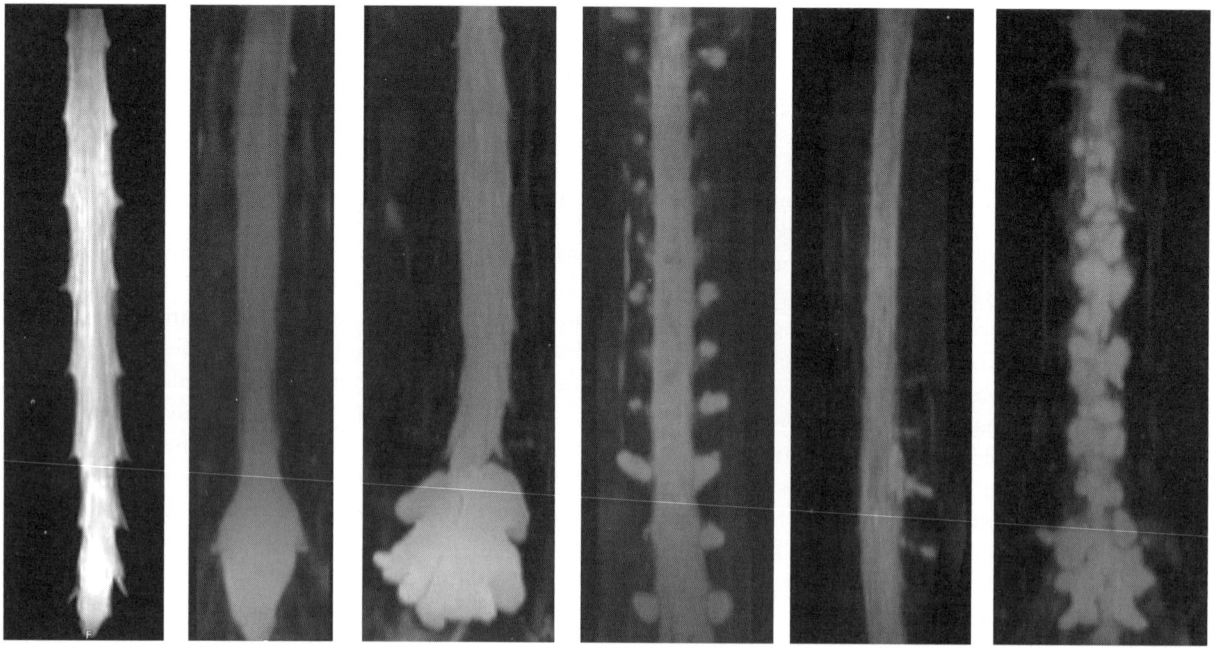

Figure 22.2 MR myelography demonstrating various examples of dural ectasia and meningeal diverticula in patients with spontaneous intracranial hypotension (normal scan is on the left).

Table 22.1 Diagnostic criteria for headache due to spontaneous spinal CSF leak and intracranial hypotension as defined by the International Classification of Headache Disorders, 2nd Edition (2004) [48]

A. Diffuse and/or dull headache that worsens within 15 minutes after sitting or standing, fulfilling criterion D and with 1 of the following:
1. Neck stiffness
2. Tinnitus
3. Hypacusia
4. Photophobia
5. Nausea
B. At least 1 of the following:
1. Evidence of low CSF pressure on MRI (e.g. pachymeningeal enhancement)
2. Evidence of CSF leakage on conventional myelography, CT myelography, or cisternography
3. CSF opening pressure 60 mmH$_2$O in sitting position
C. No history of dural puncture or other cause of CSF fistula
D. Headache resolves within 72 hours after epidural blood patching

following epidural blood patch. The second of these two sets of criteria are for those without a demonstrated spinal CSF leak or MR brain findings consistent with a leak; such patients may meet the criteria for diagnosis by meeting all three of the additional criteria noted above (low opening pressure, spinal meningeal diverticula, and improvement in symptoms after blood patch) or two of such criteria in addition to orthostatic headaches [49]. Other groups have generally seemed to agree with this newer set of diagnostic criteria, while pointing out the potential need to define specific criteria for measuring spinal meningeal diverticula and the potential need to define a 24- to 72- hour time window to allow for symptomatic improvement following a blood patch [50].

Most recently, a multi-institutional group of experts have proposed a simplified algorithm for diagnosis in which any patient with orthostatic headaches, no recent history of dural puncture, and headaches not attributable to another disorder can meet criteria for spontaneous intracranial hypotension with the addition of only one of the following additional criteria: low opening pressure (less than or equal to 60 mmH$_2$O), sustained improvement following blood patch, demonstration of active spinal CSF leak, or cranial MR changes consistent with intracranial hypotension [51]. Rigorous work analyzing the relative efficacy of these varying diagnostic criteria has yet to be undertaken.

Treatment, outcomes, and future directions

Although data are lacking, it is often stated that many cases of spontaneous intracranial hypotension resolve spontaneously without any intervention and with only conservative management at most. Conservative management has traditionally consisted of bed rest, oral hydration, and use of an abdominal binder. While this conservative management is anecdotally felt to help in most, a subset of patients may have persistent debilitating symptoms or may desire more timely resolution of symptoms. For such patients, additional interventions may include the use of steroids, intravenous caffeine, or theophylline, though the efficacy of such interventions seems limited at best.

For those patients who continue to have significant symptoms despite the conservative or relatively noninvasive approaches noted above, the mainstay of first-line interventional treatment has been the injection of 10–20 ml of autologous blood into the spinal epidural space, otherwise known as an epidural blood patch [52,53]. For those undergoing this procedure, the relief of symptoms often is instantaneous, thought to be due to a combination of replacing CSF volume loss with blood volume within the spinal canal, due to the blood patch forming a type of dural tamponade thus sealing the leak, and due to the blood restricting CSF flow within the spinal epidural space thereby interfering with CSF absorption. Although such a blood patch is effective in relieving symptoms in up to one-third of patients, those with residual significant symptoms may either have the 10–20 ml blood patch repeated or may alternatively be offered a high-volume (20–100 ml) blood patch. The largest volume we have ever given was 130 ml. Because patients with spontaneous intracranial hypotension have such a large epidural space due to the loss of intrathecal CSF, such a large volume can be accommodated. Given the high volume of such patches, a minimum of 5 days is usually advised between a regular and high-volume blood patch.

For those patients in which epidural blood patch fails, either percutaneous placement of fibrin sealant or an open/direct epidural blood patch may be advised. Generally, either of these additional approaches would necessitate that the exact site of the CSF leak be known in order to maximize the odds of successful intervention. Attempting percutaneous fibrin sealant placement remains a viable non-operative therapeutic option and may be beneficial in up to one-third of patients in whom an epidural blood patch has not been effective [54].

Surgical treatment is reserved for those in whom these nonsurgical interventions such as blood patch or fibrin glue have failed and remains a viable option for those in whom a focal structural abnormality leading to CSF leak can be identified. Leaking meningeal diverticula can be ligated with either suture or aneurysm clips, while dural tears can be repaired either directly with suture or with placement of a muscle pledget and fibrin sealant. Ventral dural tears (Figure 22.3) are best treated with suturing although placement of a dural substitute along with fibrin sealant or placement of a sling may also be effective. Headache following successful percutaneous or open treatment may indicate either a recurrent leak or rebound transient intracranial hypertension. The pattern of headaches post-intervention may help elucidate the etiology of such headaches. For instance, if the character of the headaches remains similar to initial presentation, including orthostatic headaches, then likelihood of recurrent leak may be relatively increased. However, if the patient experiences worse headaches when supine, so-called pressure headaches, the likelihood of rebound transient intracranial hypertension may be relatively increased and such patients may benefit from at least a short course of acetazolamide [55].

Overall, outcomes are good for the great majority of patients with spontaneous intracranial hypotension, but some patients are refractory to any treatment and innovative but unproven therapies should be explored

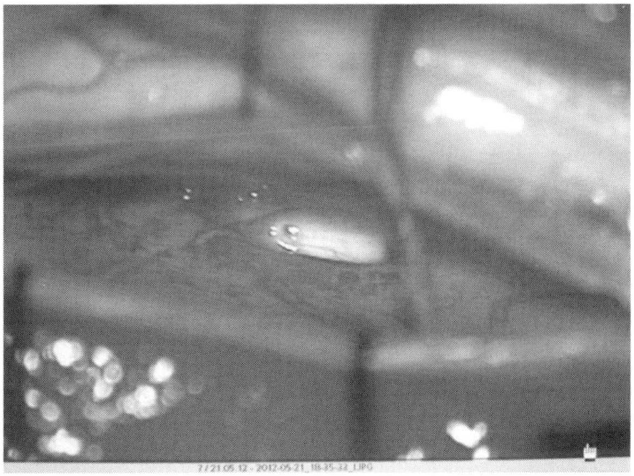

Figure 22.3 Intraoperative picture of a ventral dural tear in a patient with spontaneous intracranial hypotension. A full-color version is included in the color plate section.

[56]. Also, orthostatic headaches can be due to various other ailments and there are some patients who insist that they have a CSF leak even though extensive investigations fail to support such a diagnosis.

Much needs to be learned about the enigma of spontaneous intracranial hypotension. Radiologic methods to define a CSF leak in patients with multiple spinal meningeal diverticula but no demonstrable CSF leak are needed, a noninvasive therapy for closure of ventral dural tears is a priority, and methods of strengthening the dura need to be investigated.

References

1. Schievink WI. Spontaneous spinal cerebrospinal fluid leaks and intracranial hypotension. *JAMA* 2006;295:2286–96.
2. Beckhardt RN, Setzen M, Carras R. Primary spontaneous cerebrospinal fluid rhinorrhea. *Otolaryngol Head Neck Surg* 1991;104(4):425–32.
3. Schievink WI, Schwartz MS, Maya MM, et al. Lack of causal association between spontaneous intracranial hypotension and cranial cerebrospinal fluid leaks. *J Neurosurg* 2012;116:749–54.
4. Schievink WI, Morreale VM, Atkinson JLD, et al. Surgical treatment of spontaneous spinal cerebrospinal fluid leaks. *J Neurosurg* 1998;88:243–6.
5. Schievink WI, Roiter V. Epidemiology of cervical artery dissection. In: Baumgartner RW, Bogouss-lavsky J, Caso V, et al. (Eds.) *Handbook of Cerebral Artery Dissection*. Basel: Karger; 2005: 12–15.
6. Bell WE, Joynt RJ, Sahs AL. Low spinal fluid pressure syndromes. *Neurology* 1960;10:512–21.
7. Billings JJ, Gilford EJ, Henderson JK. The low intracranial pressure syndrome. *Proc Aust Assoc Neurol* 1975;12:31–4.
8. Chung SJ, Kim JS, Lee MC. Syndrome of cerebral spinal fluid hypovolemia: clinical and imaging features and outcome. *Neurology* 2000;55:1321–7.
9. Lasater GM. Primary intracranial hypotension: the low spinal fluid pressure syndrome. *Headache* 1970;10:63–6.
10. Lindquist T, Moberg E. Spontaneous hypoliquorrea. *Acta Med Scand* 1949;132:556–61.
11. Miyazawa K, Shiga Y, Hasegawa T, et al. CSF hypovolemia vs intracranial hypotension in "spontaneous intracranial hypotension syndrome." *Neurology* 2003;60:941–7.
12. Rando TA, Fishman RA. Spontaneous intracranial hypotension: report of two cases and review of the literature. *Neurology* 1992;42:481–7.
13. Renowden SA, Gregory R, Hyman N, et al. Spontaneous intracranial hypotension. *J Neurol Neurosurg Psychiatry* 1995;59:511–15.
14. Schievink WI, Meyer FB, Atkinson JLD, et al. Spontaneous spinal cerebrospinal fluid leaks and intracranial hypotension. *J Neurosurg* 1996;84:598–605.
15. Schievink WI. Misdiagnosis of spontaneous intracranial hypotension. *Arch Neurol* 2003;60:1713–18.
16. Teng P, Papatheodorou C. Primary cerebrospinal fluid hypotension. *Bull Los Angeles Neurol Soc* 1968;33:121–8.
17. Schievink WI, Ebersold MJ, Atkinson JLD. Rollercoaster headache due to spinal cerebrospinal fluid leak. *Lancet* 1996;347:1409.
18. Schievink WI. Spontaneous spinal cerebrospinal fluid leaks. *Neurosurg Focus* 2000;9:1–9.
19. Schievink WI, Louy C. Precipitating factors of spontaneous spinal CSF leaks and intracranial hypotension. *Neurology* 2007;69:700–2.
20. Schievink WI, Reimer R, Folger WN. Surgical treatment of spontaneous intracranial hypotension associated with a spinal arachnoid diverticulum: case report. *J Neurosurg* 1994;80:736–9.
21. Schievink WI, Jacques L. Recurrent spontaneous spinal cerebrospinal fluid leak associated with "nude nerve root" syndrome: case report. *Neurosurgery* 2003;53:1216–18.
22. Schievink WI, Gordon OK, Tourje J. Connective tissue disorders with spontaneous spinal cerebrospinal fluid leaks and intracranial hypotension: a prospective study. *Neurosurgery* 2004;54:65–70.
23. Schievink WI, Schrijver I, Meyer FB, et al. A syndrome of spontaneous spinal cerebrospinal fluid leaks and skeletal features of Marfan syndrome. *Ann Neurol* 1998;44:458.
24. Davenport RJ, Chataway SJ, Warlow CP. Spontaneous intracranial hypotension from a CSF leak in a patient with Marfan's syndrome. *J Neurol Neurosurg Psychiatry* 1995;59:516–19.
25. Schievink WI, Torres VE. Spinal meningeal diverticula in autosomal dominant polycystic kidney disease. *Lancet* 1997;349:1223–4.
26. Erkulvrawatr S, El Gammal T, Hawkins J, et al. Intrathoracic meningoceles and neurofibromatosis. *Arch Neurol* 1979;36:557–69.
27. Lehman RAW, Stears JC, Wesenberg RL, et al. Familial osteosclerosis with abnormalities of the nervous system and meninges. *J Pediatr* 1977;90:49–54.
28. Philip N, Andrac L, Moncla A, et al. Multiple lateral meningoceles, distinctive facies and skeletal anomalies: a new case of Lehman syndrome. *Clin Dysmorphol* 1995;4:347–51.

29. Levine DN, Rapalino O. The pathophysiology of lumbar puncture headache. *J Neurol Sci* 2001;192:1–8.

30. Schievink WI, Wijdicks EFM, Meyer FB, et al. Spontaneous intracranial hypotension mimicking aneurysmal subarachnoid hemorrhage. *Neurosurgery* 2001;48:513–16.

31. Portier F, deMinteguiaga C, Racy E, et al. Spontaneous intracranial hypotension: a rare cause of labyrinthine hydrops. *Ann Otol Rhinol Laryngol* 2002;111:817–20.

32. Horton JC, Fishman RA. Neurovisual findings in the syndrome of spontaneous intracranial hypotension from dural cerebrospinal fluid leak. *Ophthalmology* 1994;101:244–51.

33. Ferrante E, Savino A, Brioschi A, et al. Transient oculomotor cranial nerves palsy in spontaneous intracranial hypotension. *J Neurosurg Sci* 1998;42:177–9.

34. Warner GT. Spontaneous intracranial hypotension causing a partial third cranial nerve palsy: a novel observation. *Cephalalgia* 2002;22:822–3.

35. Brady-McCreery KM, Speidel S, Hussein MA, et al. Spontaneous intracranial hypotension with unique strabismus due to third and fourth cranial neuropathies. *Binocul Vis Strabismus Q* 2002;17:43–8.

36. Pleasure SJ, Abosch A, Friedman J, et al. Spontaneous intracranial hypotension resulting in stupor caused by diencephalic compression. *Neurology* 1998;50:1854–7.

37. Schievink WI, Moser FG, Pikul BK. Reversal of coma with an injection of glue. *Lancet* 2007;369:1402.

38. Hong M, Shah GV, Adams KM, et al. Spontaneous intracranial hypotension causing reversible frontotemporal dementia. *Neurology* 2002;58:1285–7.

39. Wicklund MR, Mokri B, Drubach DA, et al. Frontotemporal brain sagging syndrome: an SIH-like presentation mimicking FTD. *Neurology* 2011;76:1377–82.

40. Pakiam AS, Lee C, Lang AE. Intracranial hypotension with parkinsonism, ataxia, and bulbar weakness. *Arch Neurol* 1999;56:869–72.

41. Schievink WI, Maya MM, Moser FG, et al. Spectrum of subdural fluid collections in spontaneous intracranial hypotension. *J Neurosurg* 2005b;103:608–13.

42. Schoffer KL, Benstead TJ, Grant I. Spontaneous intracranial hypotension in the absence of magnetic resonance imaging abnormalities. *Can J Neurol Sci* 2002;29:253–7.

43. Schievink WI, Meyer FB, Atkinson JLD, et al. Spontaneous spinal cerebrospinal fluid leaks and intracranial hypotension. *J Neurosurg* 1996;84:598–605.

44. Hoxworth JM, Trentman TL, Kotsenas AL, et al. The role of digital subtraction myelography in the diagnosis and localization of spontaneous spinal CSF leaks. *AJR Am J Roentgenol* 2012;199:649–53.

45. Weber WE, Heidendal GA, de Krom MC. Primary intracranial hypotension and abnormal radionuclide cisternography: report of a case and review of the literature. *Clin Neurol Neurosurg* 1991;93:55–60.

46. Dillon WP. Spinal manifestations of intracranial hypotension. *AJNR Am J Neuroradiol* 2001;22:1233–4.

47. Rabin BM, Roychowdhury S, Meyer JR, et al. Spontaneous intracranial hypotension: spinal MR findings. *AJNR Am J Neuroradiol* 1998;19:1034–9.

48. Headache Classification Subcommittee of the International Headache Society. The International Classification of Headache Disorders, 2nd ed. *Cephalalgia* 2004;24(Suppl 1):1–160.

49. Schievink WI, Maya MM, Louy C, Moser FG, Tourje J. Diagnostic criteria for spontaneous spinal CSF leaks and intracranial hypotension. *AJNR Am J Neuroradiol* 2008;29(5):853–6.

50. Albayram S, Ozer H, Kara B. Diagnostic criteria for spontaneous spinal CSF leaks and intracranial hypotension. *AJNR Am J Neuroradiol* 2008;29:e94.

51. Schievink WI, Dodick DW, Mokri B, et al. Diagnostic criteria for headache due to spontaneous intracranial hypotension: a perspective. *Headache* 2011;51:1442–4.

52. Sencakova D, Mokri B, McClelland RL. The efficacy of epidural blood patch in spontaneous CSF leaks. *Neurology* 2001;57:1921–3.

53. Berroir S, Loisel B, Ducros A, et al. Early epidural blood patch in spontaneous intracranial hypotension. *Neurology* 2004;63:1950–1.

54. Schievink WI, Maya MM, Moser FM. Treatment of spontaneous intracranial hypotension with percutaneous placement of a fibrin sealant: report of four cases. *J Neurosurg* 2004;100:1098–100.

55. Berroir S, Grabli D, Heran F, et al. Cerebral sinus venous thrombosis in two patients with spontaneous intracranial hypotension. *Cerebrovasc Dis* 2004;17:9–12.

56. Schievink WI. A novel technique for treatment of intractable spontaneous intracranial hypotension: lumbar dural reduction surgery. *Headache* 2009;49:1047–51.

Chapter 23

Management of the adult with congenital hydrocephalus

Jonathan Pindrik and Edward S. Ahn

Introduction

Hydrocephalus denotes increased volume of cerebrospinal fluid (CSF) contained within the intracranial ventricular system, with concomitant elevated intracranial pressure (ICP). Increased ventricular volume results from abnormal production, flow, or absorption of CSF. The specification of congenital hydrocephalus indicates diagnosis during prenatal screening, at birth, or the perinatal period. Etiologies of congenital hydrocephalus include structural abnormalities like Dandy–Walker complex, Chiari malformation, or aqueductal stenosis; spinal dysraphism or myelomeningocele; and intraventricular (IVH) or germinal matrix hemorrhage. Hydrocephalus diagnosed early in infancy may also result from neonatal meningitis. The causes of hydrocephalus diagnosed at birth typically differ from hydrocephalus diagnosed in adulthood and require different long-term management strategies.

Management of adults with hydrocephalus treated during infancy or childhood represents a challenging process. Several factors account for this complexity, including the multiplicity of shunt revisions, the transition from pediatric to adult-centered care, potential conversion to shunt independence, management of chronic shunting with concomitant headaches, and impact on neuropsychological development. Furthermore, many patients with congenital hydrocephalus experience medical comorbidities requiring coordinated, interdisciplinary care. While pediatric neurosurgeons routinely engage in collaborative care, interdisciplinary models may not represent the routine approach for adult or general neurosurgeons [1]. Optimal neurosurgical management of adult patients with congenital hydrocephalus requires close attention to the complex issues of transitioning care, shunt management, and neuropsychological development.

Transitioning neurosurgical care

The transition of care from pediatric to adult-centered practices has received considerable attention over the last two decades. Several academic journals and medical professional organizations (Joint Section of Pediatric Neurological Surgery of the American Association of Neurological Surgeons [AANS] and Congress of Neurological Surgeons [CNS], American Academy of Pediatrics [AAP], American Society of Pediatric Neurological Surgeons [ASPN]) have supported articles, editorials, and conference presentations regarding this complex topic. To further complicate this process, many pediatric neurosurgical patients represent those with special healthcare needs (SHCN) and cognitive impairments. Children and adolescents with congenital hydrocephalus may exhibit mild or profound developmental delay that significantly impacts their progress in school, society, and independent living. The stress of transitioning between healthcare providers, especially from pediatric to adult-centered care, impacts both patients and their families. The familiarity and close bonds between patient and provider may disintegrate upon transferring care. Furthermore, the intricacies of a patient's complicated medical history and the inherent differences between pediatric and adult neurosurgical practices contribute to the complex transition process.

Given the frequent coexistence of congenital anomalies with hydrocephalus, optimal medical care of patients with congenital hydrocephalus represents a collaborative process. These children may exhibit other neurologic (spina bifida, cerebral palsy, developmental delay), ophthalmologic, or orthopedic impairments. Coordinated, multidisciplinary care has become the standard approach to care optimally for these children. In contrast, many adult or general neurosurgery practices may not employ a collaborative approach, may not

Adult Hydrocephalus, ed. Daniele Rigamonti. Published by Cambridge University Press.

have access to interdisciplinary clinics in their area of catchment, or may seek independent consultation for additional care [2]. An adult patient with congenital hydrocephalus requires continued follow-up for shunt management, but also for any medical comorbidities related to their congenital abnormalities. Maintaining continuity of collaborative care represents only one of the challenging issues facing patients and their providers upon the transition from pediatric to adult care.

Pediatric neurosurgery perspective

Prolonged continuity of care coupled with the characteristic personality and communicative practices embraced by many pediatric neurosurgeons help forge strong bonds with patients and their families. Pediatric neurosurgery teams (including attendings, physician assistants, and nurse practitioners) often care for a child from birth to adolescence given the chronicity of their disease and need for long-term follow-up [1]. However, given the constant influx of new patients, transitioning care of young adults to general neurosurgeons helps provide outflow to balance pediatric practices and help prevent over-saturation. Furthermore, children's hospitals employing pediatric neurosurgeons may discourage care of patients reaching adulthood at their facility [1].

Many general hospitals offer support for patients over a wide age range. Large academic hospitals often house facilities for both children and adults, lowering barriers for pediatric neurosurgeons to continue caring for young adults. This dual-role model allows pediatric and congenital neurosurgeons to care for children and adults with developmental or childhood disorders [1]. Furthermore, certain units primarily accommodate young adults with SHCN diagnosed during infancy or childhood [1]. These hybrid models provide adolescents with established, continuous medical care into middle-age [1]. However, they do not represent a universal approach to providing continuous care for young adults. Consequently, many pediatric neurosurgeons routinely face the issue of transitioning patients with congenital hydrocephalus from pediatric to adult-oriented care.

Adults with congenital hydrocephalus who lack cognitive or physical deficits may progress smoothly through the transition process. When only adult neurosurgical follow-up is required, pediatric neurosurgeons may serve primary roles in the transfer of care [3]. In contrast, adults with congenital hydrocephalus and SHCN, cognitive impairment, or related comorbidities may require a collaborative approach. Multidisciplinary strategies especially benefit spina bifida patients who have intricate medical profiles [3]. More complex adult patients with congenital hydrocephalus and profound developmental delay may fail to transition care. Their degree of cognitive impairment may prevent independent functional living or participation in medical decision-making. These patients may remain under the care of a willing pediatric neurosurgeon into adulthood, given their medical and social complexity [4]. Even following successful transfer of care, pediatric neurosurgeons should remain available for discussion or consult with prior patients or new healthcare providers [1].

Adult neurosurgery perspective

Given their training and style of practice, adult neurosurgeons may not be equipped optimally to handle patients transitioning from pediatric-oriented care. Staff members within adult-oriented practices often lack experience with developmentally delayed patients or child-onset diseases [4]. Furthermore, the subset of neurological disorders handled by pediatric neurosurgeons differs considerably from the range of pathologies familiar to adult or general neurosurgeons [1]. The lack of familiarity with these patients from both the medical staff and general neurosurgeon may lead to suboptimal care. Beyond general characteristics of the patient population with congenital hydrocephalus, idiosyncrasies of individual patients unbeknownst to the newly accepting adult neurosurgeon may impact care. For instance, the previously treating pediatric attending may have become familiar with a certain patient's pattern of presentation during shunt malfunction [1]. Much of this information about a patient and their neurologic profile must be relearned by the adult practitioner.

Congenital hydrocephalus differs considerably from adult-onset hydrocephalus regarding etiology and natural history. Hydrocephalus diagnosed at birth or in infancy can result from developmental malformations, myelomeningocele, hemorrhage, meningitis, tumor, or other type of obstruction. While adult neurosurgeons may have experience with obstructive, normal pressure, or tumor-related hydrocephalus, they may lack perspective on the management of a chronically shunted patient treated since birth or childhood [1]. Furthermore, patients shunted during infancy may not exhibit expected ventricular enlargement during shunt malfunction. Despite increased ICP and shunt failure, the ventricles within these children or adults may exhibit little response and misguide radiographic or clinical interpretation. This condition, referred to as normal volume hydrocephalus (NVH) or nonresponding ventricles, may affect up to 25% of patients shunted during infancy [1]. Accustomed to ventricular enlargement during shunt malfunction, general neurosurgeons may fail to recognize shunt failure in an adult with congenital hydrocephalus.

Despite the presence of guidelines, few health systems employ standard practices regarding transition of care for young adults, especially those with SHCN or cognitive impairment [4]. Without standardized practices, adult or general neurosurgeons may face a complicated task during the first consultation involving laborious review of prior medical files and operative reports. Furthermore, guidelines do not exist regarding the follow-up of adults with congenital hydrocephalus beyond the transition period [3]. Patients without significant comorbidities or cognitive impairment may simply require regularly scheduled neurosurgery clinic visits. However, adults with congenital hydrocephalus and SHCN or cognitive impairment likely require continued follow-up with rehabilitation specialists and other medical professionals [3].

Patient and family perspective

An adolescent's intellectual and behavioral development and their ability to function independently represent critical factors impacting their transition to adult care [4]. The presence of family or caretaker support also affects this process. Congenital hydrocephalus, representing both a chronic illness and potential cause of cognitive impairment or developmental delay, deserves special attention regarding the transition process from pediatric to adult-oriented care.

Adolescents may face several stressors upon transitioning care. Timing of the transition represents an important component, especially concerning other major life events (issues with school, family, friends, etc.). Additionally, patients often experience distress upon breaking the relationship with a familiar pediatric physician and visiting new, unfamiliar adult practitioners [4]. In addition to personnel changes, physical settings differ between typical children's hospitals and most general neurosurgery practices [1].

Young adults with congenital hydrocephalus may exhibit cognitive impairment, further complicating the transition process. Intellectual impairment may limit independent functioning, decision-making, executive function, and organizational skills [4]. These limitations impair the patient's ability to assume an active, independent role in their care, forcing more responsibility onto family members, caretakers, or healthcare professionals [1]. The presence of SHCN may also delay or prolong the transition process from pediatric to adult-oriented care [1]. Patients with developmental delay may require longer durations of time to feel prepared for the transfer [4]. Nevertheless, the coexistence of SHCN in a young adult with congenital hydrocephalus should not preclude that individual's contribution to medical decision-making as they reach maturity [1].

Recommendations

Most sets of recommendations regarding transition from pediatric to adult-oriented care champion standardized and collaborative approaches. General pediatric guidelines suggest having appropriately trained healthcare providers facilitate the transition process. This may help ensure that the transition occurs without lapses in medical coverage [4]. Furthermore, healthcare professionals should document the transition plan in consultation with the patient and family. Patients and caretakers should maintain accurate, updated medical summaries that are readily available [4]. In addition to this formalized approach, the transition process should be flexible and individualized based on patient needs. Relevant patient factors include chronologic and developmental age, neurocognitive function, and family dynamics and resources [4]. The healthcare providers responsible for facilitating the transfer process must consider these factors when determining an individual patient's readiness and role in the transition [4].

Adolescents with SHCN or cognitive deficits, including those with congenital hydrocephalus, may benefit from a multidisciplinary approach to transferring care. Parents or other caretakers, social workers, pediatricians, adult healthcare providers, pediatric and adult neurosurgeons, and pediatric psychologists may all provide integral roles in the successful transition to adult-oriented care [4]. Depending on their cognitive function, adults with congenital hydrocephalus may still rely upon parents or other family members for medical decision-making and coordination of care. Therefore, transfer of care into adult-oriented practices may still require the designation of a caretaker intimately involved in the process [4]. Additionally, adult neurosurgeons newly seeing a patient with congenital hydrocephalus should communicate openly with pediatricians and pediatric neurosurgeons previously responsible for that individual's care [1]. This would benefit those adults with congenital hydrocephalus and complex medical profiles due to spina bifida, cerebral palsy, or orthopedic deformities. Social workers represent integral components of the transition process as well. Their assistance may be required for case management, coordination of care, and facilitation of vocational services for patients with developmental delay [4].

For adolescents with congenital hydrocephalus and cognitive impairment, pediatric psychologists may also serve an important role in the transfer from pediatric to adult-oriented care. While neuropsychologists may help assess a patient's cognitive and adaptive skills, pediatric psychologists can translate these results into clinical practice [4]. For instance, these professionals can implement a variety of strategies (multisensory communication, frequent review and repetition, language adjustment) when communicating with and teaching cognitively impaired adolescents [4]. These tactics may assist pediatric healthcare providers, including pediatric neurosurgeons, to prepare a young adult for transition. Pediatric psychologists can assist in educating patients about their illness, reinforcing disease management and coping skills, and fostering greater independence and a stronger sense of responsibility within the patient. Finally, pediatric psychologists can assess an adolescent's readiness for transfer and whether they require longer transition periods [4].

Based on AAP guidelines, discussions regarding transition of care for adolescents should commence at age 14, with the knowledge that most children's hospitals discourage admissions beyond age 18 or 21 [1]. However, this process must be modified according to the individual needs of an adolescent with SHCN. Early initiation of the transition process at age 14 allows greater time intervals for young adults requiring more support. The transition process may begin with education and encouraging the patient to learn more about their conditions [1]. Beyond knowledge of their medical history, adolescents should become familiar with a plan of action in the setting of emergencies and understand who to contact with questions. Additionally, the designation of an individual to make medical decisions as necessary and serve as a power-of-attorney is recommended [1]. The creation of a written, stored, accessible document with this and other pertinent information may help clarify and demystify an individual's medical profile for both patient and provider [1]. These steps may also help a young adult feel more comfortable and empowered to embrace a proactive role in their care. These patient and provider efforts, along with a multidisciplinary approach, help tailor transition planning to the individual needs of a young adult with congenital hydrocephalus [3,4].

Achieving shunt independence

In certain contexts, ventricular shunting for hydrocephalus does not represent a permanent necessity. Adult patients may outgrow the necessity for CSF flow diversion, or this flow diversion may be accomplished by alternate means. In rare cases, a few adults with congenital hydrocephalus may spontaneously escape shunt dependency [3,5]. In this setting, shunts can be functionally terminated with ligature or completely removed. Alternatively, adults reliant on CSF diversion may respond favorably to endoscopic third ventriculostomy (ETV), especially in the context of obstructive hydrocephalus. Occasionally, ETV can be combined with hardware removal in the setting of recurrent shunt infection or mechanical obstruction. Additionally, ETV represents an alternative approach to avoid long-term shunt-related complications like slit ventricle syndrome, CSF overdrainage, and distal CSF malabsorption [6]. Despite numerous advantages, shunt ligature or removal and conversion to shunt independence via ETV carry considerable risks. Even following successful ETV, chronically shunted patients may exhibit transient elevations in intracranial pressure during the early postoperative period. This phenomenon suggests that adaptations in CSF absorption and circulation require prolonged time following ETV in the setting of chronic shunting [5].

Confirming shunt independence in adults with congenital hydrocephalus requires careful judgment and thorough analysis. The imaging presence of shunt disconnection or catheter fracture in an asymptomatic adult does not exclude the possibility of shunt dependence [3]. Formalized testing through radionuclide tracer shunt surveys and short trials of shunt ligature may help confirm true shunt independence. While evaluation and management styles may differ among neurosurgeons, the importance of ensuring shunt independence prior to permanent ligature or hardware removal cannot be overstated.

Endoscopic third ventriculostomy (ETV)

Endoscopic third ventriculostomy can be used to functionally convert appropriately selected hydrocephalic patients to shunt independence. Individuals with noncommunicating hydrocephalus classically represent the best candidates for ETV. Additionally, ETV has been applied to chronically shunted patients presenting with recurrent shunt malfunction [6–9]. Given the variability of and difficulty to predict outcomes in such patients, especially those with communicating hydrocephalus, considerable controversy exists regarding this treatment strategy [5]. Several case series report successful conversion of patients with chronic hydrocephalus to shunt independence via ETV. Many of these patients underwent ETV as an alternative approach to treating shunt complications like slit ventricle syndrome, mechanical obstruction, or infection. With study sizes ranging between 4 and 88 patients, including children and adults with shunted hydrocephalus, various research groups have reported rates of shunt independence following ETV between 38% and 84% [5–9].

In a large series of 88 pediatric and adult patients with hydrocephalus and shunt complications, 61% of patients responded favorably to ETV (after first or second attempts) [9]. Patients with noncommunicating hydrocephalus exhibited higher rates of shunt independence (73%) than those with communicating hydrocephalus (46%) following ETV [5,8,9]. Additionally, 73% of patients failing ETV in the setting of shunt malfunction suffered from post-hemorrhagic hydrocephalus [9]. Notably, congenital hydrocephalus represented a risk factor for ETV failure in this study. Of those patients failing ETV, 88% underwent shunt placement early during infancy [5,9].

A retrospective review of 63 patients (pediatric and adult) with shunted hydrocephalus undergoing secondary ETV for shunt malfunction showed a 70% ETV success rate [6]. Statistical analysis showed similar trends of success irrespective of the type of shunt malfunction, including mechanical obstruction and infection [6]. Regarding the original etiology of hydrocephalus, patients with spina bifida exhibited a 55% ETV success rate, while those with aqueductal stenosis displayed a 68% success rate [6]. Clinical evidence of ETV failure occurred within 1 month following neuroendoscopy in 95% of patients; however, one patient expired acutely 5 months postoperatively [6]. Patients presenting with ETV failure may undergo a repeat trial of ventriculostomy or ventricular shunt reinsertion.

In another large series of adult patients with shunt malfunction (without stratification by type of hydrocephalus), Jenkinson et al. reported an ETV success rate of 67% [7]. The authors explained the relatively high success rate of secondary ETV in the setting of shunt infection as compared to primary ETV for neonatal post-meningitic hydrocephalus based on differing pathophysiology. Meningitis frequently results in development of subarachnoid membranes and adhesions that may not be visualized during endoscopy or re-form following fenestration [7]. These obstructions to CSF flow can result in ETV failure rates of up to 45% [7]. In contrast, shunt infections do not typically propagate formation of subarachnoid adhesions, leading to higher success rates with secondary ETV. Similarly, primary ETV for post-hemorrhagic hydrocephalus may exhibit high failure rates due to blockage of CSF flow through subarachnoid spaces and arachnoid granulations by debris [6]. CSF flow diversion via shunting may alter intracranial anatomy, allowing subarachnoid CSF spaces to re-expand and the sylvian aqueduct to stenose. Such factors favor the success of secondary ETV in communicating hydrocephalus (infective or post-hemorrhagic) after shunt malfunction [6].

ETV failure and complications

In the same study by Jenkinson et al., ETV failure in adult patients with shunt malfunction occurred at a median duration of 2 weeks postoperatively [7]. While ETV success plateaued by 3 months postoperatively on Kaplan–Meier survival analysis, delayed ETV failure still occurred with potentially devastating consequences, stressing the importance of prolonged long-term follow-up [7]. Adults with congenital hydrocephalus who undergo ETV to achieve shunt independence should be educated and counseled thoroughly about the risks of acute intracranial hypertension [6].

Despite the potential benefits of shunt independence, many patients fail or are not candidates for ETV. Relative contraindications of ETV include slit ventricles or aberrant anatomy that would complicate visualization or perforation of the third ventricular floor. Other factors that increase the risk of ETV failure include subarachnoid membranes deep to the third ventricular floor, prior subarachnoid hemorrhage or intracranial infection, and narrowing of the ventriculostomy stoma [5]. Furthermore, patients with multiple shunt revisions prior to ETV in the setting of shunt malfunction exhibit higher risk of shunt reinsertion [8]. Retrospective series have reported median times to failure within 4–6 weeks following ETV for shunt malfunction [7,9]. However, case reports describing remote sudden death in the setting of acute obstructive hydrocephalus following ETV and shunt removal illustrate the importance of vigilant follow-up [6,9,10].

In addition to ETV failure requiring shunt reinsertion, several complications exist with ETV. These risks include CSF leakage, intracranial infections or hemorrhage, hypothalamic-pituitary axis abnormalities, cranial nerve palsies, transient memory or cognitive disturbances, and thalamic or anterior spinal infarcts [8,11]. A case series by Hader et al. reported elevated frequency of serious complications with ETV at the time of shunt malfunction (31%) as opposed to primary intervention for hydrocephalus (8%) [8]. In contrast, other series have reported lower serious complication rates of 1.6–5.6% for ETV in the setting of shunt malfunction [8,9]. Rates of infection following ETV (1–2%) typically fall below those of ventriculoperitoneal (VP) shunt insertion (5–10%) [6].

Complications may occur more frequently in secondary ETV due to the increased difficulty of performing neuroendoscopy in the context of chronic shunting. Distorted anatomy, lower degrees of ventricular enlargement, and thickened third ventricular floors enhance the complexity of ETV in shunted patients [8]. Furthermore, the practice of external ventricular drain (EVD) insertion following ETV in chronically shunted patients leads to higher risk of CSF leaks and infections [8]. However, this strategy also helps protect patients against temporary intracranial hypertension following ETV during adjustment to shunt independence [8]. The potential complications and risks of ETV failure necessitate careful patient selection when considering ETV in the setting of shunt malfunction.

Management of chronically shunted patients

The presence of long-term internal flow diversion likely alters intracranial CSF hydrodynamics and cerebral anatomy. For instance, down-regulation of CSF production, drift of paramedian structures (thalamus, basal ganglia) towards midline, and concave inflection of the corpus callosum all may potentially occur in chronically shunted patients [5]. Unfortunately, the precise pathophysiologic mechanisms and implications of these processes remain largely unknown. Furthermore, the likelihood of successful conversion to shunt independence often cannot be predicted adequately. Many adults with congenital hydrocephalus continue to show signs of shunt dependence due to CSF malabsorption. Additionally, shunted patients trialed with ETV may fail due to ventriculostomy site stenosis or scarring or unvisualized subarachnoid membranes within the basal cisterns [5]. In long-term follow-up series of adults with pediatric-onset hydrocephalus, up to 89% of patients still possess an implanted shunt [11]. Adults with congenital hydrocephalus who remain shunt dependent should be regularly followed to help manage and avoid potential complications associated with chronic shunting.

Slit ventricle syndrome (SVS)

Prolonged shunting since infancy or childhood frequently results in decreased ventricular compliance. Up to 20% of patients with hydrocephalus addressed during infancy may develop stiffening of the ventricles that fail to enlarge with elevated ICP [12]. This phenomenon may result from increased superior sagittal sinus (SSS) venous pressure and a type of shunt-related pseudotumor cerebri [12]. Headaches associated with chronic shunting also represent a common problem for adults with congenital hydrocephalus. Over 50% of adults treated during infancy for hydrocephalus may experience chronic or recurrent headaches [13]. The coexistence of chronic or recurrent headaches with non-dilated ventricles and a functioning shunt results in the perplexing slit ventricle syndrome (SVS). This complex phenomenon may result from various pathophysiologic mechanisms and requires careful, thorough evaluation to select the appropriate management strategy.

Ambiguity regarding accepted definitions contributes to the perplexity of SVS. The radiographic appearance of slit-like or small ventricles in a shunted individual should not be misconstrued for this clinical syndrome. Multiple authors have suggested the replacement of the term SVS with noncompliant ventricle syndrome to distinguish SVS from radiographic findings [14]. SVS involves a severe headache disorder, non-dilated or small ventricles, and delayed refill of shunt pumping devices [12,14]. Several authors have reported the existence of five subtypes of SVS, requiring different approaches and treatment modalities [12].

Headaches in shunted adults that do not significantly impair quality of life and shunt-related migraines can be treated medically [12,14]. However, adequate evaluation of ventricular size and shunt function typically proceeds in these patients presenting with headache complaints. Several prophylactic and treatment regimens exist to prevent and terminate migraine episodes. These medical options may improve quality of life without necessitating surgical manipulation of shunt systems.

SVS related to CSF overdrainage can result in intermittent proximal obstruction or low pressure headaches. In the former context, collapse of ventricular walls surrounding the proximal catheter prevents CSF diversion until ventricular volume reconstitutes. When sufficient CSF builds up around the proximal catheter, the shunt reclaims functionality only to reproduce ventricular collapse [14]. The recurrent elevations in ICP may cause troubling headaches for patients. Furthermore, collapse of ventricular walls around the proximal catheter may increase the risk of partial proximal obstruction by particulate debris. Low pressure headaches result from CSF overdrainage as well. Imaging correlates of CSF overdrainage include small or slit-like ventricles, occasional subdural hygromas, and diffuse contrast enhancement or thickening of the pachymeninges. Treatment of SVS related to CSF overdrainage involves shunt valve upgrades or addition of antisiphon devices [12,14]. Exchanging or reprogramming valves to higher resistance or pressure settings represent straightforward approaches to managing SVS. Antisiphon devices help limit CSF overdrainage by reducing the siphoning effect of flow from recumbent to standing positions.

Noncompliant ventricles fail to dilate in the setting of shunt malfunction and rising ICP. This phenomenon has also been called normal volume hydrocephalus (NVH). Shunts that access the cortical subarachnoid space, including lumboperitoneal (LP) shunts and cisterna magna shunts, represent useful treatment modalities in NVH [12]. Preoperative cisternography can help confirm communication between the cortical and intrathecal subarachnoid spaces. Successful LP shunt insertion may allow VP shunt removal or retention of only a ventricular reservoir [12]. Coupling the LP shunt with a pressure or flow valve helps lower the risk of tonsillar or hindbrain herniation [12,14]. Contraindications to LP shunting include spina bifida, achondroplasia, radiographic evidence of hindbrain herniation, Chiari I malformation, or obstructive hydrocephalus. In these patients, and in those without established communication between the intracranial and intrathecal subarachnoid compartments, a cisterna magna-ventriculoperitoneal shunt is a useful alternative [12]. Shunts that access the cortical subarachnoid space represent effective methods of managing SVS with NVH or noncompliant ventricles.

More aggressive treatment strategies for severe SVS include subtemporal decompression and cranial expansion. These surgical approaches typically are reserved for patients with noncompliant ventricles and craniofacial syndromes involving craniosynostosis and microcephaly [12,14]. Chronic shunting for neonatal or infantile hydrocephalus frequently leads to skull thickening and apparent craniosynostosis [12]. In this setting, a cephalocranial disproportion develops. Multiple authors have reported success with subtemporal decompression and cranial expansion (second-line treatment) in these patients developing SVS [12,14]. However, these aggressive surgical approaches carry increased morbidity due to their invasive nature. Furthermore, many authors argue against subtemporal decompression or cranial expansion due to insufficient data and unfavorable anecdotal experience [12].

Management strategies

Recurrent headaches and shunt malfunctions in the setting of SVS represent challenging problems for adults with congenital hydrocephalus and their care providers. These scenarios require careful consideration and planning to ultimately re-establish normal or near-normal CSF physiology [12]. Initial interventions typically include shunt valve upgrades, reprogramming, or addition of an antisiphon device [12,14]. Further evaluation typically requires data from shunt removal and temporary external ventricular drainage (EVD).

A small subset of adults with congenital hydrocephalus and severe SVS may benefit from shunt removal. Following shunt removal and insertion of an EVD, adult patients can be monitored in an intensive care unit and undergo clamping trials. Minimal or absent ventricular enlargement with stable, normal ICPs predict favorable response to shunt removal [12,14]. These patients should be followed postoperatively to confirm shunt independence.

Elevation of ICP with concomitant increase in ventricular size during EVD clamping or shunt failure may respond favorably to ETV [14]. However, these do not represent typical SVS patients with congenital hydrocephalus [12,14]. Management of traditional SVS in the setting of congenital hydrocephalus with ETV typically requires temporary shunt modifications, EVD clamping, or placement of an antisiphon device to allow safe endoscopic navigation [5,14]. Shunt removal may follow successful ETV, with vigilant postoperative follow-up.

Complexity arises when ventricles fail to dilate with concomitant rises in ICP during EVD clamping. These adults with congenital hydrocephalus exhibit the severe classical form of SVS. Elevated SSS venous pressures prevent drainage of subarachnoid CSF, causing subarachnoid compartment distension and intracranial hypertension [12]. While representing suboptimal candidates for ETV, these patients may respond favorably to shunts accessing the cortical subarachnoid space (LP or cisterna magna shunting).

Adult spina bifida patients with congenital hydrocephalus may benefit from adjunctive ICP monitoring in the context of chronic headaches. Nearly 55% of hydrocephalic adult spina bifida patients reported chronic headaches in a retrospective review performed in Great Britain [15]. Etiologies of headaches included shunt malfunction or ETV failure, Chiari malformation, tension headaches, migraines, shunt overdrainage, decompensation of previously arrested hydrocephalus, or unknown causes [15]. Baseline head CT or brain MRI, repeated every few years, represents a useful strategy to survey shunt function and maintain radiographic images for comparison in case headaches develop. Additionally, ICP monitoring via an implanted ventricular access device or temporary intraparenchymal monitor is a useful adjunct to headache evaluation in the absence of other clinical-radiographic signs of intracranial hypertension [15]. This practice can help diagnose low pressure headaches and potentially avoid unnecessary surgical shunt explorations [15]. In the same retrospective study of adult spina bifida patients with congenital hydrocephalus, increasing age represented a risk factor for developing chronic headaches. Of this cohort, 10% of patients experienced idiopathic chronic headaches that benefited from referral to a multidisciplinary pain management team [15].

Clinical and neuropsychological outcomes

Clinical outcomes

The introduction of internalized shunts in the 1960s dramatically improved mortality and morbidity of patients with hydrocephalus. While survival into adulthood previously approached 20%, children with hydrocephalus now mostly mature into adulthood with varying levels of impairment and autonomy [3]. This large shift in survival necessitates investigation of the clinical and neuropsychological outcomes of adults with congenital hydrocephalus to better appreciate their medical and social profile.

While ventriculoperitoneal (VP) shunt insertion improves survival in patients with hydrocephalus, this procedure has several associated risks and complications. Shunt infection, proximal or distal obstruction, hardware fracture or disconnection, wound breakdown, catheter migration, and shunt overdrainage all represent etiologies of shunt malfunction potentially requiring revision. Over 80% of adult patients with pediatric-onset, VP shunted hydrocephalus encounter at least one shunt malfunction during their lifetime (or 20-year follow-up period) requiring revision [11,13,16]. Of these patients, over 50% may undergo multiple shunt revisions [13,16]. Among adult transition patients with pediatric-onset hydrocephalus, those with congenital hydrocephalus fall at even greater risk (93.9%) of shunt failure during childhood and adulthood [16]. Nearly 40% of those patients experiencing shunt malfunction encountered this complication at least once during adulthood [16]. Early diagnosis and treatment of hydrocephalus correlates with higher risk of multiple future shunt revisions – patients undergoing shunt insertion within the first 6 months of life exhibited significantly higher numbers of subsequent revisions [11]. Similarly, adults with congenital hydrocephalus encountered higher median numbers of shunt revisions (3.0) over their development into maturity [16].

Despite the preponderance of shunt complications within the first 2 weeks to 6 months following shunt surgery, late shunt infection or malfunction represent important causes of morbidity and mortality in adults with congenital hydrocephalus. While the incidence of shunt malfunction remains low in adulthood, the risk never vanishes completely. Many patients may have to undergo reoperation for shunt complications in adulthood remote from their initial shunt insertion or last revision in childhood [3]. Mortality rates of congenital hydrocephalus (13–14%, excluding causes of tumor, infection, and hemorrhage) mirror those of pediatric-onset hydrocephalus reported in long-term follow-up series [11]. Deaths specifically related to shunt malfunction occur in 2–5% of patients followed long term since pediatric-onset hydrocephalus [11]. Given the risks of morbidity and mortality of shunt malfunction, patients and their caretakers should be reminded frequently about the appropriate plan of action when suspecting shunt problems [3]. Certain authors recommend routine surveillance radiographic studies (head CT, brain MRI, plain films) every 4–5 years (or more frequently) in addition to clinical follow-up to assess shunt continuity and function [11].

Beyond shunt complications, adults with congenital or infantile hydrocephalus may experience other morbidities. For instance, depression affects up to 70% of adults with hydrocephalus treated during infancy, with almost 45% requiring treatment [13]. Many adult patients exhibit some type of neurologic deficit due to hydrocephalus or underlying etiology of hydrocephalus. In a study by Vinchon et al., no adult myelomeningocele patients were free of neurologic sequelae, while only 24–27% of adult patients with congenital hydrocephalus due to hemorrhage or cerebral malformation lacked neurologic deficits [3].

Neuropsychological outcomes

Depending on the etiology of hydrocephalus, surviving neonates can ultimately mature into adulthood with varying levels of social and professional success. Vinchon et al. retrospectively studied adults with hydrocephalus diagnosed at or near birth (in the setting of myelomeningocele, hemorrhage, cerebral malformations, or meningitis) and showed them to have mean Karnofsky Performance Scale scores of 65.1–80.6 [3]. Cognitively, 41–56% of adults with congenital hydrocephalus due to myelomeningocele, meningitis, or hemorrhage exhibited intelligence quotient (IQ) scores greater than or equal to 80. Before the 1950s, less than 40% of surviving adults with hydrocephalus had an IQ score ≥85 [14]. Interestingly, over 70% of patients with malformative causes of hydrocephalus (Dandy–Walker malformation, etc.) scored an IQ ≥80 [3].

Several authors have evaluated the neuropsychological outcomes of patients with shunted congenital hydrocephalus maturing into adulthood. Debate exists regarding continuation of the nonverbal learning disabilities syndrome, frequently present in hydrocephalic children, into adulthood [17]. Older reports suggest a discrepancy between verbal and visuospatial cognition in children with congenital hydrocephalus, based on normal verbal IQ but low performance IQ scores. The impaired development of visuospatial cognitive skills could lead to a nonverbal learning disabilities syndrome characterized by deficits in visual or tactile perception, attention, and memory, as well as conceptualization and problem solving [17].

Hommet et al.'s prospective study on the neuropsychological and behavioral outcomes of young adults with congenital hydrocephalus challenged the notion of the nonverbal learning disabilities syndrome persisting into adulthood. Young adults with congenital hydrocephalus scored similarly on verbal and performance IQ examinations, in contrast to the results from other studies assessing younger patients [17]. Additionally, patients with hydrocephalus related to spina bifida exhibited greater impairment than patients with aqueductal stenosis in several cognitive and memory tasks [17]. Subnormal performance in visuospatial tasks might reflect poor motor skills, deficits in fine motor coordination, or centrally impaired visuospatial processing [17]. This finding suggests that certain elements of the nonverbal learning disabilities syndrome may continue into adulthood for congenital hydrocephalus related to spina bifida. However, these patients also exhibited deficits in verbal performance, specifically the use of oral language in pragmatic or social settings [17]. Adults with congenital hydrocephalus related to spina bifida also exhibited subnormal arithmetic and reasoning performance [17]. In contrast, adults with congenital hydrocephalus due to aqueductal stenosis did not exhibit these trends in verbal or visuospatial cognition [17].

From a behavioral and adaptive perspective, young adults with congenital hydrocephalus may perform reasonably well. However, studies have shown that these patients exhibit minor deficits in communication and autonomy compared to their chronologic age-matched counterparts [17]. Nevertheless, improved treatments of congenital hydrocephalus, along with better educational and psychological support, have allowed many affected adults to become productive members of society.

Pursuit of education and employment represent important measures to evaluate the social development and integration of adults with congenital hydrocephalus. Vinchon et al. explored clinical and functional outcomes of adults treated during childhood for hydrocephalus in a large French retrospective review [3]. For those patients with hydrocephalus originally due to hemorrhage, myelomeningocele, or malformation, 31–44% attended normal schooling while only 24% of adults with infantile hydrocephalus due to meningitis received normal education. Furthermore, 18–35% of adults with congenital hydrocephalus maintained normal employment [3]. Adults with acquired causes of hydrocephalus (tumor, arachnoid cyst) in infancy or childhood typically fared better in education and employment than did adults with congenital hydrocephalus [3]. This trend did not remain constant for adults with childhood post-traumatic hydrocephalus, likely due to diffuse brain injury [3].

Other long-term follow-up series of patients with pediatric-onset hydrocephalus have shown encouraging results applicable to adults with congenital hydrocephalus. Within a Norwegian retrospective review of adult patients treated during childhood for hydrocephalus, 76% of survey respondents completed secondary elementary education, while at least 5% pursued higher education [11]. With a 23% unemployment rate and 23% frequency of respondents still completing school, 54% of study subjects maintained employment [11]. Furthermore, nearly 60% of adults with pediatric-onset hydrocephalus reported functionally independent daily living, with 40% requiring some form of assistance from family members or nursing staff [11]. Gupta et al. reported similar results, showing that over 70% of adults shunted during infancy pursued education beyond high school, though 45% required special services in school. Almost 20% of adults with infantile hydrocephalus achieved a bachelor's degree, while 56% reported independent living arrangements and stable employment [13].

These results from long-term studies of adults developing hydrocephalus during infancy and childhood may reflect trends for the subset of adults with congenital hydrocephalus. Furthermore these encouraging rates of social development and integration reflect the beneficial roles of administrative and public support (e.g. the Norwegian welfare system) for adolescents and adults with SHCN. With individualized management from neurosurgeons and healthcare teams, along with support from caretakers and social programs (as needed), many adults with congenital hydrocephalus can lead productive and healthy lives.

References

1. Rekate HL. The pediatric neurosurgical patient: the challenge of growing up. *Semin Pediatr Neurol* 2009;16:2–8.
2. American Academy of Pediatrics: Committee on Children with Disabilities and Committee on Adolescence. Transition of care provided for adolescents with special health care needs. *Pediatrics* 1996;98(6):1203–6.
3. Vinchon M, Baroncini M, Delestret I. Adult outcome of pediatric hydrocephalus. *Childs Nerv Syst* 2012;28:847–54.
4. Herzer M, Goebel J, Cortina S. Transitioning cognitively impaired young patients with special health needs to adult oriented care: collaboration between medical providers and pediatric psychologists. *Curr Opin Pediatr* 2010;22:668–72.
5. Maldonado IL, Valery CA, Boch AL. Shunt dependence: myths and facts. *Acta Neurochir* 2010;152:1449–4.
6. O'Brien DF, Javadpour M, Collins DR, et al. Endoscopic third ventriculostomy: an outcome analysis of primary cases and procedures performed after ventriculoperitoneal shunt malfunction. *J Neurosurg (Suppl Pediatrics)* 2005;103:393–400.
7. Jenkinson MD, Hayhurst C, Al-Jumaily M, et al. The role of endoscopic third ventriculostomy in adult patients with hydrocephalus. *J Neurosurg* 2009;110:861–6.
8. Hader WJ, Walker RL, Myles ST, et al. Complications of endoscopic third ventriculostomy in previously shunted patients. *Neurosurgery* 2008;63:ONS170–7.
9. Buxton N, Macarthur D, Robertson I, et al. Neuroendoscopic third ventriculostomy for failed shunts. *Surg Neurol* 2003;60:201–4.
10. Drake J, Chumas P, Kestle J, et al. Late rapid deterioration after endoscopic third ventriculostomy: additional cases and review of the literature. *J Neurosurg* 2006;105(2 Suppl):118–26.
11. Paulsen AH, Lundar T, Lindegaard KF. Twenty-year outcome in young adults with childhood hydrocephalus: assessment of surgical outcome, work participation, and health-related quality of life. *J Neurosurg Pediatr* 2010;6:527–35.
12. Rekate HL. The slit ventricle syndrome: advances based on technology and understanding. *Pediatr Neurosurg* 2004;40:259–63.
13. Gupta N, Park J, Solomon C, et al. Long-term outcomes in patients with treated childhood hydrocephalus. *J Neurosurg (Suppl Pediatrics)* 2007;106:334–9.
14. Olson S. The problematic slit ventricle syndrome: a review of the literature and proposed algorithm for treatment. *Pediatr Neurosurg* 2004;40:264–9.
15. Edwards RJ, Witchell C, Pople IK. Chronic headaches in adults with spina bifida and associated hydrocephalus. *Eur J Pediatr Surg* 2003;13:S13–S17.

16. Reddy GK, Bollam P, Caldito G, Punt J. Ventriculoperitoneal shunt surgery outcome in adult transition patients with pediatric-onset hydrocephalus. *Neurosurgery* 2012;70(2):380–9.

17. Hommet C, Billard C, Gillet P, et al. Neuropsychologic and adaptive functioning in adolescents and young adults shunted for congenital hydrocephalus. *J Child Neurol* 1999;44:144–50.

Chapter 24

Management of hydrocephalus with associated cerebrospinal fluid pathologies

Petra Margarete Klinge

Introduction

Hydrocephalus can occur in association with other pathologies of the cerebrospinal fluid (CSF) system, e.g. cerebellar and posterior fossa anomalies (Dandy–Walker complex, Blake's pouch, and megacisterna magna), arachnoid cysts, Chiari malformation, and spina bifida. The etiology of hydrocephalus as a result of impaired CSF circulation when coexisting with these pathologies still challenges our understanding of CSF dynamics, as cerebellar anomalies and or arachnoid cysts, for example, not infrequently occur as stand-alone pathologies; in other words, they can exist with and without hydrocephalus.

The aim of this chapter is not to provide a comprehensive overview or textbook information on all these pathologies, but rather to strengthen our appreciation of how complex the treatment of hydrocephalus and associated CSF disorders can be, across ages. For despite many advances in neurosurgery, these pathologies still provide a challenging complexity for those involved in diagnosing and treating hydrocephalus in both pediatric and adult patients.

There is an element of disturbance of CSF circulation in all of these; however, the mechanism of how and why symptoms occur is still not clearly understood, and not always as obvious as it is with Chiari I and the resolution of syringomyelia after sufficient decompression. As congenital pathologies, they occur during the development of the central nervous system, and are therefore traditionally deemed incidental findings and rarely thought to be symptomatic. And yet, at the time of diagnosis, patients may exhibit symptoms that challenge the decision about clinical relevance and treatment indication, particularly in the adult or elderly population. The chronicity of the diseases is usually associated with insidious onset of a disease process, and as such, considered "benign." If symptomatic, they might have significant impact on quality of life and function in an individual. Beyond that, little is still known about pathophysiology of the CSF system in the prenatal period. Furthermore, surgical treatment is associated with a high rate of recurrence or unsatisfactory results, for example in arachnoid cysts, and contemporary approaches need to utilize multimodal concepts; traditional shunt placement and microsurgical approaches are now partnered by more contemporary and "noninvasive" endoscopic treatment. There is no state-of-the-art treatment strategy available.

Clinical scenarios will be presented that support the complex nature of the disease, the challenging decision-making about whether or not to surgically intervene, and the difficulties with choosing the most efficient type of surgical intervention. The discussion will provoke suggestions for contemporary management, e.g. the importance of interdisciplinary management of patients, the role of modern magnetic resonance imaging (MRI) in the detection of CSF circulation and pathologies, and multimodal surgical strategies. The presentation of an 86-year-old patient with hydrocephalus associated with a symptomatic cerebellar arachnoid cyst should increase awareness that these pathologies might also be becoming more prevalent in the elderly population, where aging might provide a risk factor not only for normal pressure hydrocephalus but also for hydrocephalus associated with congenital CSF pathologies.

Basic and clinical research has to address improvement in diagnosis, management, and outcome of CSF disorders. Hopefully, we will be able to establish and maintain a pool of researchers and clinicians who are keen to work in the traditionally neglected area of hydrocephalus and associated disorders. Here, the recently formed International Society of

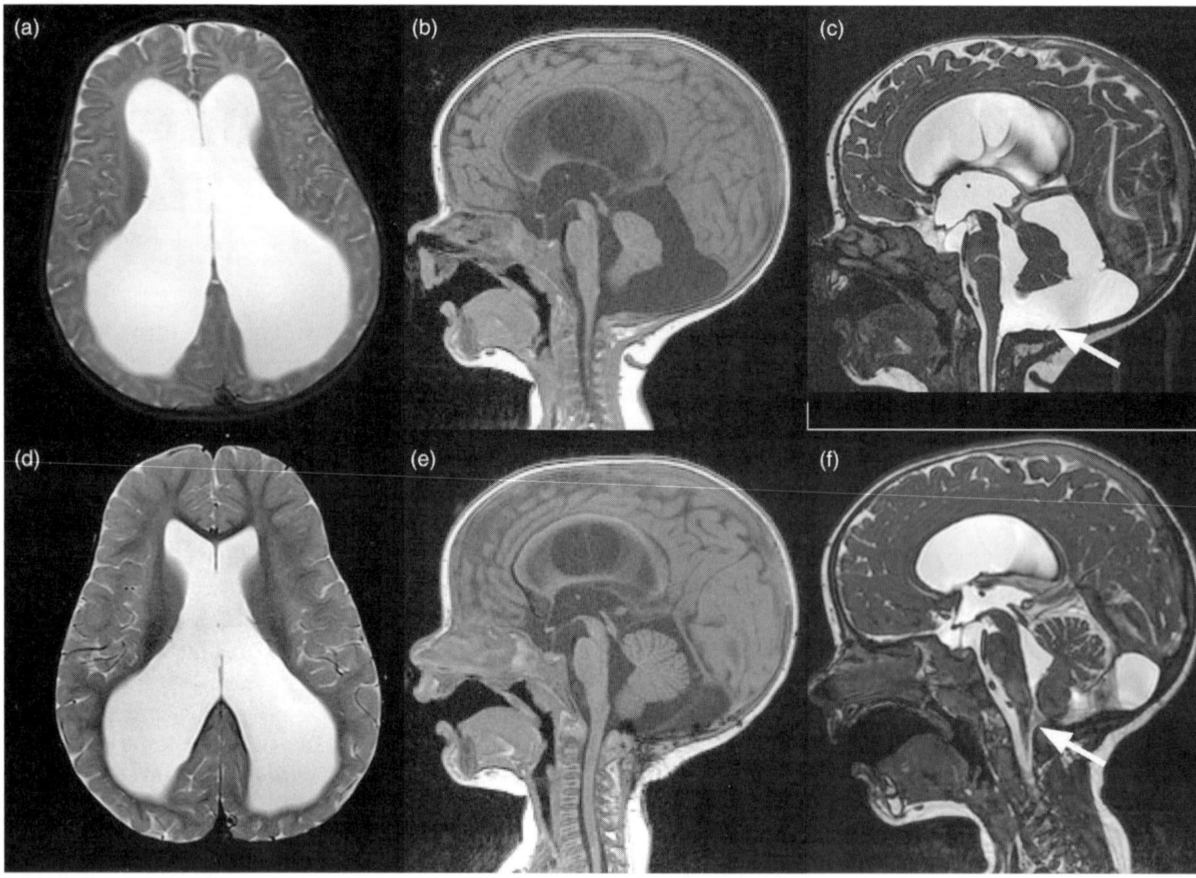

Figure 24.1 Hydrocephalus associated with posterior fossa cyst. (a–c) Preoperative MRI findings of hydrocephalus in an axial T2-weighted image (a) and a sagittal T1-weighted image showing posterior fossa pathology (b), which was suggestive of an arachnoid cyst based on web-like structures (white arrow) seen in the CISS sequence (c). (d–f) Corresponding postoperative MRI findings after microsurgical cyst fenestration with improved hydrocephalus (d) and decompression of the posterior fossa cyst and expansion of the cerebellum (e) with flow void signal at the level of the foramen of Magendie and the cisterna magna indicating restoration of CSF circulation (f; white arrow).

Hydrocephalus and Cerebrospinal Fluid disorders (ISHCSF) and the International Hydrocephalus Imaging Working Group (IHIWG) are exciting initiatives to encourage and provide platforms for young researchers. These initiatives will be introduced in the conclusion of this chapter.

Case 1. Hydrocephalus associated with a posterior fossa cyst

A 4-month-old female presented with significant change in head circumference percentiles reaching above the 97th percentile, but otherwise reaching milestones. A first child, uncomplicated term vaginal delivery of a healthy couple without contributive history. Because of the concern about the increased head circumference, a brain MRI was ordered that showed massive enlargement of the lateral and third ventricles associated with posterior fossa enlargement of the cisterna magna and atrophic cerebellum without clear mass effect. Cine flow studies indicated disrupted CSF motion at the level of the foramen magnum and additional CISS sequences were suggestive of an arachnoid cyst. The cerebral aqueduct appeared patent though narrowed in the lower segment (Figure 24.1a–c).

Notably, the parents reported that despite appropriate milestones being reached, they were always concerned with a lack of head control when comparing their daughter with others in the playgroup. However, despite the increase in head circumference, the clinical examination did not reveal any obvious signs of increased intracranial pressure. There was a full but not a tense fontanelle and absence of splayed sutures, leaving the impression of a chronic condition.

Given the clinical concern and the radiographic findings of a posterior fossa arachnoid cyst in the presence of a patent aqueduct, a midline posterior fossa craniotomy with microsurgical fenestration of the arachnoid cyst into the cisterna magna and the basolateral cisterns was selected and performed in an attempt to eventually also alleviate the hydrocephalus. A temporary external ventricular drain was placed, however, which could be weaned at postsurgical day three. The histopathological findings confirmed fragments of dense, fibrous connective tissue and adjacent pigmented arachnoid lining consistent with an arachnoid cyst, further supported by EMA (epithelial membrane antigen) positive immunohistochemistry of the specimen.

The postoperative course was uneventful and the 1-year postoperative MRI findings show resolution of posterior fossa pathology with improved but persistent hydrocephalus (Figure 24.1d, e). Clinically, the head circumference improved to the 90th percentile and seemed to plateau at that level. Pediatric neurology is following the patient bi-annually and stated that the now 2-year-old girl is developing appropriately without motor and mental delay.

Case 2. Posterior fossa cyst without hydrocephalus

A 16-year-old female was admitted emergently for failure to thrive, nausea and vomiting, and an additional history of migraines and psychiatric illness. A brain MRI showed a posterior fossa cystic lesion with mild to moderate mass effect on the cerebellum. Additional CISS sequences suggested the presence of an arachnoid cyst that had some focal communication with the spinal canal associated with CSF turbulences (Figure 24.2a–c). There was no hydrocephalus. Given the teenager's complicated and pre-existing history of migraines and psychiatric illness, the findings were initially deemed incidental. The patient continued to have excesses of headaches associated with episodes of vomiting and dry heaving during the hospital stay, and pediatric neurology was consulted and raised concerns of postural headaches associated with posterior fossa pathology.

Given the prolonged disease state despite all medical and critical care efforts, the interdisciplinary decision was made to explore the cyst. A midline craniotomy with microsurgical fenestration of the arachnoid cyst was performed, and the intraoperative finding supported a "ball-valve" mechanism possibly causing intermittent expansion of the cyst by a "jet flow" of CSF from the spinal compartment into and out of the cyst triggered by cardiac cycles (Figure 24.2f). A wide microsurgical fenestration of the cyst into the spinal compartment was performed.

Postoperatively, the patient fully recovered within 14 days; however, she developed a pseudomeningocele with recurrence of positional headaches (Figure 24.2e). The pseudomeningocele was repaired with an autologous fat graft a month later and the last postoperative MRI 3 months post-microsurgical fenestration shows resolution of the pseudomeningocele and a significantly decreased size of posterior fossa cyst and overall improved posterior fossa conditions (Figure 24.2d). The patient, 1 year after surgery, despite some occasional episodes of headaches similar to her previous baseline and history of migraines, resumed full activity without any further episodes of positional headaches and nausea and vomiting.

Case 3. Hydrocephalus associated with Chiari I malformation

A 7-year-old female with a known history of attention deficit hyperactivity disorder (ADHD) became more symptomatic with deterioration in her grades despite medical management of ADHD. For her reported "occipital headaches" she was also diagnosed with "juvenile migraines." Given the concern about her decline in grades starting from A grades now down to C and D grades as well as the increased complaints about occipital headaches, the pediatrician ordered an MRI that disclosed significant ventriculomegaly and a 7 mm Chiari malformation (Figure 24.3a–c). MRI of the spine did not show any associated syringohydromyelia or other spinal pathology. The cine flow study found absent flow signal at the level of the foramen magnum (Figure 24.3c).

Upon further evaluation it became clear that in addition to the decline in grades and the daily headaches, the girl also had a history of falls, balance problems, clumsiness, and dizziness, and the mother as well as the school teacher felt that "she spaces out" more, though it was initially attributed to her known ADHD.

The pediatric neurology department was involved and found appropriate milestones and suggested physiological intoeing as a potential cause of her clumsiness. Also, there was a positive family history of ADHD and learning disabilities on the maternal side. Her head circumference leveled at the 90th percentile.

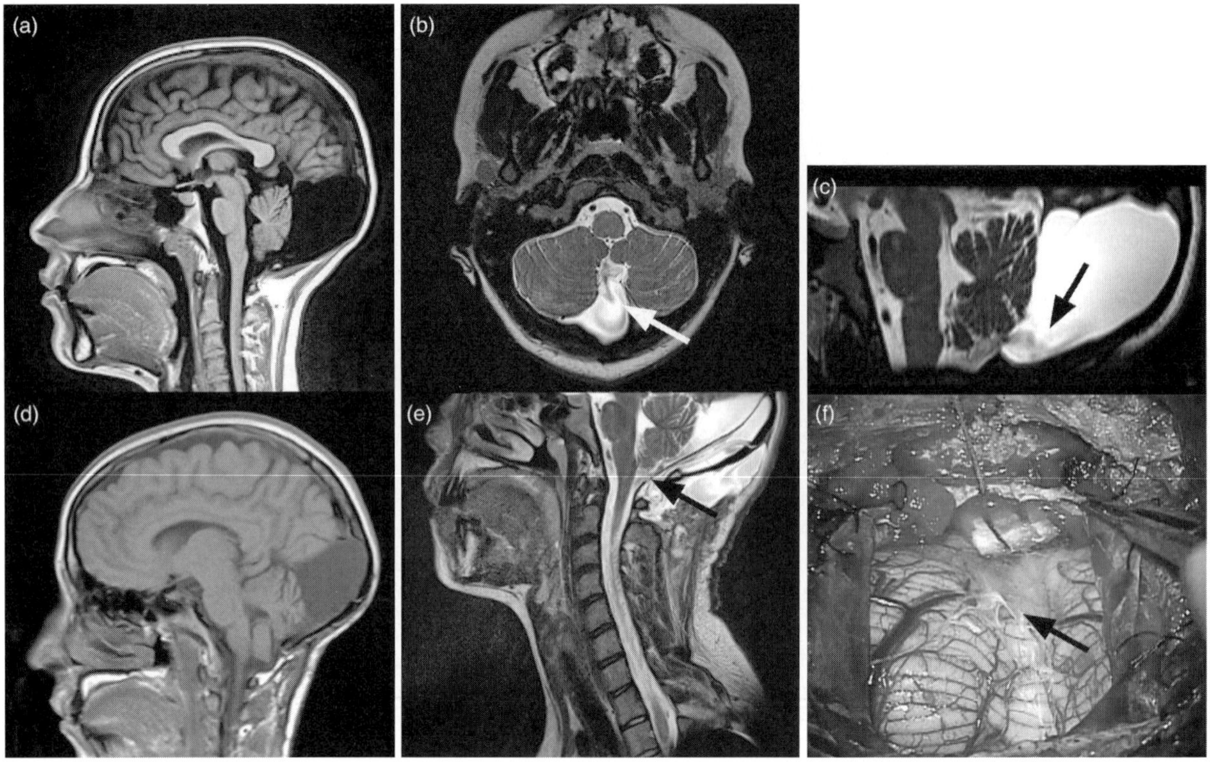

Figure 24.2 Posterior fossa cyst without hydrocephalus. (a–c) Preoperative MRI findings showing a retrocerebellar cystic lesion with some mass effect on the cerebellum as indicated in a midline sagittal T1-weighted image (a). The axial T2-weighted image (b) shows a flow void signal in the cisterna magna suggestive of CSF turbulences (white arrow), which was supported by a sagittal CISS sequence focusing on that area that indicated a focal communication inferiorly, inferior to the fourth ventricle, suggestive of a "ball-valve" mechanism causing the cyst to expand (c, black arrow). (d–e) Postoperative MRI shows reduction of the cyst and expansion of the cerebellum in a sagittal T1-weighted image as well as restored CSF flow at the level of the foramen magnum as indicated by physiological flow void signals at the foramen of Magendie, and between the cisterna magna and the cervical spinal CSF compartment (e, black arrow). The intraoperative microscopic view during microsurgical fenestration of the cyst supports the finding of an arachnoid cyst with a pre-existing focal opening (black arrow) to support the "ball-valve" mechanism as suggested by the radiographic findings (f). A full-color version is included in the color plate section.

Given the above findings, observation and neurocognitive testing was indicated in the presence of a normal neurological exam.

The neurocognitive baseline testing disclosed impairment in attention and behavioral regulation, in maintaining focus and executive function, consistent with "Attention-Deficit/Hyperactivity Disorder but R/O Specific Learning Disorder (e.g. Hydrocephalus) deficits is mandated." Despite a stable neurocognitive exam on repeated examination 6 months after initial diagnosis, there was ongoing decline in school grades and more distress with episodes of the girl holding her head for reports of headaches and "head pain." Due to the parents' as well as teachers' concern, an interdisciplinary decision was made for placement of a ventriculoperitoneal shunt with an adjustable valve system. It was felt that the progressive symptoms of cognitive and balance decline and the neurocognitive profile were attributable to the significant chronic hydrocephalus and that shunt treatment should be given priority. Though there was absent flow signal in the cine studies, the Chiari abnormality was not deemed severe enough to suggest a causal relation with the hydrocephalus, and it was felt that the Chiari I was coexisting with rather than being the cause of it. At one year after shunt placement, the girl improved remarkably with improved school performance (reports of B grades) as well as full recovery from her falling spells and significant reduction of headache episodes from daily to occasionally. The girl maintained improvement within the 2-year postoperative follow-up. However, the postoperative images at 2 years post-surgery do not show significant changes in ventriculomegaly and the Chiari I malformation (Figure 24.3d–f).

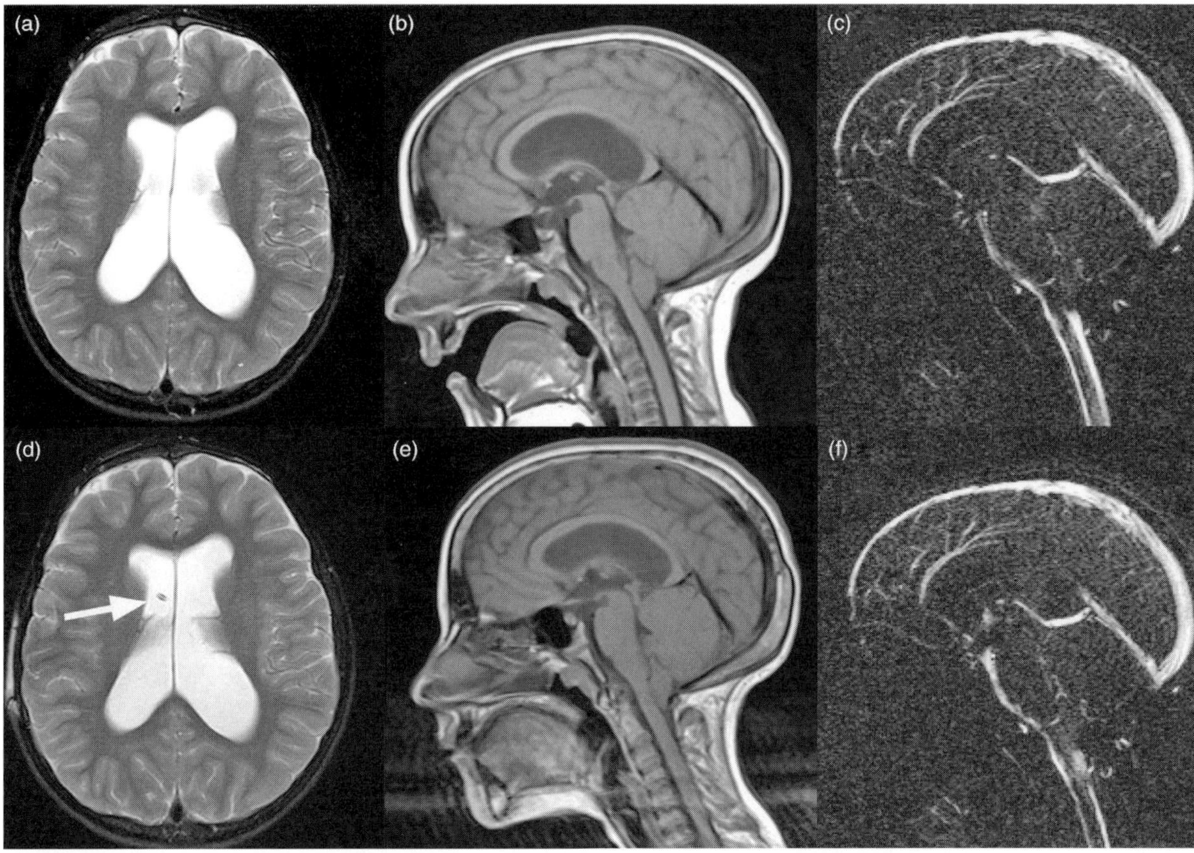

Figure 24.3 Hydrocephalus associated with Chiari I malformation. (a–c) Preoperative MRI findings show hydrocephalus in an axial T2-weighted image (a) and a 7 cm tonsillar descent in a sagittal T1-weighted image (b) with absent CSF flow signal posterior to the tonsils supported by cine flow studies (c). (d–f) Two years after shunt surgery (d, white arrow), there is slight improvement of hydrocephalus though persistent and but slightly worse appearance of Chiari malformation, now reported as 1.3 cm, with restricted CSF flow signal on cine MRI studies (e).

Case 4. Normal pressure hydrocephalus associated with cerebellar arachnoid cyst

An 86-year-old female had a history of a left-sided symptomatic cerebellar arachnoid cyst when she was 30 years old. The cyst was microsurgically fenestrated, and finally successfully shunted with one revision. She had been doing well since then though some residual balance problems remained after some difficulties with managing the cyst.

In the previous year, the patient experienced much more unsteadiness to a point where she could no longer walk independently and displayed overall weakness and lack of initiative and interest. Extensive work-up for systemic illnesses given her age was initiated by the primary care physician with negative results. A head CT scan was performed showing increase in ventricular size with transependymal signal suggestive of hydrocephalus. The ventricular size was markedly enlarged compared to previous scans performed a couple of years previously while the appearance of the cerebellar cyst was stable (Figure 24.4a, b). Due to vessel clips in the area of the posterior fossa cyst presumably applied during her first surgery with microsurgical fenestration, the patient was not able to undergo MRI assessment (Figure 24.4c).

Given the clinical and radiological findings of progressive ventriculomegaly and functional decline, ventricular shunt surgery was performed. Though it was clear that the old cyst shunt was located within a membrane that separated a small portion of the cyst indicating a non-functioning position, there was no indication of mass effect from the cyst to suggest that

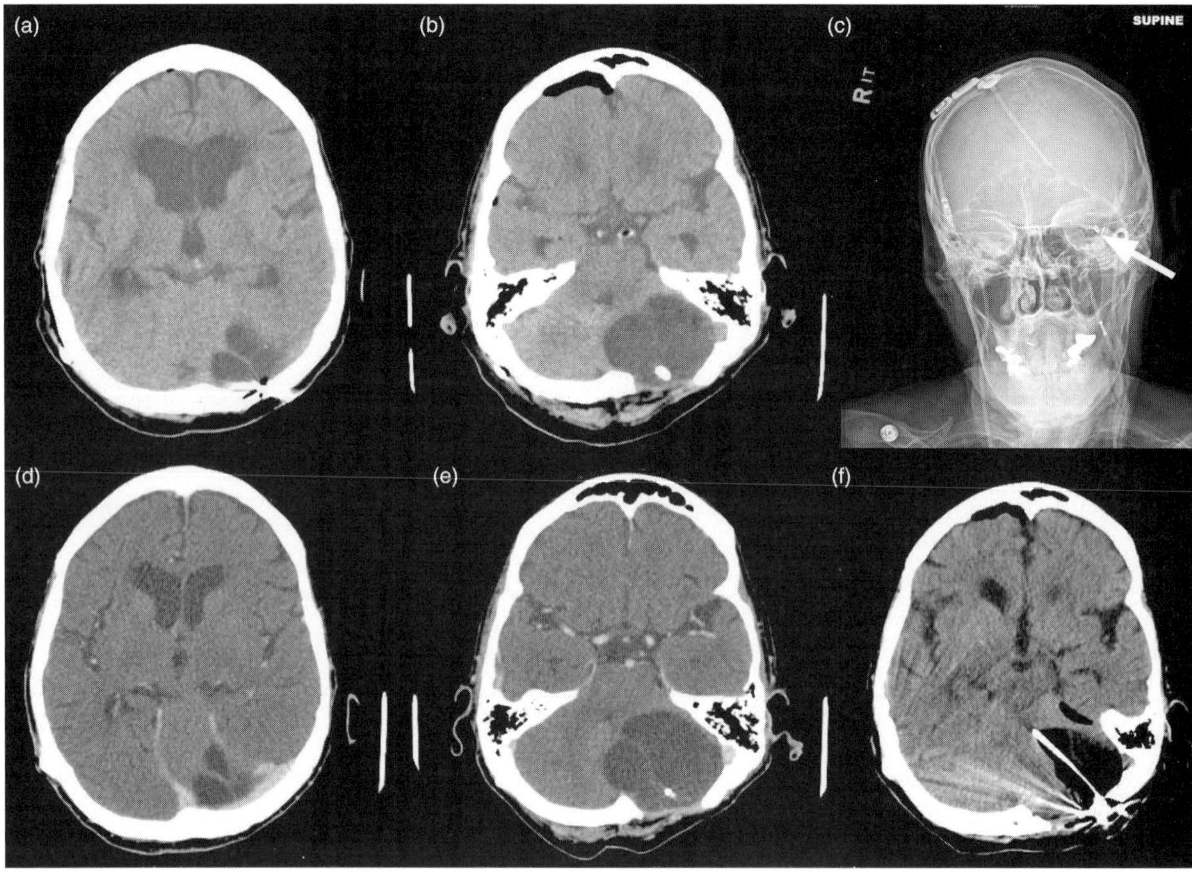

Figure 24.4 Normal pressure hydrocephalus associated with cerebellar arachnoid cyst. (a, b) A non-contrast CT scan shows findings consistent with normal pressure hydrocephalus associated with a cerebellar arachnoid cyst that was shunted 50 years previously after an unsuccessful attempt of microsurgical fenestration. It appears that the proximal catheter has moved out and is located in a cyst septum. There is no obvious mass effect from the cyst (b). (c) Anteroposterior X-ray film shows a right ventriculoperitoneal shunt placed for normal pressure hydrocephalus and also vessel clips (white arrow) that were placed 30 years ago on a first attempt to fenestrate the arachnoid cyst microsurgically. As such, an MRI was not possible. (d, e) Post-shunt placement, the hydrocephalus improved; however, the arachnoid cyst increased in size with mass effect as seen by displacement and compression of the fourth ventricle (e). CT scan after placement of a new cystoperitoneal shunt (f).

the cyst was symptomatic (Figure 24.4b). After ventriculoperitoneal shunt placement, the patient did well for about a month with improved walking and balance; however, she started to develop symptoms of loss of appetite and nausea.

Upon emergent admission to the hospital for failure to thrive, the patient was investigated again for coexisting systemic illnesses, but all tests were negative. Also, the CT scan showed resolution of hydrocephalus. However, an increase in the size of the cerebellar arachnoid cyst was noted when compared to the CT scan that was done before placement of the ventriculoperitoneal shunt 6 months prior to the onset of the above symptoms (Figure 24.4d, e). There was now a subtle mass effect on the cerebellum and fourth ventricle and brainstem. Medical management of her failure to thrive and her nausea was maximized; however, no improvement was seen and instead there was further deterioration. Given her age and the equivocal scenario, the neurology department was involved over the question of a coexisting neurodegenerative process; however, the concern with the increased size of the arachnoid cyst persisted and placement of a new cystoperitoneal shunt was performed with reduction of the cyst size and resolution of mass effect (Figure 24.4f). The patient did not show any further episodes of vomiting and nausea and had a full appetite at her 1-month and 6-month follow-up post surgery.

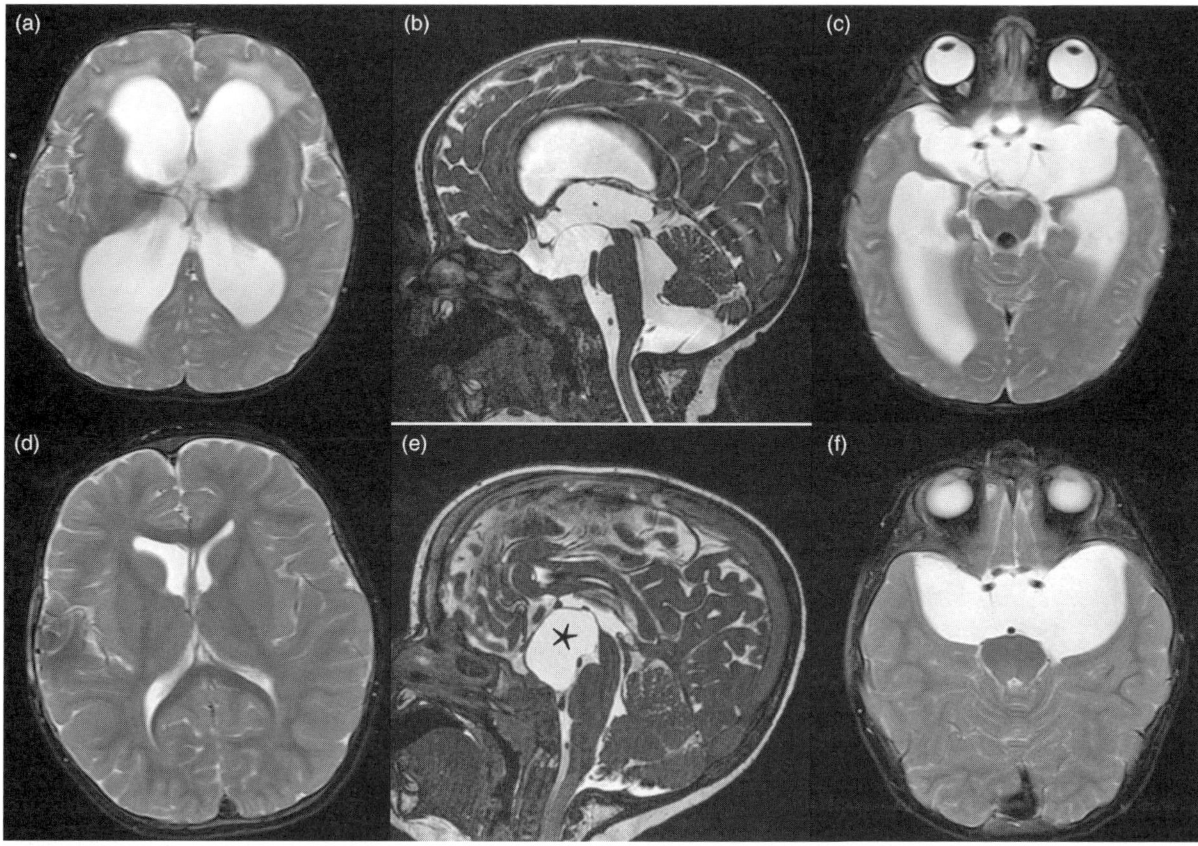

Figure 24.5 Hydrocephalus with multiple arachnoid cysts. (a–c) Preoperative T2-weighted MRI images showing severe hydrocephalus with transependymal flow signal around the frontal horns (a). A sagittal CISS sequence showed posterior fossa abnormalities suggestive of megacisterna magna or Dandy–Walker variant with a patent aqueduct (b). Additional findings were bilateral temporal arachnoid cysts (c). (d–f) Two years after shunt surgery for hydrocephalus, ventricular size has normalized as seen on T2-weighted axial MRI (d) with resolution of the posterior fossa abnormalities (e) and stable bilateral arachnoid cysts (f); however, a new finding of a suprasellar arachnoid cyst is seen in the sagittal CISS sequence (e, asterisk).

Case 5. Hydrocephalus with multiple arachnoid cysts

A 4-month-old girl was admitted emergently with failure to thrive, irritability, and lethargy along with increasing head circumference. On examination, the child displayed clear signs of increased intracranial pressure with bulging fontanelle, splayed sutures, sun setting signs, and distended scalp veins. There was no prior complicated history in this term vaginal delivery first child of a healthy couple without contributory history.

The MRI revealed massive hydrocephalus with T2 hyperintensities around the frontal and occipital horns indicating transependymal CSF signal. Of note, too, is that there were bilateral sizable temporal arachnoid cysts and enlargement of the cisterna magna. There was no indication of aqueductal stenosis as an underlying cause of the hydrocephalus (Figure 24.5a–c).

Given the clinical and radiological impression of acute hydrocephalus, shunt surgery was performed and the girl did well without signs of hydrocephalus on clinical examination and improved ventricular size on follow-up MRI scan. The girl got lost from follow-up and presented at 2.5 years of age with concerns for new irritability, headaches, and visual disturbances. A follow-up MRI ordered by the pediatrician showed sufficiently drained lateral ventricles and stable sized temporal arachnoid cysts. However, a large suprasellar arachnoid cyst as a new finding was suggestive as the cause of her new clinical symptoms of headaches and visual disturbances. Of note, the enlargement of the cisterna magna had subsided (Figure 24.5d–f). The patient recently underwent

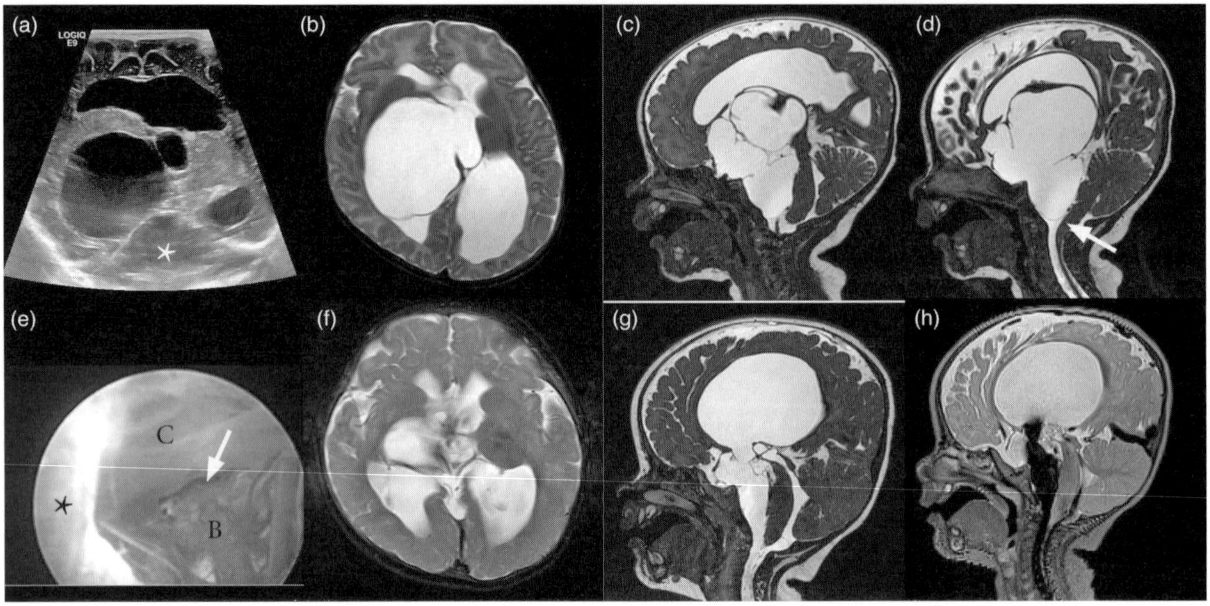

Figure 24.6 Hydrocephalus associated with a giant suprasellar arachnoid cyst diagnosed in a fetus. (a–d) Preoperative findings of a fetal ultrasound showing hydrocephalus and infratentorial pathology, suggestive of a posterior fossa cyst or Dandy–Walker malformation (a, white asterisk). T2-weighted axial MRI (B) and sagittal CISS sequences (c, d) at day 3 post-partum show a giant arachnoid cyst extending into the supra- and infratentorial compartment with multiple septi; however, the CISS sequences suggest one compartment cyst of suprasellar origin, and endoscopic fenestration into the spinal canal and opening of the caudal cyst membrane (d, white arrow) was attempted. A left frontal transventricular endoscopic approach was performed and fenestration of the cyst into the spinal compartment was accomplished as seen by the intraoperative endoscopic view (e; C = clivus, B = brainstem basilar artery, asterisk = cyst membrane, white arrow = spinal subdural space). (f–h) Postoperative corresponding MRI findings show significant reduction of cyst size and improved hydrocephalus in both axial and sagittal T2-weighted and CISS sequences (f, g) as well as CSF flow signal suggestive of communication of the lateral ventricles with the spinal compartment shown by T2 CSF space imaging (h). A full-color version is included in the color plate section.

successful endoscopic transventricular fenestration of the arachnoid cyst through a right frontal burr hole approach.

Case 6. Hydrocephalus associated with a giant suprasellar arachnoid cyst diagnosed in a fetus

A level III ultrasound revealed massive hydrocephalus associated with a posterior fossa pathology most likely an arachnoid cyst or a Dandy–Walker variant in a 24-week-old fetus of a twin gestation (Figure 24.6a). The couple have a 5-year-old healthy girl. A fetal MRI was performed that suggested hydrocephalus associated with posterior fossa arachnoid cyst.

Both fetuses were stable throughout pregnancy and cesarean section was scheduled at 38 weeks of pregnancy. The twin girls were stable, and initially, there were no signs of increase of intracranial pressure in the affected twin. An MRI of the brain and spine was done on day two, and showed a massive arachnoid cyst, likely of suprasellar origin extending into the prepontine cistern, the third ventricle, and lateral ventricles with massive displacement of midbrain, brainstem structures, and the cerebellum (Figure 24.6b–d).

Due to the stable condition and the fact that the baby was thriving, it was decided to delay treatment. Repeated MRI including dedicated CISS sequences showed that the cyst most likely consisted of one compartment, with extension into the lateral and third ventricle, as well as the potential of fenestrating the caudal portion of the cyst into the spinal CSF compartment (Figure 24.6d). Therefore endoscopic fenestration through a left frontal transventricular approach was deemed feasible. During surgery, fenestration of the inferior prepontine portions of the cyst into the spinal subarachnoid space was also accomplished (Figure 24.6e). Six months after endoscopic treatment, the child suffered from strabismus, but was otherwise well, and developmentally about 3 months behind her twin. Imaging showed improvement of the cyst size and CSF flow (Figure 24.6f–h).

Case synopsis and discussion

The above cases all demonstrate clinical scenarios in patients with congenital pathologies of the CSF system with and without hydrocephalus suggestive of disturbed CSF dynamics causing the patients' symptoms or problems. The case mix of patients shows that clinicians are confronted with these conditions at all stages of life, and that age-associated comorbidity and the individual spectrum of symptoms provides a difficult clinical scenario, e.g. in the teenager and the 86-year-old woman where despite all medical efforts and no improvement being seen, finally surgical intervention was sought by the primary care provider and the family. Sometimes treatment had to be offered in the equivocal scenario, despite incomplete understanding of how and whether the cyst ultimately caused the patient's symptoms and how surgical intervention would affect outcome. The case of the 7-year-old girl with the Chiari I and the associated normal pressure hydrocephalus type of radiological and clinical picture shows that interdisciplinary management including cognitive testing might be superior in the decision-making than the traditional methods of intracranial pressure monitoring or measurements of intracranial compliance and resistance to outflow in these complex conditions [1–3]. In particular, it is not always clear whether and how the hydrocephalus is related to the associated finding, for example in the 4-month-old girl with the posterior fossa cyst, where successful decompression and establishment of flow did not result in resolution of the hydrocephalus. It is likely that the hydrocephalus coexists with the posterior fossa cyst and will eventually need treatment once subtle symptoms that appear chronic in nature occur. This child will need thorough and close follow-up of motor and mental milestones in her young life and any decline should warrant intervention on her hydrocephalus given increasing evidence of the late life impact untreated hydrocephalus may have on cognitive outcome, e.g. as known from the LOVA concept [4,5]. Also the patient with the Chiari I plus hydrocephalus indicates that the normal pressure hydrocephalus condition with elements of the triad (i.e. slow progression of gait and balance problems, cognitive decline, and incontinence) is prevalent in toddlers and infants, and is probably still underdiagnosed in the pediatric population [6,7]. In the differential diagnosis of ADHD in this age group, hydrocephalus should be considered. The sequelae of chronic hydrocephalus with (delayed) onset of cognitive and functional decline despite stable ventriculomegaly indeed suggests a progressive neurodegenerative process associated with chronic hydrocephalus, as suggested not only by experimental studies [8–10] but also by studies of metabolism and cerebral blood flow in normal pressure hydrocephalus [10–12]. The cases also show that any intervention in the CSF spaces may unpredictably change CSF dynamics and pathology is still incompletely understood, as in the 4-month-old patient who developed a previously absent large suprasellar cyst that occurred after successful shunting of hydrocephalus associated with bilateral temporal arachnoid cysts; or the increase of the pre-existing but previously stable cerebellar arachnoid cyst in the 86-year-old woman 6 months after shunting of normal pressure hydrocephalus. Part of this might certainly indicate some of the existing limitations of imaging of hydrocephalus and the associated impairment of CSF spaces and dynamics. Ultimately, those complex scenarios also question our traditional thinking about the association of intracranial pressure, compliance and CSF absorption and hydrocephalus [13,14], and suggest that we should appreciate that our traditional and dogmatic ways of measuring ICP and CSF dynamics with compliance and R_{out} values are limited in helping our understanding of disease associated with CSF dynamic disturbances [15–19]. Also, the fact that despite enormous pathology, e.g. in the fetus with the massive suprasellar arachnoid cyst, the condition is stable, whereas in a teenager or an elderly person little pathology or only a small change in pathology can push the patient's health over the edge; age-associated susceptibility and comorbidity is probably one of the most important factors determining the disease and the outcome of pathology associated with hydrocephalus and associated CSF pathology/disorder [20–22]. Age as a complicating factor in hydrocephalus has been suggested by the LOVA concept as well as observations of congenital origin in elderly patients presenting with normal pressure hydrocephalus. However, this understanding should probably be translated to all pathologies that are associated with congenital CSF circulatory disorders. For example in Chiari I, borderline conditions more frequently seem to affect the third and fourth decades of life [23].

Needless to say that despite the difficult decision of whether to treat, the mode of treatment is very individual given the above incomplete understanding of pathology and clinical symptoms in these circumstances. Traditionally, most of the findings, particularly all kinds of arachnoid cyst as well as Chiari I, have initially been considered incidental findings when diagnosed with imaging, more or less regardless of the patient's complaints. Unless the patient exhibits focal signs that match with a potential mass effect or irritation of structures in the location of the cyst or potential CSF dynamic perturbance (e.g. in syringomyelia [24–26]), treatment is usually not offered or it is suggested that the finding has nothing to do with the patient's complaints. Particularly in non-focal or non-lesion-related signs, such as headaches, cognitive decline or decline in school performance, clumsiness, failure to thrive, behavioral outbursts, depression, and emotional problems, there is almost always for any of the above pathological circumstances and for any age group a comorbid condition at hand that might also explain and account for the patient's problem.

Only recently, again stemming from treatment of Chiari I patients, has there been more appreciation of nonspecific findings, particularly certain cognitive elements that indicate that CSF dynamic disturbances might have systemic effects on CSF homeostasis with an impact on cognitive and behavioral outcome [27,28]. Advanced concepts in the understanding of diseases associated with CSF disorders, e.g. arachnoid cysts, posterior fossa anomalies, Chiari I, and spina bifida with and without hydrocephalus, are needed including more standardized and multidisciplinary approaches [15,29]. For example, the 7-year-old girl with Chiari and hydrocephalus did show remarkable improvement in headaches, balance, and school grades, but no change in ventriculomegaly and Chiari after ventriculoperitoneal shunting. This demonstrates that, in hydrocephalus and in the CSF disorders addressed in this chapter, we often see remarkable improvement despite no or little change in pathology. This basically raises interesting research questions that have not yet been answered: (i) does shunting affect brain metabolism and CSF dynamics beyond what we can see and document by imaging; and (ii) to what extent is there a placebo effect of our interventions?

Increased accessibility and use of brain and spine imaging modalities with MRI techniques will likely discover more congenital pathology, particularly in patients at later stages in life as disability is no longer accepted due to a generally higher longevity and the demands of modern society [19,30,31].

The following paragraphs will suggest that more standardized approaches and management in those complex and sometimes exceptional conditions of hydrocephalus and associated CSF disorders across ages can be accomplished if one extrapolates recent and advanced knowledge and concepts in the diagnosis and management of hydrocephalus. The concepts include the role of cognitive testing in the diagnosis and prognosis of disease, advances in imaging of CSF physiology and pathology, multimodal and multidisciplinary neurosurgical techniques, as well as improved classification schemes of CSF disorders.

The role of cognition and cognitive assessment

In normal pressure hydrocephalus, the role of a certain cognitive profile and its importance in diagnosing the disease as well as in the understanding of the disease burden has been established and seminal work was published in the last three decades of the twentieth century. Deficits in attention, visuospatial function, visual over verbal impairment, concentration, and impaired wakefulness have been found as unique features throughout and across different investigators [30]. Despite these efforts, cognitive tests have never traditionally been used in the decision-making as to whether to shunt or not to shunt a patient or, in other words, used as predictors of shunt treatment. Mainly, neurocognitive test batteries of various origins have been used to support outcome assessment in more systematic studies. Only very few but non-systematic attempts have been made to identify prognostic values, however, and have yet not been able to identify cognitive tests with sufficient accuracy to predict the response to shunting [32,33]. Also, well-designed and systematic studies and trials from expert centers published on intracranial pressure measurement, measurement of resistance to CSF outflow and compliance, and other adjunctive testing have ultimately failed to accurately predict shunt response [19].

The recent European multicenter trial conducted on the prediction of outcome in idiopathic NPH revealed the importance of a neurocognitive test battery with accuracy of diagnosis and prognosis of shunt response and 1-year outcome of shunt treatment far superior to the high-volume CSF tap test and R_{out} measurement [34–36]. The findings showed that a battery of three cognitive tests, the Stroop test, Rey Auditory Verbal Learning Test (RAVLT), and Grooved Pegboard test, were highly discriminative and diagnostically accurate in both probable and possible NPH when comparing the performance of iNPH patients with that of 108 healthy individuals (HI). iNPH patients performed significantly worse than HI on all of the neuropsychological measures at entry. The discriminative capacities of the eight variables were similar, with areas under the curve (AUC; ROC analysis) ranging between 0.86 (Delayed Recall) and 0.95 (Grooved Pegboard). The most usable test was RAVLT (Learning and Delayed Recall), administered to ≥90% of patients on all occasions. However, the Grooved Pegboard and the Stroop test were more sensitive to treatment effects. The three neuropsychological tests used in the European iNPH study are expedient, highly diagnostically discriminative, and well suited to evaluate changes following shunt treatment [37].

Little is known about the potential of cognitive tests and their diagnostic and prognostic accuracy in other CSF pathologies with potential CSF dynamic disturbance, e.g. Chiari I, arachnoid cysts, spina bifida, and posterior fossa anomalies. As discussed above, some evidence exists for Chiari I malformation and associated cognitive decline to suggest that any abnormal anatomy of the CSF spaces in fact has an impact on cognitive function [23,27,28,38–40], e.g. behavioral and autistic problems indicating higher cognitive impairment. The above supports and stresses the importance of cognitive disorder in CSF dynamic diseases and the potential value of cognitive batteries to improve the diagnosis and prognosis. Systematic prospective studies in hydrocephalus and associated CSF disorders are encouraged to identify cognitive domains most likely affected by these disorders and which show change after treatment and intervention and have the potential to increase the diagnostic as well as prognostic accuracy of cognitive test batteries [33].

The role of neuroimaging and MRI

As stated above, invasive CSF dynamic testing, e.g. R_{out} and compliance measurements, have failed to improve selection of shunt candidates, and have not helped our understanding of disease processes and pathophysiology. For example, variable and only weak correlation of resistance to outflow or compliance and CSF biomarkers of neurodegeneration and ischemia (e.g. neurofilament and sulfatide) has been shown [41,42]. Furthermore, other metabolic studies done in chronic hydrocephalus have rarely shown any correlation with CSF dynamics. This questions the significance of those measures and of CSF dynamic testing for the disease and the pathophysiology of chronic hydrocephalus [43,44].

MRI has evolved in the past 5 to 10 years with improved dynamic imaging (e.g. MR phase-contrast imaging) enabling assessment of CSF pulsations in relation to arterial pulsation and visualization of CSF pulsation in critical areas of interest, e.g. the cerebral aqueduct or at the foramen magnum [45].

Certainly, to date, these measures, too, lack evidence as to the definitive diagnostic and prognostic value, as seen with the battle around the value of the aqueductal stroke volume in normal pressure hydrocephalus [46–48]. But aqueductal stroke volume and its evolution is also an example of encouraging and ongoing research to improve MRI techniques, accuracy, and also ways of quantifying CSF volume and CSF spaces and compartments using MR imaging [49]. An example is the research provided by Alperin et al. on the ICP-MRI [50,51]. Though still a subject of controversy it leaves one with encouragement that future diagnosis of hydrocephalus and CSF disorders will be noninvasive and superior to classical invasive CSF dynamic testing. Besides new ways of quantification it allows assessment of dynamics with anatomical details in various brain and CSF compartments in conjunction with measures of metabolism and anatomical structures, which will eventually give us a more comprehensive understanding as they might reflect both brain biomechanics and biochemistry.

With regard to anatomical detailing of CSF spaces, most exciting are the T2-weighted 3D-volume-based detailed imaging of CSF spaces as obtained by the CISS and FIESTA sequences that are increasingly being used to assess cysts, Chiari, and other types of obstruction of CSF flow in hydrocephalus [52]. They have the potential to change our understanding and classification as well as management of hydrocephalus as they might shed light on the causes of CSF flow disruption or noncommunication in conditions previously thought to be communicating hydrocephalus [53–58]. Also, the better anatomical detail of membranes and webs in association with physiological CSF spaces will eventually change and improve the reasoning behind, approaches to, and techniques of surgical treatment.

The role of multimodal surgical management

Endoscopic approaches to arachnoid cysts and hydrocephalus have dramatically increased in the past 10 years. For example, the indication of third ventriculostomy has expanded and is increasingly used with success in non-classical conditions such as normal pressure hydrocephalus as well as in post-hemorrhagic and/or post-meningitic hydrocephalus and hydrocephalus associated with spina bifida and interhemispheric arachnoid cysts [59,60]. This further challenges our full understanding of where and how CSF dynamics fail in hydrocephalus and associated CSF disorders.

Also, in arachnoid cysts, more endoscopic treatment routes and management is published in locations that were thought to be the domain of microsurgical fenestration, e.g. posterior fossa, cerebellopontine angle and/or supracerebellar cysts and spine [61].

Particularly in pediatric neurosurgery, the "minimally invasive" aspect is promoted, though in most cases and not just the complex ones, the limitations of all the available surgical approaches, e.g. shunting versus endoscopy versus microsurgical techniques, should be appreciated. A more thorough and evidence-based approach to the pros and cons and the efficacy of these measures both as stand-alone and in combination should be considered in collaborations among surgeons who are dealing with complex CSF pathology. Also, information about long-term outcome in various endoscopic approaches is still lacking. Certainly, neuronavigation and modern MR imaging techniques will allow multimodal approaches utilizing microsurgical and neuroendoscopic techniques, but knowledge about disease mechanisms, indications, and timing of treatment and outcome needs standardization in both the adult and pediatric population.

One aspects needs attention, which is the fetal aspect of intervention as recently challenged by the results of the MOMs trial, evidencing improved outcome of Chiari I and hydrocephalus as well as ambulation in the prenatal repair group. The MOMs trial was initiated in February 2003 as a multicenter trial involving the Children's Hospital of Philadelphia (CHOP), University of Vanderbilt, Tennessee, and University of San Francisco, California (UCSF). The trial aimed to assess the benefits of prenatal repair in spina bifida, and the prospective protocol applied very strict criteria on the selection of women and their fetuses diagnosed with spina bifida. One of the selection criteria was that the defect should be below L3. Here, one has to acknowledge the advances made in fetal MRI and its assessment and interpretation. Despite enormous difficulties with recruitment, one of which was the fact that families had to commit to staying in close proximity to the centers from the time that fetal surgery had been performed around week 26, and also mothers had to commit to accepting cesarean section for any future pregnancies, the trial showed clear and stunning benefits for the child and due to the significance of the benefit, the trial was halted prematurely for evidence of success; for example, at 30 months 42% of the children that had undergone prenatal repair were walking independently compared with 21% in the postnatal repair group. Furthermore, 36% in the prenatal group were free of Chiari versus only 4% in the postnatal group and, finally, only 40% of children received a shunt compared to 82% in the postnatal group [62,63]. Soon the results of MOMs II will shed further light on the long-term consequences and effects, e.g. differences in cognitive outcome or prevalence of tethered spinal cord and complications of LOVA with reluctance and potential bias to treat hydrocephalus. Despite some criticism and concerns, mainly with the maternal complications, there are important aspects with the MOMs trial that deserve attention particularly in line with the message of this chapter.

As mentioned above, difficulties with recruitment had led to skepticism that any definite result based on the calculated number of surgeries needed would ever be available anywhere in a reasonable time frame. With multicenter collaboration utilizing a well-designed prospective study protocol backed up with scientific and surgical expertise and endurance based on a multidisciplinary (e.g. prenatal team) program and hospital supports, revolutionary results can be obtained. This has happened even in rare or complex diseases and/or diseases where further advances were not thought likely, but, in the end advances came, to the surprise and excitement of an entire medical community and generation, e.g. the results of the MOMs trial of fetal repair of spina bifida.

The role of disease classification

It is important also to think about new dimensions of classification of hydrocephalus and associated abnormalities of the central nervous system (CNS) at various ages. This is even more important considering the fact that with increased knowledge of molecular science, new treatment modalities for central nervous disorders will become available (e.g. pharmacological CNS applications and stem-cell treatment). A very neat classification of posterior fossa anomalies had been proposed by King et al. in the *Journal of Neurosurgery: Pediatrics* in 2010 [61]. Due to the known uncertainties and the disease spectrum that complicates the clinical and radiological differential diagnosis of congenital posterior fossa anomalies that occur in Dandy–Walker, megacisterna magna, Blake's pouch, and posterior fossa arachnoid cysts with and without hydrocephalus, King et al. subsumed these pathologies based on their anatomical location under the term "giant retrocerebellar cysts." They identified pathological as well as distinct imaging criteria and listed the frequency of those criteria observed in each of the traditional entities, e.g. choroid plexus is absent in Dandy–Walker cyst, while ependymal lining is never seen in arachnoid cyst. While imaging does not discriminate between the anatomy of the posterior fossa and appearance of the occipital bone, all can show normal size to enlarged and thinned occipital bone, and variable mass effect is also present in all entities. Arachnoid cyst and Blake's pouch rarely show other associated CNS malformations with a preserved falx cerebelli, whereas in Dandy–Walker cyst the falx cerebelli is absent but the combination with other CNS malformations is frequent. The differentiation between Blake's pouch and arachnoid cyst on imaging is the mild vermian hypoplasia, which certainly still provides difficulties; however, the proposal from King et al. [61] is a very nice example that should encourage stepping back from traditional entities and providing classification schemes that are based on advanced molecular, pathological, and imaging criteria and on disease and pathology rather than names.

Another important step forward in this direction, though still criticized among researchers, is the recent proposal for a new classification scheme for hydrocephalus that tries to overcome the limitation of thinking in terms of communicating versus noncommunicating hydrocephalus and to clarify that diseasc classification should ultimately be linked to treatment efficacy and patient outcome and cure [17].

Conclusions

The ISHCSF (www.ishcsf.com) was founded in 2006 during an exciting meeting hosted by Carsten Wikkelsö in Gothenburg, Sweden. With HYDROCEPHALUS 2006, Carsten Wikkelsö fathered the concept and initiated a group dedicated to building an international society to provide a platform of exchange between senior and young researchers to assure continuity of education, clinical and basic research in hydrocephalus, CSF disorders and related fields. International and interdisciplinary collaboration should support guidelines, standardized research methods, and funding structures.

Since 2006, successful meetings have followed up on this. In Hanover, Germany, in 2008, the society was inaugurated, and the first "official" meeting of the ISHCSF was hosted in Baltimore, Maryland in 2009. In 2010, a meeting was held in Crete, Greece, in conjunction with the 5th International Hydrocephalus Workshop and the annual meeting of the Hellenic Neurosurgical Society. The society decided to implement the Anthony Marmarou Memorial Lecture, the first of which was held at the meeting, in Copenhagen, Denmark, in 2011.

Also, as an important step forward in this direction, Hydrocephalus 2012, held in Kyoto, Japan, is the first meeting officially combining with the bi-annual meeting of the IHIWG (International Hydrocephalus Imaging Working Group, http://ihiwg.org/).

The IHIWG was founded in 2010 to advance the study of hydrocephalus utilizing a full range of imaging modalities. As such, its members so far include a multi- and transdisciplinary team of neuroradiology, biophysics/engineering, basic science and clinical neurology and neurosurgery. The goal is to get these disciplines with special knowledge in their field to communicate to allow a more rapid evolution of the understanding in diagnosing hydrocephalus, and improve management and understanding of the neurological and pathophysiological sequelae of hydrocephalus across age groups. Meanwhile, this group consists of about 30 members of dedicated scientists. Two successful meetings have already been held, in April 2011 in Great Neck in New York, and a more recent one in association with the Annual Meeting of the American Society of Neuroradiology (ASNR) in April 2012 in Manhattan, NY, hosted by Professor William Bradley, Chairman, Department of Radiology, Professor of Radiology, UCSD School of Medicine, University of California, San Diego, USA. Yet only a few colleagues from neuroradiology usually attend focused meetings on hydrocephalus, and vice versa, hydrocephalus researchers usually do not attend neuroradiological meetings to enable face-to-face interdisciplinary contact and exchange. The main prospectus of the IHIWG meetings is implementation of evidentiary work and later guidelines for noninvasive assessment of hydrocephalus with neuroimaging, and recommendations for how to proceed and conduct clinical research studies in the field of neuroimaging of hydrocephalus.

Acknowledgments

I would like to acknowledge the collaboration with Dr. Jeffrey Rogg and Dr. Jerrold Boxermann, Department of Radiology, Division of Neuroradiology, Rhode Island Hospital and Warren Alpert Medical School of Brown University. Their contribution to imaging these patients and profound knowledge and expertise in understanding CSF diseases provided optimal diagnosis of pathology, and ultimately guided management and surgical approach in the presented patients and in many others. For collaboration in the patients' care I would like to thank Dr. David Mandelbaum, Director of Child Neurology, Hasbro Children's Hospital, Providence.

References

1. Shapiro K, Marmarou A, Shulman K. Abnormal brain biomechanics in the hydrocephalic child. *From: Concepts in Pediatric Neurosurgery*, 1982(2). *Pediatr Neurosurg* 1993;19:216–22; discussion 223.
2. Munch TN, Bech-Azeddine R, Boegeskov L, Gjerris F, Juhler M. Evaluation of the lumbar and ventricular infusion test in the diagnostic strategy of pediatric hydrocephalus and the therapeutic implications. *Childs Nerv Syst* 2007;23:67–71.
3. McCullough DC. A critical evaluation of continuous intracranial pressure monitoring in pediatric hydrocephalus. *Childs Brain* 1980;6:225–41.
4. Canu ED, Magnano I, Paulus KS, et al. Neuropsychophysiological findings in a case of long-standing overt ventriculomegaly (LOVA). *Neurosci Lett* 2005;385:24–9.
5. Oi S, Shimoda M, Shibata M, et al. Pathophysiology of long-standing overt ventriculomegaly in adults. *J Neurosurg* 2000;92:933–40.
6. Oi S, Hidaka M, Honda Y, et al. Neuroendoscopic surgery for specific forms of hydrocephalus. *Childs Nerv Syst* 1999;15:56–68.
7. Baykan N, Isbir O, Gercek A, Dagcnar A, Ozek MM. Ten years of experience with pediatric neuroendoscopic third ventriculostomy: features and perioperative complications of 210 cases. *J Neurosurg Anesthesiol* 2005;17:33–7.
8. Kondziella D, Sonnewald U, Tullberg M, Wikkelsø C. Brain metabolism in adult chronic hydrocephalus. *J Neurochem* 2008;106:1515–24.
9. Klinge PM, Samii A, Muhlendyck A, et al. Cerebral hypoperfusion and delayed hippocampal response after induction of adult kaolin hydrocephalus. *Stroke* 2003;34:193–9.
10. Luciano MG, Skarupa DJ, Booth AM, et al. Cerebrovascular adaptation in chronic hydrocephalus. *J Cereb Blood Flow Metab* 2001;21:285–94.
11. Klinge PM, Brooks DJ, Samii A, et al. Correlates of local cerebral blood flow (CBF) in normal pressure hydrocephalus patients before and after shunting – a retrospective analysis of [(15)O]H(2)O PET-CBF studies in 65 patients. *Clin Neurol Neurosurg* 2008;110:369–75.
12. Klinge P, Ruckert N, Schuhmann M, et al. Neuropsychological sequels to changes in global cerebral blood flow and cerebrovascular reserve capacity after shunt treatment in chronic hydrocephalus – a quantitative PET-study. *Acta Neurochir Suppl* 2002;81:55–7.
13. McAllister JP, 2nd, Chovan P, Steiner CP, et al. Differential ventricular expansion in hydrocephalus. *Eur J Pediatr Surg* 1998;8(Suppl 1):39–42.
14. Rekate HL. Longstanding overt ventriculomegaly in adults: pitfalls in treatment with endoscopic third ventriculostomy. *Neurosurg Focus* 2007;22:E6.
15. Jones HC, Klinge PM. Hydrocephalus 2008, 17–20th September, Hannover Germany: a conference report. *Cerebrospinal Fluid Res* 2008;5:19.
16. Marmarou A, Young HF, Aygok GA, et al. Diagnosis and management of idiopathic normal-pressure hydrocephalus: a prospective study in 151 patients. *J Neurosurg* 2005;102:987–97.
17. Rekate HL, Aygok GA, Kouzelis K, Klinge PM, Pollay M. Fifth International Hydrocephalus Workshop, Crete, Greece, May 20–23, 2010: themes and highlights. *Acta Neurochir Suppl* 2012; 113:1–7.
18. Czosnyka M, Czosnyka Z, Agarwal-Harding KJ, Pickard JD. Modeling of CSF dynamics: legacy of Professor Anthony Marmarou. *Acta Neurochir Suppl* 2012;113:9–14.
19. Marmarou A, Bergsneider M, Klinge P, Relkin N, Black PM. The value of supplemental prognostic tests for the preoperative assessment of idiopathic normal-pressure hydrocephalus. *Neurosurgery* 2005;57:S17–28; discussion ii–v.
20. Bradley WG, Jr., Bahl G, Alksne JF. Idiopathic normal pressure hydrocephalus may be a "two hit" disease: benign external hydrocephalus in infancy followed by deep white matter ischemia in late adulthood. *J Magn Reson Imaging* 2006;24:747–55.
21. Bradley WG, Jr. Idiopathic normal pressure hydrocephalus: new findings and thoughts on etiology. *AJNR Am J Neuroradiol* 2008;29:1–3.
22. Bradley WG, Safar FG, Furtado C, Ord J, Alksne JF. Increased intracranial volume: a clue to the etiology of idiopathic normal-pressure hydrocephalus? *AJNR Am J Neuroradiol* 2004;25:1479–84.

23. Riva D, Usilla A, Saletti V, Esposito S, Bulgheroni S. Can Chiari malformation negatively affect higher mental functioning in developmental age? *Neurol Sci* 2011;32(Suppl 3):S307–09.

24. Martinez-Lage JF, Almagro MJ, Ros de San Pedro J, Ruiz-Espejo A, Felipe-Murcia M. Regression of syringomyelia and tonsillar herniation after posterior fossa arachnoid cyst excision. Case report and literature review. *Neurocirugia (Astur)* 2007;18:227–31.

25. Sekula RF, Jr., Arnone GD, Crocker C, Aziz KM, Alperin N. The pathogenesis of Chiari I malformation and syringomyelia. *Neurol Res* 2011;33:232–9.

26. Apok V, Constantini S, Roth J. Microsurgical fenestration of retrocerebellar cysts as a treatment for syringomyelia. *Childs Nerv Syst* 2012;28:653–6.

27. deSouza RM, Zador Z, Frim DM. Chiari malformation type I: related conditions. *Neurol Res* 2011;33:278–84.

28. Vinck A, Maassen B, Mullaart R, Rotteveel J. Arnold-Chiari-II malformation and cognitive functioning in spina bifida. *J Neurol Neurosurg Psychiatry* 2006;77:1083–6.

29. Al-Jumaily M, Jones B, Hayhurst C, et al. Long term neuropsychological outcome and management of 'decompensated' longstanding overt ventriculomegaly in adults. *Br J Neurosurg* 2012;26:717–1.

30. Relkin N, Marmarou A, Klinge P, Bergsneider M, Black PM. Diagnosing idiopathic normal-pressure hydrocephalus. *Neurosurgery* 2005;57:S4–16; discussion ii–v.

31. Aygok G, Marmarou A, Fatouros P, Young H. Brain tissue water content in patients with idiopathic normal pressure hydrocephalus. *Acta Neurochir Suppl* 2006;96:348–51.

32. Katzen H, Ravdin LD, Assuras S, et al. Postshunt cognitive and functional improvement in idiopathic normal pressure hydrocephalus. *Neurosurgery* 2011;68:416–19.

33. Klinge P, Marmarou A, Bergsneider M, Relkin N, Black PM. Outcome of shunting in idiopathic normal-pressure hydrocephalus and the value of outcome assessment in shunted patients. *Neurosurgery* 2005;57:S40–52; discussion ii–v.

34. Klinge P, Hellström P, Tans J, Wikkelsø C. One-year outcome in the European multicentre study on iNPH. *Acta Neurol Scand* 2012;126:145–53.

35. Hellström P, Edsbagge M, Archer T, et al. The neuropsychology of patients with clinically diagnosed idiopathic normal pressure hydrocephalus. *Neurosurgery* 2007;61:1219–26; discussion 1227–8.

36. Hellström P, Klinge P, Tans J, Wikkelsø C. The neuropsychology of iNPH: findings and evaluation of tests in the European multicentre study. *Clin Neurol Neurosurg* 2012;114:130–4.

37. Hellström P, Klinge P, Tans J, Wikkelsø C. A new scale for assessment of severity and outcome in iNPH. *Acta Neurol Scand* 2012;126:229–37.

38. Jenkinson MD, Campbell S, Hayhurst C, et al. Cognitive and functional outcome in spina bifida-Chiari II malformation. *Childs Nerv Syst* 2011;27:967–74.

39. Miller E, Widjaja E, Blaser S, Dennis M, Raybaud C. The old and the new: supratentorial MR findings in Chiari II malformation. *Childs Nerv Syst* 2008;24:563–75.

40. Pearce M, Oda N, Mansour A, Bhalerao S. Cognitive Disorder NOS with Arnold-Chiari I malformation. *Psychosomatics* 2006;47:88–9.

41. Malm J, Kristensen B, Ekstedt J, Adolfsson R, Wester P. CSF monoamine metabolites, cholinesterases and lactate in the adult hydrocephalus syndrome (normal pressure hydrocephalus) related to CSF hydrodynamic parameters. *J Neurol Neurosurg Psychiatry* 1991;54:252–9.

42. Agren-Wilsson A, Lekman A, Sjöberg W, et al. CSF biomarkers in the evaluation of idiopathic normal pressure hydrocephalus. *Acta Neurol Scand* 2007;116:333–9.

43. Tisell M, Tullberg M, Mansson JE, et al. Differences in cerebrospinal fluid dynamics do not affect the levels of biochemical markers in ventricular CSF from patients with aqueductal stenosis and idiopathic normal pressure hydrocephalus. *Eur J Neurol* 2004;11:17–23.

44. Tullberg M, Blennow K, Mansson JE, et al. Cerebrospinal fluid markers before and after shunting in patients with secondary and idiopathic normal pressure hydrocephalus. *Cerebrospinal Fluid Res* 2008;5:9.

45. Alperin N, Sivaramakrishnan A, Lichtor T. Magnetic resonance imaging-based measurements of cerebrospinal fluid and blood flow as indicators of intracranial compliance in patients with Chiari malformation. *J Neurosurg* 2005;103:46–52.

46. Bradley WG, Jr., Kortman KE, Burgoyne B. Flowing cerebrospinal fluid in normal and hydrocephalic states: appearance on MR images. *Radiology* 1986;159:611–16.

47. Bradley WG, Jr. Magnetic resonance imaging in the central nervous system: comparison with computed tomography. *Magn Reson Annu* 1986:81–122.

48. Bradley WG, Jr. Magnetic resonance imaging in the evaluation of cerebrospinal fluid flow abnormalities. *Magn Reson Q* 1992;8:169–96.

49. Bradley WG, Jr., Scalzo D, Queralt J, et al. Normal-pressure hydrocephalus: evaluation with cerebrospinal fluid flow measurements at MR imaging. *Radiology* 1996;198:523–9.

50. Alperin NJ, Lee SH, Loth F, Raksin PB, Lichtor T. MR-Intracranial pressure (ICP): a method to measure intracranial elastance and pressure noninvasively by means of MR imaging: baboon and human study. *Radiology* 2000;217:877–85.

51. Alperin N, Lee SH, Sivaramakrishnan A, Lichtor T. Relationship between total cerebral blood flow and ICP measured noninvasively with dynamic MRI technique in healthy subjects. *Acta Neurochir Suppl* 2005;95:191–3.

52. Parekh ND, Prabhu SP. Aqueductal web causing obstructive hydrocephalus demonstrated on sagittal FIESTA sequence. *Pediatr Radiol* 2010;40(Suppl 1):S154.

53. Dincer A, Yildiz E, Kohan S, Memet Ozek M. Analysis of endoscopic third ventriculostomy patency by MRI: value of different pulse sequences, the sequence parameters, and the imaging planes for investigation of flow void. *Childs Nerv Syst* 2011;27:127–35.

54. Laitt RD, Mallucci CL, Jaspan T, et al. Constructive interference in steady-state 3D Fourier-transform MRI in the management of hydrocephalus and third ventriculostomy. *Neuroradiology* 1999;41: 117–23.

55. Shi J, Fu W, Wu Q, et al. Endoscopic third ventriculostomy associated 3D-constructive inference steady state MRI for obstructed hydrocephalus: a retrospective study. *Clin Neurol Neurosurg* 2013;115(7):896–901.

56. Dincer A, Kohan S, Ozek MM. Is all "communicating" hydrocephalus really communicating? Prospective study on the value of 3D-constructive interference in steady state sequence at 3T. *Am J Neuroradiol* 2009;30:1898–906.

57. Aydin K, Cokluk C, Gokce E, et al. Use of 3DFT-CISS sequences and virtual MR endoscopy for the neuroendoscopic treatment of unilateral hydrocephalus: case illustration. *Minim Invasive Neurosurg* 2007;50:239–42.

58. Aleman J, Jokura H, Higano S, et al. Value of constructive interference in steady-state three-dimensional, Fourier transformation magnetic resonance imaging for the neuroendoscopic treatment of hydrocephalus and intracranial cysts. *Neurosurgery* 2001;48:1291–5; discussion 1295–6.

59. Warf BC, Campbell JW, Riddle E. Initial experience with combined endoscopic third ventriculostomy and choroid plexus cauterization for post-hemorrhagic hydrocephalus of prematurity: the importance of prepontine cistern status and the predictive value of FIESTA MRI imaging. *Childs Nerv Syst* 2011;27:1063–71.

60. Cinalli G, Peretta P, Spennato P, et al. Neuroendoscopic management of interhemispheric cysts in children. *J Neurosurg* 2006;105:194–202.

61. King JA, Auguste KI, Halliday W, Drake JM, Kulkarni AV. Ventriculocystostomy and endoscopic third ventriculostomy/shunt placement in the management of hydrocephalus secondary to giant retrocerebellar cysts in infancy. *J Neurosurg Pediatr* 2010;5:403–7.

62. Adzick NS, Thom EA, Spong CY, et al. A randomized trial of prenatal versus postnatal repair of myelomeningocele. *N Engl J Med* 2011;364:993–1004.

63. Williams H. Questioning the rationale and conduct of the management of myelomeningocele study. *Med Hypotheses* 2011;77:101–5.

Chapter 25

Chiari malformation and hydrocephalus in adults

Aristotelis S. Filippidis and Harold L. Rekate

Introduction

Chiari malformation is a pathologic entity first described at the end of the nineteenth century by Hans Chiari [1], who was studying the pathology of babies dying with hydrocephalus. He described four different types (Chiari I–IV), with some authors also using an intermediate type Chiari 1.5 between Chiari I and Chiari II [2]. The Chiari malformation has an unfortunate name that often leads to confusion and controversy. The utilization of the term "malformation" usually refers to a pathologic entity with a single definable cause, which begins expression before birth, and leads to predictable effects on the clinical presentation of the patients and the pathology of the patient's brain. The development of magnetic resonance imaging (MRI) has led to an improved understanding of cerebellar herniation. The original studies of Hans Chiari dealt with four types of cerebellar malformation in these autopsy studies. These four types represent completely different pathologies. The Chiari III malformation (occipito-cervical encephalocele) and Chiari IV malformation (cerebellar agenesis) are extremely rare and are unlikely to be seen in the adult population. On the other hand, Chiari I (chronic tonsilar herniation, which has been called the "adult Chiari malformation") and Chiari II (essentially always associated with spina bifida) are now frequently cared for in adult settings and are the subject of this review.

What is the Chiari I malformation?

Chiari I or adult Chiari malformation is an unfortunate term as it presupposes that it is a single entity with a single cause and that it is developmental, beginning before the skull and brain are formed. Neither of these conditions is correct in a large percentage of cases. The use of terms such as hindbrain hernia or Chiari anomaly [3,4] are more appropriate but the use of the term Chiari malformation is so engrained in the parlance of neurosurgery and the literature that it is something we have to live with. Those who study and care for patients with hindbrain herniation should develop a consensus on the definition and classification of the problem to assure that we are all speaking about the same entity. In general, Chiari I malformation is a crowding of the posterior fossa with tissue primarily derived from the inferior-most part of the cerebellar hemispheres, generally called the cerebellar tonsils. The patients share an absence of the cisterna magna and by neuroradiological convention the tips of the inferior cerebellar hemispheres project below the foramen magnum by at least 5 mm.

Hindbrain herniation may occur from any of four pathogenetic mechanisms. These mechanisms are based on the physical principles of the Monro–Kellie hypothesis and are:

(1) The skull, particularly in the posterior fossa, is too small to accommodate the brain contents, which causes the herniation through the foramen magnum. Since the squamous portion of the occipital bone is made of "membranous bone" this development must occur quite early in development. This mechanism is most convincingly expressed in the case of Crouzon's and Pfeiffer's syndromes and is most dramatic in patients with Kleebaatschädl (cloverleaf skull).

(2) There is a pressure differential across the foramen magnum caused by increased pressure intracranially. This can be due to a mass within the skull or to too much fluid intracranially. In hydrocephalus this is increased cerebrospinal fluid (CSF) within the ventricles. In pseudotumor cerebri it is a combination of too much CSF in the cortical subarachnoid space and too much venous

Adult Hydrocephalus, ed. Daniele Rigamonti. Published by Cambridge University Press.

blood in the substance of the brain and in the dural venous sinuses.

(3) There is a pressure gradient across the foramen magnum due to low pressure in the spinal subarachnoid space. This can be due to spontaneous intracranial hypotension such as from a leaking perineural cyst or from overdrainage of a non-valved lumboperitoneal shunt.

(4) Finally, there is traction on the distal end of the spinal cord from severe tethering due to lipoma, thickened filum terminale, or myelomeningocele that had been previously repaired.

Hydrocephalus and Chiari I: which came first?

Based on the new consensus classification of hydrocephalus, hindbrain herniation can cause hydrocephalus in two ways. It can either block the outlet foramina of the fourth ventricle if both the foramen of Magendie and the foramina of Luschka are occluded. This would lead to severe dilatation of the fourth ventricle and would be clearly shown to be an obstructive cause of hydrocephalus using the classic classification of Dandy that a dye placed into the lateral ventricle would not be able to be recovered from the spinal subarachnoid space. The second possibility would be that the CSF that did exit the foramina into the spinal subarachnoid space would be prevented from flowing from the spinal subarachnoid space into the cortical subarachnoid space, which Dandy would classify as communicating even though there is a very clear point of obstruction.

Both of these processes are quite rare, particularly in adults. Because there is a failure of communication between the lateral ventricles and the cortical subarachnoid spaces, both of these mechanisms should respond to endoscopic third ventriculostomy (ETV).

By its very nature, hydrocephalus adds volume to an already closed intracranial skull volume and therefore may be the cause of the hydrocephalus itself. In infants it is often very difficult to discern which of the conditions is the cause and which is the result. In cases in which the question is unanswered or unanswerable performing a Chiari decompression could lead to a refractory pseudomeningocele. If one plans to do a Chiari I decompression and the patient has hydrocephalus that seems well compensated, we strongly recommend postoperative intracranial pressure monitoring for early diagnosis of decompensation of the compensated hydrocephalus. If the patient exhibits signs of increased intracranial pressure it is wise to treat the hydrocephalus first either with a shunt or with an ETV.

Hydrocephalus and the Chiari II malformation

The Chiari II malformation is a complex developmental disorder associated exclusively with open neural tube defects, most commonly spina bifida aperta but also found with encephaloceles. As demonstrated by the work of McLone [5–7], it is due to the constant leaking of CSF from the intracranial compartment via the open defect causing distortion of brain development and, at least transiently, a state of microcephaly during intrauterine development. Figure 25.1b is an artist's representation of the major findings in Chiari II malformation including a small posterior fossa, vertical and incompetent tentorium, tectal beaking, and herniation of the brainstem and cerebellar vermis into the cervical canal. This deranged anatomy causes hydrocephalus in four different ways and the patient may have any one of the specific points of obstruction or may have two, three, or all four. In the mildest forms of the condition, the manifestations of the Chiari II malformation may be so mild as to be difficult to detect. The clinical presentation and to some extent the treatment options differ depending on the point of obstruction. The specific types of hydrocephalus that depend on a specific point of obstruction are described below. They include:

(1) Closure of the aqueduct of Sylvius secondary to upward herniation of the top of the cerebellar vermis. These patients are generally found in utero by ultrasound to have severe ventriculomegaly that progresses fairly rapidly in the last trimester. Delivery here when recognized is always by cesarean section due to cephalopelvic disproportion. These babies should be delivered before the thickness of the brain at the foramen of Monro (cerebral mantle) falls below one centimeter, which may be a point of no-return implying that the brain cannot reconstitute after shunting and the babies would have severe developmental delays that could have been avoided by early intervention. At the time of shunt failure these children always will be symptomatic and show increase in ventricular size if they have ever gotten smaller.

(a)

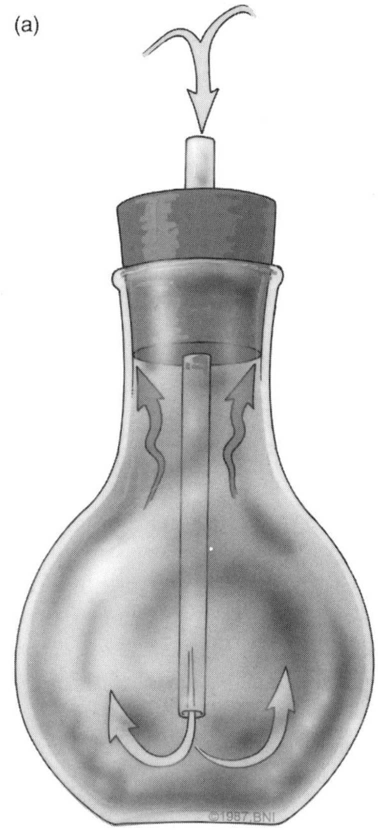

(b)

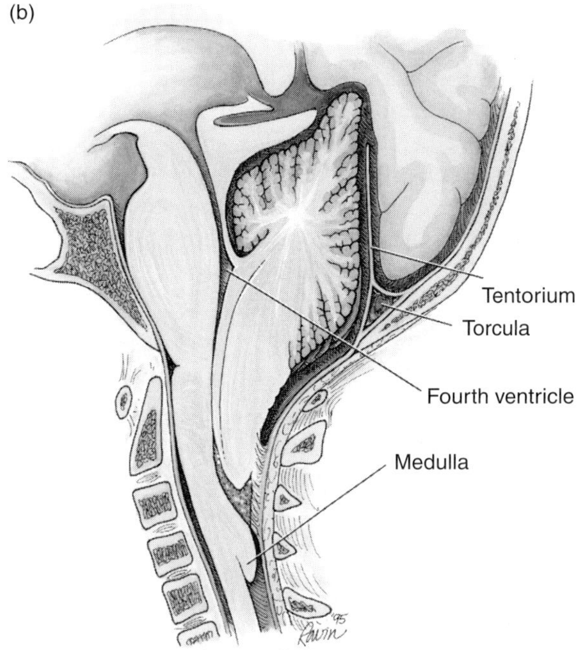

© 1998, BNI

Figure 25.1 (a) Stopper in the bottle analogy for hindbrain herniation. (b) Artist's rendition of a sagittal view of Chiari II malformation showing the overall anatomy of the posterior fossa and upper cervical spine. The four potential points of obstruction causing hydrocephalus are demonstrated as the secondary closure of the aqueduct of Sylvius, closure of the outlet foramina of the fourth ventricle, impaction of the brainstem causing poor flow from the spinal subarachnoid space and the cortical subarachnoid space, and compression of the torcula causing high venous pressure in the dural venous sinuses.

(2) Occlusion of the outlet foramina of the fourth ventricle due to the herniation of the entire fourth ventricle into the cervical spine. In this case the entire brainstem is distorted, but because the anatomy of the fourth ventricle is determined by the narrow space in which it is confined it may not be appear to be distended. These patients will frequently present with overt brainstem dysfunction at the time of shunt failure. They will be found to have a fourth ventricle that is elongated into the cervical spine, which it may not be possible to visualize on MRI when the shunt is working.

(3) The "stopper in the bottle" phenomenon. If the CSF can exit through the outlet foramina of the fourth ventricle, that fluid can mix with the remainder of the CSF in the cortical subarachnoid space but cannot get back into the intracranial compartment to access the dural venous sinuses in order to be terminally absorbed. This type of hydrocephalus typically is present early in postnatal life and progresses slowly if at all. It may be observed without shunting for a few months to make certain that the hydrocephalus has become compensated and the patient does not need a shunt. That this compensation can occur can usually be ascertained within the first half year of life [8].

(4) The final point of obstruction relates to the position of the torcula within the cervical spine seen in a significant number of patients with spina bifida. This is due to the small volume of the posterior fossa and the vertical position of the tentorium. Hydrocephalus develops somewhat

slowly in these cases and it is due to the fact that the head is still distensible and the absorption of CSF requires a pressure differential of at least 5–7 mmHg in order for CSF to be absorbed. Once a shunt is inserted the ventricles decrease in size and the skull becomes a fixed volume. When the shunt fails in such circumstances the skull cannot distend and therefore the ventricles do not enlarge. The patient now exhibits a severe form of the "slit ventricle syndrome" (SVS). This is seen in about 25% of patients with spina bifida shunted in infancy. Management here is quite difficult. One of the authors has treated such a patient in whom intracranial pressure (ICP) was measured to be over 80 mmHg with no evidence of ventricular distension [9].

Shunt dependency in this population is a severe burden. The published mortality for shunt-dependent spina bifida patients has been reported to be 1%/year into adulthood. Shunt infection in this population if it occurs within the first 6 months of life tends to result in a 25 point drop in predicted IQ.

The recent publication of the results of the "Management of Myelomeningocle Study" has led to new forms of treatment and exciting new potential for more normal lives for the affected individuals [10]. The data are quite convincing that if the neural tube defect is repaired in the 24th to 26th week of gestational life and the baby can be carried to term or near term, the radiographic appearance of the Chiari II malformation is much improved and the incidence of hydrocephalus that needs to be shunted falls to a minority of patients.

The Chiari I malformation and benign intracranial hypertension or pseudotumor cerebri

About 10% of patients seen at the Chiari Institute will be found to have pseudotumor cerebri. Sometimes this diagnosis is made prior to intervention when papilledema is found on fundoscopic examination. Usually, however, it is found when the patient develops recurrent pseudomeningocele postoperatively. Lumbar puncture or formal ICP monitoring shows them to have raised ICP.

The most likely situation in which Chiari I malformation and pseudotumor will coexist occurs in the context of morbid obesity. Morbid obesity results in increased intracranial pressure, especially in women due to the effect on the pressure in the right atrium. Acetazolamide in this situation acts as a diuretic and lowers intracranial pressure. High right atrial pressures also lead to high sagittal sinus pressures, an increase in the venous volume of the brain and therefore the total volume of the brain and in some cases may actually be the cause of the Chiari I malformation. Operating on the craniovertebral junction in morbidly obese patients is both difficult and dangerous. Bariatric surgery carries the highest likelihood of a good outcome in patients with Chiari who are morbidly obese and has been shown to be effective treatment of the increased ICP [11,12]. We strongly recommend bariatric surgery for all patients with pseudotumor, with or without Chiari I malformation, who have a body mass index of 35 or greater.

In non-obese patients pseudotumor is often overdiagnosed and while shunting may help to treat a pesky pseudomeningocele every effort should be made to get rid of the shunt as soon as possible. Often after the pseudomeningocele is healed it is possible to remove the shunt and place an external ventricular drain and record the ICP. This frequently shows that the CSF absorptive deficit either no longer exists or was not there in the first place.

In thin patients who have documented pseudotumor and a Chiari I malformation the management requires some thought. Treatment with ventriculoperitoneal shunts often leads to recurrent failure of the ventricular catheter. The absorptive deficit is in the cortical subarachnoid space and it is difficult for the CSF to flow retrograde from the cortical subarachnoid space to the ventricle to get out of the intracranial compartment via the shunt. The ventricle will frequently collapse around the catheter. There are three potential strategies that have been shown to be effective in this situation:

(1) Decompression surgery showing a reconstituted cisterna magna will allow the management of this condition with a lumboperitoneal shunt with good success.
(2) If a ventricular shunt is felt to be needed it is likely that a second catheter in the cervical subarachnoid will be needed to balance the pressure on the inside and outside of the brain and make certain that the ventricle does not collapse around the ventricular catheter.
(3) Finally, all pseudotumor is thought to be due to increased pressure in the superior sagittal sinus. If a point of restriction to flow is found, recent

studies have shown the usefulness of venous stenting in the treatment of pseudotumor without shunting [11,13,14].

Conclusion

Chiari malformation in adults is a complex disease entity with different types of pathophysiological mechanisms involved. The first and most important issue that the neurosurgeon has to face is the definition of this malformation, which meets distinct radiological, clinical, pathologico-anatomical, and physiological characteristics. All the study and treatment groups involved, from pathologists to radiologists and neurosurgeons, need to develop a common language, a consensus that fully describes this syndrome, underlines its pathophysiology, and suggests the best treatment in relation to its different types. The sure assumption is that currently there is no single best treatment not only because the Chiari malformation is complex but because it often presents with accompanying diseases such as hydrocephalus, or benign intracranial hypertension or pseudotumor cerebri. Neurosurgeons have to "dissect" each individual case in order to decide on the best approach that targets the presentation of the malformation holistically to treat the disease rather than the radiology.

References

1. Chiari H. Uber Veränderungen des Kleinhirns infolge von Hydrocephalie des Grosshirns. *Dtsch Med Wochenschr* 1891;17:1172–5.
2. Tubbs R, Hankinson T, Wellons III J. The Chiari malformations and syringomyelia. In: Ellenbogen R, Abdulrauf S, Sekhar L (Eds.) *Principles of Neurological Surgery*, 3rd edn. Philadelphia: Elsevier Saunders; 2012.
3. Di Rocco C, Velardi F. Acquired Chiari type I malformation managed by supratentorial cranial enlargement. *Childs Nerv Syst* 2003;19(12):800–7.
4. Di Rocco C, Frassanito P, Massimi L, Peraio S. Hydrocephalus and Chiari type I malformation. *Childs Nerv Syst* 2011;27(10):1653–64.
5. McLone DG, Knepper PA. The cause of Chiari II malformation: a unified theory. *Pediatr Neurosci* 1989;15(1):1–12.
6. McLone DG, Naidich TP. Developmental morphology of the subarachnoid space, brain vasculature, and contiguous structures, and the cause of the Chiari II malformation. *AJNR Am J Neuroradiol* 1992;13(2):463–82.
7. McLone DG, Dias MS. The Chiari II malformation: cause and impact. *Childs Nerv Syst* 2003;19(7–8):540–50.
8. Rekate HL. To shunt or not to shunt: hydrocephalus and dysraphism. *Clin Neurosurg* 1985;32:593–607.
9. Rekate HL, Nadkarni T, Wallace D. Severe intracranial hypertension in slit ventricle syndrome managed using a cisterna magna-ventricle-peritoneum shunt. *J Neurosurg* 2006;104(4 Suppl):240–4.
10. Adzick NS, Thom EA, Spong CY, et al. A randomized trial of prenatal versus postnatal repair of myelomeningocele. *N Engl J Med* 2011;364(11):993–1004.
11. Karahalios DG, Rekate HL, Khayata MH, Apostolides PJ. Elevated intracranial venous pressure as a universal mechanism in pseudotumor cerebri of varying etiologies. *Neurology* 1996;46(1):198–202.
12. Nadkarni T, Rekate HL, Wallace D. Resolution of pseudotumor cerebri after bariatric surgery for related obesity. Case report. *J Neurosurg* 2004;101(5):878–80.
13. Owler BK, Parker G, Halmagyi GM, et al. Pseudotumor cerebri syndrome: venous sinus obstruction and its treatment with stent placement. *J Neurosurg* 2003;98(5):1045–55.
14. Albuquerque FC, Dashti SR, Hu YC, et al. Intracranial venous sinus stenting for benign intracranial hypertension: clinical indications, technique, and preliminary results. *World Neurosurg* 2011;75(5–6):648–52; discussion 592–5.

Chapter 26

Pseudotumor cerebri syndrome

John D. Pickard and Nicholas Higgins

Pseudotumor cerebri syndrome (PTCS) and normal pressure hydrocephalus (NPH) share malabsorption of cerebrospinal fluid (CSF) as part of their respective mechanisms but their clinical pictures are very different. In general, PTCS is a disease of young people that presents as an almost pure form of raised intracranial pressure (ICP) without focal neurological disturbance and without evidence on investigation of structural abnormality. NPH is a disease of the elderly and ICP is not raised. The cortical subarachnoid space is obliterated in NPH (cortical block and ventricular reflux on isotope cisternography and air encephalography) but patent in PTCS. It is likely that the block to CSF absorption in PTCS is at the level of the arachnoid granulations.

History

The first descriptions of PTCS depended upon the development of the ophthalmoscope by Von Helmholtz in 1851 and the technique of lumbar puncture by Quincke in 1891. Although there had been descriptions of PTCS-like cases in the period 1866–1896 [1] such as "recoverable optic neuritis in young women suffering from uterine derangement" in the 1880s, it was Quincke who in 1897 defined cases of "serous meningitis" and Nonne who coined the term "pseudotumor cerebri" in 1904. The association of PTCS with middle ear disease followed in the period 1905–1936. Then came the introduction both of neuroradiology (angiography, ventriculography, and lumbar air encephalography) and of therapies such as steroids, acetazolamide, and antibiotics for otitis media and subtemporal decompression.

Nomenclature

There has been much debate about nomenclature that has led to some unthinking tautology amongst journal editors and referees. The term in vogue at present is idiopathic intracranial hypertension ("I"IH). Strictly speaking, IIH should only include cases where there is no known cause. This begs the question of how to label cases where there is a known cause – "secondary IIH" is really silly. The term IIH is too exclusive and has led to denial by some journals of the importance of venous changes: to quote one editor, "it cannot be IIH because you have found contributory factors." Many cases labeled as idiopathic have simply not been fully investigated so that case series of IIH will almost certainly include secondary causes.

The term benign intracranial hypertension (BIH) reflects the absence of sinister intracranial pathology. However, many patients deeply resent the term – their lives are often a misery even though their vision has been preserved.

Pseudotumor cerebri is long established (Nonne 1904, 1914) and is inclusive of patients with similar symptoms and signs requiring similar treatments. It highlights the exclusion of an intracranial mass and makes no assumptions about etiology or mechanism. The addition by Ian Johnston of "syndrome" to PTC (= PTCS) is very helpful and is analogous to the distinction between Cushing's disease and Cushing's syndrome [1].

Dandy criteria (modified)

The diagnostic criteria for PTCS were eponymously ascribed to Walter Dandy [2] following his detailed description of the clinical features of 22 cases in 1937, and they have subsequently been modified in the light of new knowledge:

(1) Symptoms and signs of raised intracranial pressure in a conscious patient.
(2) Measured increase in CSF pressure.

(3) Absence of focal neurological signs (except sixth cranial nerve).
(4) CSF of normal composition.
(5) Normal imaging studies (including magnetic resonance venography [MRV]) apart from possible small ventricles
    - an empty sella is allowed (see below).
(6) Not attributable to another cause.
(7) Benign clinical course except for effects on vision.

Clinical features

The headache of PTCS has no distinguishing characteristics [3] unlike the headache of raised ICP due to a brain tumor (early morning headache made worse by bending down, etc.). PTCS headache may mimic migraine without aura, chronic daily headache, and tension headache. To complicate matters, many patients may have additional headache secondary to overuse of analgesics. It is instructive to assess which components of the headache are helped by CSF withdrawal at lumbar puncture. Many patients whose visual problems have been resolved by treatment still have various forms of headache. A minority of patients learn that hyperventilation helps their headache and may present with carpopedal spasm. Headache often occurs without papilledema and vice versa.

Visual symptoms [4] occur in over half of PTCS patients and include blurring and obscurations of vision and lateral diplopia. Nausea and vomiting is common (20% of cases). Patients may present with tinnitus which is often pulsatile in character [5]. Pressure on the ipsilateral internal jugular vein may stop the tinnitus, probably because it raises the pressure within the transverse sinus and expands the area of reversible stenosis. CSF withdrawal may also reverse such tinnitus. Other ear symptoms may occur and may be attributable to raised pressure being transmitted to the inner ear through the cochlear aqueduct. A minority of patients may complain of root symptoms in the arms and legs, presumably due to dilatation of the root sleeves – CSF drainage may ameliorate such root symptoms.

CSF rhinorrhea may occur either spontaneously through an empty sella or via dehiscence of the tegmen tympani or superior semicircular canal. CSF leaks after trans-sphenoidal pituitary surgery or foramen magnum decompression for Chiari malformations may prove refractory to reoperation until the presence of PTCS is recognized and CSF pressure lowered.

PTCS certainly occurs in men where it is usually not associated with obesity. Men are more likely to lose vision early: “beware the thin man with PTCS.”

PTCS in childhood is uncommon [6] and may be overdiagnosed unless congenital abnormalities of the optic disk (e.g. drusen) are excluded and CSF pressure accurately measured under calm conditions. Children are often not overweight. Where obesity is not an issue, children must be protected against becoming anorexic.

Signs

Visual abnormalities are present in the majority of patients including papilledema, visual field changes, reduction in visual acuity, and diplopia. An expert neuro-ophthalmology review is mandatory not only to confirm the diagnosis but also to exclude congenital abnormalities and provide an objective baseline as the basis for subsequent assessment of progress.

A general physical and neurological examination is performed to identify any associated conditions, whose treatment might help to reverse the PTCS.

Associated conditions

There are many conditions that have been associated with PTCS. However, few studies of such associations pass the fundamental criterion of causality, namely that withdrawal of the condition results in reversal of PTCS; reintroduction causes recurrence of PTCS.

- Female-specific factors: obesity, pregnancy, exogenous estrogens, polycystic ovary.
- Pregnancy may precipitate or ameliorate PTCS.
- Obstructive sleep apnea.
- Familial – some families include members with both PTCS and hydrocephalus.
- Cranial venous outflow: congenital, compression/obstruction (extracranial and intracranial).
- Hematological abnormality: hypercoagulation, iron deficiency anemia, myeloma, leukemia, polycythemia, etc.
- Endocrine disorders: thyroid, Cushing’s, parathyroid, acromegaly, growth hormone replacement, miscellaneous.
- Infections: middle ear, chronic meningitis, etc.
- Head injury including fractures over the major venous sinuses.
- Systemic lupus erythematosus, Behçet’s, Pickwickian syndrome, etc.

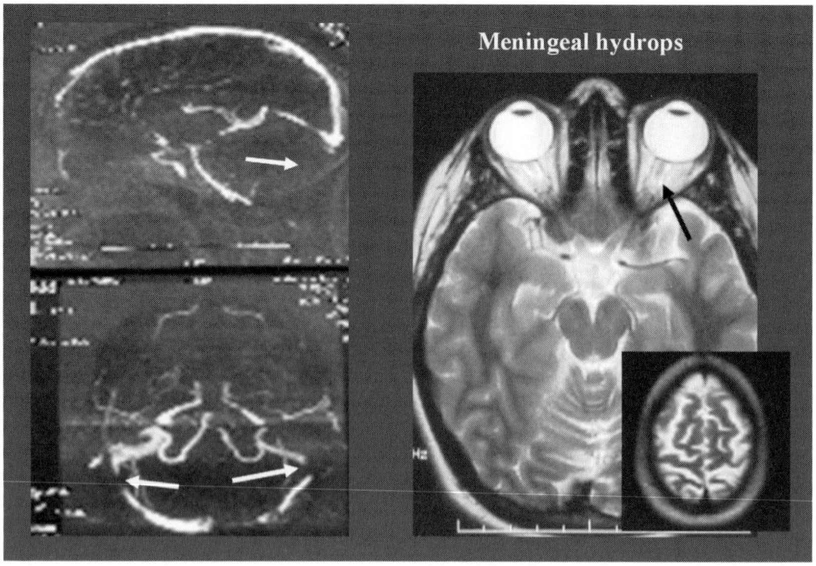

Figure 26.1 MR scan showing the features of PTCS.

- Drugs and chemicals: vitamin A, steroids (administration and withdrawal), tetracycline, nalidixic acid, etc.
- Nutritional disorders: rickets, malnutrition.
- Space flight.

Investigations

Neuroradiology

Computed tomography (CT) scanning will exclude a mass lesion and hydrocephalus but will not detect the subtle features of PTCS that a magnetic resonance (MR) scan will display. These include dilatation of the optic nerve sheaths (Figure 26.1, black arrow) with flattening of the posterior part of the globe of the eye, dilatation of the cortical sulci (meningeal hydrops), empty sella, and narrowing of the transverse sinuses (Figure 26.1, white arrows). The MRV changes have often been dismissed as normal variants but a careful controlled study with headache-free control subjects demonstrated that the venous changes should not be dismissed as MR flow artifacts [7].

Lumbar puncture

CSF pressure measurement should be performed by an experienced operator, preferably under X-ray control and with electronic recording of the pressure for 20 minutes or more. Children may require sedation or a general anesthetic – hyperventilation will reduce CSF pressure through lowering of arterial carbon dioxide levels. Traumatic lumbar punctures and use of a simple manometer may underestimate the true CSF pressure.

There has been much debate about what should be the threshold for raised CSF pressure, particularly in the presence of morbid obesity and obstructive sleep apnea. It is essential to appreciate that CSF pressure can fluctuate considerably. In various series, single measurements at lumbar puncture have demonstrated pressures of 10–20 mmHg in a minority of patients with all the other features of PTCS – subsequent continuous monitoring has revealed pressures of >20 mmHg. It is therefore misleading to insist on, say, a pressure of over 25 cmH_2O (18 mmHg) in adults and 28 cmH_2O (20 mmHg) in children before making the diagnosis. If there is doubt, continuous monitoring is required [8,9]. The presence of waves of pressure on electronic recordings are also valuable indicators of raised CSF pressure. There are a small number of patients (~2%) who have symptoms and signs of PTCS at CSF pressures of less than 10 mmHg. Where a Chiari malformation is present, ICP monitoring may be required to confirm the diagnosis although characteristic narrowing of the transverse sinuses on CT venography is indicative of raised pressure.

CT venography (CTV) is superior to MRV in defining any changes in the venous sinuses. Partial reversal of the narrowing of the transverse sinuses and other intracranial venous sinuses by CSF withdrawal may be documented by CTV (Figure 26.2).

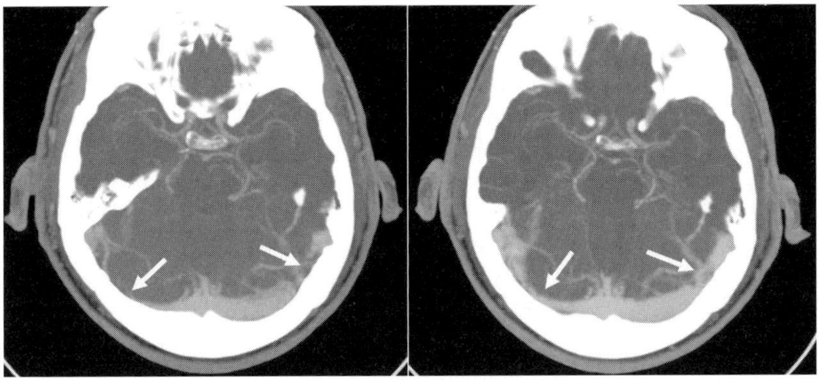

Figure 26.2 CT venogram in a case of PTCS with compressible veins: the narrowing of the transverse sinuses is immediately improved by CSF withdrawal by lumbar puncture.

Angiography with retrograde venography may be indicated not only to exclude a dural fistula but also to quantify the importance of venous sinus narrowing.

CSF composition

CSF in PTCS has a normal level of protein and glucose. There is a trend to protein levels that are slightly lower than normal. There may prove to be changes in specific peptides but such refined measurements are still at the research stage [10].

Pathophysiology

The absorption of CSF is a passive phenomenon and described by Davson's equation [11]:

$$P_{csf} - P_{sss} = I_f \times R_{out}$$

where P_{csf} is the CSF pressure, P_{sss} is the pressure in the superior sagittal sinus, I_f is the CSF formation rate, and R_{out} is the CSF outflow resistance.

It has been assumed that, in adults, P_{sss} remains constant in the face of increasing CSF pressure. As will be shown later, this assumption may not be valid in PTCS patients.

A number of mechanisms have been proposed as the basis for PTCS. More than one mechanism may of course be operating.

(1) Excess CSF production. This is unlikely as the sole mechanism: the only cases of raised ICP due to excess CSF production are choroid plexus villous hypertrophy and choroid plexus papilloma where there are gross increases in size of the choroid plexus which is seen in PTCS. A doubling of CSF production rate by itself would only increase ICP by 3 mmHg, according to Davson's equation.

(2) Cerebral edema. Early studies with brain biopsies were complicated by methodological artifact. Modern diffusion-weighted MR scanning [12] has confirmed that there is no evidence for cytotoxic or vasogenic cerebral edema in PTCS. This was always unlikely given the depth of the subarachnoid space in PTCS at operation and on isotope cisternography and MR.

(3) Abnormal CSF absorption. There is considerable experimental and clinical evidence for impairment of CSF absorption in PTCS but recent findings with measurement of superior sagittal sinus pressure in PTCS have complicated the interpretation of CSF infusion studies (see below) [13]. It appears that CSF absorption via the arachnoid granulations in the intracranial venous sinuses may be inadequate but that spinal arachnoid granulations and other routes of absorption may then be recruited but only at higher baseline pressures [14]. Interestingly, phase-contrast MR has demonstrated increased CSF movement through the foramen magnum in PTCS [15].

(4) Cerebral venous narrowing. The venous sinuses adjacent to infected ears were always thought to be the link to raised ICP in otitic hydrocephalus. Pierre Janny et al. demonstrated narrowing in the superior sagittal sinus of patients with PTCS using direct pressure measurements through a burr hole [16]. The advent of MR scanning with MRV misled the subject – MRV changes were often dismissed as MR flow artifacts. Very careful methodological studies using headache-free control subjects then confirmed that these venous changes on MRV in PTCS were not artifacts [9].

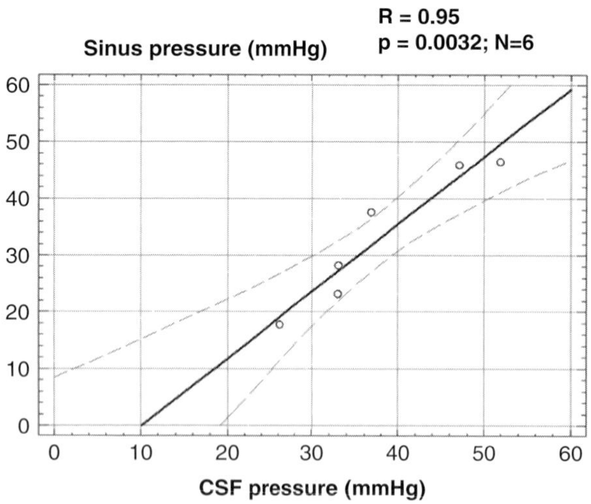

Figure 26.3 Results from a study of six patients in which pressure in the superior sagittal sinus was measured simultaneously with CSF pressure during retrograde venography. Pressure in the superior sagittal sinus changed pari passu with CSF pressure.

The introduction of retrograde cerebral venography [17,18] then demonstrated that there was often a significant pressure gradient across transverse sinus narrowings. Venous stenting of such narrowing has helped resolve the papilledema in many patients (see below [19,20]) but the issue now is the distinction between fixed stenoses and stenoses that reverse at least in part with reduction in CSF pressure at lumbar puncture. It is now clear that sagittal sinus pressure in typical PTCS (obese young females) is not independent of CSF pressure [13]. In a study of six patients in which P_{sss} was measured simultaneously with CSF pressure during retrograde venography, P_{sss} changed pari passu with P_{csf} (Figure 26.3).

One of the many phenomena surrounding PTCS that remains unexplained is why lumbar puncture provides symptomatic relief often for weeks or months despite the fact that CSF is turned over three times each day. It has been suggested that collapsible venous sinuses may introduce a positive feedback loop into the usual linkage between CSF pressure and drainage. If the narrowing of the venous sinuses is relieved by CSF drainage, the sinuses may remain fully open until a critical CSF pressure is again reached but that may take weeks or months.

(5) Steroid metabolism, inflammation, hypercoagulopathy, and obesity. The venous story alone cannot explain why CSF pressure initially increases, or the relationship to obesity. Intriguing possibilities are emerging that link obesity to altered steroid metabolism and inflammation. For example, obesity may be linked to abnormalities of 11β-hydroxysteroid dehydrogenase type 1, which is present in both the choroid plexus and endothelial cap of arachnoid granulations. Sinclair et al. [20] have suggested that there may be dual effects on the choroid plexus with an increase in CSF production coupled with impaired absorption through the arachnoid granulations. Experimentally, administration of steroids and then withdrawal increases CSF outflow resistance. Hypercoagulability and connective tissue disorders may alter the properties of the endothelial cap of the arachnoid granulations.

Management

It is essential that patients with PTCS are managed in a multidisciplinary team setting with clearly defined care pathways.

Medical interventions

- If a causative agent can be identified, then clearly it should be withdrawn or treated. Effective weight reduction through dieting has been confirmed in a randomized controlled trial to improve vision and reduce the severity of headaches [21]. Unfortunately, many patients cannot maintain their diets long term.
- Drugs. A randomized controlled trial (RCT) has confirmed that acetazolamide will help patients with the less severe forms of PTCS but many cannot tolerate the side effects [22]. Regular blood chemistry measurements should be made. Topiramate has the advantage of a modest carbonic anhydrase blocking effect plus appetite suppression. Again, it has to be used with care because of potential side effects and some patients just feel awful on it. Conventional diuretics are little used. Glucocorticoids are now restricted to cases where there is very rapid visual deterioration in combination with an urgent CSF drainage procedure. Octreotide [23] has been used in a few cases but great care has to be used in supervising its administration in the light of experience with its use in acromegaly – it is not simple to use.

- Repeated lumbar punctures. Neurosurgeons are often referred patients who have been psychologically traumatized by multiple lumbar punctures, often poorly performed. Apart from the often increasing difficulty of performing such punctures, there is a risk of inducing arachnoiditis. The poor quality of life of patients managed by prolonged use of ineffectual drugs and multiple lumbar punctures should not be underestimated.

Surgical interventions

- Subtemporal decompression was the first procedure to be used prior to the introduction of shunts. It has to be performed with care to avoid the risk of temporal lobe epilepsy. It should not be offered if a prior foramen magnum decompression has been performed for fear of precipitating brain slump in its various manifestations including further tonsillar herniation, syrinx formation, and midbrain distortion.
- CSF diversion is not straightforward [24–26]. The ventricles are small or normal in size so that image-guided placement of the ventricular catheter is required. There is a tendency for ventricular catheters to intermittently block, possibly because of intermittent exacerbations of the underlying condition. Placement of the peritoneal catheter into a grossly obese abdomen is not easy and either migration of the catheter or variable absorption of CSF may occur.
    - Lumboperitoneal shunts are often followed by problems with kinking and overdrainage with secondary descent of the tonsils unless a valve with antisiphon properties is used.
    - Personally, I (JDP) currently use a lumbopleural shunt that incorporates an adjustable valve and siphon control device. This approach has the advantage of connecting two large spaces with the added advantage of negative pleural pressures with each breath to hopefully keep the shunt patent. A minority of patients develop a refractory pleural effusion and a careful watch has to be kept for secondary Chiari formation.
- Optic nerve sheath fenestration. This technique continues to be used in expert hands [27]. Many ophthalmic surgeons have stopped using it because they have experienced complications and it cannot be expected to resolve headaches. Complications that have been described include ocular motility problems, optic nerve hematoma, optic disk infarcts, central and branch retinal artery occlusion, sudden postoperative blindness, dacryocystitis, and fibrosis [1].
- Bariatric surgery has been used for morbid obesity, particularly where vision is not under immediate threat [28]. An RCT is at the planning stage in the UK.
- Venous stenting was the logical development of the common finding of transverse sinus stenoses. The first case report was published in

Table 26.1 Current published experience of stenting for PTCS

Higgins et al. 2003 (Cambridge) [29]	12 patients: 5 asymptomatic, 2 improved and 5 unchanged
Owler et al. 2003 (Sydney) [31]	4 patients: headaches improved in all; vision improved in 3
Case reports: Ogungbo et al. 2003 (Newcastle) [32]; Rajpal et al. 2005 (Wisconsin) [33]; Paquet et al. 2008 (Poitiers) [34]	All improved
Donnet et al. 2008 (Marseille) [35]	10 patients: papilledema resolved in all; headache 6 asymptomatic; 2 less; 2 no change
Bussière et al. 2010 (Ottawa) [36]	10 patients: papilledema resolved in 8
Ahmed et al. 2011 (Sydney) [30]	52 patients: papilledema, tinnitus, diplopia and headache resolved in 49; 2 deaths
Albuquerque et al. 2011 (Phoenix) [37]	18 patients: safe
Higgins et al. (Cambridge, in preparation)	53 patients: safe – transient headache, transient arm weakness; in-stent thrombosis that resolved with rTPA Papilledema resolved/improved in 77%; no visual deterioration

2002 [19] and attracted considerable skepticism and foreboding about the potential risks. In practice and in expert hands, it has proven safe when used for PTCS including pulsatile tinnitus [29]. Stent migration, venous sinus perforation, in-stent thrombosis, and subdural hemorrhage have certainly been described [30]. Such complications are more likely to occur when more difficult lesions are tackled such as areas of thrombosis. The controversial concept of chronic cerebrospinal venous insufficiency in multiple sclerosis has confused the literature (Table 26.1).

Conclusions

The etiology of PTCS remains a mystery but new management techniques are being developed that are achieving sufficient maturity for RCTs to be viable. Multidisciplinary team working is essential. Patients need access to a carefully audited care pathway and to have access to and be part of research. The formation of specific charities devoted to "I"IH in the UK and USA is to be applauded.

Acknowledgments

JDP is supported by an NIHR Senior Investigator Award and by the Cambridge NIHR Biomedical Research Centre Neurosciences Theme.

Conflict of interest

JDP receives occasional royalties from sale of the monograph *The Pseudotumor Cerebri Syndrome* that was co-authored with Ian Johnston and Brian Owler (Cambridge University Press 2007).

References

1. Johnston I, Owler B, Pickard J. *Pseudotumor Cerebri Syndrome*. Cambridge University Press; 2007.
2. Dandy WE. Intracranial pressure without brain tumour: diagnosis and treatment. *Ann Surg* 1937;106:492–513.
3. Friedman DI, Rausch EA. Headache diagnoses in patients with treated idiopathic intracranial hypertension. *Neurology* 2002;58:1551–3.
4. Corbett JJ, Savino PJ, Thompson HS, et al. Visual loss in pseudotumor cerebri. *Arch Neurol* 1982;39:461–74.
5. Sismanis A. Pulsatile tinnitus. A 15 year experience. *Am J Otol* 1998;19:472–7.
6. Brara SM, Koebnick C, Porter AH, et al. Pediatric idiopathic intracranial hypertension and extreme childhood obesity. *J Pediatr* 2012;161:602–7.
7. Higgins JN, Gillard JG, Owler B, et al. MR venography in idiopathic intracranial hypertension: unappreciated and misunderstood. *J Neurol Neurosurg Psychiatry* 2004;75:621–5.
8. Johnston IH, Paterson A. Benign intracranial hypertension. II CSF pressure and circulation. *Brain* 1974;97:301–12.
9. Weisberg LA, Chutorian AM. Pseudotumor cerebri of childhood. *Am J Dis Child* 1977;131:1243–8.
10. Brettschneider J, Hartmann N, Lehmensiek V, et al. Cerebrospinal fluid markers of idiopathic intracranial hypertension: is the rennin-angiotensinogen system involved? *Cephalalgia* 2011;31:116–21.
11. Davson H, Hollinsworth JR, Segal MD. The mechanism of drainage of the cerebrospinal fluid. *Brain* 1970;96:329–36.
12. Owler BK, Higgins JN, Pena A, et al. Diffusion tensor imaging of benign intracranial hypertension: absence of cerebral oedema. *Br J Neurosurg* 2006;20:79–81.
13. Pickard JD, Czosnyka Z, Czosnyka M, et al. Coupling of sagittal sinus pressure and cerebrospinal fluid pressure in idiopathic intracranial hypertension – a preliminary analysis. *Acta Neurochir Suppl* 2008;102:283–5.
14. Pickard JD, Csoznyka M, Czosnyka Z, Higgins JN. CSF dynamics in idiopathic intracranial hypertension: how to estimate the resistance to CSF outflow? Paper presented at the meeting of the International Society for Hydrocephalus and CSF Disorders in Kyoto, Japan, on October 21, 2012.
15. Alperin N, Ranganathan S, Bagci AM, et al. MRI evidence of impaired CSF homeostasis in obesity-associated idiopathic intracranial hypertension. *AJNR Am J Neuroradiol* 2013;34:29–34.
16. Janny P, Chazal J, Colnet G, et al. Benign intracranial hypertension and disorders of CSF absorption. *Surg Neurol* 1981;15:168–74.
17. Karahalios DG, Rekate HL, Khataya MH, et al. Elevated intracranial venous pressure as a universal mechanism in pseudotumor cerebri of varying aetiologies. *Neurology* 1996;46:198–202.
18. King JO, Mitchell PJ, Thomson KR, et al. Cerebral venography and manometry in idiopathic intracranial hypertension. *Neurology* 1995;45:2224–8.
19. Higgins JN, Owler B, Cousins C, et al. Venous sinus stenting for refractory benign intracranial hypertension. *Lancet* 2002;359:228–30.
20. Sinclair AJ, Walker EA, Burdon MA, et al. Cerebrospinal fluid corticosteroid levels and cortisol metabolism in patients with idiopathic intracranial

hypertension: a link between 11beta-HSD1 and intracranial pressure regulation. *J Clin Endocrinol Metab* 2010;95:5348–56.

21. Sinclair AJ, Burdon MA, Nightingale PG, et al. Low energy diet and intracranial pressure in women with idiopathic intracranial hypertension. *BMJ* 2010;341:c2701.
22. Ball AK, Howman A, Wheatley K, et al. A randomised controlled trial of treatment for idiopathic intracranial hypertension. *J Neurol* 2011;258:874–81.
23. Deftereos SN, Panagopoulos G, Georgonikou D, et al. Treatment of idiopathic intracranial hypertension: is there a place for octreotide? *Cephalalgia* 2011;31:1679–80.
24. Sinclair AJ, Kuruvath S, Sen D. Is cerebrospinal fluid shunting in idiopathic intracranial hypertension worthwhile? A 10 year experience. *Cephalalgia* 2011:1627–33.
25. Abubaker K, Ali Z, Raza K, et al. Idiopathic intracranial hypertension: lumboperitoneal shunts versus ventriculoperitoneal shunts – case series and literature review. *Br J Neurosurg* 2011;25:94–9.
26. Tarnaris A, Toma AK, Watkins LD, et al. Is there a difference in outcomes of patients with idiopathic intracranial hypertension with the choice of cerebrospinal fluid diversion site: a single centre experience. *Clin Neurol Neurosurg* 2011;113:477–9.
27. Alsuhaibani AH, Carter KD, Nerad JA, et al. Effect of optic nerve sheath fenestration on papilloedema of the operated and the contralateral nonoperated eyes in idiopathic intracranial hypertension. *Ophthalmology* 2011;118:412–14.
28. Sugerman HJ, Felton WL, Sismanis A, et al. Gastric surgery for pseudotumor cerebri associated with severe obesity. *Ann Surg* 1999;229:634–42.
29. Higgins JN, Cousins C, Owler B, et al. Idiopathic intracranial hypertension: 12 cases treated with venous sinus stenting. *J Neurol Neurosurg Psychiatry* 2003;74:1662–6.
30. Ahmed RM, Wilkinson M, Parker GD, et al. Transverse sinus stenting for idiopathic intracranial hypertension: a review of 52 patients and of model predictions. *AJNR Am J Neuroradiol* 2011;32:1408–14.
31. Owler BK, Parker G, Halmagyi GM, et al. Pseudotumor cerebri syndrome: venous sinus obstruction and its treatment with stent placement. *J Neurosurg* 2003;98(5):1045–55.
32. Ogungbo B, Roy D, Gholkar A, Mendelow AD. Endovascular stenting of the transverse sinus in a patient presenting with benign intracranial hypertension. *Br J Neurosurg* 2003;17(6):565–8.
33. Rajpal S, Niemann DB, Turk AS. Transverse venous sinus stent placement as treatment for benign intracranial hypertension in a young male: case report and review of the literature. *J Neurosurg* 2005;102(3 Suppl):342–6.
34. Paquet C, Poupardin M, Boissonnot M, Neau JP, Drouineau J. Efficacy of unilateral stenting in idiopathic intracranial hypertension with bilateral venous sinus stenosis: a case report. *Eur Neurol* 2008;60(1):47–8.
35. Donnet A, Metellus P, Levrier O, et al. Endovascular treatment of idiopathic intracranial hypertension: clinical and radiologic outcome of 10 consecutive patients. *Neurology* 2008;70(8):641–7.
36. Bussière M, Falero R, Nicolle D, Proulx A, Patel V, Pelz D. Unilateral transverse sinus stenting of patients with idiopathic intracranial hypertension. *AJNR Am J Neuroradiol* 2010;31(4):645–50.
37. Albuquerque FC, Dashti SR, Hu YC, et al. Intracranial venous sinus stenting for benign intracranial hypertension: clinical indications, technique, and preliminary results. *World Neurosurg* 2011;75(5–6):648–52.

Epilogue

Almost 50 years ago Solomon Hakim and his colleagues described the syndrome of normal pressure hydrocephalus (NPH). The three patients described had obstructive hydrocephalus demonstrated on pneumo-encephalography, secondary to a colloid cyst in one case, and to blockage of the subarachnoid space (SAS) at the cervicomedullary junction in the other two cases. By definition the original cases were secondary, because a cause was found.

Hydrocephalus is defined as idiopathic when an obvious cause is missing.

Idiopathic normal pressure hydrocephalus (iNPH) is a syndrome of "chronic" ventricular dilatation, without obvious obstruction, that may lead eventually to the clinical development of the classic triad of cognitive, gait, and urinary symptoms.

Today, thanks to a phenomenal improvement in imaging techniques, we are able to visualize many more cases of "obstructive" hydrocephalus than before. Our Japanese colleagues have described what they believe is the radiological trademark of iNPH: the disproportionately enlarged subarachnoid space hydrocephalus (DESH). Other imaging techniques looking at aqueductal stroke volume and diffusion tensor imaging, although intriguing, have yet to demonstrate an unequivocal clinical usefulness.

Because iNPH is a disease affecting the elderly, the presence of comorbidities will always obscure the picture and make the selection criteria difficult until we better quantify the relative weight of other conditions in the development of the clinical picture.

A better understanding of iNPH will occur through better characterization of patients at their different stages of the disease, through the insight that animal studies provide, and by the identification of specific biomarkers.

There is increasing supportive evidence pointing to the efficacy of endoscopic third ventriculostomy (ETV) in the management of obstructive hydrocephalus secondary to aqueductal stenosis. There is anecdotal evidence of efficacy of other endoscopic procedures in the management of other types of obstructive hydrocephalus.

In truly nonobstructive "communicating" hydrocephalus, the efficacy of ETV is lacking in spite of several initial reports. In this latter condition, shunting remains the main treatment tool to stop and even reverse the functional decline.

Unfortunately the success of shunting is not guaranteed.

Reasons for the failure of the shunt to produce satisfactory recovery are many: a wrong diagnosis, selection of the wrong hardware, a surgical complication, and lack of recognition of a shunt malfunction.

It is our communal responsibility to improve our understanding of hydrocephalus and the effect of comorbidities, to reach earlier diagnosis, to standardize the surgical procedures (shunting and ETV), to reduce complications, to develop proper monitoring guidelines of the postoperative course, and recognize shunt failure. If we succeed in these efforts, we will all bring about a substantial increase in positive outcomes.

Index

Note:
All index entries relate to NPH unless otherwise stated.
vs denotes differential diagnosis, or comparisons.

Abbreviations:
CBF –cerebral blood flow
ETV –endoscopic third ventriculostomy
NPH –normal pressure hydrocephalus
PTCS –pseudotumor cerebri syndrome
SAH –subarachnoid hemorrhage
SHYMA –syndrome of hydrocephalus in young and middle-aged adults

abdominal shunt, CT, 114, 116
abdominal X-ray, 110, 111
acetazolamide, 261, 294, 300
acquired hydrocephalus, 36, 38
see also idiopathic NPH (iNPH)
adolescents, care transitioning, 265, 266–267
age/aging (hydrocephalus and), 16–17, 283
blood and CSF flow, 127
experimental animals, 29
iNPH and, 59, 207
SHYMA, 247–248
see also elderly
aleuronate granules, 31
Alzheimer's disease (AD), 71, 101
biomarkers, 101, 164, 165
cognitive dysfunction, 72, 101
iNPH differential diagnosis, 77, 103
biomarker use, 165–167, 169
neuropsychological deficits, iNPH *vs*, 74
NPH coexistence, 16–17, 71, 76, 101
case study, 108
urinary incontinence, 80, 81
amyloid, soluble precursor protein (sAPP), 166, 168, 169
amyloid beta protein, as iNPH biomarker, 164, 169
Alzheimer's disease *vs*, 165, 166, 169
Parkinson's disease *vs*, 168
prognostic biomarker, 168, 169
amyloid plaques, 165
anatomy, CSF system, 1–2
spinal, 3
animal models (hydrocephalus), 28–33, 48
animals used, 30
classification, 30
CSF shunting techniques, 33
ethics, 28–29
EU legislation, 28
existing/preferred (for hydrocephalus), 30–32
genetically determined, 32
physical/chemical agents inducing, 31, 33
formal (general) requirements, 29–30
genes for hydrocephalus, *see* genes/loci
genetic models, *see* genetic models
interstitial edema (brain), 71
NPH, 33
principles (ethical), 28–29
questions needing clarification, 30
recent/current research areas, 32–33, 48
requirements/challenges, 30
validity evaluation, 29–30
see also experimental hydrocephalus
animal(s), naturally occurring hydrocephalus, 30, 31
antibiotic(s)
intravenous, in shunt infections, 186–187
perioperative, 186
prophylactic, for ETV, 224
antibiotic-impregnated shunts (AIS), 186, 213
costs and cost/benefits, 215
decreased infection rates, 213–214
pathogens/infections despite, 214–215
antisiphon devices (ASD), 176, 193–194, 241
external pressure effect, 199
indications and functions, 176
membrane construction, 194
positioning, 176
types, 193–194
Apaf1 protein, 46
ApoE e3 allele, 38
ApoE e4 allele, 38
apoptotic pathways, disrupted, 46
aquaporin(s), 6–7, 8
aquaporin-1 (AQP1), 6, 8, 46
knockout (KO) mice, 7
pathophysiological role, 46
aquaporin-1 channel, 4, 46
aquaporin-4 (AQP4), 6, 7, 8, 46
astrocytic endfeet, 6, 7
knockout mice/deficiency, 7, 32, 46
up-regulation/increased, 46
aqueductal stenosis, *see under* cerebral aqueduct (of Sylvius)
arachnoid barrier cells, 6
arachnoid cell layer, 5–6
arachnoid cyst, 275
cerebellar, NPH with, 279–280, 283
in elderly, 275, 279–280, 283
giant suprasellar, in fetus, 282
management, 285, 286
multiple, hydrocephalus management, 281
posterior fossa, 276–277
arachnoid fibrosis, 14
arachnoid granulations, 8–9
anatomy, 8–9
CSF reabsorption, 8, 150, 296
in PTCS, 296, 299, 300
in newborn infants, 219
spinal, CSF drainage, 10
arachnoid trabecular cells, 6
arachnoid villi, 8, 9, 150
arterial blood flow energy, CSF pulsation and, 10, 71
ASPP2, and *ASPP2*, 46
astrocytes, reactive, 23
astrocytoma, 250
asymptomatic ventriculomegaly, *see* ventricular enlargement, asymptomatic
atrial catheter insertion, 180–182
complications, 181
procedure, 181

atrial pressure, right, 294
attention deficit, 73–74, 76
attention deficit hyperactivity disorder (ADHD), 277–278
autoregulation, cerebral, 159–160
autosomal dominant inheritance, 38
autosomal recessive congenital hydrocephalus mice, 39–40
autosomal recessive hemorrhagic hydrocephalus (hhy) mouse, 40
autosomal recessive hydrocephalus with hop gait (hyh) mouse, 40

B waves, 70, 154–155, 159
B9d2 protein, 46
balance, grading scale, 95, 240
balance control, 63, 67
  impaired, gait dysfunction, 67
bariatric surgery, 294, 301
Barthel ADL Index, 242
basilar artery, in ETV, 224, 225
"bedside to bench" concept, 29
behavioral outcome, congenital hydrocephalus, 272
bioactive peptides, 5
biofilm, 186, 213
biomarkers (CSF), 164–170
  Alzheimer's disease, 101, 164, 165
  CSF sample requirements, 170
  definition, 164
  experimental problems, 169–170
  idiopathic NPH
    Alzheimer's disease *vs*, 165–167, 169
    historical perspective, 164, 170
    Parkinson's disease *vs*, 167–169
    rationale for use, 164–165
    summary of current evidence, 169
    vascular dementia *vs*, 167
  prognostic, 165, 168–169
  study requirements and limitations, 170
Black outcome scale, 242
Black's classification, 91, 93
bladder (urinary), 82
  contraction, control, 82
  filling, sensation, 23
  overactive, 81, 82, 84, 85
  sensation, terminology, 83
Blake's pouch cysts, 286–287
blood flow, cerebral, *see* cerebral blood flow
blood–brain barrier, aquaporins role, 7
body position, *see* posture
brain
  atrophy, 147, 158, 159
  damage, pathogenesis in NPH, 15
  equilibrium pressure, 126
  sagging, in intracranial hypotension, 257, 258–259
  tumors, 102, 248–251
  volume, 1
  water distribution, 1
burr holes, for ETV, 224, 225

carbon dioxide (CO_2) reactivity, 160
carcinomatous meningitis, 249
cardiac cycle
  CSF and blood flow interactions, 126, 129
  CSF flow affected by, 5, 6, 71, 124, 128, 150
    CSF flow parameters, 124
    temporal normalization of PC-MRI, 124
    Windkessel effect, 10, 153, 154
  intracranial pressure fluctuations, 127–128, 152
  intracranial volume change, 128
cardiac gating, MRI, 121–122
cardiac pulsation, recording (ECG, plethysmography), 121–122
caregiver burden, urinary incontinence and, 80, 85
caregiver burden scale, 94
  case studies, 105, 106, 108
  see also management, of hydrocephalus in CSF pathologies
caspases, 46
caudate nucleus, 68
CD68, 47
CDO protein, 47
cerebellar arachnoid cyst, NPH with, 279–280, 283
cerebellar herniation, 291
cerebellar tonsils, 291
cerebral aneurysms, 60, 251, 252
cerebral aqueduct (of Sylvius), 1
  anatomy, 2
  closure, Chiari II malformation and, 292
  defective development, 40
  fast CSF flow-induced artifact (flow void), 121, 133
  flow normalization, cognition improvement, 73
  hyperdynamic CSF flow, 71
  MRI scans, 114
  obstruction, 17
  secondary closure in development, 46, 292, 293
  stenosis, 17, 40, 45, 130
    ETV outcome, 218, 219, 227
    HTX and LEW/Jms rat models, 40, 44
    incomplete, PC-MRI, 130
    late-onset idiopathic, 247–248
    in LOVA, 247–248
    PC-MRI, 115–117, 130–131
  stroke volume in NPH, 285
  subcommissural organ role, 40
cerebral autoregulation, 159–160
cerebral blood flow (CBF), 23, 125, 160–161
  arterio-venous flow difference, 126–128
  CSF flow and, *see* cerebrospinal fluid (CSF) flow
  experimental hydrocephalus, 15
  global decrease, iNPH mechanism, 71, 72
  healthy *vs* NPH patients, 127
  hypoperfusion, NPH and, 15, 23, 127, 160
  inflow calculation, 126
  mean, normal, 126, 127
  pulsation, disorder, 154
  regional, 160
    decrease, effects, 68, 71
  shunting effect, 160–161
  in white matter, 160, 161
cerebral blood pressure, 147
cerebral convexity CSF spaces, 3
cerebral edema, 71, 299
cerebral elasticity, 152
cerebral vein, engorgement, 257
cerebral venography, retrograde, 300
cerebral venous narrowing, PTCS, 299–300
cerebral venous outflow, 126, 133
cerebrospinal dynamic compensation, law, 152
cerebrospinal fluid (CSF), 2, 139–147
  absorption/reabsorption, 8, 14, 139, 143, 150, 151, 299
    arachnoid villi, 8, 9, 14
    cerebral autoregulation and, 159
    lymphatic drainage, 9–10
    pressures, 141
    production balance, 139, 151
    production imbalance, 72, 130
    in PTCS, 296, 299
    rate, 140
    spinal lymphatics, 9–10
    Windkessel effect, 10
  biomarkers, *see* biomarkers (CSF)
  circulation/flow, *see* cerebrospinal fluid (CSF) flow
  cleansing role of choroid plexus, 5, 16
  composition, 1, 31, 299
  density, 1
  diversion, *see* shunt(s); shunting
  drainage (normal), *see* cerebrospinal fluid (CSF), absorption/reabsorption
  drainage (surgical), *see* shunt(s); shunting

dynamics, 139–141, 150–152, 176, 190
applications, 150
B wave assessment, 154–155
brain atrophy, 158, 159
cerebrovascular pressure reactivity (PRx), 155–156
infusion tests, 155–156
long-term shunts, 269
normal, 159
pathophysiology not correlated, 285
in persistent symptoms, 190
quantitative assessment, 150–161
shunt indication, 159, 190, 284, 285
shunts effect on, 191
unpredictable nature, 283
see also specific parameters
fistulae, 256
functions, 1, 14, 71, 128, 150
hypovolemia, pathogenesis, 256
leaks, 256–262
detection, 262
diagnostic criteria, 259–260
etiology, 256
ETV complication, 227
imaging, *see under* intracranial hypotension, spontaneous
management and outcome, 261–262
pathogenesis, 256
spinal, headaches, 257
see also intracranial hypotension, spontaneous
opening pressure, 259
outflow resistance, 139, 143, 146
R_{out}, *see* R_{out} (CSF outflow resistance)
physiology, NPH differential diagnosis, 103–104
pressure–volume compensation, 150–152
pressure–volume compensatory reserve, 155, 158–159
pressure–volume curve, 139–140
production and rate of, 1, 3, 14, 139, 150
average rate, 143, 204
choroid plexectomy effect, 8
choroid plexus role, 4, 128
clearance balance, 139, 151
clearance imbalance, 72, 130
drugs reducing, 4
excess, pseudotumor cerebri, 299
increased, in tumors, 249
interstitial fluid role, 3, 5
measurement, 144
reduced, toxin accumulation, 71, 72
protein, 1
pulsation, 5, 10, 150, 220
pulsation energy, dissipation, 10, 71
pulse pressure, 147
pulse pressure amplitude, monitoring, 146
replacement, hypovolemia, 261
rhinorrhea, 297
secretion, 4, 139
shunting, *see* shunt procedures; shunting
siphoning into distal compartment, 176
storage rate, 140, 151, 152
stroke volume, 124, 125, 128, 133, 285
turnover, aquaporins and ion channels, 6–8
ventricular pulsation amplitude, 154
volume, 1, 128
cerebrospinal fluid (CSF) disorders, 275
cerebrospinal fluid (CSF) flow, 3, 5, 139, 150, 191
aquaporins role, 6, 46
blood flow interaction, 125–129, 133
arterio-venous flow difference, 126–128
cardiac cycle effect, 126, 129, 128
healthy adults, 126–129
protocol, regions explored, 126
cardiac cycle affecting, *see* cardiac cycle
cells influencing, 5
cervical *vs* ventricular, 126, 133–134
Chiari malformation, 135, 134
curve, PC-MRI, 125
electrical model, 139, 141, 151, 191
healthy *vs* NPH case, 132, 133–134
hydrocephalus with CSF pathologies, 275
hyperdynamic, 71, 133
imaging, 121–136
flow parameters, 124
flow rate estimation, 124
inflow/outflow artifacts, 121, 133
MRI, before ETV, 223–224
MRI impact, 285
temporal normalization, 124
time-of-flight MRA, 121
see also phase-contrast MRI (PC-MRI)
imaging of disorders, 129–134
after ETV, 131, 131
aqueductal stenosis, 130–131
Chiari malformation, 135, 134
NPH, 129–134
syringomyelia, 135
impairment, causes, 6, 14
mechanisms and models, 150–152
normal, dynamics, 159
oscillation quantification, 127, 128, 131, 133
outflow resistance, infusion test, 103
perivascular, 6
posterior fossa cyst without hydrocephalus, 277
pulsatile, 5, 10, 150, 220
rate, diagnosis of NPH, 131–133
rate estimation, 124
regulation, 125
routes, 1–2, 6–8
spinal, 6
subarachnoid cisterns, 5–6
through ventricles, 5
venous sinuses, 9
Virchow–Robin spaces, 5–6
vascular components, 159
cerebrospinal fluid (CSF) spaces, 1–3, 285
cerebral convexity, 3
spinal, 3
see also cisterns (subarachnoid); subarachnoid space (SAS); *specific ventricles*
cerebrospinal fluid (CSF) system, 1–10
anatomy, 1–2
spinal, anatomy, 3
see also cerebrospinal fluid (CSF) spaces
cerebrovascular disease, 15–16, 17, 101
cerebrovascular pressure reactivity (PRx), 155–156
Certas valve, 196
cervical lymphatics, 9
cervical spondylotic myelopathy, 101
chest ultrasound, 112
chest X-ray, 110, 111, 177
Chiari I malformation, 277–278, 284, 285, 291
anatomy, 291
benign intracranial hypertension, 294–295
decompression, 292, 294
description/features, 291–292
hydrocephalus relationship, 292
management, 278, 279, 283
prenatal surgery, 286
pseudotumor cerebri and, 294–295
Chiari II malformation, 291–294
Chiari malformation, 291–295
adult, *see* Chiari I malformation
CSF flow, 135, 134
types, 291
children
closed fontanelle, ventricular catheter insertion, 179
ETV in, 218–219, 222
PTCS in, 297
shunt infection rates, 212

choroid plexectomy, 8
choroid plexus, 2, 4–5
  CSF production/secretion, 3, 4, 128
    PTCS pathophysiology and, 299, 300
  functions, 4, 5
  ion channels and CSF turnover, 7
  structure, 4
  tumors, 249, 251
chromosome 8q12–2–q21.2 microdeletion, 38
chromosome 19q12–13.31, 38
chronic subdural hematoma, 102
cilia, 5, 44
  receptor signaling, defects, 45–46
ciliopathies, 44–46
cisterns (subarachnoid), 1, 3
  anatomy, 3, 223
  CSF flow, 5–6
  CSF flow blockage, 6, 220
classification (human hydrocephalus), 36, 91, 287
  based on symptomatology, 104
  CSF pathologies with, 286–287
  see also grading scales (NPH)
closing pressure, 196
Codman Certas Valve, 199
Codman Hakim Adjustable Valve, 176, 194, 196, 199–200
cognitive changes, 23
cognitive function, in walking/gait, 65–66
cognitive impairment (in CSF pathologies), 285
cognitive impairment (in iNPH), 72–73, 101–102
  adolescents/young adults, 266
  CSF drainage effect, 75–77
  differential diagnosis, 101–102
  evaluation, 72, 73, 95, 101, 284–285
    iNPH scale, 239, 284–285
    patient selection, outcome improvement, 233, 242, 284–285
  features, 72–73, 74, 77, 99, 284–285
  grading, *see* grading scales (NPH)
  pathophysiology, 70–77
    putative pathogenic mechanisms, 70–72
    see also under pathophysiology (of iNPH)
  transitional care (pediatric to adult), 265
  see also dementia; neuropsychological deficits (in iNPH)
communicating hydrocephalus, 190, 220–221
  choroid plexus tumors and, 249
  CSF dynamics, 159, 220–221
  ETV in, 218–222, 304
  experimental, 31, 33
  intracranial CBF pulsation disorder, 154, 220–221
  pathogenesis, 3, 6
  shunt type, 185
comorbid diseases, 76, 77, 100, 304
  Alzheimer's disease, *see* Alzheimer's disease (AD)
  biomarker use in, 165, 170
  cerebrovascular disease, 15–16, 17, 101
  grading scales and, 94, 96
  impact on NPH outcome, 244
  VP shunt complications, 210
comorbidity index, 94, 96, 244
compensated hydrocephalus, 247, 248, 292, 293
compliance, 125, 133, 152
  decreased, communicating hydrocephalus, 220–221
  decreased in prolonged shunting, 269, 270
    see also normal volume hydrocephalus (NVH)
  definition, 139–140
compliance curve, 139–140
computed tomography (CT), 103, 110–114
  abdominal shunt evaluation, 114, 116
  chest, 115
  CSF leak, 257
  diagnosis of NPH, 110–113, 113
  postoperative management, 113–114
  pre- *vs* postoperative image comparison, 113, 114
  pseudotumor cerebri syndrome, 298
  risks, 114
  shunt assessment, 209
  shunt malfunction detection, 113–114, 115, 116
  ventricular catheter insertion, 179
  ventriculoperitoneal shunt, 209
  volumetric analysis by, 113
computed tomography (CT) venography, 298, 299
computerized infusion test, 155–156
congenital hydrocephalus, 36
  adult hydrocephalus differences, 265
  clinical outcome, 271–272
  complications/morbidities, 271–272
  education and employment, 272–273
  epidemiology, 38, 57
  etiologies, 264
  genetic epidemiology, 37
  genetics, and inheritance, 38–39
  monogenic (animal models), 39–40
  neuropsychological outcome, 272–273
  pathophysiology, *see* pathophysiology, genetic basis
  recurrence risk ratios (RRRs), 37
  risk rates, 38
  shunt independence, 267–269
    see also endoscopic third ventriculostomy (ETV)
  transition of care (to adult centers), *see* management
  twin studies, 36–37
  uncomplicated (third ventricle obstruction), 38
  X-linked, 38
congenital malformations, prevalence, 57
connective tissue disorders, 256
constant flow infusion method, 144–145
constant pressure infusion method, 145
construct validity, animal models, 29
continuous spinal/ventricular drainage, 103
cooperative studies, differences, grading scale role, 96
core imaging, 103, 110–119
corpus callosum, 15, 17
cortical dysfunction, gait dysfunction theories, 65–66
cortical-subcortical circuit defects, 67
corticobasal degeneration, 102
cranial compartments, 125, 128–129
craniosynostosis, 270
Creutzfeldt–Jakob disease (CJD), 102
cribriform plate, 9
CYP2J2 transgene, 44

Dandy criteria, 292, 296–297
Dandy–Walker cyst, 286–287
Davson's equation, 299
DBI ($GABA_A$ receptor modulator), 48
deep white matter ischemia (DWMI), 240–241
dementia
  Alzheimer's, *see* Alzheimer's disease (AD)
  dual-tasking and gait dysfunction, 66
  falls, 81
  frontotemporal, 101–102, 106
  grading scales, iNPH, 92
  iNPH differential diagnosis, 77, 99, 101
  iNPH epidemiology, 59
  multi-infarct, 80, 81
  in NPH, assessment, 92
  NPH outcome, 244
  post-stroke, 80

urinary incontinence, 80–81
vascular, 101, 167
see also cognitive impairment (in iNPH)
dementia with Lewy bodies (DLB), 101, 102
depression, 101, 272
DESH, 99, 115, 117, 233, 304
detrusor overactivity, 85–87, 102
shunt surgery results, 87–88
development
abnormal, hydrocephalus pathophysiology, 48, 275
CSF and blood flow, 125
early, enhanced gene expression, 47–48
loss of molecular cues during, 40–46, 47
developmental delay, 264, 266
diagnosis (of NPH), 99–104
criteria in iNPH, 59
delay in, 100, 104
difficulties, 60–61, 99, 100
imaging, *see individual imaging modalities*
infusion tests, *see* infusion techniques/tests
iNPH, for outcome improvement, 232–233
lack of awareness reducing, 60–61, 99, 100, 104, 215
neurological examination, 99–100
universal criteria, lack of, 61
see also differential diagnosis (of NPH)
diagnostic work-up, 100–101
DIAPPER mnemonic, 82
diaschisis, 72
differential diagnosis (of NPH), 76–77, 99–104, 207
Alzheimer's disease, *see* Alzheimer's disease (AD)
case studies, 105, 106, 108
dementia syndromes, 77, 99, 101–102
by imaging, 102–103, 233
iNPH, 233
Parkinson's disease *vs*, biomarkers, 167–169
by pathology, 169–170
R_{out} use, 158
by symptoms
cognitive impairment, 101–102
gait dysfunction, 100–101
urinary dysfunction, 81–82, 102
vascular dementia, biomarkers, 167
disproportionately enlarged subarachnoid space hydrocephalus (DESH), 99, 115, 117, 233, 304
Dlg5 protein, 44
dopamine, 23
dopamine D2 receptor, hypoactivity, 23, 68
dopamine signaling abnormalities, 68
dual-tasking, gait dysfunction, 66, 67
duplex ultrasound, 110, 112, 181
dural sinus pressure, 141, 143
Dutch NPH Scale, 242
dynein, 45

education, congenital hydrocephalus, 272–273
Eide's classification, 91, 93
elastance coefficient (elasticity), 158, 159
ELD, *see* external lumbar drainage (ELD)
elderly
arachnoid cyst and hydrocephalus, 275, 279–280, 283
case study, NPH diagnosis, 108
iNPH symptoms, 61, 100, 147
NPH and cerebrovascular disease, 15–16
NPH prevalence, 59, 104, 207
symptom onset, pathogenesis, 15
urinary tract symptoms, 82
electrical circuit analogy, CSF circulation, 139, 141, 151, 191
electrocardiography (ECG), 121–122
En1 (*Engrailed 1*), 47
En2 gene, 47
endoscopic third ventriculostomy (ETV), 218–228, 268, 304
adult patients, 218, 268
advantages/disadvantages, 222, 267
anatomic eligibility, 222–224
cerebral blood flow, 126
in children (age/etiology-dependence), 218–219, 222
communicating hydrocephalus, 218–222, 228, 304
complications, 226–227, 268–269
frequency and type, 269
contraindications, 223, 268
CSF flow, 126, 222
PC-MRI, 131, 223–224
CSF leaks after, 227
endoscope size, 222–224
failure, 225, 227, 268–269
causes/risk factors, 222, 268
diagnosis, 221–222
management, 222, 268
timing, 222, 227, 268, 269
failure rates
adult patients, 218
previously shunted patients, 220
young infants, 219
grading system for eligibility, 223
hemorrhage and vascular injuries, 226–227
hypothalamic disorders after, 227
indications, 218–221, 268, 285
hydrodynamic concept and, 220–221
iNPH, 220–221
navigation systems, 223, 224
obstructive hydrocephalus, 218, 219, 221
outcome, 304
children, 218–219
factors influencing, 218
iNPH, 220, 221
intraoperative factors affecting, 221
nonobstructive hydrocephalus, 218, 220, 222
obstructive hydrocephalus, 218, 227
post-hemorrhagic hydrocephalus, 268
previously shunted patients, 219–220, 268
patency, MRI/PC-MRI detection, 117, 131, 223
postoperative care and follow-up, 227–228
preoperative planning, 222–224
repeated, 219, 222
stoma obstruction, 221, 222, 225, 227
stoma size, 221
success, definition of, 221–222
surgical technique, 224–226
ventricular reservoir placement, 225
ventricular bowing for, 218
ventriculoperitoneal shunt *vs*, 222
energy transfer, Windkessel effect, 10, 153, 154
ependymal cells, 5, 44
atrophy, ventricular enlargement causing, 15
cilia and ciliopathies, 44–46
ependymoma, 250
epidemiology (of hydrocephalus), 57–61, 207
age relationship, 59, 207
congenital and infantile hydrocephalus, 57
genetic, *see* genetic epidemiology
idiopathic NPH, 57–60, 104
incidence/prevalence of NPH (unclassified), 58, 59, 207
shunt insertion criterion, 59
secondary NPH, 60
summary of studies, 58
surgery frequency, 60–61
epidural blood patch, 261

essential tremor-idiopathic NPH (ETINPH) disorder, 38
ethics, animal models, 28–29
etiology of hydrocephalus, 36, 103, 190, 264, 275
ETV success score (ETVSS), 223
Evans ratio, 111, 113
executive function, in gait, 65–66
  impaired, 66, 73–74
experimental hydrocephalus
  cerebral blood flow changes, 15
  obstructive, kaolin injection and, 31, 33
  physical/chemical agents inducing, 31, 33
  see also animal models
external lumbar drainage (ELD), 145–146
  biomarkers as prognostic indicator for, 168
  cognitive and gait response to, 75
  outcome in iNPH, prediction, 233
  shunt responder prediction, 146
external ventricular drain (EVD), 252, 269, 270
extracellular fluid, 16
extracellular space, enlargement, 16

FAC gene mutation, 37
falls, 81
  familial hydrocephalus, 36, 37, 38
  see also genetics (of hydrocephalus)
Fas, 46
FGFR3, 46
fibrin sealant, 261
"fifth ventricle", 204
fine motor coordination deficits, 75
flow–pressure test, 195, 197
flow-regulating antisiphon devices, 194
follow-up, 207–215
  ETV, 227–228
  idiopathic NPH, 232, 243
  time frame, 243
foramen magnum, 291
foramen of Luschka, 2
foramen of Magendie, 2
foramen of Monro, 1, 2
forkhead genes, 40
fornix, of brain, atrophy, 15
fourth ventricle, 1
  anatomy, 2
  cellular composition, 5
  compensated hydrocephalus, 293
  occlusion of outlet foramina, 292, 293
  small, 247
FOXC1 gene, 38, 40
frontal lobe defects, gait dysfunction, 66, 67
frontotemporal dementia (FTD), 101–102, 106

gait, 65–66
  in SHYMA, 248
  speed, 66, 92
gait dysfunction in NPH, 63–68, 81
  characteristic features, 63, 64, 99, 100, 167
  CSF drainage improving, *see* shunting
  diagnosis of NPH, 100–101
  differential diagnosis of NPH, 100–101
  evaluation, 92, 100, 242
    iNPH MCV scale, 241
    iNPH scale, 239
    patient selection and outcome, 233
  grading, *see* grading scales (NPH)
  neurodegenerative disease similarity, 64–66, 100–101, 167
  objective measures, 63–64
  older theories on, 63
  pathogenesis, 23
  presenting symptom, 63, 100
  tentative theories on pathophysiology, 63, 64–68
    see also midbrain, diameter
gender, experimental animals, 29
genes/loci, 36, 39
  animal models (summary), 41
  FOXC1 and ch mouse, 40
  hhy mouse, 40
  HTX rat model, 39
  human hydrocephalus (summary), 39
  hyh gene (α-SNAP), 40
  mouse models, 39
  transgenic mouse OVE459, 39
  see also pathophysiology, genetic basis
genetic epidemiology, 36–37
  see also genetics (of hydrocephalus)
genetic models, 39–40
  enhanced expression of genes, 47–48
  inbred strains/genetic manipulation, 32
  monogenic congenital hydrocephalus, 39–40
  mutant genes, *see* genes/loci
  quantitative trait locus (QTL), 39
genetics (of hydrocephalus), 36–48
  congenital hydrocephalus, 38–39
  essential tremor-idiopathic NPH disorder, 38
  idiopathic NPH, 38
  loci/genes associated, *see* genes/loci
  maternal component, 37
  pathophysiology, *see* pathophysiology, genetic basis
  see also genetic epidemiology
giant retrocerebellar cysts, 286–287
giant suprasellar arachnoid cyst, 282
gky mouse, 45
Gli1 and Gli3 proteins, 45
glucocorticoids, 300
grading scales (NPH), 91–96, 104
  caregiver burden, 94
  comparisons between, 96
  for ETV eligibility, 223
  general activity, 91, 92
  iNPH, for outcome improvement, 233–240, 242–243
  requirements, types and criticisms, 91
  symptomatology assessment, 91–93, 242–243
    balance, 95, 240
    Black's classification, 91, 93
    comorbidity, 94, 96
    dementia, 92
    Eide's classification, 91, 93
    gait, 94, 233, 239, 241, 242
    Hellström's classification, 92, 94
    INPH scale, 239, 240, 242–243
    Krauss's classification, 91, 93
    Kubo's scale, 92, 94, 233–240
    neuropsychological, 72, 73, 95, 239, 284–285
    for outcome assessment, 233–240
    qualitative, 91–93
    qualitative with quantitative, 92–93
    quantitative, 91, 92
    semiquantitative, 92
    urinary incontinence, 92, 95, 240
gravitational antisiphon devices, 194
gray matter, distortion and cognitive defects, 70
Grooved Pegboard test, 95, 284, 285
guidelines, 61, 131–133
  diagnosis/management of iNPH, 99, 232, 240
  Japanese, 99
  outcome assessment scales, 243

Hakim's triad, 91, 99, 232
head circumference, posterior fossa cyst, 276
head size, 15
headache
  Chiari malformation and hydrocephalus, 277–278
  chronic shunting, 269, 270
  CSF leak surgery, 261
  early morning, 201–202

intermittent, spinal CSF leaks, 257
low-pressure, 256–257, 270, 271
positional, intracranial hypotension, 256–257, 259, 262
posterior fossa cyst without hydrocephalus, 277
pressure (supine), 261
pseudotumor cerebri syndrome, 297
slit ventricle syndrome, 269, 270
spina bifida, management, 271
hedgehog signaling, 45
Hellström's grading scale, 92, 94
herniation, 291
cerebellar vermis, top, 292
ETV complication, 226
fourth ventricle, 293
hindbrain, 291–292
in myelography, 259
hhy mouse, 40
Hif-1α, 47
high pressure hydrocephalus, experimental, 31
hindbrain herniation, 291–292
histopathology, ventriculomegaly, brain damage, 15
historical perspectives, 31, 304
HIV/AIDS, 253
HTX rat, 32, 33, 39, 46
subcommissural organ development, 40
Huntingtin (htt) protein, 44
Huntington's disease, 72, 102
hy1 mouse, 39
hy2 mouse, 39
hy3 mouse, 39–40, 44
hydin (protein), 44–45
Hydin exons/mutants, 39, 45
hydrocephalus, definition, 14
hydrodynamic concept, iNPH, 220–221
hydrodynamic resistance (shunts), *see* shunt(s)
hydrophilic mice, 47
hydrostatic pressure, 176
hyh gene, 40
hyh mouse, 40
hypercoagulopathy, 300
hypovascularization, 47
hypoxic-ischemic stress/injury, 15, 23
hysteresis, valves, 198

idiopathic intracranial hypertension (IIH), 151, 296
idiopathic NPH (iNPH), 14, 17, 91, 99, 207
ApoE e3/e4 alleles and, 38
autopsy findings, 18
biomarkers, *see* biomarkers (CSF)
cognitive defects, *see* cognitive impairment (in iNPH)
definition, 304
diagnostic guidelines, 99, 232
epidemiology, 57–60, 104
ETV in, *see* endoscopic third ventriculostomy (ETV)
follow-up, 232, 243
genetics, 38
outcome, *see* outcome
selection criteria for improved outcome, 232–233
surgery frequency, 60–61
symptoms, 232
in elderly, 61, 100, 147
as "two hit" disease, 240–241
Ift88 gene mutations, 45
imaging, 103, 110–119, 304
CSF pathologies with hydrocephalus, 285
differential diagnostic role, 102–103
modalities used, 110
in PTCS, 298–299
shunt assessment, 209, 210, 242
immune response, changes, 47
impaired executive function (IEF), 66, 73–74
incontinence, *see* urinary incontinence
infantile hydrocephalus, epidemiology, 57
infections/infectious disease
cognitive dysfunction due to, 102
hydrocephalus after, 252–254
shunt, *see* shunt infections
inflammation, 31
infusion techniques/tests, 103, 104, 141–144, 146, 147, 155–156
bolus, 141–144, 146, 156
brain atrophy and, 147
Marmarou's model, 142, 144
procedure, 142–143, 146
results, 143
bolus *vs* gradual, comparisons, 144, 146–147
applications, 146
baseline pressures and, 157–158
R_{out} values, 157–158
clinical prognostic applications, 146
computerized infusion test, 155–156
constant, 141, 144–145, 157
gradual (steady-state), 144, 146, 156, 157
constant flow, 144–145
constant pressure, 145
constant pressure constant infusion rate, 144–145
herniation risk, 159
intraventricular, 155–156
periodic pulse pressure (CSF), 147
principles, 141, 142
shunt functioning assessment, 200–202
slow waves, analysis, 158–159
time-dependent pressure, responses, 141–144
volume removal (bolus withdrawal), 143–144
inheritance of hydrocephalus, 36–38
INPH scale, 239, 240, 242–243
β8-integrin, 45
interleukin-1 (IL-1), 166
International Consultation on Incontinence Modular Questionnaires (ICIq), 84, 86
International Hydrocephalus Imaging Working Group (IHIWG), 275, 287
International Society of Hydrocephalus and Cerebrospinal Fluid Disorders (ISHCSF), 275, 287
interstitial edema, NPH pathogenesis, 71, 72
interstitial fluid, CSF production, 3, 5
intracerebral hemorrhage, 114
intracisternal obstructive hydrocephalus, ETV in, 221
intracortical circuit defects, 67
intracranial hemorrhage, ETV complication, 226–227
intracranial hypertension
active obstructive hydrocephalus, 159
benign, 294–296
Chiari I malformation and, 294–295
cognitive impairment in iNPH and, 70–71
idiopathic, 151, 296
in morbid obesity, 294
pseudotumor cerebri, 296, 298
threshold, 298
tolerance, 150
transient, in ETV, 267
ventricular enlargement failure, chronic shunts, 269
intracranial hypotension, spontaneous, 256
clinical presentation, 256–257
positional headaches, 256–257, 259, 262
diagnosis, three-step approach, 259–260
diagnostic algorithm, 260
diagnostic criteria, 259–260
diagnostic imaging, 257–259
outcome, 261–262
pathogenesis, 256
surgical treatment, 261
treatment, 261–262
see also cerebrospinal fluid (CSF), leaks

intracranial pressure (ICP), 139, 147
baseline, 156–159
bolus infusion technique, 141–143, 157–158
brain atrophy, 159
elevated, *see* intracranial hypertension
fluctuations in cardiac cycle, 127, 128, 128, 152
iNPH pathophysiology and ETV mechanism, 220–221
measurements, 103, 298–299
monitoring, 150–161, 283
CSF flow changes, 128–129
headaches in spina bifida, 271
method, 152
pediatric hydrocephalus, 155, 156
prognostic biomarkers, 169
pulse waveform, 152–154
normal values, 103
optimal, 152
posture effects, 154
pressure reactivity index (PRx), 155–156, 158–159
pulse wave, in vivo shunt testing, 201
pulse wave amplitude, 152, 153, 159
peak-to-peak values, 154
reference (P_o), 152, 191
intracranial space, 1
intracranial volume change (IVC), 128
intraflagellar transport (IFT) genes, 44
intraspinal tumors, 249–250
intraventricular hemorrhage, 180, 218, 251
ion channels, CSF turnover, 7–8
IQ scores, 272
isotope cisternography, 102

kaolin, 46, 154
experimental hydrocephalus, 31, 33
Kiefer's Comorbidity Index, 94, 96
Kocher's point, 177
Krauss's classification, 91, 93
Kruppel-like factor 4 (KLF4), 47
Kubo's grading scale, 92, 94

L1CAM gene, 36, 38
lactate, 166
lamina terminalis, fenestration, 252
late-onset idiopathic aqueductal stenosis (LIAS), 247–248
lateral ventricles, 1
anatomy, 2
cellular composition, 5
CT imaging in NPH, 110
frontal horns, 111
hydrocephalus pathophysiology, 292
occipital horn, 2
temporal horn, 2, 110, 113
tumors, 249
volume reduction after ETV, 222
leptomeningeal spread, cancer, 102, 250
leucine-rich repeat kinase 2 (LRRK2), 168
leucine-rich α2-glycoprotein (LGR), 169
LEW/Jms rat model, 39, 44
Lewy body disease, 101, 102
LOTTA® rod-lens ventriculoscopic system, 224
LOVA (longstanding overt ventriculomegaly in adults), 100, 247–248, 283
low-pressure syndromes, 256–262
see also cerebrospinal fluid (CSF), leaks; intracranial hypotension, spontaneous
lower urinary tract symptoms (LUTS), *see* urinary tract symptoms
lumbar catheter insertion, 183–185
lumbar puncture, 259
multiple, 300–301
pseudotumor cerebri syndrome, 298–301
lumbar stenosis, 101, 185
lumboperitoneal shunt insertion, 184, 192
complications, in PTCS, 301
contraindications, 270
indications, 249
in normal volume hydrocephalus, 270
lumbopleural shunt, in PTCS, 301
lymphatic drainage, 9–10

macrophage, activation, 47
magnetic fields, effect on valve settings, 199–200
magnetic resonance angiography, time-of-flight, 121
magnetic resonance imaging (MRI), 103, 114–117
advantages and preferred sequence, 114–115
cardiac gating, 121–122
CSF flow studies, 121–124
CSF leak, 257–259
CSF pathologies with hydrocephalus, 285
CSF spaces, 285
diagnosis of NPH, 115, 116
disadvantages, 115
ETV, 223–224
gadolinium enhancement, 117, 118
NPH differential diagnosis, 103
phase-contrast ("cine"), *see* phase-contrast MRI (PC-MRI)
pseudotumor cerebri syndrome, 298
shunt complications, 209, 210
signal to noise ratio (SNR), 123
spinal, CSF leaks, 259
supra/infratentorial meningeal enhancement, 257
ventricular catheter insertion, 179
ventriculomegaly detection before symptom triad, 100
volumetric analysis by, 113
malignancies, and hydrocephalus, 248–251
mammillary body, 224
management, of congenital hydrocephalus in adults, 264–273
chronically shunted patients, 269–271
strategies, 270–271
see also slit ventricle syndrome
difficulties, 264
outcomes, 271–273
clinical, 271–272
neuropsychological, 272–273
shunt independence, 267–269
see also endoscopic third ventriculostomy (ETV)
transitioning neurosurgical care, 264–267
adolescents and hybrid models, 265
adult neurosurgery perspective, 265–266
cognitive impairment impact, 265, 266
difficulties, 265
dual-role care model, 265
lack of guidelines, 266
multidisciplinary care, 264–265, 266–267
patient/family perspective, 266
pediatric perspective, 265
plan/documentation, 266
recommendations, 266–267
management, of hydrocephalus in CSF pathologies, 275–287
case studies, 283–284
cerebellar arachnoid cyst with NPH, 279–280, 283
Chiari I malformation and NPH, 277–278, 279, 283
giant suprasellar arachnoid cyst (fetal), 282
multiple arachnoid cysts, 281
posterior fossa cyst, 276–277, 278, 283
cognition/cognitive assessment, 284–285
decision-making, 283–284
disease classification role, 286–287
multimodal surgery, 285–286
neuroimaging and MRI role, 285

Marfan syndrome, 256
Marmarou, Professor Anthony, 80–88, 287
Marmarou's model/theory, 139–141, 142, 144, 151–152, 190
  bolus infusion, 142, 144
  pressure/flow linear relationship, 145
Marmarou's monoexponential function, 128
Mdnah5 protein, 45
memory deficits, iNPH, 74, 76
meningitis, 252–253, 268
  carcinomatous, 249
mental status evaluation, extended, 73
mesencephalic locomotor region (MLR), 64–65
metabolic diseases, cognitive dysfunction and, 102
"Mickey Mouse" ventricles, 111
micturition, 82, 83
midbrain
  compression/atrophy, gait dysfunction, 64–65
  diameter, gait defects and, 64, 65
  volume loss, chemical/mechanical mechanisms, 65
mini-mental state examination (MMSE), 101
MOMs trial, 286
monoamine neurotransmitters, 23
Monro–Kellie doctrine, 10, 291–292
motor cortex, aberrant circuits, 67
motor skill impairment, 75, 76
Msi1 (Musashi 1), 44
MSM mouse strain, 40
Msx1 gene, 44
Mtf2 and *Mtf2* mutants, 45
myelography, CSF leaks, 259, 260
myelomeningocele, 294

neonates, post-infective hydrocephalus, 252
neural tube defects, 46–47
neurochemical disturbances, 71
neurocysticercosis, 253–254
neurodegenerative diseases
  biomarkers (CSF), 164
  cognitive dysfunction, 72
  gait dysfunction, 64–66, 100–101, 167
neurofilament protein (NFL), 167, 169
neurological examination, 99–100
neuronal death, 23
neurons, altered connections, 23
neuropathology (of hydrocephalus), 14–23
  immature/young animals as model, 14
  see also ventricular enlargement
neuropsychological deficits (in iNPH), 72
  Alzheimer's disease comparison, 74
  comorbidities, 76, 77
  differential diagnosis, 76–77
  localization, 73–75
  response to CSF drainage, 75–76
  see also cognitive impairment (in iNPH)
neuropsychological examination (in iNPH), 72, 73, 95, 239, 284–285
neuropsychological outcomes, in chronic shunting, 272–273
neurotransmission, disturbances, 71
nocturia, 85
non-canonical Wnt pathway, 45
noncommunicating hydrocephalus, *see* obstructive (noncommunicating) hydrocephalus
nonobstructive hydrocephalus, *see* communicating hydrocephalus
  nonsyndromic hydrocephalus, 36, 38
  see also congenital hydrocephalus
nonverbal learning disabilities syndrome, 272
normal pressure hydrocephalus (NPH), 14, 91, 304
  definition, and terminology, 131, 139
  see also specific aspects/topics
normal volume hydrocephalus (NVH), 265–266, 270
  treatment, 270

obesity
  Chiari I malformation and pseudotumor, 294
  PTCS and, 294, 300, 301
obstructive (noncommunicating) hydrocephalus, 159, 190, 218, 292, 304
  brain tumors and, 248–249
  CSF dynamics, 159
  ETV in, *see* endoscopic third ventriculostomy (ETV)
  intraventricular and extraventricular, 220
octreotide, 300
opening pressure, *see under* shunt(s)
OPHN1 (oligophrenin 1) protein, 46
optic nerve sheath fenestration, 301
organ failure, 102
ouabain, 8
outcome (of iNPH), 200, 232–245
  case study, 106
  comorbidities impact, 244
  congenital hydrocephalus, 271–273
  deficiencies in impairment identification, 233–240
  grading, *see* grading scales (NPH)
  difficulties in assessing, 232
  pre-/postoperative score comparison, 240, 242
  prediction
    comorbid diseases, 244
    CSF dynamics, 159
    ELD use, 233
    neurocognitive tests, 284–285
    preoperative factors, 244
    R_{out} role, 157–158
    shunt independence, 269
    see also shunting, patient selection
  publications (summary), 234
  selection criteria for iNPH diagnosis, 232–233
  shunt complications impact, 244, 271–272
  standardized management protocols, 240–243
    clinical judgment and, 243
    outcome assessment (standardized), 242–243
    shunt management, 240–242
    time period, short/long term, 243
    valve selection/use, 241
  by symptoms, 232, 242
outcome scales, 242
overdrainage (shunting), 175–176, 190, 208–209
  causes, 199, 201
  differential pressure valves, 192
  lumbar catheter placement, 185
  management and assessment, 208–209
  MRI, 209
  postural, 201
  rates, 211
  slit ventricle syndrome, 270
  symptoms, 208, 270

p57 gene, 44
PAC1 receptor, 47
Pacrg (Parkin-coregulated gene), 45
pad tests, 81
Parkinsonism, 17, 58, 167
Parkinson's disease, 167–169
  cognitive dysfunction, 72
  gait and executive function impairment, 66, 100–101
Pascal's law, 125
pathology, *see* neuropathology (of hydrocephalus); ventricular enlargement
pathophysiology, 36
  Chiari I malformation and hydrocephalus, 292

pathophysiology (*cont.*)
Chiari II malformation and hydrocephalus, 292–294
hindbrain herniation role, 292
hydrocephalus in intraspinal tumors, 250
late-onset idiopathic aqueductal stenosis, 247
pseudotumor cerebri syndrome, 299–300
urinary incontinence, *see* urinary incontinence
pathophysiology (of iNPH), 70
abnormal brain development, 48
cognitive defects, *see* cognitive impairment (in iNPH)
gait dysfunction, *see* gait dysfunction in NPH
putative pathogenic mechanisms, 70–72, 220–221, 240–241
cerebrovascular compromise, 71, 72
hyperdynamic CSF flow, 71, 133
interstitial edema, 71, 72
mechanical distortion, 70
neurochemical disturbances, 71
pressure effects, 70–71, 220–221
synthesis of mechanisms, 72, 220–221, 240–241
toxin accumulation, 71, 72
pathophysiology, genetic basis, 40–48
enhanced expression of genes, 47–48
immune response changes, 47
molecular cue loss during development, 40–46, 47
neural tube defects, 46–47
unknown causes (mouse lines), 47
see also genes/loci
pax6, 44
PC-MRI, *see* phase-contrast MRI (PC-MRI)
Pcdp1 (primary ciliary dyskinesia protein 1), 45
pediatric psychologists, 267
pedunculopontine nucleus (PPN), 65
peptide transporters, choroid plexus, 5
peripheral neuropathy, 101
peritoneal catheter insertion, 178, 180
complications, and variations, 180, 209
procedure, 177, 180
see also ventriculoperitoneal shunt
phase-contrast MRI (PC-MRI), 115–117
acceleration methods, 122
aliasing correction, 124
aqueductal stenosis, 130–131, 247
cautions/limitations, 131
cerebral venous flows, 133
CSF and blood flow interactions, 125–129, 133
healthy adults, 126, 128
CSF flow, 121, 125
after ETV, 131
CSF disorders, 129–134
before ETV, 223–224
CSF flow parameters, 124, 125
diagnosis of NPH, 131–133
ICP changes during cardiac cycle, 128–129
late-onset idiopathic aqueductal stenosis, 247
parameters affecting quality/accuracy, 122–123
parameters summary, 122
phase encoding, 122
post-processing and software, 123–125
principle and gray scale, 121, 122
quantitative *vs* qualitative, 122
questions to ask, 123
study results, 123, 124
temporal normalization, 124
pineal gland, "spiritus animalis" dogma and, 31
pituitary hyperemia, 257–258
planar cell polarity (PCP) signaling, 45
plethysmography, 121–122
pleural catheter insertion, 181–183
complications, 176, 182
Polaris valve, 196
PolL (DNA polymerase λ), 45
polycystin-1 (PC-1) protein, 45
pontine micturition center, 82
post-infective hydrocephalus, 252–254
posterior fossa anomalies, 291
classification, 286–287
posterior fossa cyst, 277, 278
hydrocephalus with, 276–277, 283
postoperative care, 176–177
postural control, 63, 67
postural instability, gait dysfunction due to, 67
posture, 154
differential-pressure valves, effect on, 192
headache in intracranial hypotension, 256–257, 259, 262
lumboperitoneal shunts, 192
postural overdrainage, 201
siphoning and, 191
predictive validity, animal models, 29
prenatal surgery, 286
preoperative planning, ETV, 222–224
preoperative preparation, 176–177, 186
presenilin-1 (PS-1) gene, 38, 44
pressure–flow performance (of shunts), 195, 198–199
pressure–flow test, 195, 197
pressure reactivity index (PRx), 155–156, 158–159
pressure–volume compensation, 150–152, 190
pressure–volume compensatory reserve, 155, 158–159
pressure–volume curve, 152
see also Marmarou's model/theory
pressure–volume index (PVI), 139–140, 142, 143, 147, 158
presymptomatic stages of NPH, threshold effect, 15
preterm infants, post-infective hydrocephalus, 252
primary ciliary dyskinesia, 46
ProGav valve, 196
progressive supranuclear palsy (PSP), 102
protein, CSF, 1
pseudomeningocele, 277, 292, 294
pseudotumor cerebri (PTC)
Chiari I malformation and, 294–295
lumbar catheter insertion complications, 185
lumbar *vs* ventricular catheterization, 185, 301
overdiagnosis, 294
pathophysiology, 291
pseudotumor cerebri syndrome (PTCS), 296–302
associated conditions, 297–298
in children, 297
clinical features, 297
Dandy criteria, 296–297
history, 296
investigations, 298–299, 300
in males, 297
management, 300–302
medical, 300–301
in obesity, 294, 300, 301
surgical, 301–302
thin patients, 294–295
nomenclature, 296
NPH *vs*, 296
pathophysiology, 299–300
psychologists, pediatric, 267
psychomotor dysfunction, localization, 73–74
ptch1 deficiency, 45
putamen, dorsal, 68
pyogenic infections, 252–253
pyramidal tracts, gait dysfunction, 63

quantitative trait locus (QTL), 39

radiation therapy, hydrocephalus after, 249
radionuclide cisternography, 259
radionuclide shunt patency test, 118–119
Rankin Scale, modified, 91, 92, 242
RAP index, 155

RAVLT (Learning and Delayed Recall test), 285
recurrence risk ratios (RRRs), 37
reduction principle, animal models, 28–29
reference pressure (P_o), 152, 191
refinement principle, animal models, 29
relative replacement principle, 28
replacement principle, animal models, 28
RFX3 (regulatory factor X3), 44
RFX4 (regulatory factor X4), 44
rhinorrhea, CSF, 297
Rickham reservoir use, 179–180
rodents, 30, 32
rostral tumor cyst, 250
R_{out} (CSF outflow resistance), 103, 151, 154, 158, 283
  bolus *vs* steady-state infusion, 157–158
  cerebral autoregulation and, 159
  elevation, 156, 159
  physiologic, 157
  pressure reactivity (PRx) and, 158
  shunt improvement prediction, 156–158

sagittal sinus pressure (P_{ss}), 133, 151, 269, 299, 300
  CSF pressure relationship, 299, 300
secondary NPH (sNPH), 14, 17, 91, 247–254
  after brain tumors, 248–251
  after infections, 252–254
  after spinal cord tumors, 249–250
  after subarachnoid hemorrhage, 251–252
  causes, 248
  epidemiology, 60
  R_{out} (CSF outflow resistance), 158
  surgery frequency, 60–61
  urinary incontinence, 85
senile plaques, 16, 17
shunt(s), 190–205
  closing pressure, 196
  distal pressure, 201
  effective operating pressure, 201
  future prospects, 204–205
  hardware, 192–194
    see also antisiphon devices; valves (shunts)
  hydrodynamic parameters tested, 191–192
  hydrodynamic properties, 196–200
  hydrodynamic resistance, 196, 199
    long distal catheters, 199
    low, overdrainage, 201–202
    specific shunts, 193
    ventricular catheters, 199
  ideal, 190
  imaging/assessment, 209, 210, 242
  long-term, CSF hydrodynamics, 269
  management standardization, outcome, 240–242
  negative outlet pressure, 199
  operating (opening) pressure, 118, 196, 199, 201
    specific valves, 200
  patency testing, *see* shunt testing
  proximal pressure, 200
  recent developments, 192
  removal, severe slit ventricle syndrome, 270
  revision, risk identification, 271
  role/aims, 190
  temperature effect, 200
  types, hydrodynamic resistances, 193
  see also shunt procedures; shunting; *specific shunt types*
shunt complications, 204, 207–215
  catheter migration, 209
  imaging, 209, 210
  impact on outcome, 244, 271–272
  major/minor, 244
  prevention, improved outcome, 244
  rates, 209–212, 244
  treatment of, 244
  types, 208, 211
  see also shunt infections; shunt malfunction
shunt failure, 208, 304
  ETV after, 219–220
  rate, 190, 211
  symptoms, 213
shunt independence, 267–269
  monitoring/evaluation, 267
  see also endoscopic third ventriculostomy (ETV)
shunt infections, 185–187, 212–215
  causative organisms, 185–186, 213–215
  costs and hospital stay duration, 187
  diagnosis, 213
  frequency, and timing, 185
  mechanisms and causes, 212–213
  rates, 209–210, 212
    adult *vs* children, 212
  secondary ETV outcome, 268
  sequelae, 212, 213
  shunt insertion protocol to reduce, 186
  symptoms, 209, 213
  treatment/preventative strategies, 213–215
    antibiotic management, 186–187
    see also antibiotic-impregnated shunts (AIS)
shunt malfunction, 190, 271–272
  adjustable valve use to reduce, 241
  blocking by particles, 200
  catheter tip obstruction, 179
  in chronically shunted patients, 265–266, 271–272
  CT detection, 113–115
  diagnosis, 200, 242
  ETV after, 268
  imaging, 242
  incidence and outcome, 271–272
  obstruction, lumbar catheter, 185
  outflow resistance, infusion tests, 146
  radionuclide detection, 118–119
  site, evaluation, 118
  ventricular catheter, 178
  VP shunts, frequency, 271
  X-ray detection, 110, 111, 112
shunt outcome, *see* outcome
shunt procedures, 175–187
  closure techniques, 177
  for communicating hydrocephalus, 185
  distal catheter insertion, 180–183
    resistance increase, 199
    see also specific catheter types
  general surgical principles, 176–177
  hardware, 192–194
  lumbar catheter insertion, *see* lumbar catheter insertion
  optimal settings, 175–176
  planning, duplex ultrasound, 110, 112
  postoperative care, 176–177
  protocol to reduce infections, 186
  proximal catheter placement, 177–180
    see also ventricular catheter insertion
shunt registry, 202–204
shunt testing
  in vivo, 190, 200–202
  laboratory, 194–197
  radionuclide, 118–119
shunt valves, *see* valves
shunting
  cognitive response, *see* cognitive impairment (in iNPH)
  evaluation, X-rays, 110
  experimental hydrocephalus, 33
  follow-up, 207–215
  frequency in iNPH and sNPH, 60–61, 104
  gait improvement, 63, 64, 73, 88
    dual-tasking and cognitive function, 66
    increased regional CBF, 68
    intracortical circuits and, 67
    midbrain diameter and, 64, 65
  incontinence improvement, *see* urinary incontinence

shunting (*cont.*)
  indications, 190
  outcome, *see* outcome
  overdrainage, *see* overdrainage (shunting)
  as "patch" not cure, 30
  patient selection, 190, 207, 210, 215
    CSF dynamics role, 159
    for improved iNPH outcome, 232–233
    tests for, 103, 146
    see also outcome (of iNPH), prediction
  pseudotumor cerebri syndrome, 301
  response prediction, 16, 165
  risk-to-benefit ratio, 207–208, 215
  underdrainage, 175–176, 208
  white matter changes, 16
  see also shunt(s); shunt procedures
"shuntogram", 118
SHYMA (syndrome of hydrocephalus in young and middle-aged adults), 247–249
SINPHONI study, 233, 244
siphoning (CSF) into distal compartment, 176
  devices to prevent, *see* antisiphon devices (ASD)
siphoning pressure, 191
slit ventricle syndrome (SVS), 192, 202, 294
  characteristics, 269
  CSF overdrainage, 270
  definitions, 269
  management, 269–271
  severe classical form, 271
  shunt removal in, 270
slow waves, 154, 158–159
α-SNAP, 40
social development, 272–273
SOCS7, 47
sodium-potassium-ATPase pump, 7, 8
soluble amyloid precursor protein (sAPP), 166, 168, 169
"solute-coupled" transport, 8
somatostatin-like immunoreactivity, 168
sonic hedgehog (Shh) signaling, 45
Sophy Adjustable valve, 194, 196, 199–200
Sox3, overexpression, 47
special healthcare needs (SHCN), 264–267
sperm associated antigen 6 (Spag6), 45
spina bifida, 292, 294
  ETV outcome, 268
  headache management, 271
  neuropsychological impairment, 272
  prenatal repair, MOMs trial, 286
  shunt dependency, 294
spinal central canal, CSF flow, 6
spinal cord tumors, 249–251
spinal CSF anatomy, 3
spinal lymphatic drainage, 9–10
spinal tap test (STT), 103, 104, 145–146
  method, and outcome evaluation, 146
Stein–Langfitt classification, 91, 92, 242
steroid metabolism, 300
Strata valve, 196, 202
stroke, 244
stroke volume, CSF, 124, 125, 128, 133, 285
stroke volume ratio, 133
Stroop Color Word Test, 73, 75, 95, 239, 284, 285
Stumpy mouse, 46
subarachnoid cisterns, *see* cisterns (subarachnoid)
subarachnoid hemorrhage (SAH)
  CSF movement impairment, 14
  ETV complication, 226–227
  hydrocephalus after, 251–252
    acute, 251
    subacute and chronic, 251–252
subarachnoid space (SAS)
  arachnoid granulations, 8–9
  cortical, in PTCS, 296
  CSF flow, 5, 127
    poor, Chiari II malformation and, 293
  DESH, 99, 115, 117, 233, 304
  enlargement, 14
  leaky epithelium, 8
  obstruction, 99, 102, 292
  spinal, CSF flow, 6
  volumetric analysis by CT/MRI, 113
subcommissural organ (SCO), 40
  abnormal development, 40–44
  defects, proteins/factors involved, 40–44, 46, 47
subcortical vascular dementia, 101, 167
subdural fluid collection, 257, 258
subdural hematoma (SDH), 102, 211, 227
subdural hygroma, 114, 115, 211
substantia nigra, damage, 71
subtemporal decompression, 301
sulfatide, as biomarker, 167
superior sagittal sinus
  narrowing, 299, 300
  pressure, *see* sagittal sinus pressure (P_{ss})
suprasellar arachnoid cyst, giant, 282
supraspinal pathways, micturition control, 82–83
surgery
  CSF leak management, 261
  minimally invasive, 286
  multimodal, 285–286
  shunt, *see* shunt procedures; shunting
Sylvius, cerebral aqueduct, *see* cerebral aqueduct (of Sylvius)
symbol digit modalities (SDMT), 73, 75, 76
symptoms, of NPH, 63, 91, 92, 99
  classification based on, 104
  duration, outcome affected by, 76, 100
  early to progressive stages, 72–73, 104
  grading scales, *see* grading scales (NPH)
  Hakim's description, 91, 99, 232
  ventriculomegaly detection before, 100
  see also cognitive impairment; gait dysfunction in NPH; urinary incontinence
syndrome of hydrocephalus in young and middle-aged adults (SHYMA), 247–249
syndromic hydrocephalus, 36
syringomyelia, 135

$T_{1/2}$ time, 118
Taenia solium, 253–254
tanycytes, 5
tap test, *see* spinal tap test (STT)
tau protein
  in Alzheimer's disease, 165
  as iNPH biomarker, 164, 168, 169
    Alzheimer's disease *vs*, 165, 166
    prognostic marker, 168, 169
    vascular dementia *vs*, 167
  in Parkinson's disease, 168
  phosphorylated (p-tau), 165, 168, 169
tauopathy, 102
temperature, shunt functioning, 200
ten-meter walk test, 92, 100
tension hydrothorax, 182
Texas strain, rat model, *see* HTX rat
thalamostriate vein, 2
third ventricle, 1
  anatomy, 2
  cellular composition, 5
  dilatation, gait dysfunction, 63
  obstruction, MRI, 114
  volume reduction after ETV, 222
tight junctions, 4
timed up and go test (TUG), 92, 100
tinnitus, 297
topiramate, 300
torcula position, and compression, 293–294
toxin accumulation, reduced CSF production, 71, 72
toxoplasmosis, 253

Trail Making tests, 73, 76
transcranial Doppler-derived pressure autoregulation, 159–160
transferrin, isoforms, 166
β2-transferrin, 1
transforming growth factor-β1 (TGF-β1), 32, 48
transgenic animals, 32
  OVE459 mouse line, 39–40
  TGF-β1 overexpression in mice, 32, 48
traumatic encephalopathy, chronic, 102
triventricular hydrocephalus, ETV in, 222
twin studies, 36–37

UK Shunt Evaluation Laboratory, 194
UK Shunt Registry, 204
ultrasonography, 110, 112, 181
uncomplicated hydrocephalus, 36
underdrainage (shunting), 175–176, 208
upper limb motor control, 63
urinary incontinence, 80–88
  caregiver distress, 80, 85
  definition, 80, 81
  in dementia, 80–81
  differential diagnosis, 102
  etiologic theories, 82
  evaluation, 92, 240, 242
    grading scales, 92, 95, 240
    see also urinary tract symptoms
  measurement, 81
  pathophysiology, 82–83, 86
  prevalence and significance, 80, 81, 85
  secondary NPH, 85
  shunting, outcome, 85–87
  stress, 82, 86
  treatment, 87–88
  urge, 85
  urologic history, 83
urinary sphincter, 82
urinary tract function, normal, 82
urinary tract symptoms, 80–88, 102
  characterization, 85–86
    Virginia Commonwealth University, 85–87
  differential diagnosis, 81–82, 102
  in elderly, 82
  evaluation, 83–85, 92
    diagnostic testing, 84
    examination, 84
    urodynamic testing, 84–85
    urologic history, 83
    validated questionnaires, 83–84, 86, 240
  grading scales, *see* grading scales (NPH)
  incontinence, *see* urinary incontinence
  pathophysiology, 63, 82–83, 85
  post-void, 83
  prevalence, 85
  shunting effect, 85–88
  SHYMA, 248
  storage (irritative), 81, 83
  terminology, 83
  types, 81
  urinary frequency, 85
  urinary urgency, 81, 85
  voiding (obstructive), 81, 83
urodynamic testing, 84–85

VACTERL with hydrocephalus, 37
valves (shunts), 175–176, 194, 198
  active, future prospects, 204
  adjustable, 175, 176, 192–194
    comparisons, 196
    magnetic field effect, 199–200
    outcome improvement, 241
    re-setting, 199, 244
  antisiphon, 175, 176
  ball on spring, 194, 198
  differential pressure, 175, 176, 192, 201, 241
    complications, 192
    long distal catheters, resistance, 199
    position effect, 192
    principles, 192
  flow-regulated, 175, 176, 194, 204
  horizontal-vertical, 175
  hydrodynamic resistances, 542/110, 193
  overdrainage, 201–202
  types, outcome improvement, 241
vascular dementia, 101, 167
vasoactive intestinal peptide (VIP), 167
vasopressin, 166
V_{enc} (velocity encoding parameter), 122, 131
venous sinuses, CSF flow, 9
venous stenting, in PTCS, 301–302
ventral dural tears, 261
ventricles, 3
  anatomy, 2, 32
  cellular composition, 5
  CSF flow, 5
  size, ETV selection, 222–223
  see also specific ventricles
ventricular catheter insertion, 177–180
  antisiphon device use, 176
  catheter tip obstruction, 179
  children, closed fontanelles, 179
  complications and advice, 178–180
  endoscopic visualization, 179
  frontal approach, 177, 178
  lumbar catheterization *vs*, 184–185
  parieto-occipital approach, 177, 179
  procedure, 177–180
  pseudotumor cerebri syndrome, 301
  resistance, 199
  stereotactic guidance, 179
  see also ventriculoperitoneal shunt
ventricular enlargement, 14
  asymptomatic, 15, 104
    prevalence, 104
    white matter changes, 16
  consequences, 15
    altered neurons/connections, 23
    atrophy and brain damage, 15
    autopsy findings, 17, 18
    blood flow reduction, 15, 23
    extracellular fluid changes, 16
    fornix and corpus callosum atrophy, 15, 17
    secondary reactive changes, 23
    white matter changes, 15–17
  factors leading to, 14–15, 220–221
  failure, in slit ventricle syndrome, 269–271
    see also slit ventricle syndrome
  increased ICP pulse amplitude, 153
  measurement, CT, 110–113
  pathophysiology, *see* pathophysiology (of iNPH)
  rate, 23
  threshold effect for tolerance to, 15
ventricular system, 1
  ventriculoatrial shunt, 182, 207
  see also atrial catheter insertion
ventriculomegaly, *see* ventricular enlargement
ventriculoperitoneal shunt, 207, 271
  brain tumors, 249
  Chiari I malformation with hydrocephalus, 278
  Chiari I malformation with pseudotumor, 294–295
  complication rate, 209–212
  complications, 210–212, 271
  CT, 114, 116, 209
  ETV *vs*, 222
  insertion, 178
  risks, 210
  see also peritoneal catheter insertion; ventricular catheter insertion
ventriculopleural shunt insertion, 183
ventriculostomy
  catheter placement/removal, 180
  ETV, *see* endoscopic third ventriculostomy (ETV)
  hydrocephalus after subarachnoid hemorrhage, 252
verbal memory, 74
vestibular schwannoma, 60

Virchow–Robin spaces, 6
visual memory, 74, 76
visual symptoms, in PTCS, 297
visuospatial skills, 74–76, 272
void diaries, 81
volume removal (bolus withdrawal), 143–144

water
  CSF production, 4, 7, 8, 14
  distribution in brain, 1
  "solute-coupled" transport, 8
  water channels, deficient, 46
  see also specific aquaporins
weight, experimental animals, 29
white matter
  cerebral blood flow reduction, 160, 161
  in NPH, 15–17, 74, 101
    distortion and cognitive defects, 70
    outcome of shunting, 240
Windkessel effect, 10, 153, 154
winged helix family, transcription factors, 45
Wistar-Lewis rat model (LEW/Jms), 39, 44
Wnt signaling, 45, 47
Wnt1 cell lineage, 44
word list learning tasks, 74

X-linked inheritance, 37
X-rays, 110, 111
  shunt assessment, 177, 209

Zarit Caregiver Burden Scale, 94
Zic5 gene, 47
zona adherens, 5
zona occludens, 4